ALZHEIMER'S AND PARKINSON'S DISEASES

Strategies for Research and Development

ADVANCES IN BEHAVIORAL BIOLOGY

Recent Volumes in this Series

Volume 17 ENVIRONMENTS AS THERAPY FOR BRAIN DYSFUNCTION
Edited by Roger N. Walsh and William T. Greenough

Volume 18 NEURAL CONTROL OF LOCOMOTION
Edited by Richard M. Herman, Sten Grillner, Paul S. G. Stein, and Douglas G. Stuart

Volume 19 THE BIOLOGY OF THE SCHIZOPHRENIC PROCESS
Edited by Stewart Wolf and Beatrice Bishop Berle

Volume 20 THE SEPTAL NUCLEI
Edited by Jon F. DeFrance

Volume 21 COCAINE AND OTHER STIMULANTS
Edited by Everett H. Ellinwood, Jr. and M. Marlyne Kilbey

Volume 22 DISCRIMINATIVE STIMULUS PROPERTIES OF DRUGS
Edited by Harbans Lal

Volume 23 THE AGING BRAIN AND SENILE DEMENTIA
Edited by Kalidas Nandy and Ira Sherwin

Volume 24 CHOLINERGIC MECHANISMS AND PSYCHOPHARMACOLOGY
Edited by Donald J. Jenden

Volume 25 CHOLINERGIC MECHANISMS: Phylogenetic Aspects, Central and Peripheral Synapses, and Clinical Significance
Edited by Giancarlo Pepeu and Herbert Ladinsky

Volume 26 CONDITIONING: Representation of Involved Neural Functions
Edited by Charles D. Woody

Volume 27 THE BASAL GANGLIA: Structure and Function
Edited by John S. McKenzie, Robert E. Kemm, and Lynette N. Wilcock,

Volume 28 BRAIN PLASTICITY, LEARNING, AND MEMORY
Edited by B. E. Will, P. Schmitt, and J. C. Dalrymple-Alford

Volume 29 ALZHEIMER'S AND PARKINSON'S DISEASES: Strategies for Research and Development
Edited by Abraham Fisher, Israel Hanin, and Chaim Lachman

ALZHEIMER'S AND PARKINSON'S DISEASES

Strategies for Research and Development

Edited by

Abraham Fisher

Israel Institute for Biological Research
Ness-Ziona, Israel

Israel Hanin

Loyola University Stritch School of Medicine
Chicago, Illinois

and

Chaim Lachman

Israel Institute for Biological Research
Ness-Ziona, Israel

PLENUM PRESS • NEW YORK AND LONDON

Library of Congress Cataloging in Publication Data

OHOLO Conference on Basic and Therapeutic Strategies in Alzheimer's and Other Related Neuropsychiatric Disorders (1985: Eilat, Israel)
Alzheimer's and Parkinson's diseases.
(Advances in behavioral biology; v. 29)

"Proceedings of the thirtieth OHOLO Conference on Basic and Therapeutic Strategies in Alzheimer's and Other Related Neuropsychiatric Disorders, held in March 24–27, 1985, in Eilat, Israel"—T.p. verso.
Includes bibliographies and index.
1. Parkinsonism—Congresses. 2. Alzheimer's disease—Congresses. I. Fisher, Abraham. II. Hanin, Israel. III. Lachman, Chaim. IV. Title. V. Series. [DNLM: 1. Alzheimer's Disease—congresses. 2. Parkinson Disease—congresses. WM 220 038 1985a]
RC382.047 1985 616.8′3 85-32056
ISBN 0-306-42232-8

First Printing—July 1986
Second Printing—November 1987

Proceedings of the thirtieth OHOLO Conference on Basic and Therapeutic Strategies in Alzheimer's and Other Related Neuropsychiatric Disorders, held March 24–27, 1985, in Eilat, Israel

A Division of Plenum Publishing Corporation
233 Spring Street, New York, N.Y. 10013

Printed in the United States of America

OHOLO BIOLOGICAL CONFERENCES COMMITTEE

Permanent Committee:

S. Cohen, M. Feldman, N. Grossowicz, I. Hertman
A. Keynan, A. Kohn, M. Sela, and G.A. Simon

Scientific Organizing Committee (30th Conference):
A. Fisher (Chairman), S. Cohen, I. Hanin, C. Lachman,
A. Levy, M. Segal, and M. Weinstock-Rozin

Technical Management:

R. Pniel and M. Navon

Secretary:

Ilana Turner

PREFACE

This book is the outcome of an international conference, held at the Aviya Sonesta Hotel in Eilat, Israel, on March 24-27, 1985. This was the 30th in a series of the annual OHOLO Conferences, sponsored by the Israel Institute for Biological Research.

Participants in this Conference consisted of scientists from fourteen countries; represented a broad spectrum of research interests; and included a well-balanced representation from academia, clinical institutions and pharmaceutical industry. The book includes talks, poster sessions, and a comprehensive general discussion, all from the proceedings of this conference.

In the interest of assuring a rapid publication of the novel information reviewed, this book has been prepared in camera-ready format. We are cognizant of the fact that several typographical errors may exist in the text, and that there are variations in style and typeface of the various chapters. This, we felt, was a reasonable compromise for the sake of speed and efficient transmission of valuable scientific information. Nobody is perfect.....

The success of the conference, and hence the quality of this book are attributable to the extensive efforts of a large number of extremely capable individuals. These include members of the Scientific Organizing Committee, and the Technical staff of the OHOLO Organization. Of course, the conference could not have succeeded without the high quality of the presentations, and the enthusiastic participation of the contributing scientists.

This book should serve as a valuable resource of information regarding current research in Alzheimer's and Parkinson's Disease. It spans a broad spectrum of topics, and bridges preclinical with clinical concepts related to these deseases states. It reviews old material, emphasizes new findings, and poses important questions which have yet to be answered. As such, it will hopefully be a valuable addition to the libraries of many students of these two crippling disease entities.

Abraham Fisher
Israel Hanin
Chaim Lachman

ACKNOWLEDGEMENTS

The Organizing Committee of the 30th OHOLO Conference gratefully acknowledges the generous support of the following organizations (in alphabetical order):

American Cyanamid Company, Pearl River, N.Y. U.S.A.
Astra Lakemedel AB, Sodertalje, Sweden
Boehringer Ingelheim KG, Ingelheim/Rhein, Germany
Center of Brain Sciences & Metabolism Charitalbe Trust, U.S.A.
E.I. du Pont de Nemours & Co., Wilmington, DE, U.S.A.
Fidia Research Laboratories, Abano Terme, Italy
Glaxo, London, England
Hoechst-Roussel Pharmaceuticals Inc., Somerville, NJ, U.S.A.
Hoffman-La Roche Inc., Nutley, NJ, U.S.A.
The Israel Academy of Sciences and Humanities, Jerusalem, Israel
Kopel Tours - Conventions Ltd., Tel-Aviv, Israel
Merck, Sharp & Dohme Research Laboratories, Rahway, NJ, U.S.A.
Ministry of Science and Development, Israel
Monsanto Company, St. Louis, MO, U.S.A.
National Council for Research and Development, Israel
Pharmacaps, Elizabeth, NJ, U.S.A.
Research Biochemical Inc., Wayland, MA, U.S.A.
Rhone-Poulenc Sante, Paris, France
Dr. R.H. Rogge, Chapel Hill, NC, U.S.A.
Sandoz Ltd., Basle, Switzerland
Snow Brand, Tokyo, Japan
Stuart Pharmaceuticals, Division of ICI Americas, Inc., Wilmington, DE, U.S.A.
Technad Inc., Belleville, NJ, U.S.A.
The Upjohn Company, Kalamazoo, MI, U.S.A.
Weizmann Institute of Science, Rehovot, Israel

CONTENTS

CLINICAL ASPECTS AND NONINVASIVE DIAGNOSTIC APPROACHES

ETIOLOGICAL AND GENETIC ASPECTS OF ALZHEIMER'S AND PARKINSON'S DISEASE

BIOLOGICAL MARKERS IN ALZHEIMER'S AND PARKINSON'S DISEASE

WELCOMING ADDRESS

I. Hertman

Director of the Israel Institute
for Biological Research

Ladies and gentlemen, participants of the 30th. OHOLO Conference; dear friends and colleagues.

It is a priviledge and honor to welcome you all here in Eilat, as we gather for the Conference on:

"Basic and Therapeutic Strategies in Alzheimer's and Other Age Related Neuropsychiatric Disorders".

The Israel Institute for Biological Research considers it a great achievement to be instrumental in organizing 30 consecutive yearly meetings on outstanding research topics pursued in Israel and throughout the world. The history of the OHOLO Conferences is in fact a mini-reflection of the changes that scientific research has undergone in this country during the last 30 years.

These conferences were initiated 30 years ago by a group of biologists from our Institute and the Hebrew University in Jerusalem, which was then the "Alma Mater" of most Israeli scientists. The purpose of these meetings was, at their initiation, "to foster interdisciplinary communication between scientists in Israel and to provide added stimulus by the participation of invited scientists from abroad". The emphasis was on informal contact between young (we were all young in those years) Israeli and prominent scientists from abroad. The expected benefits from the conferences were to enrich basic research in Israel in the Life Sciences, which were considered of great intellectual challenge and of extreme promise for the future of the society.

The site initialy chosen for the conferences was OHOLO, a seminar center of the Zionist labour movement, on the shores of the Lake of Galilee. The pioneers of OHOLO meetings believed, like most of the Israelis in those times, that scientific achievements are the propriety of the society, and that the duty of the state is to foster science and technology. Thus the first conferences were rather like a family business among Israeli scientists with highly motivated prominent friends from abroad.

During the next two decades, the academic establishment of Israel changed, and universities and research institutes with thousands of students were established. Extensive basic research was supported by the state. In this "Golden Age" of scientific research, the family atmosphere was slowly replaced by friendly institutional connections, and the uniqueness of the OHOLO Conferences was preserved.

In the third decade, the Government came to the conclusion that there are no financial means to support the ever-growing research. The academic research institutions started to look for foreign capital and collaboration with industry. This trend became more intensive in the recent years, and culminated in the present tough competition for joint ventures and industrial contacts.

The present conference reflects this trend and the participation of industrial sponsors is impressive; demonstrating that after 30 years, we have tried not to lose ground.

While considering these developments, inevitable and positive, we still must remember that the strength of our research and development (R & D) potential originates from roots planted in the "Golden Age" of basic research. It should thus be clear that bringing the present trend to an extreme standstill in independent basic research will have disastrous consequences on the quality of the Israeli scientific and technological potential.

The first premises of the OHOLO seminar center were extremely modest, but the illustrious guests (many of them Nobel prize laureates in later years) did not attach any attention to such trivialities. This was the romantic period, which only later was followed by increasing concern for convenience and luxury by our guests and our own people. So we went over to more modern and spacious hostels, like those in Maalot, Zfat and Zichron Yaakov, all of them still connected with the Israeli Labour movement. The highest sophistication was reached this year by choosing this five star resort for the conference site.

I hope that the original and unique atmosphere of the OHOLO meetings can still be preserved in these beautiful, leisurely surroundings.

To those who are newcomers to the OHOLO Conferences, let me introduce briefly, the host organization - The Israel Institute for Biological Research. We have made during the last decade considerable efforts to create an a unique R & D organization which can face the changing economic reality. We have built up an integrative R & D potential, covering the disciplines of Chemistry, Pharmacology and modern Biotechnology. We have established an industrial toxicology testing laboratory which is a company, owned by our Institute. In the management of our R & D, we are well aware of the necessity of ongoing research activities by viable scientific teams and we are therefore trying to support them from commercial benefits. Some products of our R & D activities are exhibited in the hall, and we hope that some of our guests will find them of interest.

The topic of the present conference is a research subject actively pursued in our Departments of Organic Chemistry and Pharmacology. This research involves basic explorations, drug design and first stages of commercialization. Parts of this R & D are sponsored by Japanese Industry, and we are sure that this collaboration will be of mutual benefit.

Age related neuropsychiatric disorders are of increasing concern in industrialized societies, and we believe therefore that the present conference is a timely conference of extreme importance. We very much appreciate the participation of so many prominent scientists in this field. We are most thankful for the generous contributions of the indus-trial sponsors listed in the program.

I wish to express my personal thanks to members of the Scientific Organizing Committee, chaired by Dr. Fisher of our Institute, for their untiring efforts in the organization of this conference, and to the technical staff for their marvellous work in preparing this conference.

It is with great warmth that I welcome the participants of the 30th. OHOLO Conference, and wish our guests a very pleasant and memorable stay in Eilat.

CHOLINERGIC SYSTEMS IN THE BRAIN AND SPINAL CORD: ANATOMIC ORGANIZATION AND OVERVIEW OF FUNCTIONS

Larry L. Butcher and Nancy J. Woolf

Department of Psychology and Brain Research Institute
University of California
Los Angeles, California 90024, U.S.A.

INTRODUCTION

A cartoon in a recent issue of the Los Angeles Times newspaper bore the interesting caption "How the brain works." A cut-away depiction of a human head was shown, and, inside it, a workman was busily plugging and unplugging various wires and cords. What the cartoonist was suggesting, we believe, is that when we understand how the brain is wired, we will have taken a necessary step in understanding how it works, and this viewpoint, in our opinion, has considerable merit. Regardless of the particular communication system under consideration, information transmission always occurs within a physical framework consisting essentially of a sender, a communication channel, and a receiver (Shannon, 1948). In the nervous system the sender may be a neuron, the communication channel a synaptic cleft or other conduit of information (e.g., circulatory system) between two or more cells, and the receiver a particular target structure such as another neuron or a gland or muscle cell. The data neuroanatomy provides is relevant to understanding the matrix within which information transmission in the nervous system occurs, and, if neurons containing particular transmitters are demonstrated, neuroanatomy can indicate what chemical messengers are used to transmit information at certain loci.

Although we realize that the issue of how different neurotransmitter systems interact, both structurally and functionally, must be increasingly addressed, we will focus in this paper on only one transmitter network, namely that in which acetylcholine is used. We do so not only because cholinergic mechanisms have been importantly implicated in Alzheimer's disease and related dementias but also because cholinergic neuroanatomy, until recently, has been incompletely specified. The recent development of specific and histochemically useful antibodies against choline-O-acetyltransferase (ChAT), however, has permitted more valid mapping of presumed cholinergic neurons than previously possible, and it is this immunohistochemical methodology, in combination with fluorescent tracer histology, that we have used to chart the distribution and projection patterns of cells thought to use acetylcholine as a neurotransmitter.

METHODS

For most of our experiments, rats or cats were used. Intracerebral infusions of propidium iodide, True Blue, or both fluorescent tracers were made stereotaxically 48 hours before the animals were anesthesized and sacrificed subsequently by cardiac perfusion with cold phosphate buffered saline (PBS; pH, 7.4) followed by cold 4% paraformaldehyde in 0.1 M phosphate buffer (pH, 7.4). Brains were post-fixed at 4° C for 90 minutes in the latter fixative before being transferred to cold 30% sucrose in 0.1 M phosphate buffer (pH, 7.4) for an additional 3-14 days. The tissue was then blocked, frozen onto a brass specimen holder, and cut at 15 µm intervals in a cryostat maintained at -20° C or at 30 µm intervals on a sliding microtome. The resulting cryostat sections were mounted on glass slides precoated with 0.5% gelatin in 0.05% chromium potassium sulfate, whereas microtome sections were mounted onto coated slides after staining was completed.

Tissue sections mounted on glass slides and free floating sections were preincubated in a 4° C solution of 0.3% Triton-X 100 in PBS for 24 hours with gentle agitation followed by a 48-hour incubation with agitation in a 4° C PBS solution containing a monoclonal antibody against ChAT (code 11/255; for characterization, see Eckenstein and Thoenen, 1982), diluted 1:50 or 1:100. At the end of the incubation period, the sections were rinsed twice in PBS for 10 minutes each before being reacted with a solution of affinity purified IgG conjugated with fluorescein isothiocyanate, diluted 1:100 in PBS with 0.3% Triton-X 100, for 2 hours at room temperature. The sections were then rinsed with several changes of PBS and coverslipped under a medium of glycerine and PBS (3:1, v/v) containing 0.1 M n-propyl gallate to retard photobleaching. Control brain sections were treated in the same manner except that incubation with the primary antibody was omitted.

Orange-red to red neuronal somata labeled with propidium iodide and light blue cell bodies labeled with True Blue were visualized with transmitted illumination. The yellow-green fluorescein isothiocyanate label was examined with epi-illumination. Double- and triple-labeled cells on the same tissue section were identified sequentially by changing the filter combinations. Further details of the combined ChAT-immunohistochemical and fluorescent-tracer procedure are contained in Woolf et al. (1983, 1984) and Woolf and Butcher (1985).

OVERVIEW OF CENTRAL CHOLINERGIC SYSTEMS

Application to the study of the rat and cat central nervous systems of the histochemical methodology detailed in the immediately preceding section has revealed that cholinergic neurons evince two general organizational schemata: those that are local-circuit cells and those that are projection neurons. Local-circuit neurons are found in the caudate-putamen complex, nucleus accumbens, olfactory tubercle, and probably also the hippocampus and cerebral cortex. Four separable, but not necessarily mutually exclusive, major cholinergic projection systems have been delimited: (1) the basal forebrain cholinergic system consisting of ChAT-positive cells in the medial septal nucleus, vertical and horizontal limbs of the diagonal band, the magnocellular preoptic area, the subpallidal substantia innominata and its rostral extension into the ventral pallidal area (substriatal gray), the nucleus basalis, and the so-called nucleus of the ansa lenticularis projecting to the amygdala, hippocampus, all limbic cortical and neocortical fields, habenula, and interpeduncular nucleus (Figs. 1-3), (2) the pontine cholinergic system composed prominently of ChAT-positive neurons in the pedunculopontine tegmental region and the dorsolateral (laterodorsal) tegmental nucleus projecting rostrally to the thalamus, tectum, pretectal nucleus, habenula, interpeduncular nucleus, globus pallidus, lateral hypothalamus, and basal forebrain (Figs. 3-4) and probably caudally to various loci in the caudal brainstem, including the nucleus raphe magnus, the nucleus of cranial nerve VII, and nucleus reticularis pontis oralis (Fig. 5), (3) the somatic motor and parasympathetic neurons of cranial nerves III-VII and IX-XII, and (4) the ChAT-positive alpha- and gamma- motor neurons and cells of the intermediolateral column and sacral division of the parasympathetic nervous system in the spinal cord.

A schematic representation of the major cholinergic systems in the brain is displayed in Fig. 6. It is noteworthy that the basal forebrain cholinergic system and the pontine tegmental cholinergic system essentially innervate different regions of the brain with one exception: the interpeduncular nucleus and possibly also the habenular complex receive cholinergic afferents from both the forebrain and brainstem systems (Figs. 3, 6).

THE BASAL FOREBRAIN CHOLINERGIC SYSTEM: ORGANIZATIONAL PRINCIPLES AND FUNCTIONS

It appears clear from the foregoing discourse that the basal forebrain contains a neuroanatomically complex constellation of cholinergic neurons that projects significantly to virtually all of the neural structures in the non-striatal telencephalon and to certain brainstem loci, at least insofar as is currently known. As discussed in Bigl et al. (1982), Woolf et al. (1984), and Woolf and Butcher (1985), it is possible that this system can be parcelled into two different, but not necessarily mutually exclusive, components: (1) a rostral, predominantly medial, portion composed of ChAT-positive cells associated with the medial septal nucleus, vertical and horizontal limbs of the diagonal band, the magnocellular preoptic area, and the rostral substantia innominata that provides cholinergic afferents primarily to limbic structures in the telencephalon and brainstem, and (2) a caudal, essentially lateral, segment consisting of cholinergic neurons in the subpallidal substantia innominata, nucleus basalis, and so-called nucleus of the ansa lenticularis that are the source of cholinergic fibers preferentially innervating neocortical regions.

Despite the fact that the neuroanatomy of the basal forebrain cholinergic system is becoming increasingly understood, there is presently a relative paucity of information concerning its physiology. Nonetheless, various experimental findings suggest that this system is involved in neuronal processes operating at the highest levels of brain function and integration. In 1945, Murphy and Gellhorn reported that the pyramidal discharge produced by electrical stimulation of the motor cortex could be enhanced by simultaneous stimulation of sites that, in part, would now be included in the basal forebrain as conceived in this manuscript. Stimulation of those basal forebrain loci alone did not evoke muscular responses. Clemente et al. (1963) further showed that electroencephalographic synchronization and sleep produced by stimulation of the basal forebrain could, after several conditioning trials, come to be elicited by a tone paired with that stimulation, a result all the more interesting in view of the results of Hernandez-Peon and Chavez-Ibarra (1963) that acetylcholine applied to the preoptic area induced sleep. In other behavioral studies, Sterman and Fairchild (1966) demonstrated that the running velocity of cats could be decreased by electrical stimulation of diagonal band nuclei and the rostral preoptic area, and, five years later, DeLong (1971) observed that neurons in the medullary lamina of the globus pallidus and in the substantia innominata of monkeys displayed altered activity primarily in relation to the delivery of positive reinforcement. Similarly, Linseman and Olds (1973) and Linseman (1974) found that neurons in the basal forebrain of rats decreased their rates of firing as a function of pairing an auditory stimulus with food reward.

Additional, but again only suggestive, evidence that the basal forebrain cholinergic system might be involved in complex behavioral functions comes from various pharmacologic and neuropathologic investigations (Table 1). Drugs influencing cholinergic mechanisms, for example, have been found to have significant effects on memory (for review, see Squire

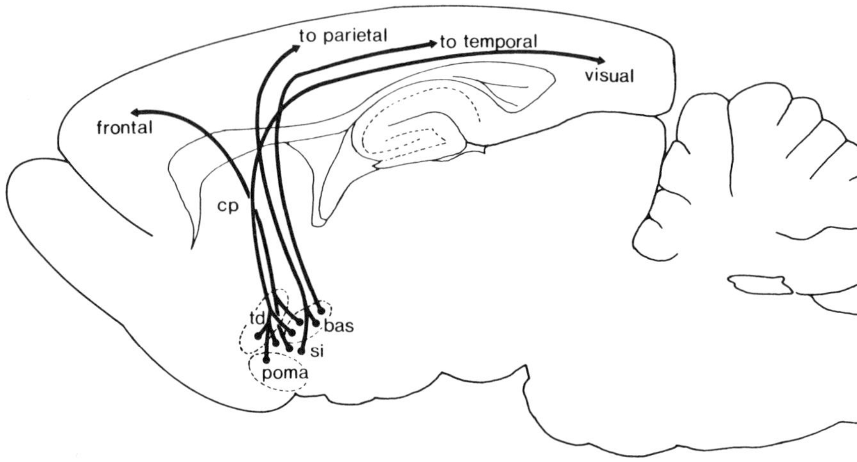

Fig. 1. Schematic representation of the cholinergic innervation of neocortical fields. Abbreviations: **bas**, nucleus basalis; **cp**, caudate-putamen complex; **frontal**, frontal cortex; **parietal**, parietal cortex; **poma**, magnocellular preoptic area; **si**, substantia innominata; **temporal**, temporal cortex; **td**, diagonal band; **visual**, visual cortex.

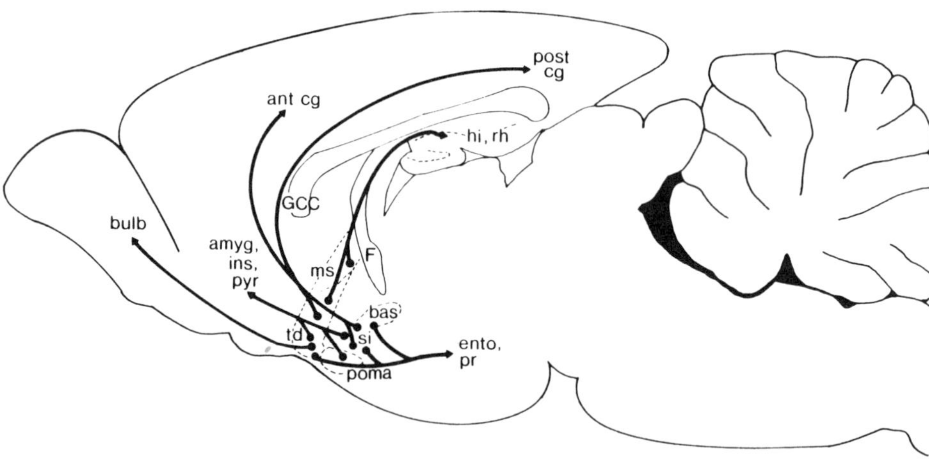

Fig. 2. Schematic representation of the cholinergic innervation of the limbic telencephalon. Abbreviations: **amyg**, amygdala; **ant cg**, anterior cingulate cortex; **bulb**, olfactory bulb; **ento**, entorhinal cortex; **F**, fornix; **GCC**, genu of corpus callosum; **hi**, hippocampus; **ins**, insular cortex; **ms**, medial septal nucleus; **post cg**, posterior cingulate cortex; **pr**, perirhinal cortex; **pyr**, pyriform cortex; **rh**, retrohippocampal region. For other symbols, see legend of Fig. 1.

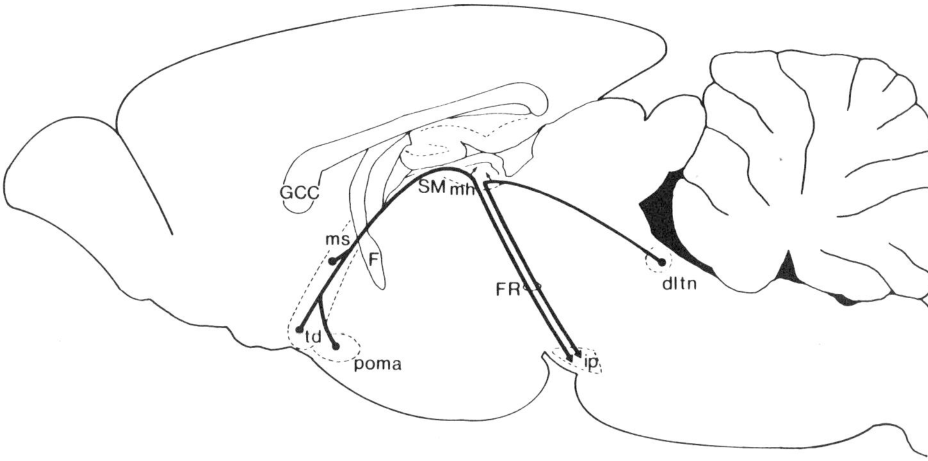

Fig. 3. Schematic representation of the cholinergic innervation of the interpeduncular nucleus. Abbreviations: **dltn**, dorsolateral (laterodorsal) tegmental nucleus; **FR**, fasciculus retroflexus; **ip**, interpeduncular nucleus; **mh**, medial habenula; **SM**, stria medullaris. For other symbols, see legends of Figs. 1 and 2.

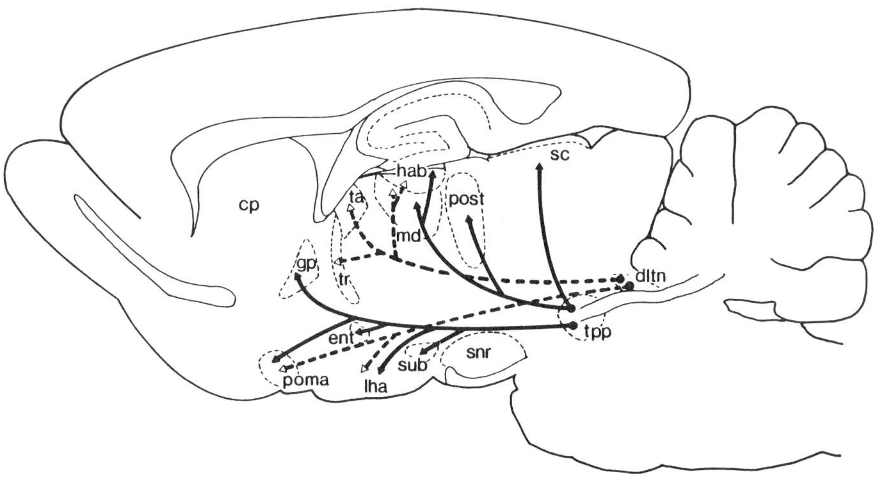

Fig. 4. Schematic representation of the ascending projections of the pontine tegmental cholinergic system. Abbreviations: **ent**, entopeduncular nucleus; **gp**, globus pallidus; **hab**, habenula; **lha**, lateral hypothalamic area; **md**, thalamic medial dorsal nucleus; **post**, posterior thalamic nucleus; **sc**, superior colliculus; **snr**, substantia nigra, pars reticularis; **sub**, subthalamic nucleus; **ta**, anterior thalamic nucleus; **tpp**, pedunculopontine tegmental nucleus; **tr**, thalamic reticular nucleus. For other symbols, see legends of Figs. 1-3.

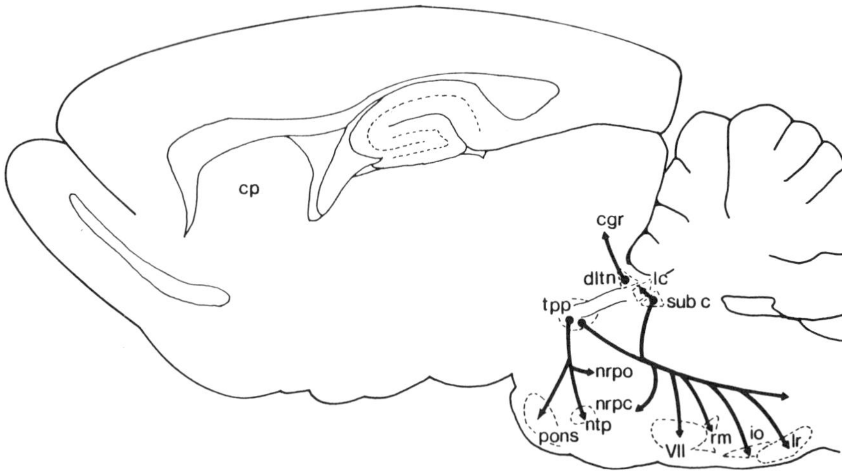

Fig. 5. Schematic representation of the essentially descending projections of the pontine tegmental cholinergic system. Abbreviations: **cgr**, central gray area; **io**, inferior olive; **lc**, locus ceruleus; **lr**, lateral reticular nucleus; **nrpc**, nucleus reticularis pontis caudalis; **nrpo**, nucleus reticularis pontis oralis; **ntp**, nucleus reticularis tegmenti pontis; **rm**, raphe magnus; **sub c**, subcerulear region (probably a part of the tpp); **VII**, facial nucleus. For other symbols, see legends of Figs. 3-4.

and Davis, 1981), and the acetylcholinesterase inhibitor physostigmine has been used to ameliorate the symptoms of schizophrenia (Lloyd, 1978) and to control manic episodes (Davis et al., 1978) in humans. Loss of neurons in the sublenticular substantia innominata has been reported in normal aging (Hassler, 1938), and decrements in cholinergic indices have been observed in the basal forebrain, hippocampus, and cerebral cortex of patients with Alzheimer's disease or with senile dementia of the Alzheimer type (for reviews, see Terry and Davies, 1980; Bartus et al., 1982; Price et al., 1982).

BRAINSTEM CHOLINERGIC SYSTEMS

Based on currently available evidence, the brainstem appears to contain two major systems of cholinergic neurons: (1) the various somatic and parasympathetic somata of cranial nerves III-VII and IX-XII and (2) the pontine tegmental cholinergic system composed prominently of ChAT-

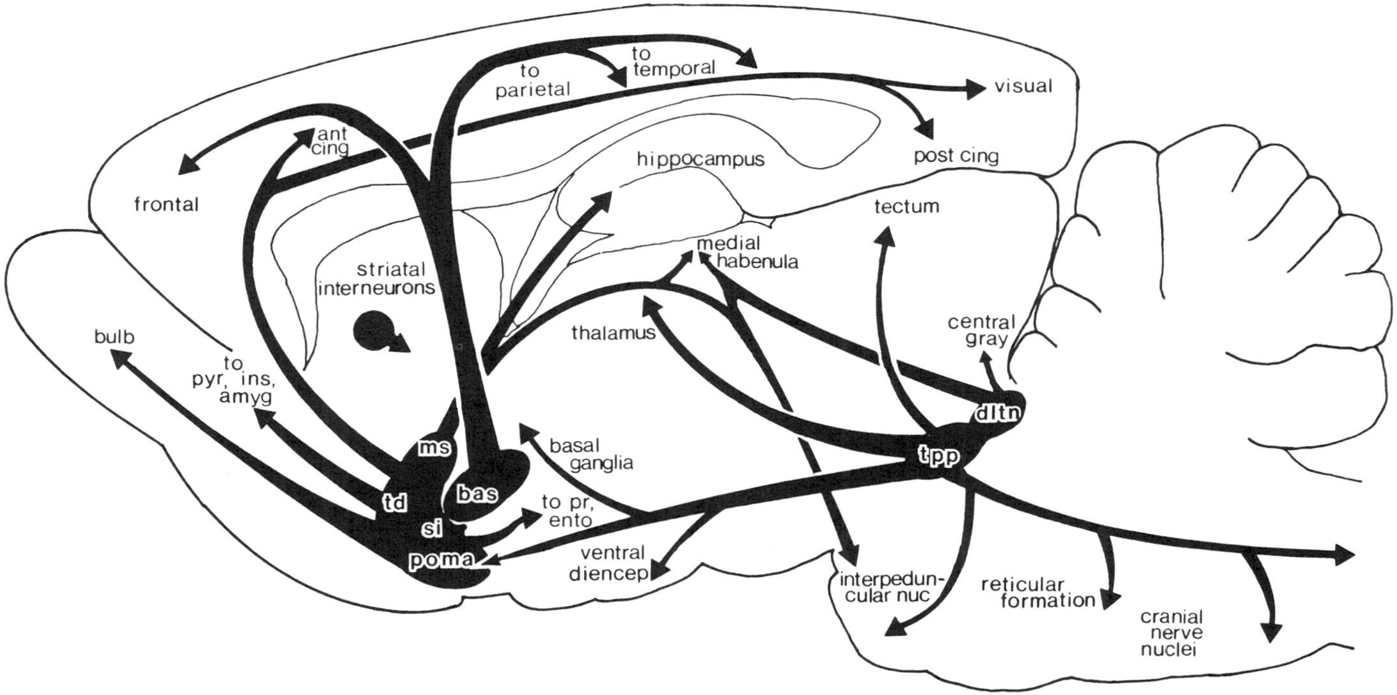

Fig. 6. Schematic representation (facing page) of the major cholinergic systems in the rat brain. Abbreviations: **ant cing**, anterior cingulate cortex; **post cing**, posterior cingulate cortex; **ventral diencep**, ventral diencephalon. For other abbreviations and symbols, see legends of Figs. 1-4.

Table 1. Some Normal and Pathologic Behaviors and Physiologic Processes in which Acetylcholine has been Implicated

Function/Dysfunction	Selected Experimental Evidence
Motor Activity	
(a) Posture, reflexes, and gait	Spinal neurons are cholinergic (Phillis, 1970); intrathecal injections of acetylcholine or neostigmine depress spinal reflexes (Kremer, 1942); oxotremorine produces ataxia and and spasticity (George et al., 1962).
(b) Catalepsy	Systemic administration of arecoline produces catalepsy (Costall and Olley, 1971).
(c) Tremor	Intracaudate infusions of carbachol, eserine, and DFP and systemic injection of oxotremorine elicit tremors (George et al., 1962; Lalley et al., 1970).
(d) Circling	Intracarotid injections of DFP produce contralateral circling (Freedman and Himwich, 1949).
Temperature Regulation	Infusions of carbachol or acetylcholine and eserine into the hypothalamus produce hyperthermia in monkeys (Myers and Yaksh, 1969).
Nociception	Oxotremorine, DFP, and pilocarpine produce analgesia (George et al., 1962; Karczmar, 1978).
Ingestive Behavior	
(a) Drinking	Injections of carbachol into the hypothalamus, preoptic area, septum, and hippocampus elicit drinking in rats (Levitt and Boley, 1970).
(b) Feeding	Intrahypothalamic infusions of carbachol elicit feeding in rabbits (Sommer et al., 1967).
Aggression	Neostigmine injections into the lateral hypothalamus increase mouse-killing by rats (Bandler, 1969); "rage" is produced in cats by infusions of carbachol into the anteromedial hypothalamus (Baxter, 1966); ChAT inhibition reduces isolation-induced aggression in mice (see Russell, 1978); oxotremorine produces a rage-like state state in cats and monkeys (George et al., 1962).
Sleep and Wakefulness	Depletion of acetylcholine with hemicholinium-3 decreases amounts of REM sleep (Domino et al., 1968); acetylcholine release from cortex is greatest during EEG desynchrony of wakefulness and REM sleep (Jasper and Tessier, 1971).
Learning and Memory	Cerebroventricular injections of hemicholinium-3 increase number of trials to criterion in a conditioned avoidance task (Russell, 1978); physostigmine produces retrograde amnesia (Hamburg, 1967); scopolamine impairs recall in humans (Drachman and Leavitt, 1974).
Disease States	
(a) Parkinsonism	Atropine ameliorates tremor (Friedman and Everett, 1964).
(b) Huntington's Chorea	Physostigmine and choline decrease involuntary movements (Davis et al., 1978); benztropine exacerbates those movements (Weiner and Klawans, 1978).
(c) Schizophrenia	Physostigmine and arecoline ameliorate symptoms (Lloyd, 1978).
(d) Mania	Predominantly euphoric manics become less manic after physostigmine (Davis et al., 1978).
(e) Alzheimer's Disease and Senile Dementia of the Alzheimer Type	ChAT and AChE are reduced in the cerebral cortex and hippocampus (for review, see Terry and Davies, 1980); cholinergic neurons in the basal forebrain project to the cortex, hippocampus and amygdala (e.g., see Bigl et al., 1982; Woolf et al., 1983, 1984); neurons in the basal forebrain cholinergic system undergo degeneration (e.g., see Whitehouse et al., 1981; Jabobs et al., 1985).

positive cells associated with the pedunculopontine tegmental and dorsolateral tegmental nuclei (Figs. 3-6). Of these, the latter system is incompletely specified at present. Although the existence of cholinergic projections to the thalamus appears well established, knowledge concerning the remaining pathways is either controversial or in a nascent state.

With the exception of the cholinergic neurons associated with cranial nerve nuclei, the functions of the remaining brainstem cholinergic pathways are poorly understood. Although DeFeudis (1974) has argued admirably that brainstem cholinergic neurons are involved in arousal and consciousness, in some motor and motivated behaviors, and in certain homeostatic and regulatory mechanisms (see also Table 1), the evidence is far from complete, and the methodologies employed in the studies cited by him invite alternative explanations for the results obtained.

SPINAL CORD CHOLINERGIC NEURONS

In the spinal cord, large neurons demonstrating ChAT-like immunoreactivity are found in the ventral horns at all levels, probably alpha-motor neurons, and in the intermediolateral column at thoracic and lumbar levels and the intermediate zone at sacral levels, where, in the latter two instances, they comprise the preganglionic neurons of the sympathetic nervous system and the sacral division of the parasymapthetic nervous system, respectively. Smaller ChAT-positive somata are seen in the region of the ventral horn as well, and it is conceivable that some of them are gamma-motor neurons. The functions of these sets of cholinergic cells are reasonably well established (see, for example, Table 1; DeFeudis, 1974; and Silver, 1974).

A few ChAT-positive somata are also scattered throughout non-autonomic intermediate zones of the spinal cord gray matter and in ventral aspects of the dorsal horns, but their functions are unknown.

CONCLUDING COMMENTARY

Until recently, the anatomy of central cholinergic systems, with the exception of the septo-hippocampal projection, was largely unknown. Formulations and findings based on the use of acetylcholinesterase histochemistry were dismissed cursorily by many students of the nervous system because the mere presence of the cholinergic degradative enzyme in a given neuron, as is well appreciated by careful workers, is not a sufficient criterion to label that cell cholinergic. Indeed, in a recent compendium of psychopharmacology (Lipton et al., 1978), extensive coverage of monoaminergic and peptidergic neuroanatomy is given, but cholinergic systems in the brain and spinal cord are scarcely mentioned, an inglorious fate for the first neurotransmitter to be described. Fortunately, the situation has now changed dramatically. Much of the impetus for this renewed interest in cholinergic neuroanatomy can be traced, we believe, to three major breakthroughs: (1) the development and use of the pharmacohistochemical regimen for acetylcholinesterase (Butcher et al., 1975; Butcher, 1978, 1983), (2) the development and use of morphologically acceptable and specific methods for the immunohistochemical demonstration of ChAT (Eckenstein and Thoenen, 1982; Houser et al., 1983; Levey et al., 1983), and (3) the development and use of methods based on the combination of acetylcholinesterase and ChAT histochemistry with anterograde and retrograde tract-tracing procedures, other histologic and histochemical techniques, and chemical and biochemical methods for ChAT and acetylcholine (see, for example, Butcher, 1977, 1978, 1983; Woolf et al., 1983, 1984; Woolf and Butcher, 1985). Use of these procedures has permitted confirmation of a cholinergic component to the septo-hippocampal pathway and has allowed the discovery, description, and delineation of major cholinergic projection systems deriving from the basal forebrain and pontine tegmentum, among others, as well as detailed analyses of the intrinsically organized constellation of cholinergic cells in the caudate-putamen complex. No doubt additional cholinergic systems and refinements in the descriptions of existing cellular aggregates and pathways will be ascertained and delimited as more data become available. The linking of cholinergic mechanisms with human neuropathologic disorders such as Alzheimer's disease further suggests that the study of cholinergic neuroanatomy will remain an exciting and fruitful area of investigation for many years to come, both in its own right and in relation to analyses of the functions of central cholinergic systems.

ACKNOWLEDGEMENTS

This research was supported by USPHS grant NS-10928 to L.L.B. We thank all of those individuals who are or were members of our laboratory and who contributed to the ideas and data presented in this paper.

REFERENCES

Bandler, R.J., 1969, Facilitation of aggressive behaviour in the rat by direct cholinergic stimulation of the hypothalamus, Nature (London), 224: 1035-1036.

Bartus, R.T., Dean, R.L. III, Beer, B., and Lippa, A.S., 1982, The cholinergic hypothesis of geriatric memory dysfunction, Science, 217: 408-417.

Baxter, B.L., 1966, Chemical and electrical stimulation of hypothalamic sites mediating "emotional" behavior, Pharmacologist, 8: 205.

Bigl, V., Woolf, N.J., and Butcher, L.L., 1982, Cholinergic projections from the basal forebrain to frontal, parietal, temporal, occipital, and cingulate cortices: a combined fluorescent tracer and acetylcholinesterase analysis, Brain Res. Bull., 8: 727-749.

Butcher, L.L., 1977, Nature and mechanisms of cholinergic-monoaminergic interactions in the brain, Life Sci., 21: 1207-1226.

Butcher, L.L., 1978, Recent advances in histochemical techniques for the study of central cholinergic mechanisms, in: "Cholinergic Mechanisms and Psychopharmacology," D.J. Jenden, ed., Plenum Press, New York, pp. 93-124.

Butcher, L.L., 1983, Acetylcholinesterase histochemistry, in: "Handbook of Chemical Neuroanatomy, Vol. 1, Methods in Chemical Neuroanatomy," A. Björklund and T. Hökfelt, eds., Elsevier Press, Amsterdam, pp. 1-49.

Butcher, L.L., Talbot, K., and Bilezikjian, L., 1975, Acetylcholinesterase neurons in dopamine-containing regions of the brain, J. Neural Transm., 37: 127-153.

Clemente, C.D., Sterman, M.B., and Wyrwicka, W., 1963, Forebrain inhibitory mechanisms: conditioning of basal forebrain induced EEG synchronization and sleep, Exp. Neurol., 7: 404-417.

Costall, B., and Olley, J.E., 1971, Cholinergic and neuroleptic induced catalepsy: modifications by lesions in the caudate-putamen, Neuropharmacology, 10: 297-306.

Davis, K.L., Berger, P.A., Hollister, L.E., DoAmaral, J.R., and Barchas, J.D., 1978, Cholinergic dysfunction in mania and movement diseases, in: "Cholinergic Mechanisms and Psychopharmacology," D.J. Jenden, ed., Plenum Press, New York, pp. 755-779.

DeFeudis, F.V., 1974, "Central Cholinergic Systems and Behaviour," Academic Press, New York.

DeLong, M., 1971, Activity of pallidal neurons during movement, J. Neurophysiol., 34: 414-427.

Domino, E.F., Yamamoto, K., and Dren, A.T., 1968, Role of cholinergic mechanisms in states of wakefulness and sleep, in: "Progress in Brain Research, Vol. 28," P.B. Bradley and M. Fink, eds., Elsevier Press, Amsterdam, pp. 113-133.

Drachman, D.A., and Leavitt, J.L., 1974, Human memory and the cholinergic system. A relationship to aging?, Arch. Neurol., 30: 113-121.

Eckenstein, F., and Thoenen, H., 1982, Production of specific antisera and monoclonal antibodies to choline acetyltransferase: characterization and use for identification of cholinergic neurons, EMBO J., 1: 363-368.

Freedman, A.M., and Himwich, H.E., 1949, DFP: site of injection and variation in response, Amer. J. Physiol., 156: 125-128.

Friedman, A.H., and Everett, G.M., 1964, Pharmacological aspects of parkinsonism, in: "Advances in Pharmacology, Vol. 3," S. Garattini and P.A. Shore, eds., Academic Press, New York, pp. 83-127.

George, R., Haslett, W.L., and Jenden, D.J., 1962, The central action of a metabolite of tremorine, Life Sci., 8: 361-363.

Hamburg, M.D., 1967, Retrograde amnesia produced by intraperitoneal injection of physostigmine, Science, 156: 973-974.

Hassler, R., 1938, Zur pathologie der paralysis agitans und des postenzephalitischen parkinsonismus, J. Psychol. Neurol. (Leipzig), 48: 387-476.

Hernandez-Peon, R., and Chavez-Ibarra, G., 1963, Sleep induced by electrical or chemical stimulation of the forebrain, Electroenceph. Clin. Neurophysiol., Suppl., 24: 188-198.

Houser, C.R., Crawford, G.D., Barber, R.P., Salvaterra, P.M., and Vaughn, J.E., 1983, Organization and morphological characteristics of cholinergic neurons: an immunocytochemical study with a monoclonal antibody to choline acetyltransferase, Brain Res., 266: 97-119.

Jacobs, R.W., Farivar, N., and Butcher, L.L., 1985, Alzheimer dementia and reduced nicotinamide adenine dinucleotide (NADH)-diaphorase activity in senile plaques and the basal forebrain, Neurosci. Lett., 53: 39-44.

Jasper, H.H., and Tessier, J., 1971, Acetylcholine liberation from cerebral cortex during paradoxical (REM) sleep, Science, 172: 601-602.

Karczmar, A.G., 1978, Exploitable aspects of central cholinergic functions, particularly with respect to the EEG, motor, analgesic and mental functions, in: "Cholinergic Mechanisms and Psychopharmacology," D.J. Jenden, ed., Plenum Press, New York, pp. 679-708.

Kremer, M., 1942, Action of intrathecally injected physostigmine, acetylcholine, and eserine, on the central nervous system in man, Quart. J. exp. Physiol., 31: 337-357.

Lalley, P.M., Rossi, G.V., and Baker, W.W., 1970, Analysis of local cholinergic tremor mechanisms following selective neurochemical lesions, Exp. Neurol., 27: 258-275.

Levey, A.I., Wainer, B.H., Mufson, E.J., and Mesulam, M.-M., 1983, Co-localization of acetylcholinesterase and choline acetyltransferase in the rat cerebrum, Neuroscience, 9: 9-22.

Levitt, R.A., and Boley, R.P., 1970, Drinking elicited by injection of eserine or carbachol into rat brain, Physiol. Behav., 5: 693-695.

Linseman, M.A., 1974, Inhibitory unit activity of the ventral forebrain during both appetitive and aversive Pavlovian conditioning, Brain Res., 80: 146-151.

Linseman, M.A., and Olds, J., 1973, Activity changes in rat hypothalamus, preoptic area, and striatum associated with Pavlovian conditioning, Brain Res., 36: 1038-1050.

Lipton, M.A., DiMascio, A., and Killam, K.F., eds., 1978, "Psychopharmacology: A Generation of Progess," Raven Press, New York.

Lloyd, K.G., 1978, Observations concerning neurotransmitter interaction in schizophrenia, in: "Cholinergic-monoaminergic Interactions in the Brain," L.L. Butcher, ed., Academic Press, New York, pp. 363-392.

Murphy, J.P., and Gellhorn, E., 1945, The influence of hypothalamic stimulation on cortically induced movements and on action potentials of the cortex, J. Neurophysiol., 8: 341-364.

Myers, R.D., and Yaksh, T.L., 1969, Control of body temperature in the unanesthetized monkey by cholinergic and aminergic systems in the hypothalamus, J. Physiol. (London), 202: 483-500.

Phillis, J.W., 1970, "The Pharmacology of Synapses," Pergamon Press, Oxford.

Price, D.L., Whitehouse, P.J., Struble, R.G., Clark, A.W., Coyle, J.T., DeLong, M.R., and Hedreen, J.C., 1982, Basal forebrain cholinergic systems in Alzheimer's disease and related dementias, Neurosci. Comment., 1: 84-92.

Russell, R.W., 1978, Cholinergic substrates of behavior, in: "Cholinergic Mechanisms and Psychopharmacology," D.J. Jenden, ed., Plenum Press, New York, pp. 709-731.

Shannon, C.E., 1948, A mathematical theory of communication, Bell Syst. Tech. J., 27: 379-423 and 623-656.

Silver, A., 1974, "The Biology of Cholinesterases," North-Holland Publ. Co., Amsterdam.

Sommer, S.R., Novin, D., and Levine, M., 1967, Food and water intake after intrahypothalamic injections of carbachol in the rabbit, Science, 156: 983-984.

Squire, L.R., and Davis, H.P., 1981, The pharmacology of memory: a neurobiological perspective, Annu. Rev. Pharmacol. Toxicol., 21: 323-356.

Sterman, M.B., and Fairchild, M.D., 1966, Modification of locomotor performance by reticular formation and basal forebrain stimulation in the cat: evidence for reciprocal systems, Brain Res., 2: 205-217.

Terry, R.D., and Davies, P., 1980, Dementia of the Alzheimer type, Annu. Rev. Neurosci., 3: 77-95.

Weiner, W.J., and Klawans, H.L., 1978, Cholinergic-monoaminergic interactions in the striatum: implications for choreiform disorders, in: "Cholinergic-monoaminergic Interactions in the Brain," L.L. Butcher, ed., Academic Press, New York, pp. 335-362.

Whitehouse, P.J., Price, D.L., Clark, A.W., Coyle, J.T., and DeLong, M.R., 1981, Alzheimer disease: evidence for selective loss of cholinergic neurons in the nucleus basalis, Ann. Neurol., 10: 122-126.

Woolf, N.J., and Butcher, L.L., 1985, Cholinergic systems in the rat brain: II. Projections to the interpeduncular nucleus, Brain Res. Bull., 14: in press.

Woolf, N.J., Eckenstein, F., and Butcher, L.L., 1983, Cholinergic projections from the basal forebrain to the frontal cortex: a combined fluorescent tracer and immunohistochemical analysis, Neurosci. Lett., 40: 93-98.

Woolf, N.J., Eckenstein, F., and Butcher, L.L., 1984, Cholinergic systems in the rat brain: I. Projections to the limbic telencephalon, Brain Res. Bull., 13: in press.

HISTOPATHOLOGY OF THE BASAL FOREBRAIN AND ITS TARGETS IN ALZHEIMER DEMENTIA

Roland W. Jacobs and Larry L. Butcher

Department of Psychology and Brain Research Institute
University of California
Los Angeles, California 90024, U.S.A.

INTRODUCTION

The age-old problem of senility has been the subject of increasing scientific inquiry in recent years and for a good reason. When the proportion of aged individuals in a population rises, as is currently the situation in many Western societies, so does the incidence of age-related disorders. Prominent among these maladies have been diseases of the Alzheimer type, which have been estimated to account for approximately 60% of all senile dementias and for the vast majority of presenile dementias (Schneck et al., 1982). Although a "unified theory," if such exists, of the etiology of Alzheimer dementias has yet to emerge, reasearch efforts have focused on various causal factors including increased aluminum concentrations in affected neurons, the presence of immunoglobulins, possible slow virus and/or subviral (prion) encephalopathies, microvasculature derangements, genetic susceptability, and involvement of specific neurotransmitter systems (for review, see Wurtman, 1985). In this report, we will concentrate on the role of one set of transmitter systems in the brain, namely those using acetylcholine as a chemical messenger, in the pathogenesis of Alzheimer's disease (AD, clinical onset of symptoms before age 65) and senile dementia of the Alzheimer type (SDAT, clinical onset of symptoms at age 65 or later). In particular, we will consider the relationships between pathologic involvement of the basal forebrain cholinergic system in AD/SDAT and certain aspects of the clinical and classic neuropathologic profiles of those two disorders.

METHODS

Brain samples having autolysis times of 24 hours or less were analyzed from 27 autopsied patients. The tissue, either fresh or frozen (-70° C), was received in coronally sectioned slabs, 5-8 mm thick, from the National Neurological Research Brain Bank (Wadsworth Veteran's Administration Hospital, Los Angeles, CA) or from the Department of Pathology, University of California, Los Angeles (UCLA). Diagnosis was independently confirmed histologically by the Department of Neuropathology, Harbor-UCLA Medical Center (Los Angeles, CA). Six patients (mean age at death, 78 years; range, 74-86) were diagnosed with SDAT; seven were afflicted with AD (mean age at death, 66.5 years; range, 64-69); four were neuropsychiatrically intact, non-demented aged controls (mean age at death, 82 years; range, 60-98); and five were non-demented, young controls (mean age at death, 24 years; range, 18-30). In addition, two patients were diagnosed with Pick's disease (ages at death, 63 and 80 years), and one was afflicted with multi-infarct dementia (age at death, 69 years). One senile (age at death, 78 years) and one presenile (age at death, 68 years) case, both with no morphologic changes, completed the patient population.

The parts of the brain slabs analyzed included unilateral or bilateral portions of the frontal, parietal, temporal, insular, and cingulate cortices; amygdala; hippocampus; and the sublenticular substantia innominata (SI), also referred to as the nucleus basalis of Meynert by some investigators (e.g., Whitehouse et al., 1981).

The tissue was fixed in 10% neutral buffered formalin at 4° C for one week before being placed into a cold 30% sucrose solution for an additional seven days. The brain slabs were then cut on a freezing microtome at 60-μm intervals. Under optimal conditions, successive sections were processed for Nissl substance (cresyl violet stain; Woolf and Butcher, 1981), acetylcholinesterase (Butcher et al., 1974), NADH-diaphorase (Butcher et al., 1974), senile plaques and neurofibrillary tangles (silver protargol stain; Bodian, 1936), amyloid (Congo Red stain; Lillie, 1965), and astrocytes (variation of Hortega's silver carbonate stain; Friede and Magee, 1962). Additional sections were stained with hematoxylin (Lillie, 1965). Not all sections from a particular brain slab, however, were necessarily stained for all of the indices indicated.

Three sets of quantitative measurements were generated. First, cell counts in the SI were performed by two independent blind raters in cresyl violet stained material from all 27 patients. These data were compared with adjacent sections stained for acetylcholinesterase. Second, senile plaque counts were made in silver stained sections containing portions of the frontal, parietal, temporal, insular, and cingulate cortices and the amygdala. Finally, clinical histories were available on each patient. Often these included various diagnostic tests, outpatient clinical notes by private physicians, and hospital records with admission and discharge summaries that spanned several years in some cases. In the patients histologically and histochemically processed by us, the duration of AD/SDAT ranged from 2.5 to 11 years with a mean of seven years. Each index case was clinically staged from 1 to 4 depending on the severity of dementia just prior to death. Medical records, including mental status examinations, were also available on the age-matched controls, and, because they were not demented, they were assigned a dementia score of zero. The criteria for assigning a particular dementia score were derived from the systems of Schneck et al. (1982) and Jervis (1971). Stage 1 dementia is characterized by difficulty in remembering names and appointments, often accompanied by an increase in anxiety. In Stage 2, there are loss of memory for recent events, lability of mood, changes in personality, disinhibition, paranoia, anomia, and dysarthria. Stage 3 is exemplified by worsening of memory, confabulations and vague delusions, depression, restlessness, compulsive crying and laughing, clang associations, agnosias and apraxias, tremors, paresis, rigidity, and grand mal seizures. In Stage 4, the patient is deeply demented, displaying a purely vegetative existence with recurrent infections.

RESULTS AND DISCUSSION

General Observations and Acetylcholinesterase Staining

The number of somata in the SI of aged but non-demented patients and AD/SDAT patients was 60.2% ($p < 0.01$) and 34.6% ($p < 0.01$), repectivley, of that found in young controls. Significant negative correlations existed between the number of cells in the SI and the mean number of plaques in the various cortical fields and amygdala ($r = -0.93$, $p < 0.01$; Fig. 1) and between SI neuron counts and the severity of clinically assessed dementia ($\eta = -0.88$, $p < 0.01$; Fig. 2). That some of the neuronal loss in

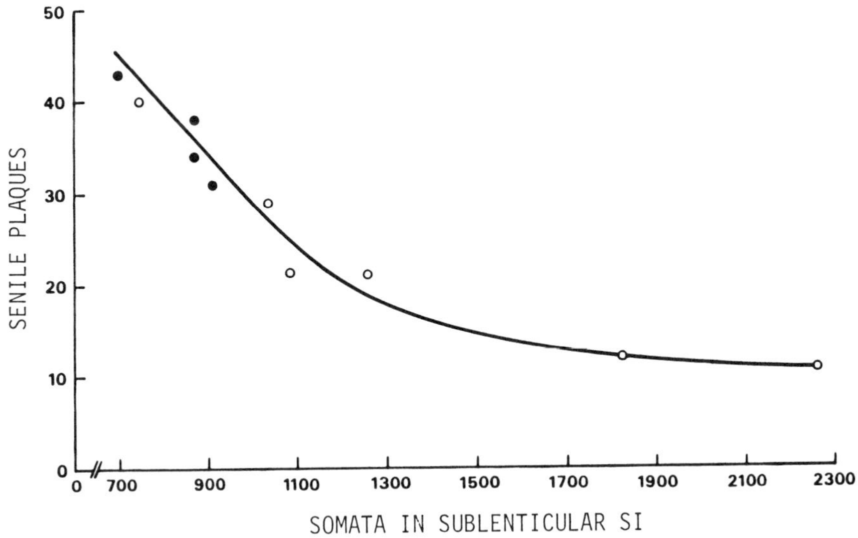

Fig. 1. Relationship between number of cells in the sublenticular substantia innominata (SI) and the mean number of senile plaques in the cerebral cortex and amygdala, considered together. Open and solid black circles represent, respectively, senile and presenile cases of Alzheimer dementia.

the basal forebrain may have been attributable to pathologic involvement of cholinergic cells is suggested by decreases in acetylcholinesterase staining in the SI in AD/SDAT (Fig. 3). Compared to SDAT cases, AD patients displayed a 21% greater reduction in the number of SI cells ($p < 0.01$), a 17% increase in the number of senile plaques ($p < 0.01$), and a 63% longer duration of the disease ($p < 0.01$). Furthermore, 71% of all AD cases reached Stage 4 dementia at death, whereas the corresponding proportion for SDAT patients was approximately 40%. We conclude from these data that individuals contacting Alzheimer dementia at an earlier age tend to suffer from the disorder longer, reach profounder stages of dementia, and manifest greater decrements in the number of cells, at least some of which are cholinergic, in the SI accompanied by increased senile plaques in the telencephalon.

NADH-diaphorase Staining

Six brain samples were prepared for NADH-diaphorase. Two cases, one a 76-year old female and the other an 82-year old male, were clinically and neuropathologically diagnosed as having severe SDAT, which had a duration of approximately five years in both individuals. Two additional patients were first diagnosed in the presenium with Alzheimer dementia, a diagnosis confirmed at autopsy. One was an 69-year old male with a 10-year history of the disorder, and the other was a 67-year old male with a 2 to 3-year course of dementing illnes. A 22-year old male and a 69-year old female with no history of dementia served as controls.

Although comparatively few senile plaques were found in the brains of the control cases (range, 0-16 plaques/square cm), numerous telencephalic plaques (range, 309-1236 plaques/square cm) were observed in the

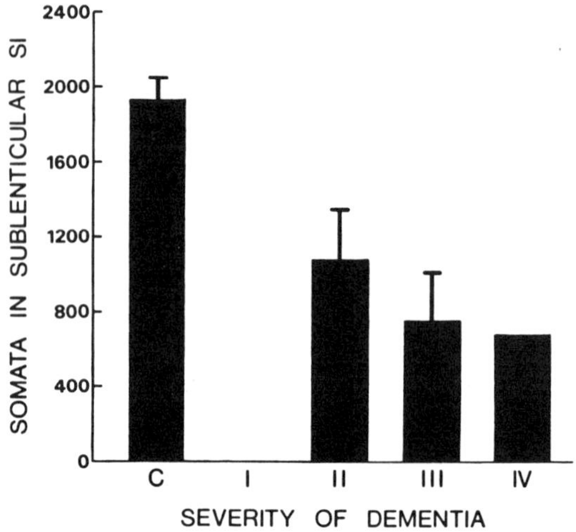

Fig. 2. Relationship between number of cells in the sublenticular substantia innominata (SI) and the severity of dementia. For further explanation, see text.

four cases of AD/SDAT, and many of them demonstrated appreciable NADH-diaphorase activity (cf., Friede, 1965; see also Jacobs et al., 1985). In addition, a number of hypertrophied astrocytes highly reactive for NADH-diaphorase were observed throughout and at the peripheries of the plaques. This latter finding was correlated in AD/SDAT patients with a loss of neurons positive for NADH-diaphorase in the SI, as well as with an increase in the number of astrocytes in that region of the basal forebrain. It is tentatively suggested that senile plaques may show augmented metabolic activity at some stage during their development and that the increased NADH-diaphorase associated with senile plaques and their accompanying astrocytes may be linked, in part, to the increased astrogliosis and decrease of NADH-positive neurons in the SI in AD/SDAT.

Plaque-like Lesions in the Basal Forebrain

All 27 brain samples were stained with Bodian's silver procedure (Bodian, 1936), and numerous senile plaques and neurofibrillary tangles were found in the cortices, amygdalas, and hippocampi of all AD/SDAT patients. Granulovacular degeneration was also seen in association with hippocampal pyramidal cells. Examination of the SI revealed, however, not only the expected loss of neurons but also the presence of numerous plaque-like lesions and a moderate increase in background argentophilia. These lesions, scattered throughout the SI among intact cells, were characterized by increased silver avidity and the presence of glial cells and neurites or neurite-like elements. Contrasted to "classic" senile plaques in the telencephalon, however, SI plaques were somewhat less argentophilic and generally smaller (30-50 µm in diameter). Furthermore, they did not appear to accumulate as the dementia progressed (i.e.,

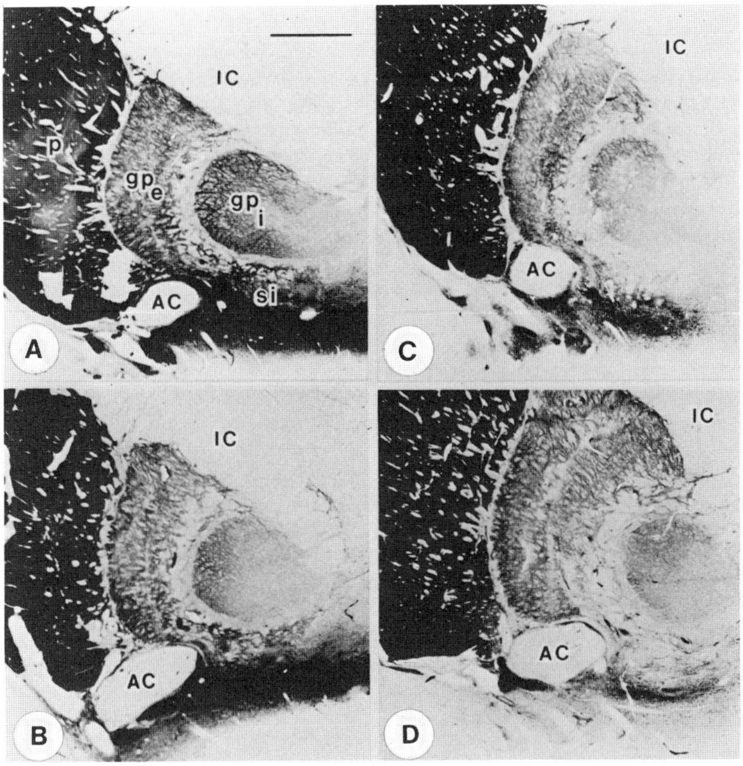

Fig. 3. Acetylcholinesterase staining in the sublenticular substantia innominata (si) of a 30-year old young control (A), a 69-year old age-matched control (B), an 81-year old patient with senile dementia of Alzheimer type (C), and a 67-year old individual with Alzheimer's disease (D). Abbreviations: **AC**, anterior commissure; **gpe**, globus pallidus, external segment; **gpi**, globus pallidus, internal segment; **IC**, internal capsule; **p**, putamen. Scale, 5 mm.

greater numbers were not found in more advanced forms of the disorder). The significance of these plaque-like lesions is not known, but, because they approximate the size of intact large cells in the SI, it is possible they represent pathologic processes associated with degenerating neuronal somata.

Amyloid and Astrocytes

Twenty-five brain samples were processed with Congo Red and hematoxylin. As with previous histologic and histochemical findings, the AD/SDAT patients distinguished themselves by certain persistent features not found in the control or the non-Alzheimer dementia groups. In addition to the deposition of amyloid in a majority of telencephalic senile plaques visualized in the fluorescence microscope, amyloid deposits were also observed in association with SI neurons. This Congo Red staining was seen in approximately one-third of the SI cells in AD/SDAT, either within the cytoplasm as possible tangle material or as an extracytoplasmic veil enveloping the soma. Neither the control nor the non-Alzheimer dementia cases, with the exception of one Pick's disease patient, contained any appreciable amounts of amyloid in the SI, either within neurons or in the neuropil.

Silver carbonate staining performed on several samples highlighted hypertrophied astrocytes within the SI in the AD/SDAT cases. Unlike the astrocytes revealed by NADH-diaphorase staining, however, the astrocytes demonstrated by silver carbonate histology appeared larger with long filamentous processes extending for considerable distances forming, in some instances, a reticular network. When tissue was processed with both silver carbonate and Congo Red, astrocytes were found in close communication with SI neurons, especially those with amyloid deposits. Often their fine tentacular processes were directly apposed to the neuronal surface and, in some cases, simultaneously to the surface of a blood vessel.

CONCLUDING COMMENTARY

The present data are consistent with previous findings suggesting a link between the basal forebrain, including its cholinergic components, and certain of the neuropathologies associated with AD/SDAT (Bowen et al., 1976; Davies, et al., 1976; Perry et al., 1977; Price et al., 1982; Arendt et al., 1983). Although cholinergic systems are not the only transmitter networks affected in AD/SDAT, they appear to be consistently involved. Future research in dementing illnesses may well be directed to determining how different neurotransmitter systems interact, both structurally and functionally and in both normal and disease states. Clues to the essential gestalt of AD/SDAT may thereby be obtained.

ACKNOWLEDGEMENTS

This research was supported by post-doctoral fellowship MH-08969 to R.W.J. and by NIH grant NS-10928 to L.L.B. Dr. W.W. Tourtelotte and his staff at the National Neurological Research Brain Bank are thanked for their assistance in obtaining samples of human brain material.

REFERENCES

Arendt, T., Bigl, V., Arendt, A., and Tennstedt, A., 1983, Loss of neurons in the nucleus basalis of Meynert in Alzheimer's disease, paralysis agitans, and Korsakoff's disease, Acta Neuropathol. (Berlin), 61: 101-108.

Bodian, D., 1936, A new method for staining nerve fibers and nerve endings in mounted paraffin sections, Anat. Rec., 63: 89-97.

Bowen, D.M., Smith, C.B., White, P., and Davison, A.N., 1976, Neurotransmitter-related enzymes and indices of hypoxia in senile dementia and other abiotrophies, Brain, 99: 459-495.

Butcher, L.L., Eastgate, S.M., and Hodge, G.K., 1974, Evidence that punctate intracerebral administration of 6-hydroxydopamine fails to produce selective neuronal degeneration, Naunyn-Schmiedeberg's Arch. Pharmacol., 285: 31-70.

Davies, P., and Maloney, A.J.R., 1976, Selective loss of central cholinergic neurons in Alzheimer's disease, Lancet, 2: 1403.

Friede, R.L., Enzyme histochemical studies of senile plaques, J. Neuropathol. exp. Neurol., 24: 477-491.

Friede, R.L., and Magee, K.R., Alzheimer's disease. Presentation of a case with pathologic and enzyme histochemical observations, Neurology, 12: 213-222.

Jacobs, R.W., Farivar, N., and Butcher, L.L., 1985, Alzheimer dementia and reduced nicotinamide adenine dinucleotide (NADH)-diaphorase activity in senile plaques and the basal forebrain, Neurosci. Lett., 53: 39-44.

Jervis, G.A., 1971, Alzheimer's disease, in: "Pathology of the Nervous System, Vol. 2," J. Minckler, ed., McGraw-Hill Co., New York, pp. 1385-1404.

Lillie, R.D., 1965, "Histopathologic Technic and Practical Histochemistry, 3rd Ed.," McGraw-Hill Co., New York.

Perry, E.K., Perry, R.H., Blessed, G., and Tomlinson, B.E., 1977, Necropsy evidence of central cholinergic deficits in senile dementia, Lancet, 1: 189.

Price, D.L., Whitehouse, P.J., Struble, R.G., Clark, A.W., Coyle, J.T., DeLong, M.R., and Hedreen, J.C., 1982, Basal forebrain cholinergic systems in Alzheimer's disease and related dementias, Neurosci. Comment., 1: 84-92.

Schneck, M.K., Reisberg, B., and Ferris, S.H., 1982, An overview of current concepts of Alzheimer's disease, Am. J. Psychiat., 139: 165-173.

Whitehouse, P.J., Price, D.L., Clark, A.W., Coyle, J.T., and DeLong, M.R., 1981, Alzheimer disease: evidence for selective loss of cholinergic neurons in the nucleus basalis, Ann. Neurol., 10: 122-126.

Woolf, N.J., and Butcher, L.L., 1981, Cholinergic neurons in the caudate-putamen complex are intrinsically organized: a combined Evans Blue and acetylcholinesterase analysis, Brain Res. Bull., 7: 487-507.

Wurtman, R.J., 1985, Alzheimer's disease, Sci. Am., 252: 62-74.

CLINICAL, PATHOLOGICAL AND BIOCHEMICAL ASPECTS OF ALZHEIMER'S DISEASE

Henryk M. Wisniewski

New York State Office of Mental Retardation and Developmental Disabilities, Institute for Basic Research in Developmental Disabilities, 1050 Forest Hill Road Staten Island, NY 10314

Clinical diagnosis of Alzheimer's disease/senile dementia of the Alzheimer's type (AD/SDAT) is based on progressive loss of mental faculties, often beginning with memory, learning, attention and judgment. According to Sinex and Myers (1982) the following are the stages of AD:

TABLE 1

1.	Early stages -	change in mood and loss of judgment, spatial orientation and memory
2.	Intermediate stages -	anxiety, uncooperativeness and loss of ability to communicate
3.	Late stages -	apathy, loss of response to most stimuli, incontinence, seizures, and difficulties in swallowing

Cohen et al. (1984) divides the signs and symptoms of AD/SDAT into the following phases:

TABLE 2

PHASES	PATIENT'S EXPRESSION
Recognition and concern	"Something is wrong"
Denial	"Not me."
Anger/guilt/sadness	"Why me?"
Coping	"In order to function I must do ..."
Maturation	"Living each day until I die."
Separation from self	.....

Today, the geriatric centers are using several tests to assess the mental status of AD/SDAT patients such as the Global Deterioration Scale (GDS) for Age-Associated Cognitive and Alzheimer's Disease and Brief Cognitive Rating Scale (BCRS) (Reisberg 1983) or Mental Status Testing (Katzman 1981) questionnaire.

According to the criteria specified in DSM-III (Diagnostic and Statistical Manual of Mental Disorder III of the American Psychiatric Association), Alzheimer's disease can be viewed as consisting of three components: a) memory and other cognitive impairment--the core features of dementia; b) functional and structural impairment of the brain; and c) behavioral manifestations that affect the patient's ability for self-care, interpersonal relationships, and adjustment in the community. While these three components are closely related, they do not closely parallel each other. For example, in some cases, memory and other cognitive impairment is rather severe, although there may be minimal or no evidence of other cerebral dysfunctions. In other cases, the reverse may happen--there is little memory and cognitive impairment in the presence of significant manifestations of brain dysfunction (Alzheimer's Disease. Report of the Secretary's Task Force on Alzheimer's Disease, 1984, Department of Health and Human Services Publication No. (ADM) 84-1323).

Neuropathological diagnosis of AD/SDAT is based on the presence of neurofibrillary changes and neuritic (senile) plaques. However, the plaques and tangles found in AD/SDAT are also found in much lower numbers in normal old individuals. Until recently neuropathologists had not determined how many plaques and/or neurons with tangles should be considered as a "normal" age-associated process and at which point the diagnosis of SDAT should be made.

During the recent National Institutes of Health/American Association of Retired Persons (NIH/AARP) sponsored "Workshop on the Diagnosis of Alzheimer's Disease," it was agreed that in any microscopic field encompassing 1 mm^2 of tissue, the following are the neuropathological criteria for the diagnosis of Alzheimer disease (Wisniewski and Merz 1985):

1. In any patient less than 50 years of age, the number of neuritic plaques and neurofibrillary tangles seen anywhere in the neocortex should be greater than 2-5 per field. This enables the anatomical pathologist to establish a very firm diagnosis, even in medicolegal cases and in the absence of any helpful clinical history.

2. In any patient between age 50 and 65 years, there will be some tangles, but the number of plaques must be 8 or greater per field. This will again permit a diagnosis with a very high degree of confidence ($\pm$95%).

3. For any patient between 66 and 75 years of age, some tangles will still be present, but the number of neuritic plaques must be greater than 10 per field.

4. In any patient older than 75 years, tangles may sometimes not be found in the neocortex, but the number of plaques should exceed 15 per microscopic field.

Implicit in the neuropathological criteria listed above is the view that the presence of neurons with neurofibrillary changes and plaques in small numbers is accepted as "normal" in older people.

Studies carried out by Ball and Nuttall (1977), Roth et al. (1966) and Tomlinson et al. (1970), revealed that with an increased number of neurofibrillary changes and neuritic plaques, the chance of showing clinical signs and symptoms of dementia increase. However, from the above neuropathological criteria of AD/SDAT it appears that with increased age one can tolerate more plaques and tangles without developing clinical signs of Alzheimer dementia. It appears also that in Down syndrome with Alzheimer type of neuropathology there is no direct correlation between the number of plaques and tangles and cognitive deficiency (Ropper and Williams 1980; Wisniewski et al. 1985).

Since quantimetric studies are done on post-mortem material with long clinical histories of the disease, it is possible that at the early stage of the disease in spite of the presence of cognitive deficiency the number of plaques and tangles is low. Therefore at the beginning of AD, not the structural, but biochemical abnormalities such as neurotransmitters deficiency (Bowen 1983) and blood-brain barrier changes (Wisniewski and Kozlowski 1982) could be responsible for the dementia. At the later stages the structural pathology contributes to the global and massive dementia seen in these patients. In this respect quantimetric studies of plaques and tangles on biopsy material obtained at the early stages of Alzheimer's dementia will be of great importance.

Morphological studies of AD/SDAT victims' brains showed that not all areas of the cortex and subcortical structures are affected by Alzheimer's type of pathology. The most affected are the hippocampus, amygdala and certain areas of the frontal, parietal and temporal cortex (Kemper 1984). The list of pathological findings in AD/SDAT is long (Wisniewski and Terry 1973a; Kemper 1984). However, as indicated above the neuropathological diagnosis of this disease is based on the presence of primitive (immature), classical (mature) and amyloid or burned out plaques and neurons with neurofibrillary changes.

NEUROFIBRILLARY CHANGES (Reprinted with permission of Springer-Verlag, New York from Aging 2000: Our Health Care Destiny, edited by C.M. Gaitz and T. Samorajski, Volume I, Biomedical Issues, 1985.)

Neurofibrillary changes refer to an excessive accumulation of fibrous profiles in the perikarya of neurons. Neurons with neurofibrillary changes are found, in varying numbers, in many and unrelated human diseases (Wisniewski et al. 1979). In the light microscope the affected nerve cells are best visualized by silver staining techniques. Ultrastructural studies of the neurons with neurofibrillary tangles reveal that, in the majority of human diseases, the tangles are composed of abnormal structures called paired helical filaments (PHF) (Wisniewski et al. 1976). Each filament in the pair is 10-12 nm in diameter and is helically wound around its partner thereby giving an overall PHF profile that is 20-24 nm in diameter. The helical feature of the PHF results in the repeating "nodes" at regular 80 nm intervals. Recent negative staining studies of PHF and supra-ultrathin sections of the PHF revealed that each of the 10 nm filaments making the PHF is made of four protofilaments (Wisniewski etal 1984). However, the ultrastructure of the PHF protofilaments and those of the 10 nm normal neurofilaments is different (Wisniewski and Wen, in press). The PHF are uniquely pathological and as indicated above their morphology is quite unlike the normal neurofilaments, neurotubules and microfilaments that are typical of the normal neuron.

One of the remarkable features of PHF is their resistance to various fixatives and post-mortem autolysis. Although the basis for this is not known it is probably related to another characteristic of the PHF. When the neurofibrillary tangles are stained with congo red they exhibit a characteristic green-red birefringence when viewed with polarized light. This is also a property of amyloid, another pathologic fiber. In the case of the systemic amyloid it is known that this property is a consequence of a β-pleated configuration of the constituent proteins (Glenner 1980). Although a β-pleated configuration has not yet been established for the PHF, it seems likely to be the case. Another feature probably contributing to the stability of the tangle is seen in recent studies which show that in some neurons the PHF are tightly packed into what are described as paracrystalline arrays in which the individual PHF are connected by "crossbridges" (Metuzals et al. 1982).

Administration of various chemicals such as aluminum salts in some animal species and spindle inhibitors in all animal species leads to the formation of neurofibrillary changes that, in the light microscope, resemble those seen in SDAT. However, electron microscopy revealed that these induced tangles are composed of 10 nm unpaired, straight filaments that are indistinguishable from normal neurofilaments (Wisniewski et al. 1968; Wisniewski et al. 1970; Wisniewski et al. 1981a).

Biochemical studies of the purified PHF confirms the morphological observation that such profiles are very resistant to various degradation conditions (Selkoe 1982). They can, however, be degraded by a combination of sonication and repeated cycles of heating to 100° C in sodium dodecyl sulfate and B-mercaptoethanol (Iqbal et al. 1984). Polyacrylamide gel electrophoresis of this material revealed a high molecular weight polypeptide band and several bands in the 45,000-60,000 dalton range. These bands are also found in normal control preparations but in much lower amounts. The origin of these polypeptides is not known but it appears that they are not new or novel (Iqbal et al. 1982). Rather it is likely that they are the product of an impaired degradation process in which a normal cellular component accumulates perhaps as a result of incomplete degradation of cell protein(s). This could well be the result of a quantitative or qualitative abnormality in protein degrading enzymes which leads to the polymerization of proteins and their storage in a manner analogous to the formation of lipofuscin granules from lipids and amyloid fibers in the systemic amyloidosis.

Immunohistochemical studies have shown that antisera prepared against microtubule preparations crossreacts with antigens present in neurofibrillary tangles (Grundke-Iqbal et al. 1979; Yen et al. 1981). Other work has shown that some antisera prepared against neurofilament components also immunostain AD/SDAT neurofibrillary tangles (Gambetti et al. 1980; Dahl et al. 1982). These immunohistochemical studies must be interpreted with caution because of what appears to be the trapping of nonconstituent proteins within the tangle. Evidence for this comes from recent work showing that (1) the blood brain barrier is compromised in SDAT such that the tangles (and plaques) contain both albumin and gamma globulins, and (2) both tangles and plaques are stained with antibodies to prealbumin (Wisniewski and Kozlowski 1982; Shirahama et al. 1982). Thus light microscopic immunocytochemistry alone is unlikely to provide an unequivocal candidate for the PHF precursor protein.

NEURITIC (SENILE) PLAQUES

Neuritic (senile) plaques are complex structures made of both neuronal and non-neuronal elements. They were first observed by Blocq and Marinesco in 1892, and named senile plaques by Simchowicz (1911). Since Bielschowsky's (1911) and Divry's (1934) reports, it has been known that amyloid is present in these plaques. The metallic impregnation methods show also that the glia elements, particularly the microglia and astrocytes, are part of the plaque structure. However, because of the limitations of light microscope techniques in identifying the various elements of the neuropil the origin and nature of the silver positive rods and granules seen in the plaques was not known. Subsequent ultrastructural studies showed that the granular structures were the dystrophic, regenerating and degenerating unmyelinated neuronal processes (neurites). At this point it should be recalled that early investigators like Fisher (1907) were of the opinion that nerve cell processes are involved in plaque formation. Bouman (1934), influenced by the silver staining methodology, postulated that the buds and knots represented regenerating neurites. As already mentioned these observations were confirmed by electron microscopic studies as well as recent examination of the plaques using the Golgi method (Probst et al. 1983). Many varieties of plaques have been described, but in general the following types are recognized: (1) typical, classical or mature plaques with a central core of amyloid surrounded by microglia, phagocytes and astrocytes and silver positive rods and granules which represent dystrophic regenerating and degenerating neurites; (2) primitive, atypical or immature plaques in which the amyloid is dispersed between the reactive cells and regenerating and dystrophic neurites; and (3) compact, burned-out or amyloid plaques that are made almost entirely by the deposits of amyloid.

One of the unanswered questions of plaque pathogenesis concerns the relationship between the amyloid deposition and the neuritic pathology. According to one hypothesis the first change which leads to plaque formation is the deposition of a "thread-like substance" (i.e., amyloid fibers) in the brain tissue. The second phase of the process is characterized by a reaction on the part of the nerve fibers (Marinesco and Minea 1912; Divry 1934; Schwartz 1970). A second hypothesis states that pathologic changes in other CNS components (e.g., blood vessels, glia, and neurons with neurofibrillary change) were responsible for the initiation of plaque formation. According to this view the amyloid originated either from the disintegration of the nerve cells or necrobiosis of neurologia (Simchowicz 1911; Ferraro 1931; Bouman 1934). The observation that, in the cortex, dystrophic neurites (in clusters no larger than 2-3) were found without amyloid lent to the belief that amyloid is not the initiator of plaque formation (Terry and Wisniewski 1970; Wisniewski and Terry 1973b). On the strength of this observation we proposed that the primary dystrophic and degenerative changes in neurites attracted microglia which, activated by the local pathology of the neuropil, started to produce amyloid. Subsequent studies of the pattern of degeneration of cortical terminals undergoing Wallerian degeneration due to undercutting or spindle inhibitor induced terminal pathology revealed that none of these changes led to amyloid deposition and plaque formation (Wisniewski and Terry 1970; Ghetti and Wisniewski 1972). Also in studies of infantile neuroaxonal dystrophy in humans in which there are many dystrophic neurities in the cortex, amyloid deposition has not been observed as a component of the pathology (Seitelberger 1971; Jellinger 1973). Thus, neuritic dystrophy and degeneration per se is not sufficient to initiate plaque formation.

Another approach to plaque pathogenesis was suggested by the finding that infection of genetically susceptible strains of mice with selected scrapie agents leads to the formation of neuritic and amyloid plaques in the central nervous system (CNS) (Wisniewski et al. 1975; Bruce et al. 1976). Because of a suggestion of an immune response to scrapie infection (Collis et al. 1979) it was proposed that the formation of a neurotoxic immune complex might be responsible for the dystrophic and degenerative changes in neuropil and the formation of amyloid fibers (Wisniewski et al. 1975). Furthermore observation of alterations in the blood brain barrier (BBB) of scrapie infected mice (Wisniewski et al. 1981b) provided the means by which such complexes might gain access to the CNS. Subsequent studies, however, showed that the BBB is also changed in scrapie infected mice that do not form plaques. Therefore chronic change in the BBB was not sufficient to explain plaque formation. Regardless of the role of BBB changes and/or presumed immune complexes ultrastructural studies revealed that the first changes appear to be related to hypersecretory activity of microglia which release proteinacious material into the extracellular space (Wisniewski et al.

1982; Moretz et al. 1983). It is in this milieu that assembly of amyloid fibers takes place. This concept envisions that the primary etiological and pathogenetic events are associated with the CNS amyloidogenesis and that the neuritic abnormalities are a secondary phenomenon. At this point the factor(s) leading to the formation of the amyloidogenic protein are not known. One possibility is that etiological factors such as an infectious agent might alter the biology of microglia/pericytes such that they become "producer cells" in which amyloidogenic protein arise as a new protein not normally expressed or as an overproduction of a native protein normally present in the cell. A second option is that the amyloidogenic protein is derived from either the blood stream or elsewhere in the brain. In this case the microglia behave as "processor" cells and alter the protein(s) in such a way that it now polymerizes into fibers that are deposited locally.

Studies have shown that in SDAT there is a cortical cholinergic deficiency (Davies and Maloney 1976) which is a consequence of the destruction of the cholinergic neurons of the diagonal band of Broca (dbB) and the nucleus basalis of Meynert (nbM) that project into the cortex (Whitehouse et al. 1981, 1982).

The studies of the nuclei of the basal forebrain led to the belief that the neuronal loss in these nuclei may play a role in the pathogenesis of neuritic plaques (Struble et al. 1982). It was postulated that "due to an unidentified pathogenetic process (for example, a toxin, transmissible agent, genetic factor, or age related event) a dbB or nbM neuron first begins to show abnormalities in distal intracortical axons; these acetylcholine esterase (AChE) rich neurites form immature plaques. With time some of these neurites degenerate; these polypeptides, liberated into the microenvironment of the neuropil, may contribute to the amyloid core. Thus, the mature plaque shows argentophilic AChE-positive neurites and amyloid. Eventually, the AChE-containing neurites disappear, leaving an amyloid plaque as the only evidence of this process" (Price et al. 1982). However, if this is really the case one would expect to find that, in the endstage of the disease, most if not all of the plaques would be of the burned-out or amyloid type. In fact, this type of plaque is not very common in the cortex of SDAT victims. What one sees is the predominance of the primitive (or immature), and classical (or mature) plaques. In other words at the time of death there are many abnormal neurites in spite of all the extensive loss of cholinergic terminals.

Other evidence pointing to the fact that dbB or nbM neurites are not necessary for initiation of the plaque formation is the presence of neuritic plaques in the cerebellar cortex where these nuclei do not project (Pro et al 1980). Our recent study shows that plaques occur more frequently than expected not only within defined subcortical nuclei including nucleus basalis of Meynert but also within the subcortical fiber system (Rudelli et al. 1984). This study showed also that the peripheral "halo" portion of the plaque where the abnormal neurites are found is determined by the neuropil response to the amyloid deposits, irrespective of the presence or absence of the cholinergic terminals. There are also cases with predominant perivascular distribution of plaques and there is no evidence of selective perivascular projection from nbM or dbB. Finally, data from the scrapie experiments show that the formation of plaques is closely associated not with the distribution of the cholinergic terminals but with the distribution of the infective agent. This conclusion is derived from several studies showing that in experimental scrapie in mice the distribution of plaques in brain with different inoculation routes is similar to the distribution of infectivity. For example, there are considerably more plaques in the inoculated hemisphere than in the contralateral hemisphere (Bruce and Fraser 1981). A relation betweem amyloid formation and infectivity is also implied by finding that large masses of amyloid are found in the needle track formed by the intracerebral inoculation of scrapie into mice (Wisniewski et al. 1981c). These data have led us to propose the following sequence of events in the pathogenesis of neuritic and amyloid plaque formation.

1. Microglia and pericytes produce and/or process amyloidogenic protein(s) which are subsequently assembled into amyloid fibers.

2. In areas rich in terminals Wallerian-like and dystrophic changes in the neurites occur due to the neurotoxic effect of certain enzymes associated with the amyloidogenic proteins and/or compressive neuropil degeneration.

3. Regenerative changes in the neuropil lead to the formation of many sprouting strongly silver positive neurites.

4. A healing process leads to the removal of the dystrophic neurites and the disappearance of reactive cells leaving behind the amyloid deposits which constitute to "burned out" or amyloid plaques.

According to this hypothesis the presence of amyloid deposits (plaques) without the abnormal neuritic component in areas rich in terminals can either be the result of the finished healing process (burned-out plaques) or the result of rapidly formed amyloid deposits. In the latter situation, the host neuropil has had no chance or for reasons not clear, did not respond to the toxic and/or compressive amyloid deposits with the formation of the dystrophic and regenerating neurites.

As indicated above in SDAT there is a cortical cholinergic deficiency. This is believed to be a consequence of the destruction of the cholinergic neurons of the dbB and the nbM that project into the cortex (Whitehouse et al. 1981; Price et al. 1982). In the authors' opinion "the clear association between loss of cholinergic innervation and most, if not all, of the symptoms of Alzheimer's disease has significant implications for diagnosis, treatment, and, one may hope, ultimately prevention of the disease" (Coyle et al. 1982). The authors further point out that this view suggests that in SDAT there is a defect paralleling that seen in Parkinson's disease. In our view such a primary "monotransmitter" pathology is not likely to be the case in SDAT. The topography of the SDAT lesions is much broader than in Parkinson's disease where, by and large, only pigmented nuclei are affected. In contrast SDAT involves the neocortex, hippocampal formation, amygdala and basal forebrain nuclei. This broader distribution of lesions obviously affects more than one transmitter system. Recent studies show that somatostatin mediated and noradrenegic systems are also affected in SDAT (Davies et al. 1980; Wood et al. 1982; Adolfsson et al. 1979; Mann et al. 1980). Therefore if one were to find a way to overcome the cholinergic deficiency in SDAT one might see some improvement in cognitive function but not full recovery of their mental functions. Thus, one should not expect a repetition of the success of L-dopa therapy seen in Parkinson's disease. Besides it is now evident that the L-dopa therapy did not stop the progress of Parkinson's disease. Concentration on how to treat the symptoms of Parkinson's disease appeared to detract the scientist and the funding agencies from the studies into causes of Parkinson's disease. This mistake should not be repeated with Alzheimer disease.

CURRENT HYPOTHESIS OF THE ETIOLOGY AND PATHOGENESIS OF SENILE DEMENTIA OF THE ALZHEIMER TYPE

At the moment there are three hypotheses regarding the etiology of SDAT. The aluminum hypothesis postulates that the disease is caused by the accumulation of toxic amounts of aluminum in the central nervous system (Crapper et al. 1981). While it is clear that elevated aluminum levels can affect cognitive function (as in dialysis dementia) there is little evidence to support the idea that aluminum is responsible for the Alzheimer type of pathology and dementia (Wisniewski et al. 1980; Wisniewski et al. 1985, in press)

TABLE 3

ALUMINUM IS NOT THE CAUSE OF AD BECAUSE

AL^{+3} intoxication affects neurons in the spinal cord, AD does not
Al^{+3} induced tangles are composed of 10 nm straight filaments.
AD tangles are composed of paired helical filaments.
Proteins comprising the 10 nm filaments are different from the proteins that make up the paired helical filaments.
Dialysis dementia (which is associated with high levels of Al^{+3}) does not exhibit the same pathology or clinical signs as AD.

The second hypothesis has it that SDAT is a genetic disorder. As indicated in Table 4, while there appears to be a genetic predisposition, it is not likely that a genetic defect is sufficient to explain the etiology of SDAT.

TABLE 4

A GENETIC COMPONENT IS NECESSARY BUT NOT SUFFICIENT TO CAUSE ALZHEIMER'S DISEASE

A high proportion of AD cases have no affected parent or sib
Few cases have pedigrees with a clear-cut Mendelian mode of inheritance (i.e., autosomal dominant trait)
Slow virus infection in man (e.g., CJD) have a similar mixture of cases exhibiting sporadic, familial and Mendelian inheritance.
AD type lesions (in lower numbers) are found in 100% of individuals over age 80.

The third hypothesis (Table 5) suggests that the disease is caused by an infectious agent and that both the agent and the pathogenesis of the disease are similar to those described for diseases caused by unconventional infectious agents. These diseases include Creutzfeldt-Jakob (CJD) and kuru of humans as well as scrapie, transmissible mink encephalopathy and chronic wasting disease (CWD) of lower animals. This hypothesis includes the concept that the genetic susceptibility of the individual plays a role in the development of disease.

TABLE 5

BASIS OF AD/SDAT SLOW VIRUS HYPOTHESIS

1. Presence of neuritic and amyloid plaques in scrapie, Kuru, CJD and AD/SDAT
2. Compromised blood-brain barrier in scrapie and AD/SDAT
3. Polyetiology of paired helical filaments includes virus infection
4. Both scrapie and AD/SDAT are characterized by the spectrum of clinical expression and pathological changes
5. Role of genetics in the expression of scrapie and SDAT

It is our view that the most viable hypothesis (both in conceptual and practical terms) is the third. This view is based on several observations. First, the genetics of SDAT has much in common with the genetics of other transmissible encephalopathies such as Creutzfeldt-Jakob disease (CJD), Gerstmann-Straussler syndrome (GSS), and scrapie in sheep, goats and mice. Second, there are associations between SDAT and known genetic conditions such as Down syndrome. Third, one of the two hallmark lesions of SDAT, the amyloid and neuritic plaque, occurs in scrapie, CJD, kuru and CWD. It is interesting that the development of plaques is under genetic control. In summary it appears that AD/SDAT is caused by an infectious agent in genetically susceptible individuals.

ACKNOWLEDGMENT

Supported in part by Grant No. 5P01-AG0-4220-02 from the National Institute on Aging. The author wishes to thank Marjorie Agoglia for her excellent secretarial assistance.

REFERENCES

Adolfsson R., Gottfries, C.G., Roos, B.E., and Winblad, B., Changes in the brain catecholamines in patients with dementia of the Alzheimer type, Br. J. Psychiat. 135:216-223 (1979).

Alzheimer's Disease, Report of the Secretary's Task Force on Alzheimer's Disease, U.S. Department of Health and Human Services, Publication No. (ADM) 84-1323 (1984).

Ball, M.J., and Nuttall, K., Neurofibrillary tangles, granulovascuolar degeneration in the hippocampus with ageing and dementia. Acta Neuropathol. (Berl) 37:111-118 (1977).

Bielschowski, M., Zur Kenntnis de Alzheimerischen Krankheit (prasenilen Demenz mit Herdsymptomen), J. Psychol. Neurol. 18:273-292 (1911).

Blocq, P., and Marinesco, G., Sur les lesions et la pathogenie de l'epilepsie dite essentielle, Sem. Med. 12:445-446 (1892).

Bouman, L., Senile plaques, Brain 57:128-142 (1934).

Bowen, D.M., Biochemical assessment of neurotransmitter and metabolic dysfunction and cerebral atrophy in Alzheimer's disease, Banbury Report 15: Biological Aspects of Alzheimer's Disease, Cold Spring Harbor Laboratory, pp. 219-231 (1983).

Bruce, M.E., Dickinson, A.G., and Fraser, H., Cerebral amyloidosis in scrapie in the mouse: Effect of agent strain and mouse genotype, Neuropathol. Appl. Neurobiol. 2:471-478 (1976).Cohen, D., Kennedy, G., and Eisdorfer, C., Phases of change in the apatient with Alzheimer's dementia: A conceptual dimension for defining health care management. J. Amer. Geriatrics Soc. 32(1):11-15 (1984).

Bruce, M.E., and Fraser, H., Effect of route of inoculation on the frequency and distribution of cerebral amyloid plaques in scrapie mice, Neuropathol. Appl. Neurobiol. 7:289-298 (1981).

Collis, S.C., Kimberlin, R.H., and Millson, G.C., Immunoglobulin G concentration in the sera of Hardwick sheep with natural scrapie, J. Comp. Pathol. 89:389-396 (1979).

Coyle, J.T., Price, D.L., and DeLong, M.R., Brain mechanisms in Alzheimer's disease, Hosp. Practice 17:55-63 (1982).

Crapper, D.R., Dalton, A.J., Karlik, S.J., DeBoni, U., Role of aluminum in Alzheimer's disease, in, "Electrolytes and Neuropsychiatric Disorders," P.E. Alexander, ed., S.P. Medical and Scientific Books, New York, pp. 89-111 (1981).

Dahl, D., Selkoe, D.J., Pero, R.T., and Bignami, A., Immunostaining of neurofibrillary tangles in Alzheimer's senile dementia with a neurofilament antiserum, J. Neurosci. 2:113-119 (1982).

Davies, P., Katzman, R., and Terry, R.D., Reduced somatostatin-like

immunoreactivity in cerebral cortex from cases of Alzheimer's disease and Alzheimer senile dementia, Nature 288:279-280 (1980).
Davies, P., and Maloney, A.J.F., Selective loss of central cholinergic neurons in Alzheimer's disease, Lancet 2, 1403 (1976).
Divry, P., De la nature de l'alteration fibrillaire d'Alzheimer, J. Belge Neurol. Psychiatr. 34:197-201 (1934).
Ferraro, A., The origin and formation of senile plaques, Arch. Neurol. Psych. 25:1042 (1931).
Fisher, O., Miliare Nekrosen mit drusigen Wuckerunger der Neurofibrillen, eine regelmassige Veranderung der Hirnrinde bei senile Demenz, Monatsschr. Psychiat. Neurol. 22:361-372 (1907).
Gambetti, P., Velasco, M.E., Dahl, D., Bignami, A., Roessmann, U., and Sindley, S.D., Alzheimer neurofibrillary tangles: An immunohistochemical study, in, "Aging of the Brain and Dementia," L. Amaducci, A.N. Davison, and P. Antuono, eds., Raven Press, New York, pp. 55-63 (1980).
Ghetti, B., and Wisniewski, H.M., On degeneration of terminals in the cat striatal cortex, Brain Res. 44:630-635 (1972).
Glenner, G., Amyloid deposits and amyloidosis, New Eng. J. Med. 302:1283-1292; 1333-1343 (1980).
Grundke-Iqbal, I., Johnson, A.B., Wisniewski, H.M., Terry, R.D., and Iqbal, K., Evidence that Alzheimer neurofibrillary tangles originate from neurotubules. Lancet 1: 578-580 (1979).
Iqbal, K., Grundke-Iqbal, I., Merz, P.A., and Wisniewski, H.M., Alzheimer neurofibrillary tangle: Morphology and biochemistry, Exp. Brain Res. (Suppl.) 5:10-14 (1982).
Iqbal, K., Zaidi, T., Thompson, C.H., Merz, P.A., and Wisniewski, H.M., Alzheimer paired helical filaments: Bulk isolation, solubility and protein composition, Acta Neuropathol. (Berl) 62: 167-177 (1984).
Jellinger, K., Neuroaxonal dystrophy: Its natural history and related disorders, in, "Progress in Neuropathology," H.M. Zimmerman, ed., Grune and Stratton, New York, Vol. II, pp. 129-180 (1973).
Katzman, R., Early detection of senile dementia, Hosp. Practice, 16:61-76 (1981).
Kemper, T., Neuroanatomical and neuropathological changes in normal aging and dementia, in, "Clinical Neurology of Aging," M.L. Albert, ed., Oxford University Press, New York-Oxford, pp. 9-52 (1984).
Mann, D.M.A., Lincoln, J., Yates, P.U., Stamp,J.E., and Toper, S., Changesin the monoamine containing neurons of the human CNS in senile dementia, Br. J. Psychiat. 136:533-542 (1980).
Marinesco, G., and Minea, J., Untersuchungen uber die senilen plaques, Monatasshi f. Psych. u. Neuc. 31, Eng. H. 79 (1912).
Metuzals, J., Montpetit, V., Clapin, D.F., and Nelson, R.F., Arrays of paired helical filaments in Alzheimer's disease, in, "Proc. of the Electron Microscopy Socity of America," Washington, D.C., Claitor's Publ. Div., Baton Rouge, pp. 348-349 (1982).
Moretz, R.C., Wisniewski, H.M., and Lossinsky, A.S., Pathogenesis of neuritic and amyloid plaques in scrapie - ultrastructural study of early changes in the cortical neuropil. In "Aging of the Brain," D. Samuel, S. Algeri, S. Gershon, V.E. Grimm, and G. Toffano, eds., Raven Press, New York, pp. 61-79 (1983).
Price, D.L., Whitehouse, P.J., Struble, R.G., Clark, A.W., Coyle, J.T., DeLong, M.R., and Hedreen, J.C., Basal forebrain cholinergic systems in Alzheimer's disease and related dementias, Neurosci. Commentaries 1:84-92 (1982).
Pro, J.D., Smith, Maj. C.H., and Sumi, S.M., Presenile Alzheimer's disease: Amyloid plaques in the cerebellum, Neurology 30:820-825 (1980).
Probst, A., Basler, V., Bron, B., and Ulrich, J., Neuritic plaques in senile dementia of the Alzheimer type: A Golgi analysis in the hippocampal region, Brain Res. 268:249-254 (1983).

Reisberg, B., Clinical presentation, diagnosis and symptomatology of age-associated cognitive decline and Alzheimer's disease, in, "Alzheimer's Disease," B. Reisberg, ed., The Free Press, New York, pp 173-187, (1983).

Ropper, A.H., and Williams, R.S., Relationship between plaques, tangles and dementia in Down syndrome, Neurology 30:639-644 (1980).

Roth, M., Tomlinson, B.E., and Blessed, G., Correlation between scores for dementia and counts of senile plaques in cerebral gray matter of elderly subjects, Nature 206:109-110 (1966).

Rudelli, R.D., Ambler, M.W., and Wisniewski, H.M., Morphology and distribution of Alzheimer neuritic (senile) and amyloid plaques in striatum and diencephalon, Acta Neuropathol. (Berl) 64:273-281 (1984).

Schwartz, P., Amyloidosis: Cause and Manifestations of Senile Deteriorations, Charles C. Thomas, Springfield, Illinois (1970).

Seitelberger, F., Neuropathological conditions related to neuroaxonal dystrophy, Acta Neuropathol. (Berl) (Suppl V), 17-29 (1971).

Selkoe, D.J., Molecular pathology of the aging human brain, Trends in Neuroscience 5:332-336 (1982).

Shirahama, T., Skinner, M., Westermark, P., Rubinow, A., Cohen, A.S., Brun, A., and Kemper, T.L., Senile cerebral amyloid: Prealbumin as a common constituent in the neuritic plaque, in the neurofibrillary tangle, and in microangiopathic lesion, Amer. J. Pathol. 107:41-50 (1982).

Simchowicz, T., Histologische studien uber die senile demenz. Nissl-Alzheimer's Arbeiten 4:267-444 (1911).

Sinex, F. Marrott, and Myers, R.H., Alzheimer's disease, Down's syndrome and aging: The genetic approach, Annals NY Acad. Sci. 396:3-13, (1982).

Struble, R.G., Cork, L.C., Whitehouse, P.J., and Price, D.L., Cholinergic innervation in neuritic plaques, Science 216:413-415 (1982).

Terry, R.D., and Wisniewski, H.M., The ultrastructure of the neurofibrillary tangle and the senile plaque, in, "Alzheimer's Diseases and Related Conditions," G.E. Wolstenholme and M. O'Connor, eds., Ciba Foundation Symposium, London, Churchill, London, pp. 145-168 (1970).

Tomlinson, B.E., Blessed, G., and Roth, M., Observations on the brains of demented old people. J. Neurol. Sci. 11:205-242 (1970).

Whitehouse, P.J., Price, D.L., Clark, A.W., Coyle, J.T., and DeLong, M.R., Alzheimer's disease: Evidence for selective loss of cholinergic neurons in the nucleus basalis, Ann. Neurol. 10:122-126 (1981).

Whitehouse, P.J., Price, D.L., Struble, R.G., Clark, A.W., Coyle, J.T., and DeLong, M.R., Alzheimer's disease and senile dementia: Loss of neurons in the basal forebrain, Science 215:1237-1239 (1982).

Wisniewski, H.M., Bruce, M.E., and Fraser, H., Infectious etiology of neuritic (senile) plaques in mice, Science, 190:1108-1110 (1975).

Wisniewski, H.M., Iqbal, K., and McDermott, J.R., Aluminum-induced neurofibrillary changes: Its relationship to senile dementia of the Alzheimer's type, Neurotoxicology 1:121-124 (1980).

Wisniewski, H.M., and Kozlowski, P.B., Evidence for blood-brain barrier changes in senile dementia of the Alzheimer type (SDAT), Ann. New York Acad. Sci. 396:119-129 (1982).

Wisniewski, H.M., Lossinsky, A.S., Moretz, R.C., and Vorbrodt, A.W., Neuritic plaque formation and blood-brain barrier (BBB) changes in scrapie, J. Neuropathol. Exp. Neurol. 40:1342 (1981b).

Wisniewski, H.M., and Merz, G.S., Neuropathology of the aging brain and dementia of the Alzheimer type, in, "Aging 2000: Our Health Care Destiny," C.M. Gaitz and T. Samorajski, eds., Volume I, Biomedical Issues, Springer-Verlag, New York, pp. 231-243 (1985).

Wisniewski, H.M., Merz, P.A., and Iqbal, K., Ultrastructure of paired

helical filaments of Alzheimer's neurofibrillary tangle, J. Neuropath. Exp. Neurol. 43:643-656 (1984).
Wisniewski, H.M., Moretz, R.C., and Lossinsky, A.S., Evidence for induction of localized amyloid deposits and neuritic plaques by an infectious agent, Ann. Neurol. 10:517-522 (1981c).
Wisniewski, H.M., Narang, H.K., and Terry, R.D., Neurofibrillary tangles of paired helical filaments, J. Neurol. Sci. 27:173-181 (1976).
Wisniewski, H.M., Shelanski, M.L., and Terry, R.D., Effects of miotic spindle inhibitors on neurotubules and neurofilaments in anterior horn cells, J. Cell Biol. 38:224-229 (1968).
Wisniewski, H.M., Sinatra, R.S., Iqbal, K., and Grundke-Iqbal, I., Neurofibrillary and synaptic pathology in the aged brain, in, "Aging and Cell Structure," J.E.Johnson, Jr., ed., Vol. 1, Plenum Press, New York, pp. 104-142 (1981a).
Wisniewski, H.M., Sturman, J.A., Shek, J.W., and Iqbal, K., Aluminum and the central nervous system, in, "Clinical Implication of Aluminum Neurotoxicity," L. Liss, ed., Chem-Orbital, Park Forest South, Illinois, in press.
Wisniewski, H.M., and Terry, R.D., An experimental approach to the morphogenesis of neurofibrillary degeneration and the argyrophilic plaque, in, "Alzheimer's Diseases and Related Conditions," G.E. Wolstenholme and M. O'Connor, eds., Ciba Foundation Symposium, London, Churchill, London, pp. 223-243 (1970).
Wisniewski, H.M., and Terry, R.D., Morphology of the aging brain, human and animal, Progress in Brain Research 40:167-186 (1973a).
Wisniewski, H.M., and Terry, R.D., Reexamination of the pathogenesis of the senile plaque, in "Progress in Neuropathology," H.M. Zimmerman, ed., Vol. II, Grune and Stratton, New York, pp. 1-26 (1973b).
Wisniewski, H.M., Terry, R.D., and Hirano, A., Neurofibrillary pathology. J. Neuropathol. Exp. Neurol. 29:163-176 (1970).
Wisniewski, H.M., Vorbrodt, A.W., Moretz, R.C., Lossinsky, A.S., and Grundke-Iqbal, I., Pathogenesis of neuritic (senile) and amyloid plaque formation, in, "The Aging Brain - Physiological and Pathological Aspects," S. Hoyer, ed., Experimental Brain Research Supplementum 5, Springer-Verlag, New York, pp. 3-9, (1982).
Wisniewski, H.M., and Wen, G.Y., Substructures of paired helical filaments from Alzheimer's disease neurofibrillary tangles. Acta Neuropathol. (Berl) in press.
Wisniewski, K., Jervis, G.A., Moretz, R.C., and Wisniewski, H.M., Alzheimer neurofibrillary tangles in diseases other than senile and presenile dementia, Ann. Neurol. 5:288-294 (1979).
Wisniewski, K.E., Wisniewski, H.M., and Wen, G.Y., Occurrence of neuropathological changes and dementia of Alzheimer's disease in Down's syndrome, Ann. Neurol. 17:278-282 (1985).
Wood, P.L., Etienne, P., Lal, S., Gauthier, S., Cajal, S., and Nair, N.P.V., Reduced lumbar CSF somatostatin levels in Alzheimer's disease, Life Sci. 31:2073-2079 (1982).
Yen, S.C., Gaskin, G., and Terry, R.D., Immunocytochemical studies of neurofibrillary tangles, Am. J. Pathol. 104:77-89 (1981).

MOLECULAR PROPERTIES OF PAIRED HELICAL FILAMENTS AND SENILE PLAQUE AMYLOID FIBERS IN ALZHEIMER'S DISEASE

Dennis J. Selkoe, Carmela Abraham, and C. G. Rasool

Harvard Medical School, McLean Hospital, and
Brigham and Women's Hospital, Boston, MA

Introduction

In a disorder as complex and enigmatic as Alzheimer' disease, numerous distinct research strategies must be applied simultaneously. While some experimental approaches will provide information about secondary events in the disease process, it is hoped that other strategies will yield clues to the fundamental biological process that initiates the neuronal degeneration. Most current investigations of the biological aspects of Alzheimer's disease address one or more of three broad questions. The first question regards the etiologic event(s) that initiate the progressive loss of selected brain neurons. Research strategies in this area include molecular genetic investigations of the chromosomal locus and identity of an abnormal gene in hereditary forms of Alzheimer's disease; the search for an infectious pathogen; and the study of the role of environmental toxins in this disease. The second broad question concerns the molecular mechanism of cell death, once the initiating event(s) have taken place, whether they are genetic, infectious and/or toxic. The third question is that of the identity of the degenerating neurons as to location, functional class and neurotransmitter status. This latter question in Alzheimer's disease has received the most experimental attention during the past decade since it appears to offer the earliest chance of developing a therapy that could ameliorate symptoms of the disease. With the rapid development of molecular genetics and neurovirology in recent years, experiments aimed at the first question are also accelerating.

Experiments focusing on the second question, that is, the sequence of molecular events that occurs during the dysfunction and death of neurons in Alzheimer's disease, have received relatively less attention than the other two questions. Information about the precise mechanism of neuronal degeneration could obviously provide clues to earlier events in the disease process, whether they be genetic, infectious or both.

Protein Chemical Approaches to the Nature of Paired Helical Filaments

During the past several years, our laboratory has sought information about molecular changes that lead to cell death in Alzheimer's disease by studying the protein chemistry and antigenic structure of paired helical filaments (PHF) and, more recently, senile plaque amyloid fibers. If the process that allows formation and massive accumulation of abnormal fibers in neuronal cell bodies and neurites could be understood, events that precede the formation of these fibers could come under study. We began our analysis by partially purifying PHF from postmortem human cerebral cortex and comparing them to similarly isolated fractions from normal aged human brain.[1-3] Numerous one- and two-dimensional gel electrophoretic experiments failed to demonstrate specifically augmented or altered neuronal proteins as a constituent of PHF-enriched fractions. Consequently, we hypothesized that PHF might have unusual molecular properties that did not allow their analysis by conventional electrophoretic techniques. We then examined the detergent-insoluble fraction of our PHF preparations by electron microscopy and found that the PHF remained intact following extensive extraction and heating in sodium dodecyl sulfate (SDS) and other denaturants used to solubilize proteins for analytical separation.[3]

This observation indicated that PHF were assembled by many strong non-covalent bonds, by covalent crosslinks, or by both. We subsequently found that the PHF were also resistant to quantitative digestion by specific or non-specific proteases.[4] As a candidate for the crosslinking reaction that could bind normal fibers (e.g., neurofilaments [NF]) into insoluble polymers, we proposed the transglutaminase-catalyzed formation of glutamyl-lysine intermolecular bonds.[5] This reaction is one of the most common known mechanisms for the crosslinking of intracellular and extracellular mammalian proteins. Although NF proteins can be crosslinked _in vitro_ by the action of transglutaminase,[5] it has not been possible to demonstrate such glu-lys crosslinks directly in PHF because of the resistance of the fibers to the sequential enzymatic digestion required for detecting these dipeptides.

The highly inert nature of PHF allowed development of new methods for their purification that included extraction in SDS and reducing agents.[6,7] Although such techniques markedly enrich brain preparations in PHF and remove many proteinaceous contaminants, biochemical purification strategies have not produced complete purification of PHF. Furthermore, the use of any extraction procedure, including SDS, has the disadvantage of removing non-covalently associated proteins of the PHF, knowledge of which may be important for understanding the composition and assembly of the fibers. We have therefore recently concentrated on various immunochemical strategies for PHF and plaque amyloid purification (see below).

We have determined the amino acid composition of considerably but not completely purified PHF.[4] These analyses demonstrate abundant glycine and other non-polar, hydrophobic residues in the protein, comprising approximately 55% of all residues. There is very little proline (that present may actually derive from contaminants in the preparation) and a small amount of methionine. The amino acid analysis of PHF is distinct from that published for the NF triplet proteins.

In collaboration with Daniel Kirschner at Harvard Medical School, we have recently studied the tertiary structure of the PHF polymer using x-ray diffraction analysis.[8] A molecular spacing pattern consistent with a protein containing extensive cross-β-pleated sheet conformation was observed. This work represents the first direct demonstration of the presence of β-pleated sheet structure in a CNS amyloid. Such a structure has long been postulated on the basis of studies of systemic amyloid deposits. The presence of β-pleated sheet structure may explain, at least in part, the resistance of PHF to solubilization and their hydrophobic behavior in aqueous solutions.

Immunochemical Approaches to PHF Analysis

Since conventional protein chemical techniques that are applied to soluble polypeptides cannot be used on the insoluble, polymeric PHF and since complete purification by biochemical strategies has not been achieved, we turned to immunochemical approaches both as a method of analysis and for the purpose of purification.

Rabbits injected with extensively purified PHF fractions (prepared in SDS) produced antisera that reacted at high titer with neurofibrillary tangles (NFT) and senile plaque neurites *in situ* as well as with tangles isolated in either physiologic or denaturant buffers.[6] Unexpectedly, these polyclonal PHF antibodies failed to react with normal NF either in tissue sections or by western blot analysis.[6] They also do not react with other normal brain proteins tested to date. This finding indicates that PHF contain unique antigens not shared with normal brain NF, which had heretofore been considered the best candidate for the precursor proteins of the pathological fibers. On the other hand, several laboratories have reported that certain polyclonal or monoclonal antibodies to NF do indeed cross-react with NFT in tissue sections.[9-13] Incollaborative studies with Brian Anderton and colleagues, we showed that their monoclonal antibodies RT97 and BF10, to the 200,000 and 160,000 M.W. NF proteins, respectively, labeled the same tangle-bearing neurons that are identified by our PHF-specific antibodies.[14] Following denaturant extraction, most of the immunoactivity of these NF monoclonals with NFT is lost, while PHF antibodies continued to be reactive.[14] However, under certain conditions of prolonged denaturant incubation of isolated NFT, at least a portion of the NF epitopes apparently become exposed on the PHF fiber and are again identifiable by labeling with monoclonal RT97 or BF10.[15] Such results indicate a complex antigenic structure of the PHF, including epitopes shared with NF that are partially buried in the fiber and epitopes that are quite distinct or at least highly modified from normal fibrous proteins. We have also recently produced several monoclonal antibodies to SDS-insoluble PHF fibers.[16] These similarly show complex antigenic cross-reactivities: some react solely with PHF, while others demonstrate shared epitopes with certain normal brain proteins, including NF, glial filaments and proteins that are presumed not to be involved in PHF formation, e.g., myelin basic protein.

The availability of PHF-specific antibodies has been useful in several ways. It has been possible to carry out double-labeling studies of certain brain areas markedly affected in Alzheimer's disease, e.g., the cholinergic neurons of the basal forebrain. We carried out PHF immunolabeling and acetylcholinesterase histochemistry simultaneously on sections of nucleus basalis of Meynert (nbM) and found that a large number of NFT were present in the nbM and that many tangles existed in loci where AChE-reactivity had disappeared.[17] It thus appears that, as in the cerebral cortex, NFT formation occurs extensively in the nbM and could explain, in part, the dysfunction and death of these important cholinergic neurons.

PHF antibodies have also demonstrated the presence of apparently extracellular ("ghost") tangles in both the cerebral neocortex and nbM.[14] These light-microscopically identifiable structures appear more loose and open than the classical compacted intracellular tangles and are not associated with any recognizable cell structure. We have observed apparently cell-free bundles of either PHF or straight 12-16nm fibers in some cases of Alzheimer's disease by electron microscopy; presumably, these correlate with the "ghost" tangles demonstrated by light microscopy using our PHF antibodies. This finding would be consistent with the highly inert nature of PHF *in vitro* and would suggest that the neuron and the surrounding extracellular milieu in the brain are not able to catabolize the PHF fibers quickly and efficiently once they are formed, so that they may remain for a time as residual bodies following cell death.

The fact that the antibodies to PHF are specific and do not react with normal brain proteins allows one to examine non-Alzheimer fibrillary degenerative diseases to detect cross-reacting pathological fibers. An example of such work is provided by our observation that the characteristic Pick bodies in degenerating neurons in Pick's disease cross-react strongly with PHF.[18] The Pick bodies in such cases usually contain abnormal 10-20nm straight filaments (usually 12-16 nm) and only rarely contain PHF or unconventional helically wound filaments. Thus, despite their ultrastructural distinction, the abnormal fibers that comprise the Pick bodies and the Alzheimer NFT, respectively, appear to share specific antigens. This work confirms earlier work by Probst and colleagues demonstrating specific labeling of Pick bodies by monoclonal NF antibodies that recognize NFT but not by NF antibodies that fail to react with NFT.[19]

Studies of Senile Plaque Amyloid

In attempts to use PHF antibodies for immunopurification of the fibers to homogeneity, we found that traditional strategies such as immunoaffinity chromatography on a solid matrix do not work well with the insoluble, rigid PHF fibers. We therefore decided to attempt a somewhat unusual strategy for isolation of a cerebral organelle, namely fluorescence-activated cell sorting (FACS). In our initial attempts to use flow cytometry for purification, we took advantage of the dense, roughly spherical nature of SDS-isolated amyloid plaque cores to purify these by FACS[20] prior to turning to the more difficult problem of NFT purification by this method.

We have developed a protocol for preparation of considerably enriched amyloid core fractions using standard techniques of solvent extraction, differential centrifugation, and sucrose gradient fractionation. Such core-enriched fractions are then analyzed and sorted on a FACS instrument so that autofluorescent lipofuscin granules are largely separated from the non-fluorescent cores. We subsequently raised a rat polyclonal antiserum to partially purified amyloid cores and used this to immunolabel the cores following an initial FACS sort. The rhodamine-tagged cores were then sorted a second time through the FACS and produced highly purified core fractions. By both light- and electron-microscopic particle counting, these fractions are greater than 90% amyloid cores and contain only small numbers of contaminating aggregates of lipofuscin and occasional irregular sheets of densely packed amyloid fibrils, the origin of which is unclear.[20,21]

The purification of the amyloid cores to near homogeneity has now allowed their compositional analysis.[21] Their amino acid compositions are quite similar but not identical to that of partially purified PHF fractions. Again, the amyloid cores differ in their composition from normal NF. X-ray diffraction analysis of FACS-purified cores has also demonstrated the presence of β-pleated sheet structure in these fibers.[8]

The core amyloid fibers share with PHF a high degree of insolubility and resistance to enzymatic digestion. We have attempted to quantitatively depolymerize the amyloid fibers and detect their protein subunits by solubilization in strong chaotropic salts (e.g., guanidine SCN) or in formic acid. Although these reagents immediately clarify core suspensions and birefringent cores are no longer seen by polarization microscopy, altered filamentous material can be pelleted and viewed by electron microscopy after such treatments. Furthermore, several kinds of assays, including gel electrophoresis, high performance liquid chromatography, and amino acid analysis of guanidine SCN- or formic acid-treated cores, have not revealed specific solubilized protein subunits. The reasons for the apparent resistance of cores purified by our method to solubilization are currently being studied. We are currently carrying out protein sequencing experiments on the purified cores using the intact polymeric fibers or fibers digested by limited acid hydrolysis. Such analyses should determine more precisely the protein origin of amyloid fibers and, following similar analyses on

PHF, their relationship to the intraneuronal fibers that accumulate in Alzheimer's disease.

Conclusions

The results of our studies to date on paired helical filaments and senile plaque amyloid fibrils can be summarized as follows.

1. Both the intraneuronal PHF and the extracellular amyloid fibrils of senile plaques are highly stable protein polymers that are insoluble in most denaturants and resist enzymatic digestion.

2. NFT-bearing neurons may also contain abnormal straight filaments (10-20 nm), either alone or in combination with PHF. Such straight filaments are antigenically related to PHF.

3. The observation that PHF are insoluble in SDS and other solvents has led to considerable but not complete purification.

   The insolubility and spherical form of isolated amyloid cores has enabled their purification as intact particles using fluorescence-activated cell sorting.

4. The amino acid composition of purified cores is similar to that of partially purified PHF; both are distinct from that of neurofilaments (NF).

5. Antibodies that specifically label PHF also react with purified amyloid cores. These antibodies do not react with NF. On the other hand, certain polyclonal and monoclonal antibodies to NF do label NFT.

6. X-ray diffraction analysis reveals an apparent β-pleated sheet conformation for both PHF and plaque amyloid fibers.

7. Thus, senile plaque amyloid proteins and PHF, although ultrastructurally distinct, share solubility properties, β-pleated sheet structure, similar amino acid compositions and certain antigenic determinants.

   Sequence analysis should determine whether these unusual fibers derive from highly modified NF or represent newly genetically expressed proteins.

References

1. D. J. Selkoe, Altered protein composition of isolated human cortical neurons in Alzheimer disease, Ann. Neurol. 5:468 (1980).
2. D. J. Selkoe, B. A. Brown, F. J. Salazar, and C. A. Marotta, Myelin basic protein in Alzheimer disease neuronal fractions and mammalian neurofilament preparations, Ann. Neurol. 10:429 (1981).
3. D. J. Selkoe, Y. Ihara, and F. J. Salazar, Alzheimer's disease: Insolubility of partially purified paired helical filaments in sodium dodecyl sulfate and urea, Science 215:1243 (1982).
4. D. J. Selkoe, Y. Ihara, C. Abraham, C. G. Rasool, and A. H. McCluskey, Biochemical and immunocytochemical studies of Alzheimer paired helical filaments, in: "Banbury Report 15: Biological Aspects of Alzheimer's Disease," R. Katzman, ed., Cold Spring Harbor Laboratory, Cold Spring Harbor, N. Y. (1983).
5. D. J. Selkoe, C. Abraham, and Y. Ihara, Brain transglutaminase: In

vitro crosslinking of human neurofilament proteins into insoluble polymers, Proc. Natl. Acad. Sci. USA 79:6070 (1982).

6. Y. Ihara, C. Abraham, and D. J. Selkoe, Antibodies to paired helical filaments in Alzheimer's disease do not recognize normal brain proteins, Nature 304:727 (1983).

7. K. Iqbal, T. Zaidi, C. H. Thompson, P. A. Merz, and H. M. Wisniewski, Alzheimer paired helical filaments: Bulk isolation, solubility, and protein composition, Acta Neuropathol. (Berl.) 62:167 (1984).

8. D. Kirschner, C. Abraham, and D. J. Selkoe, Structure of Alzheimer paired helical filaments by x-ray diffraction (abstract), Amer. Soc. Neurochem., Baltimore, MD, March 1985.

9. P. Gambetti, M. E. Velasco, D. Dahl, A. Bignami, U. Roessmann, and S. D. Sindely, Alzheimer neurofibrillary tangles: An immunohistochemical study, in: "Aging of the Brain and Dementia," L. Amaducci, A. N. Davison, and P. Antuono, eds., Raven Press, New York (1980).

10. Y. Ihara, N. Nukina, H. Sugita, and Y. Toyokura, Staining of Alzheimer's neurofibrillary tangles with antiserum against 200K component of neurofilament, Proc. Jap. Acad., 57:152 (1981).

11. B. H. Anderton, D. Breinburg, M. J. Downes, P. J. Green, B. E. Tomlinson, J. Ulrich, J. N. Wood, and J. Kahn, Monoclonal antibodies show that neurofibrillary tangles and neurofilaments share antigenic determinants, Nature 298:84 (1982).

12. L. Autilio-Gambetti, P. Gambetti, and R. C. Crane, Paired helical filaments: Relatedness to neurofilaments shown by silver staining and reactivity with monoclonal antibodies, in "Banbury Report 15: Biological Aspects of Alzheimer's Disease," R. Katzman, ed., Cold Spring Harbor Laboratory, Cold Spring Harbor, N. Y. (1983).

13. S.-H. Yen, H. Reding, P. Davies, and G. Ciment, The compositions of neurofibrillary tangles of senile dementia of the Alzheimer type: An immunological study, Ann. N. Y. Acad. Sci. 1984 (in press).

14. C. G. Rasool, C. Abraham, B. H. Anderton, M. Haugh, J. Kahn, and D. J. Selkoe, Alzheimer's disease: Immunoreactivity of neurofibrillary tangles with anti-neurofilament and anti-paired helical filament antibodies, Brain Res. 310:249 (1984).

15. C. G. Rasool and D. J. Selkoe, Alzheimer's disease: Exposure of neurofilament immunoreactivity in SDS-insoluble paired helical filaments, Brain Res. 322:194 (1984).

16. D. J. Selkoe, C. Abraham, C. G. Rasool, A. McCluskey, and L. K. Duffy, Production and characterization of monoclonal antibodies to Alzheimer paired helical filaments, Ann. N. Y. Acad. Sci. 1984 (in press).

17. C. Svendsen, C. G. Rasool, and D. J. Selkoe, Neurofibrillary degeneration in cholinergic and non-cholinergic neurons of the basal forebrain in Alzheimer's disease (AD) (abstract), J. Neuropath. Exp. Neurol. 43:307 (1984).

18. C. G. Rasool and D. J. Selkoe, Sharing of specific antigens by degenerating neurons in Pick's disease and Alzheimer's disease, New Engl. J. Med., March 14, 1985.

19. A. Probst, J. Ulrich, and Ph. U. Heitz, Senile dementia of Alzheimer type: Astroglial reaction to extracellular neurofibrillary tangles in the hippocampus, Acta Neuropathol. (Berl.) 57:75 (1982).

20. D. J. Selkoe, C. Abraha, and C. G. Rasool, A new method of purification of neurofibrillary tangles and senile plaque amyloid using fluorescence-activated cell sorting (abstract), IV International Symposium on Amyloidosis, Harriman, NY, November 1984.

21. D. J. Selkoe and C. Abraham, Amyloid plaques in Alzheimer's disease: purification by flow cytometry and protein characterization (submitted).

STRUCTURAL AND CHEMICAL ASPECTS OF CORTICAL PATHOLOGY IN ALZHEIMER'S DISEASE

James Edwardson, Robert Perry, John Candy, Arthur Oakley and Elaine Perry*

MRC Neuroendocrinology Unit and *Dept of Neuropathology
Newcastle General Hospital
Westgate Road
Newcastle upon Tyne NE4 6BE, U.K.

SUMMARY

In Alzheimer's disease, which primarily involves memory disturbance, the neuropathological changes that occur may disrupt normal synaptic function. The presence of dystrophic nerve terminals associated with senile plaques in cortical areas involved with learning (especially the hippocampus and temporal neocortex) provides evidence of significant presynaptic disruption which increases with increasing plaque density. Such presynaptic abnormalities are reflected in the neurochemical deficits that occur in at least three extrinsic neurotransmitter systems in the cerebral cortex (cholinergic, noradrenergic and serotoninergic) in Alzheimer's disease. The cholinergic deficit appears to be most closely correlated with the memory disturbance observed in both Alzheimer's disease and Parkinson's disease with dementia. Currently available evidence suggests that retrograde degeneration of the cortical cholinergic input may occur as a result of the neuropathological changes in Alzheimer's disease, while in Parkinson's disease with dementia where there are no marked neuropathological changes in the cortex, anterograde degeneration of the cholinergic system may occur. This focusses attention on the nature of senile plaques in relation to their ability to induce presynaptic dysfunction in Alzheimer's disease. Elemental analysis shows that aluminium and silicon are present as aluminosilicates in the centre of plaque cores. Chemically active aluminosilicate species may be responsible for at least some of the presynaptic changes observed.

CORTICAL PATHOLOGY

Whilst the histological features of Alzheimer's disease (AD) were originally described in the cortex, interest in the anatomy of the disease has recently turned to certain subcortical nuclei as the possible site of early pathological change. In particular neuronal loss from such areas as the Meynert nucleus, which innervate the cortex, raised the possibility that the disease might involve primary degeneration in key subcortical areas. More recent findings that in some AD cases the Meynert neuron population is normal (Perry et al, 1982; Pearson et al,

1983) and that in some cases of Parkinson's Disease (PD) substantial Meynert neuronal loss is not accompanied by dementia (Candy et al, 1983; Perry et al, 1983b; Pendlebury and Perl, 1984; Perry et al, 1985) have cast considerable doubt on the importance of subcortical damage in AD. The principle areas invariably affected by the identifying features of AD (numerous senile plaques and neurofibrillary tangles) include the majority of the archi - and neo-cortices (Tomlinson, 1982). Whether plaque or tangle formation occurs first and which is the more important pathological abnormality is still unclear. The presence of moderate numbers of plaques but not tangles in the neocortex of some non-demented old people and, in some demented cases (including both AD and PD) the occurrence of numerous plaques but few tangles suggest the plaque as the earlier change. Further, observations in both aged human and monkey brains, indicating a close correlation between increasing plaque density and impairment of cognitive function during life (Blessed et al, 1968; Struble et al, 1982) suggest that the plaque may be the more important in terms of functional abnormality. Since so little is known of the origin, nature and functional significance of cortical plaques that further studies are clearly warranted. As Tomlinson (1982) has pointed out: "Until their role is precisely defined, knowledge of an important area of neuropathology and human aging will be incomplete".

TRANSMITTER ACTIVITIES

Evidence for neurotransmitter involvement in AD has accrued less from detailed neuroanatomical investigation of the plaque itself but more from biochemical studies of homogenized tissue. Despite the obvious limitations of such crude analyses, these studies have, in conjunction with neuropathological observations, pointed to particular neuronal populations which may be defective in transmitter function (see Table 1). Thus substantial reductions in presynaptic activities related to the three classical transmitters - acetylcholine, noradrenaline and serotonin (Table 1) - are compatible with degeneration of axonal processes projecting to the cortex from subcortical nuclei containing the respective cell bodies, known to be affected neuropathologically (Perry, 1984). Amongst transmitter system intrinsic to the cortex evidence so far clearly implicates a change - in only one - somatostatin - although it is not yet clear whether cortical neurons which degenerate or develop neurofibrillary tangles are specifically those which contain this peptide (Roberts et al, 1985). This latter possibility is rendered unlikely by the similar reduction in somatostatin in PD (Agid and Javoy Agid, 1985) where tangles are rarely observed. Comparisons between AD and PD have been of further value in assessing the involvement of the other transmitter abnormalities in AD in the formation of plaques. Thus, although the presynaptic cholinergic enzyme choline acetyltransferase is reduced in relation to the dementia of both AD and PD (Perry et al, 1985) the absence of excessive plaque numbers in the latter suggests that a close or direct relation between cholinergic axonal degeneration and plaque development may not exist. Curiously, post-synaptic receptor activity relating to two of the three transmitter cortical projecting systems which degenerate in AD are not apparently affected by the disease process (Table 1). This situation contrasts with the pattern of receptor super-sensitivity which develops in many tissues deprived of their neuronal input and may reflect the inability of biochemical binding studies to distinguish between receptor sub-populations which, in brain, may be situated on capillaries and glial cells as well as neurons. The finding of a reduction of somatostatin receptor binding in AD (Gulya et al, 1985) whilst requiring confirmation should encourage more detailed investigation of these receptors at the structural and functional level.

TABLE 1. CORTICAL TRANSMITTER INVOLVEMENT IN ALZHEIMER'S DISEASE+

SYSTEM*	BIOCHEMISTRY pre-synaptic	BIOCHEMISTRY post-synaptic°	MORPHOLOGY
Cholinergic	reduced choline acetyl-transferase and 10S form of acetylcholinesterase	normal muscarinic receptor binding	degeneration of Meynert neurones in some cases; acetylcholinesterase-reactive neurites, present in early plaques, are lost in AD
Noradrenergic	reduced dopamine β-hydroxylase and metabolite (MHPG)	normal binding of α_1, α_2 and βreceptor ligands	degeneration of pigmented neurones in locus coeruleus in some cases
Serotonergic	reduced metabolite (5HIAA)	reduced binding to S_1 and S_2 receptor sub-types	high density of neuro-fibrillary tangles in dorsal raphe-nucleus
Somatostatin	reduced peptide immuno-reactivity in some areas	reduced binding of the peptide analogue	loss of reactive cell bodies and neurites from cortex; astroglial reactivity in plaque region

+ observations made in collaboration with the following: BE Tomlinson, TJ Crow, AJ Cross, JR Atack, D Irving, H Yamamura and K Gulya.

* only systems for which clearcut evidence of abnormalities in AD included. Glutamatergic neurones projecting to striatum may also be involved (Pearce et al, 1984).

o receptor binding, in some instances, also pre-synaptic.

Similar reductions in somatostatin receptor binding in demented cases of PD again suggest that there may be a dissociation between neurochemical changes and cortical pathology in AD. In fact comparing pre- and post-synaptic transmitter activities in the two diseases, the only neurochemical feature so far detected which is confined to AD is a loss of the serotoninergic receptor sub-type S2 (Cross et al, 1984; Perry et al, 1984), a feature which may relate more closely to tangle formation (Perry et al, 1984). A further receptor abnormality which may be associated with cortical tangle formation is an increase in caudate L-^{3}H-glutamate binding (Pearce et al, 1984). This abnormality is compatible with degeneration of the larger pyramidal neurons affected by tangles which are known to project to the striatum and which may also contribute processes to the plaque.

Whilst elucidation of key transmitters involved in AD is of great importance in terms of developing a useful therapeutic strategy involving transmitter replacement, research has not so far shed much light on the aetiology of the disease nor even the mechanisms of for example plaque formation. In this respect examination of key plaque constituents such as amyloid is likely to be more illuminating.

PLAQUE MORPHOLOGY

This subject has been reviewed in detail by Tomlinson (1982) and it seems that all cortical plaques, regardless of their locus or stage in development, include distended nerve terminals although occasional plaques in white matter tracts are apparently devoid of neurites (Rudelli et al, 1984). The strong histochemical reactivity of the plaque for acid phosphatase indicates the presence of increased numbers of lysosomes which, together with swollen mitochondria and paired helical filaments within the neurites, are presumably associated with axonal terminal dystrophy. Other components of the plaque include astrocytic processes, microglia and a central fibrillary amyloid core. The latter feature is said to occur preferentially in larger more highly developed plaques although the presence of smaller cores, not readily identified at the light microscopic level cannot be excluded.

The presence of structurally abnormal nerve terminals suggests that neurotransmission within and around the plaque is defective and it is worth considering, whether particular neuronal cell types are selectively involved in plaque formation. Increasing evidence suggests that not one but several different neuronal populations contribute processes to the plaque region. Thus the presence of acetylcholinesterase activity in fibres in the plaques in the human and monkey cerebral cortex (Perry et al, 1980; Struble et al, 1982) and the anterograde labelling of plaques from basal forebrain Meynert neurons of the monkey (Kitt et al, 1984) strongly implicate cholinergic processes; monoamine fluorescent varicosities around the plaque (Berger er al, 1976) implicate noradrenergic processes derived from the locus coeruleus; and a Golgi analysis of the AD hippocampus implicates local circuit neurons (Probst et al, 1983). It is in fact probable that some neuronal processes will be found in the plaque region "en passant" without any particular involvement and such myelinated axons have been observed in cortical plaques (Perry et al, unpublished observations). However, acetylcholinesterase staining and choline acetyltransferase immunostaining of plaque neurites shows them to be distinctly abnormal both in their distribution and morphology compared with normal cortical acetylcholinesterase- and choline acetyltransferase-containing fibres in human and monkey cerebral cortex (Perry et al, 1980; Kitt et al, 1984). In addition, in some plaques considered to be at an early developmental stage, acetylcholinesterase-positive axonal varicosities (Struble et al, 1982) or increased fibre reactivity (Perry et al, 1980) are evident. Although these features probably do reflect functional changes in cholinergic axons confirmation in the human brain using a specific cholinergic marker is now required. In contrast to these findings on acetylcholinesterase, the region in and around the senile plaque is apparently normal with respect to muscarinic receptor density and distribution, as judged by autoradiographic analysis (Palacios, 1982).

In relation to the largely unexplored immunohistochemistry of neuropeptides in AD, the finding of somatostatin neurite immunoreactivity within the plaque (Morrison et al, 1985) is not confirmed by other groups and the observation (Perry et al, 1983a) of high somatostatin-like immunoreactivity in astroglia present in and around the plaque remains to be explained. A possible link with the neuronotrophic function of glial cells in secreting hormone or oligopeptide factors for the maintenance of neuronal processes may be worth considering.

COMPOSITION OF PLAQUE CORES

The origin and nature of the dense core of amyloid fibrils seen at the centre of many plaques are still largely unclear. The possibility that the constituents of the plaque core may provide the original stimulus for plaque formation provides a strong incentive for determining their nature. Speculations on the origin of plaque amyloid have - included: viral or other infective agents, neuroactive peptides, trophic factors, glial or serum proteins and inorganic elements such as aluminium and silicon (see below). Although, by analogy with other types of amyloid, it has generally been assumed that the major component of plaque amyloid is protein, accumulating evidence suggests this may not be the case. An amino acid composition of plaque core protein has been published (Allsop et al, 1983) and recent evidence suggests that the vascular amyloid found in congophilic angiopathy contains a peptide of 40 or so amino acids which is identical to the protein extracted from senile plaque cores (Masters et al, 1985). However, it seems likely that protein may account for only a small proportion of the actual core (Candy et al, 1984). Another organic constituent which may be present, as judged by histological staining characteristics of the amyloid, is carbohydrate, and the presence of either nucleic acids or lipids cannot yet be excluded without complete quantitative analyses of the isolated material. Recent x-ray microanalyses of both isolated and in situ plaque cores have demonstrated the colocalisation of aluminium and silicon in the centre of plaque cores (Fig 1) and solid state NMR shows that these elements exist as aluminosilicates.

IMPLICATIONS OF ALUMINOSILICATE DEPOSITS IN SENILE PLAQUES

This is the first report of the presence of aluminosilicates in the nervous system and, although possibly reflecting some form of dystrophic mineralization, the focal concentration of such material at the centre of the plaque core strongly suggests that it may be an early or initiating factor in plaque formation. Marinesco in 1928 first proposed that deposition of an argyrophilic substance initiated plaque formation and the silver binding properties of aluminosilicates are consistent with this hypothesis. Previous reports that aluminium (Duckett and Galle, 1976; Duckett and Galle, 1980) and silicon (Nikaido et al, 1972) are associated with senile plaques did not show the concentration and colocalization of these elements at the centre of the core, probably reflecting technical limitations in the instruments used. Raised

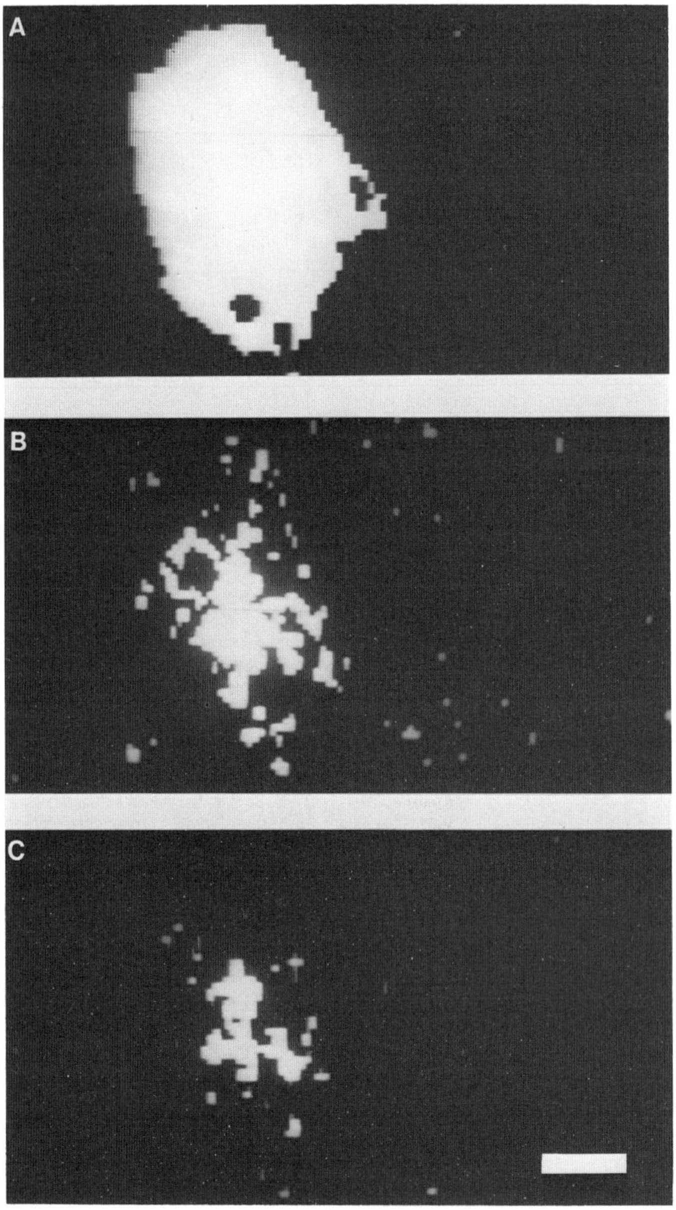

Figure 1. The presence and co-localisation of aluminium and silicon in senile plaque cores _in situ_ in the cerebral cortex in Alzheimer's disease. Maps of elemental distribution in senile plaques in silver stained, formalin fixed, cryostat sections of cerebral cortex were produced using a scanning electron microscope with an energy dispersive x-ray microanalytical system. A) shows the digimap distribution of silver in a senile plaque in the frontal cortex in a case of senile dementia of Alzheimer type. B) and C) show the digimap distribution of silicon and aluminium, respectively in the area shown in A), and demonstrate a coincident distribution of silicon and aluminium within the plaque core. A), B) and C) are all at the same magnification. Marker bar represents 10µm.

intracellular concentrations of both aluminium and silicon have been reported in neurofibrillary tangle bearing neurones in Alzheimer's disease (Perl and Brody, 1980) and the association of high concentrations of these elements with both major neuropathological features of this disorder raises the possibility of their involvement in its aetiology.

A previous hypothesis that aluminium is implicated in Alzheimer type dementia was based on the reported increased in the total level of aluminium in brains of Alzheimer patients (Crapper et al, 1973; Crapper et al, 1976) and the ability of aluminium salts to induce tangles, (Terry and Pena, 1965; Klatzo et al, 1965) similar but not identical to those seen in AD, and also produce cognitive deficits in susceptible species (Crapper, 1976; Petit et al, 1980). Age-related increases in brain aluminium (McDermott et al, 1979) and silicon (Austin et al, 1973) have been reported in the non-demented elderly and it has been claimed that the increase in Alzheimer's disease is not significant (McDermott et al, 1979; Markesbury et al, 1981; Traub et al, 1981). However, the high focal concentrations of aluminium in senile plaque cores and neurofibrillary tangle-bearing neurones suggest that the total brain level, as opposed to focal concentrations may be misleading. Lack of corresponding neuropathological features in the brains of patients with dialysis encephalopathy (Burks et al, 1976) suggests that chronic exposure to high aluminium *per se*, for up to 2 or 3 years at least, is not sufficient to induce Alzheimer-type changes. Other possible aetiological mechanism are suggested by recent studies on the Parkinsonian-dementia complex of Guam where a high content of aluminium occurs in hippocampal tangle-bearing neurones (Perl et al, 1982; Garruto et al, 1984). This accumulation is thought to be consequent to secondary hyperparathyroidism resulting from an environment low in calcium and magnesium but rich in aluminium (Garruto et al, 1984). The increased incidence of Alzheimer-type pathological changes in the elderly may similarly reflect changes in mineral homeostasis - including calcium - which occur in late life (Bullamore et al, 1970). Such mechanisms would not exclude the possibility that other factors increase vulnerability in this disease and is consistent with epidemiological findings which show geographical variations in the incidence of dementia.

CONCLUSION

Transmitter studies have clearly pointed to the involvement of specific neuronal systems in AD which may provide some directive for therapeutic strategies. In this respect the dementias of both AD and PD appear to involve pre-synaptic defects in cholinergic, noradrenergic and serotonergic cortical projections and both pre- and post-synaptic defects in the intrinsic somatostatin containing neurons. Changes in the serotoninergic S2 receptor sub-type appear to be confined to AD and may reflect intrinsic cortical pathology unique to this disorder. Fundamental research into the pathogenesis of AD may however be more fruitful in focussing on key pathological features such as the senile plaque. The nature of plaque amyloid and the role of aluminium and silicon in the formation of senile plaques merit further investigation.

REFERENCES

Agid, Y., and Javoy Agid, F., 1985, Peptides and Parkinson's disease, *Trends Neurosci.*, 8:30-35.

Allsop, D., Landon, M., and Kidd, M., 1983, Isolation and amino acid composition of senile plaque core protein, *Brain Res.*, 259:348-352.

Austin, J. H., Rinehart, R., Williamson, R. J., Burcar, P., Russ, K., Nikaido, T., and Lafrance, M., Studies in ageing of the brain. III. Silicon levels in postmortem tissues and body fluids, *in:* "Progress in Brain Research," D. H. Ford, ed., 40:485-495, Elsevier, Amsterdam (1973).

Berger, B., Escourolle, R., and Moyne, M. A., 1976, Axones caticholaminergues du cortex cerebral humain, *Rev Neurobiol.*, 136:183-191.

Blessed, G., Tomlinson, B. E., and Roth, M. 1968, The association between quantitative measures of dementia and of senile change in the cerebral grety matter of elderly subjects, *Brit. J. Psychiat.*, 114:797-811.

Bullamore, J. R., Wilkinson, R., Gallagher, J. C., Nordin, B. E. C., and Marshall, D. H., 1970, Effect of age on calcium absorption, *Lancet*, 2:535-537.

Burks, J. S., Alfrey, A. C., Huddlestone, J., Norenberg, M. D., and Lewin, E., 1976, A fatal encephalopathy in chronic haemodialysis patients, *Lancet*, 1:764-768.

Candy, J. M., Oakley, A. E., Perry, R. H., Perry, E. K., and Edwardson, J. A., New observations on the nature of the senile plaque, *in:* "Regulation of transmitter function," E. S. Vizi, and K. Magyar, eds., pp301-306, Academia, Kiado (1984).

Candy, J. M., Perry, R. H., Perry, E. K., Irving, D., Blessed, G., Fairbairn, A. F., and Tomlinson, B. E., 1983, Pathological changes in the nucleus of Meynert in Alzheimer's and Parkinson's diseases, *J. Neurol. Sci.*, 54:277-289.

Crapper, D. R., Functional consequences of neurofibrillary degeneration, *in:* "Neurobiology of Aging," R. D. Terry, and S, Gershon, eds., pp405-432, Raven Press, New York (1976).

Crapper, D. R., Krishman, S. S., and Dalton, A. J., 1973, Brain aluminium distribution in Alzheimer's disease and experimental neurofibrillary degeneration, *Science*, 180:511-513.

Crapper, D. R., Krishman, S. S., and Quittkat, S., 1976, Aluminium neurofibrillary degeneration and Alzheimer's disease, *Brain*, 99:67-80.

Cross, A. J., Crow, T. J., Ferrier, I. N., Johnson, A., Bloom, S. R., and Corsellis, J. A. N., 1984, Serotonin receptor changes in dementia of the Alzheimer type, *J. Neurochem.*, 43:1574-1581.

Duckett, S., and Galle, P., 1976, Mise en evidence de l'aluminium dans les plaques seniles de la maladie d'Alzheimer: etude de la microsonde de castaing, *C.R. Acad. Sci. (Paris)*, 282:393-395.

Duckett, S., and Galle, P., 1980, Electron microscope microprobe studies of aluminium in the brains of cases of Alzheimer's disease and ageing patients, *J. Neuropath. Exp. Neurol.*, 39:350 (Abst.).

Garruto, R. M., Fukatsu, R., Yanagihara, R., Gajdusek, D. C., Hook, G., and Fiori, C. E., 1984, Imaging of calcium and aluminium in neurofibrillary tangle bearing neurones in Parkinsonism - dementia of Guam, *Proc. Natl. Acad. Sci. USA*, 81:1875-1870.

Gulya, K., Watson, M., Vickroy, T. W., Rocske, W. R., Perry, R. H., Perry, E. K., Duckles, S. P., Wamsley, J. K., Gehlert, D., and Yamamura, H. I., 1985, Examination of cholinergic and neuropeptide receptor alterations in Alzheimer's disease (SDAT), Abstracts, Oholo Biological Conference.

Kitt, C. A., Price, D.L., Struble, R. G., Cork, L. C., Wainer, B. H., Becher, M. W., and Mobley, W. C., 1984, Evidence for cholinergic neurites in senile plaques, *Science*, 226:1443-1444.

Klatzo, I., Wisniewski, H. M., and Streiker, E., 1965, Experimental production of neurofibrillary degeneration. I. Light microscopic observations, *J. Neuropath. Exp. Neurol.*, 24:187-199.

Marinesco, G., 1928, Recherches sur les plaques seniles, *Bull. Sect. Scient de l'Acad roumaine*, 7:1.

Markesbery, W. R., Ehmann, W. D., Hassain, T. I. M., Alauddin, M., and Goodin, D. T., 1981, Instrumental neutron activation analysis of brain aluminium in Alzheimer's disease and aging, Arch. Neurol., 10:512-516.

Masters, C. L., Simms, G., Weinman, N. A., Beyreuther, K., Multhaup, G., and McDonald, B. L., 1985, Amyloid plaque core protein in Alzheimer's disease and Down's Syndrome, Proc. Natl. Acad. Sci., in press.

McDermott, J. R., Smith, A. I., Iqbal, K., and Wisniewski, H. M., 1979, Brain aluminium in aging and Alzheimer's disease, Neurology, 29:809-814.

Morrison, J. H., Rogers, J., Scherr, S., Benoit, R., and Bloom, F. E., 1985, Somatostatin immunoreactivity in neuritic plaques in Alzheimer's patients, Nature, 314:90-92.

Nikaido, T., Austin, J., Trueb, L., and Rinehart, R., 1972, Studies in ageing of the brain. II. Microchemical analyses of the nervous system in Alzheimer patients, Arch. Neurol, 27:549-554.

Palacios, J. M., 1982, Autoradiographic localization of muscarinic cholinergic receptors in the hippocampus of patients with senile dementia, Brain Res., 243:173-178.

Pearce, B. R., Palmer, A. M., Bowen, D. M., Wilcock, G. K., Esiri, M. M., and Davison, A. N., 1984, Neurotransmitter dysfunction and atrophy of the caudate nucleus in Alzheimer's disease, Neurochemical Pathology, 221-232.

Pearson, R. C. A., Sofroniew, M. V., Cuello, A. C., Powell, T. P. S., Eckenstein, F., Esiri, M. M., and Wilcock, G. K., 1983, Persistence of cholinergic neurones in the basal nucleus in a brain with senile dementia of Alzheimer type demonstrated by immunohistochemical staining for choline acetyltransferase, Brain Res., 289:375-379.

Pendlebury, W. W., and Perl, D. P., 1984, Nucleus basalis of Meynert: severe cell loss in Parkinson's disease without dementia, Ann Neurol., 16:63.

Perl, D. P., and Brody, A. R., 1980, Alzheimer's disease: X-ray spectrometric evidence of aluminium accumulation in neurofibrillary tangle-bearing neurones, Science, 208:297-299.

Perl, D. P., Gajdusek, D. C., Garruto, R. M., Yanagihara, R. T., and Gibbs, C. J., 1982, Intraneuronal aluminium accumulation in amyotrophic lateral sclerosis and Parkinsonism - dementia of Guam, Science, 217: 1053-1055.

Perry, R. H., Neuropathology of dementia, in: "Dementia, a clinical approach," J. M. S. Pearce, ed., pp89-116, Blackwell Scientific Publications, Oxford (1984).

Perry, R. H., Blessed, G., Perry, E. K., and Tomlinson, B. E., 1980, Histochemical observations on cholinesterase activities in the brains of elderly normal and demented (Alzheimer type) patients, Age and Aging, 9:9-16.

Perry, R. H., Candy, J. M., and Perry, E. K., Some observations and speculations concerning the cholinergic system and neuropeptides in Alzheimer's disease, in: "Banbury Report 15: Biological aspects of Alzheimer's disease," R. D. Terry, and R. Katzman, eds., pp351-361, Cold Spring Laboratory, New York (1983a).

Perry R. H., Candy, J. M., Perry, E. K., Irving, D., Blessed, G., Fairbairn, A. F., and Tomlinson, B. E., 1982, Extensive loss of choline acetyltransferase activity is not reflected by neuronal loss in the nucleus of Meynert in Alzheimer's disease, Neurosci. Lett., 33:311-315.

Perry, E. K., Curtis, M., Dick, D. J., Candy, J. M., Atack, J. R., Bloxham, C. A., Blessed, G., Fairbairn, A., Tomlinson, B. E., and Perry, R. H., 1985, Cholinergic correlates of cognitive impairment in Parkinson's disease: comparisons with Alzheimer's disease, J. Neurol. Neurosurg. Psychiat., in press.

Perry, E. K., Perry, R. H., Candy, J. M., Fairbairn, A. F., Blessed, G., Dick, D. J., and Tomlinson, B. E., 1984, Cortical serotonin-S_2 receptor binding abnormalities in Alzheimer's disease: comparisons with Parkinson's disease, Neuosci. Lett., 51:353-357.

Perry, R. H., Tomlinson, B. E., Candy, J. M., Blessed, G., Foster, J. F., Bloxham, C. A., and Perry, E. K., 1983b, Cortical cholinergic deficit in mentally impaired Parkinsonian patients, Lancet, 2:789-790.

Petit, T. L., Biederman, G. B., and McMullen, P. A., 1980, Neurofibrillary degeneration, dendritic dying back and learning memory deficits after aluminium administration: implications for brain aging, Exp. Neurol., 67:152-162.

Probst, A., Baster, V., Bron, B., and Ulrich, J., 1983, Neuritic plaques in senile dementia of Alzheimer type: a Golgi analysis in the hippocampal region, Brain Res., 268:249-254.

Roberts, G. W., Crow, T. J., and Polak, J. M., 1985, Location of neuronal tangles in somatostatin neurones in Alzheimer's disease, Nature, 314:92-94.

Rudelli, R. D., Ambler, M. W., and Wisniewski, H. M., 1984, Morphology and distribution of Alzheimer neuritic (senile) and amyloid plaques in striatum and diencephalin, Acta Neuropath., 64:273-281.

Struble, R. G., Cork, L. C., Whitehouse, P. J., and Price, D. L., 1982, Cholinergic innervation in neuritic plaques, Science, 216:413-415.

Struble, R. G., Hedreen, J. C., Cork, L. C. and Price, D. L., 1984, Acetylcholinesterase activity in senile plaques of aged macaques, Neurobiol. Aging, 5:191-198.

Terry, R. D., and Pena, C., 1965, Experimental production of neurofibrillary degeneration. 2. Electronmicroscopy, phosphatase histochemistry and electron probe microanalysis, J. Neuropath. Exp. Neurol., 24:200-210.

Tomlinson, B. E., 1982, Plauqes, tangles and Alzheimer's disease, Psychol. Medicine, 12:449-459.

Traub, R. D., Rains, T. C., Garruto, R. M., Gajdusek, D. C., and Gibbs, C. J., 1981, Brain distruction alone does not elevate brain aluminium, Neurology, 31:986-989.

CHOLINERGIC AND NON-CHOLINERGIC NEUROTRANSMITTER HYPOTHESES FOR ALZHEIMER'S DISEASE

D.M. Bowen, P.T. Francis and A.M. Palmer

Department of Neurochemistry
Institute of Neurology
University of London, U.K.

INTRODUCTION

Together with Parkinson's disease, Alzheimer's disease (AD) is one of a group of disorders that Gowers called abiotrophies [1], in which unexplained nerve cell loss appears to occur in selected areas (that is substantia nigra and cortex, respectively). During the last decade there has been considerable debate as to the importance and extent of neuronal loss in AD. The early studies of Kety, as well as recent *in situ* tomography [2] reveals some evidence for depressed brain energy metabolism. As we will show biochemical studies have made a contribution to these problems and give indications of the types of neurone and metabolic processes affected. Whenever possible we interpret changes in biochemical constituents in terms of their supposed cellular or subcellular identity and probable physiological action, although it is realized that this is an oversimplification, particularly for excitatory amino acid transmitters. A distinction has often been made between presenile and senile forms of AD but this division is not retained as similiar histological changes are seen in the cortex (neurofibrillary tangles within pyramidal neurones and senile or neuritic plaques in neuropil, composed of amyloid surrounded by fragments of enlarged axons and nerve terminals).

BIOCHEMISTRY OF BIOPSY SAMPLES AND CEREBROSPINAL FLUID

Methods. Choline acetyltransferase (ChAT) activity probably does not control the rate of acetylcholine formation. Thus, acetylcholine synthesis has been measured directly (in depolarized tissue prisms or mini-slices), with samples removed at diagnostic craniotomy from young AD patients [3-6]. "High affinity" choline uptake has been measured for comparison [5,7]. [U-^{14}C] glucose was used to measure acetylcholine synthesis so an indication of overall glucose oxidation has been obtained (by trapping the $^{14}CO_2$ produced) [3-5,8]. An attempt has been made to directly examine the energy balance of mini-slices [8] and oxygen uptake by mitochondria in homogenates [9]. It has been difficult to study serotonin (5-HT) neurones in humans because of the inability to demonstrate tryptophan hydroxylase so this neurone type has been assessed in mini-slices by non-enzymatic methods

[6,10,11]. Similar methods have been used to assess noradrenergic, dopaminergic and somatostatin-14-containing neurones as reported [11,12] and in more recent studies (Francis, P.T. and Bowen, D.M., unpublished observations). Most techniques used for studying amino-acid transmitter systems in animals are difficult to apply to human brain. The K^+-evoked release of amino acids from mini-slices has been used to examine neurosurgical samples [13]. Cerebrospinal fluid from biopsy-confirmed AD patients has been analyzed for content of transmitter metabolites [14], free amino-acids [15] and somatostatin [12,16].

Results. The differences between demented and control subjects in Table 1 are thought to be those which occur some 3½ years [6] after onset of cognitive decline whereas the differences detected in autopsy samples are those which typically occur a further 3-4 years later. The overall results in Table 1 clearly lay emphasis on the deficit in cholinergic neurones but also suggest that 5-HT neurones are markedly affected in AD, in both frontal and temporal lobe. 5-HT cells in the raphe nucleus innervate the caudate nucleus as well as the cerebral cortex and 5-HT was markedly reduced in the caudate nucleus [17]. Noradrenaline and dopamine were not reduced in the caudate nucleus [17,18] laying emphasis on the presynaptic serotonergic deficit. Noradrenaline innervation of the caudate nucleus seems to arise from the lateral tegmental noradrenaline system so these cells appear spared [18]. Cortical release of noradrenaline and content of 3-methyoxy-4-hydroxyphenylglycol in spinal fluid are not significantly reduced and catecholamine uptake is less affected than 5-HT uptake so coeruleocortical and coeruleospinal noradrenaline neurones also seem relatively spared. In the cerebral cortex the activity of the γ-aminobutyrate synthetic enzyme (glutamate decarboxylase), release of the transmitter as well as release of somatostatin and aspartate are not reduced suggesting that several types of intrinsic neurone are unaffected, (aspartate release may not be a good indicator of change [13]). Somatostatin was reduced only in lumbar fluid, consistent with a selective alteration in spinal somatostatin-containing terminals.

GLUTAMERGIC NEURONES IN THE CEREBRAL CORTEX

Glucose oxidation and ADP stimulated oxygen uptake were significantly increased in AD (Table 1), consistent with partial uncoupling of mitochondria in the cerebral cortex [8,9]. Glucose oxidation by depolarized mini-slices of AD samples correlates ($r = -0.98$) with the glutamate they release [13]. This finding seems specific for glutamate as there were no correlations between glucose oxidation and either acetylcholine synthesis or release of aspartate and γ-aminobutyrate. The new evidence [9] that increased glucose oxidation is due to uncoupling of oxidative phosphorylation suggests that glutamate release from AD samples reflects altered energy metabolism and so release may not be a reliable index of the density of glutamergic nerve endings in the neocortex. Mitochondria surrounding the core of neuritic plaques appear to be undergoing a change similar to that caused by a reduced ATP/ADP ratio [19], so at least some plaques may represent a previously unsuspected disease-related change in glutamergic terminals associated with intrinsic neurones in the neocortex.

Several other observations also indicate a role for cortical glutamergic neurones in AD. Firstly, large cortical neurones are lost in normal ageing and more so in AD [20], particularly in the superior

Table 1: Neurochemical Variables in Living Alzheimer Patients Compared With Control Samples.

Neurochemical Measure (content or activity)	Biopsy Brain Tissue or Spinal Fluid Assayed (TL, temporal lobe; FL, frontal lobe)			AD (% of Control)
	TL	FL	CSF	
[^{3}H] 5-HT Uptake (8)	+	-	-	29*
5-HT Release (5)	-	+	-	35*
ChAT Activity (20)	+	+	-	41*
Acetylcholine Synthesis (22)	+	+	-	50*
[^{3}H] Catecholamine Uptake (9)	+	-	-	55*
[^{3}H] Choline Uptake (6)	+	-	-	57*
Homovanillate (25)	-	-	+	72*
Adenine Nuc. Monophosphate (12)	+	-	-	72*
Noradrenaline Release (5)	-	+	-	74
5-Hydroxyindoleacetate (16)	-	-	+	75*
Somatostatin-14 (26)	-	-	+	75*
Glutamine (11)	-	-	+	78*
Adenine Nuc. Triphosphate (12)	+	-	-	79*
Adenine Nuc. Diphosphate (12)	+	-	-	79
Dopamine Release (6)	-	+	-	90
[^{3}H] 5-HT Binding (5)	+	-	-	90
γ-Aminobutyrate Release (7)	+	-	-	93
Glutamate (11)	-	-	+	96
Aspartate (11)	-	-	+	97
Glutamate Decarboxylase (4)	-	+	-	97
"Amino-Acid Synthesis" (12)	+	-	-	100
Energy Charge (12)	+	-	-	101
Somatostatin-14 Release (6)	-	+	-	107
3-Methoxy-4-Hydroxyphenylglycol (25)	-	-	+	115
Somatostatin-14 (8)	-	-	+ v	118
Aspartate Release (7)	+	-	-	118
ADP-Stimulated Oxygen Uptake (5)	-	+	-	122*
Glucose Oxidation (22)	+	+	-	126*
Glutamate Release (7)	+	-	-	141

( ), AD sample number (6-34 controls, usually at least 12); CSF, lumbar cerebrospinal fluid (except for + v, which is for ventricular fluid).

Both brain lobes were examined for only a few variables (identified by ++) and uniform results were obtained. K^+-stimulated release of the endogenous transmitter and "high-affinity" uptake were measured. Nuc., nucleotide. Energy charge is the adenylate energy charge. "Amino acid synthesis" is [U-^{14}C] glucose incorporation into total free amino acids [8].

*Significantly different from control (p usually < 0.01).

temporal gyrus and hippocampus. Since these large cells resemble in many respects the pyramidal hippocampal cells thought to utilize glutamate as transmitter we have argued [21] that regional differences in involvement of glutamergic neurones in the cerebral cortex accounts for variation in cortical glucose hypometabolism in AD [2]. Secondly, out of numerous free amino acids measured in lumbar cerebrospinal fluid from Alzheimer patients, only glutamate content correlated with measures of cognitive impairment and glutamine concentration was reduced [15]. Finally, our study of the specific binding of L-[^{3}H] glutamate to representative membranes of the entire AD caudate nucleus provides evidence of a difference from control in glutamergic neurotransmission possibly related to tangle-formation (or cell loss) in corticofugal neurones [18] and leading to atrophy of the caudate nucleus in AD [18] and perhaps in normal ageing [22]. Other brain regions may be similarly affected as corticofugal glutamergic neurones seem to innervate the amygdala and thalamus which in AD are reduced in size, part of the amygdala being one of the most severely affected regions of the brain [21]. Nigral neurones regulated by corticofugal glutamergic neurones may also be affected as the homovanillate content of cerebrospinal fluid [14] and of the entire caudate nucleus [17] are substantially reduced. Other indices of striatal and cortical dopaminergic terminals are unaltered, including the dopamine content of the entire caudate nucleus [17], release of the transmitter from the neocortex (Table 1) and the concentrations of dopamine and homovanillic acid in frontal and temporal cortex from the autopsy brains (Palmer, A.M. and Bowen, D.M., unpublished data). Greater loss of homovanillate compared with dopamine conforms with most other studies on AD but contrasts with Parkinson's disease [23]. This indicates that, whereas the few remaining nerve endings of nigral neurones in Parkinson's disease become functionally more effective, those in AD are probably not markedly reduced in number, but may not be fully operating. Cholinergic interneurones as well as corticofugal glutamergic cells normally seem to regulate dopamine release in the neostriatum but it is not known whether both types of regulation are affected in AD. Reduced striatal ChAT activity is an inconsistent finding in AD and normal ageing. Our studies on the entire caudate nucleus suggest that the enzyme is reduced only in younger patients compared with age-matched controls but by other criteria striatal interneurones appear relatively intact [18,24]. Selective loss of dopamine D_2 receptors occurs in the striatum in AD, also consistent with a loss of corticofugal fibres [25].

As methods for the localization of glutamergic neurones and their connections improve, it should be possible to test our proposal that cortical glutamergic neurones are affected in AD. It will be important to investigate glutamergic pyramidal cells in the hippocampus, association cortices and olfactory areas of brain as it is emerging that nerve cell specific pathology within large neurones in these regions (Pearson, R.C.A., Esiri, M.M., Hiorns, R.W., Wilcock, G.K. and Powell, T.P.S., personal communication) may contribute to the memory disorder of AD (Neary, D., Snowden, J.S., Bowen, D.M., Sims, N.R., Mann, D.M.A., Northern, B., Yates, P.O. and Davison, A.N., unpublished observations).

THERAPEUTIC IMPLICATIONS

Presynaptic Cholinergic Deficit. Cell-free homogenate activity determinations of ChAT, have been widely used as a basis of rational therapy for AD. Such predictions remained equivocal until a sensitive physiologically relevant *in vitro* assay for acetylcholine synthesis in fresh biopsy samples indicated that reductions in ChAT provided a reliable estimate of the deficit in synthesis [3-5]. There is good evidence that the radiolabelled acetylcholine formed by mini-slices (Table 1) provides a representative measure of the mass of transmitter synthesized [5]. The transmitter is almost certainly produced in pinched off nerve-endings (synaptosomes) free from the influence of cell bodies [4]. The mini-slices exhibit the characteristics of cholinergic terminals as, for example synthesis is correlated with another presynaptic cholinergic function ("high affinity" choline uptake) [5] and is altered by muscarinic agents, which is expected as these terminals possess muscarinic autoreceptors [26]. The mini-slices mimic the *in vivo* response to stimlation since acetylcholine synthesis shows a marked increase in response to depolarisation by potassium [3,4]. The synthesis values probably accurately reflect the conditions *in situ* as the mini-slices are prepared using a rapid technique, in the presence of physiological buffers. Extensive manipulation is avoided and some structural integrity is maintained. The validity of the biopsy procedure was checked using animal models which indicate that acetylcholine synthesis is unaffected by the anaesthetic procedure and either stagnant or oligaemic hypoxia. The synthesis values obtained for samples of rat brain are similar to *in vivo* estimates of acetylcholine turnover rate [4]. We have concluded [6] that in a group of young patients with AD an *in vitro* estimate of acetylcholine synthesis *in vivo* decreases with increasing cognitive impairment. In the most severely affected patient synthesis was reduced to only 33% of control [6].

Other Transmitter-Related Differences. By contrast, to Rossor et al [27], our larger necropsy series [6] showed reduced noradrenaline concentration in old AD patients (> 80 years) compared with matched controls. The noradrenaline metabolite 3-methoxy-4-hydroxyphenyl-glycol, was not significantly altered in these patients. Thus, a major compensatory increase in noradrenaline turnover is not evident in older AD subjects so "simple cholinergic replacement" [27] therapy may not succeed in the elderly patient. Increased turnover appears to be a feature of noradrenergic neurones in AD of earlier onset (<80 years) as it was shown that the amount of 3-methyoxy-4-hydroxyphenyl-glycol is increased in such subjects [6] (see also Gottfries et al [28]). This might be expected to ameliorate the effects of the possible loss of noradrenergic terminals.

5-HT receptors are reduced [29-31] and our working hypothesis [20,21] is that these receptors are associated with tangle-forming glutamergic neurones in the cerebral cortex as well as with the glutamergic pyramidal cells that are lost. 5-HT concentration is not significantly reduced in frontal cortex [31] of autopsy samples, which we confirm (Palmer, A.M. and Bowen, D.M., unpublished data). By contrast 5-HT concentration in the more severely affected temporal cortex [32] and limbic areas is markedly reduced [6,28], although neither the concentration nor 5-HT receptor binding were related to disease severity [6,30]. Since the lobes are not uniformly affected 5-HT dysfunction in the cerebral cortex may not be primarily the result of an intrinsic defect in the raphe nucleus, see also Pearson and colleagues [33]. It will be clearly important to extend these observations to detailed analysis of biopsy tissue. Even so investigation of non-cholinergic synaptosomes in mini-slices of AD biopsy samples shows significant reduction of depolarization-induced release of endogenous 5-HT but not catecholamines (Table 1) and greatly reduced uptake of radiolabelled 5-HT (Table 1). Moreover, new methods for the measurement of 5-HT synapses [34], now applied to autopsy samples (Table 2), confirm that both pre- and post-synaptic components of these synapses are affected in AD. No clear changes have been detected in biopsy samples of biochemical markers of intrinsic cortical neurones, although glutamate terminated somatostatin-28(1-12) [35-36] needs to be measured. These observations suggest that degeneration of postsynaptic cortical receptors and damage to noradrenergic and most intrinsic cortical neurones, are not primary events in AD and further emphasize the importance of the well-established defects in the cholinergic system. Not all clinically suspected examples of AD show the microscopic changes of AD or a presynaptic cholinergic deficit and some can be anticipated to have a selective postsynaptic cholinergic deficit. So it is important to establish non-invasive methods for excluding such patients from drug trials [6].

Table 2: Neocortical Serotonergic Neurones in Alzheimer's Disease.

Neurochemical Substance or Activity	AD (n = 15-20)	Control (n = 15-18)
Putative Presynaptic 5-HT Receptor		
(5-HT 1B receptor binding[a])		
2 nM[b]	23.3 (15.2)***	40.0 (18.4)
8 nM[b]	49.2 (24.8)**	79.2 (41.6)
Putative Postsynaptic 5-HT Receptor		
([^{3}H] 8-OH-DPAT binding[a])		
1 nM[b]	18.4 (13.4)**	30.2 (16.5)
4 nM[b]	42.9 (25.3)*	68.9 (37.0)
5-HT concentration (HPLC-ECD [6])	550 (483)**	1079 (924)
ChAT (Fonnum method [32])	3.5 (2.5)***	10.2 (3.3)

fmol/mg protein, (SD); enzyme in nmol/min/100 mg protein.
*p < 0.05, **p < 0.03, ***p < 0.01 (Mann-Whitney U-test).
[a]Methods of Middlemiss and Fozard [34].
[b]Ligand concentration in medium.

Treatment Strategies and Limitations. The correlation of acetylcholine synthesis with cognitive impairment in young patients suggests a relatively early involvement of the presynaptic cholinergic system in AD [6]. Taken together with the extensive observations implicating cholinergic activity in memory function, this correlation is consistent with involvement of the cholinergic changes in producing cognitive impairment in this disease. Thus it might be predicted that a substance acting on the cholinergic system, perhaps complemented by pharmacological activity towards the 5-HT system, would be beneficial in early onset patients. Dietary choline may not be effective [26] and major improvements could require the development of novel centrally acting agonists. However, even if the appropiate impulse generations were achieved, suspected disease-related abnormality in cortical glutamergic neurones and mitochondria may remain uncorrected.

SUMMARY AND CONCLUSIONS

The importance of the well-established presynaptic cholinergic deficit in Alzheimer's disease is emphasized. Loss of serotonin receptors, another consistently found change, could be related to suspected alterations in corticofugal and intrinsic cortical glutamergic neurones. Important changes may occur in at least certain corticopetal serotonergic pathways whereas corticopetal and coeruleospinal noradrenergic tracts, dopaminergic and γ-aminobutyric neurones and somatostatin-containing cells may not be primarily involved.

ACKNOWLEDGEMENTS

We thank Dr D.N.Middlemiss for measuring the $5\text{-}HT_{1B}$ receptor and the binding of 8-OH-DPAT and Daksha Gandhi for help in preparing the manuscript. This work was supported by the Medical Research Council, Miriam Marks Charitable Trust and Brain Research Trust.

REFERENCES

1. D. M. Bowen, C. B. Smith, P. White, and A. N. Davison, Neurotransmitter-related enzymes and indices of hypoxia in senile dementia and other abiotrophies. Brain 99:459-496 (1976).
2. N. L. Foster, T. N. Chase, P. Fedio, N. A. Patronas, R. A. Brooks, and G. DiChiro, Alzheimer's disease: focal cortical changes shown by positron emission tomography. Neurology N.Y., 33: 961-965 (1983).
3. N. R. Sims, D. M. Bowen, C. C. T. Smith, R. H. Flack, A. N. Davison, J. S. Snowden, and D. Neary, Glucose metabolism acetylcholine synthesis in relation to neuronal activity in Alzheimer's disease. Lancet i: 333-336 (1980).
4. N. R. Sims, D. M. Bowen, and A. N. Davison. [^{14}C]-acetylcholine synthesis and ^{14}C-carbon dioxide production from U-[^{14}C]-glucose by tissue prisms from human neocortex. Biochem.J. 196:867-876 (1981).
5. N. R. Sims, D. M. Bowen, S. J. Allen, C. C. T. Smith, D. Neary, D. J. Thomas, and A. N. Davison, Presynaptic cholinergic dysfunction in patients with dementia. J.Neurochem. 40: 503-509 (1983).

6. P. T. Francis, A. M. Palmer, N. R. Sims, D. M. Bowen, A. N. Davison, M. Esiri, D. Neary, J. S. Snowden, and G. K. Wilcock, Neurochemical studies suggest treatment strategies for early-onset Alzheimer's disease. New Eng.J.Med. in press.
7. D. M. Bowen, J. S. Benton, J. A. Spillane, C. C. T. Smith, and S. J. Allen, Choline acetyltransferase activity and histopathology of frontal neocortex from biopsies of demented patients. J.Neurol.Sci. 57:191-202 (1982).
8. N. R. Sims, D. M. Bowen, D. Neary, and A. N. Davison, Metabolic processes in Alzheimer's disease: Adenine nucleotide content and product of $^{14}CO_2$ from [U-^{14}C] glucose in vitro in human neocortex. J.Neurochem. 41:1329-1334 (1983).
9. N. R. Sims, J. M. Finegan, D. M. Bowen, and J. M. Blass, Mitochondrial function in Alzheimer's disease measured in vitro using neocortical tissue homogenates. J.Neurochem. in press.
10. D. M. Bowen, S. J. Allen, J. S. Benton, M. J. Goodhardt, E. A. Haan, A. M. Palmer, N. R. Sims, C. C. T. Smith, J. A. Spillane, M. M. Esiri, D. Neary, J. S. Snowdon, G. K. Wilcock, and A. N. Davison, Biochemical assessment of serotonergic and cholinergic dysfunction and cerebral atrophy in Alzheimer's disease. J.Neurochem. 41:266-272 (1983).
11. J. S. Benton, D. M. Bowen, S. J. Allen, E. A. Haan, R. R. Murphy, and J. S. Snowden, Alzheimer's disease as a disorder of isodendritic core. Lancet i:456 (1982).
12. P. T. Francis, and D. M. Bowen. Relevance of reduced concentrations of somatostatin in Alzheimer's disease. Biochem.Soc. Trans. 13:170-171 (1985).
13. C. C. T. Smith, D. M. Bowen, N. R. Sims, D. Neary, and A. N. Davison, Amino acids release from biopsy samples of temporal neocortex from patients with Alzheimer's disease. Brain Res. 264:138-141 (1983).
14. A. M. Palmer, N. R. Sims, D. M. Bowen, D. Neary, J. Palo, J. Wikstrom, and A. N. Davison, Monoamine metabolite concentrations in lumbar cerebrospinal fluid of patients with histologically verified Alzheimer's dementia. J.Neurol.Neurosurg.Psychiat. 47:481-484 (1984).
15. C. C. T. Smith, D. M. Bowen, P. T. Francis, J. S. Snowden, and D. Neary, Putative amino acid transmitters in lumbar cerebrospinal fluid of patients with histologically verified Alzheimer's dementia. J.Neurol.Neurosurg.Psychiat. in press.
16. P. T. Francis, D. M. Bowen, D. Neary, J. Palo, J. Wikstrom, and J. Olney, Somatostatin-like immunoreactivity in lumbar cerebrospinal fluid from neurohistologically examined demented patients. Neurobiol.Aging 5:183-186 (1984).
17. A. M. Palmer, and D. M. Bowen. 5-Hydroxyindoleacetic acid and homovanillic acid in the CSF and caudate nucleus of histologically verified samples of Alzheimer's disease. Biochem.Soc.Trans. 13: 167-168 (1985).
18. B. R. Pearce, A. M. Palmer, D. M. Bowen, G. K. Wilcock, M. Esiri, and A. N. Davison, Neurotransmitter dysfunction and atrophy of the caudate nucleus in Alzheimer's disease. Neurochem.Pathol. 2:221-232 (1984).
19. R. D. Terry, Ultrastructural alterations in senile dementia. In: Alzheimer's Disease: Senile Dementia and Related Disorders, R. Katzman R. D. Terry, K. L. Bick, ed., Raven Press, New York, 375-382 (1978).
20. D. M. Bowen. Alzheimer disease. In: Molecular Basis of Neuropathology, R. H. S. Thompson, A. N. Davison ed., Edward Arnold, London, 649-665 (1981).

21. D. M. Bowen, A. N. Davison, P. T. Francis, A. M. Palmer, and B. R. Pearce, Neurotransmitter and metabolism dysfunction in Alzheimer's dementia: Relationship to histopathological features. FEBEL, Interdiscipl Topics Geront. 19: in press.
22. S. J. Allen, J. S. Benton, M. J. Goodhardt, E. A. Haan, N. R. Sims, C. C. T. Smith, J. A. Spillane, D. M. Bowen, and A. N. Davison, Biochemical evidence of selective nerve cell changes in the normal ageing human and rat brain. J.Neurochem. 41:256-265 (1983).
23. C. D. Marsden, Extrapyramidal diseases. In: Molecular Basis of Neuropathology, A. N. Davison, R. H. S. Thompson eds., Edward Arnold, London, 345-383 (1981).
24. B. R. Pearce, and D. M. Bowen. [^{3}H] kainic acid binding and choline acetyltransferase activity in Alzheimer's dementia. Brain Res. 310:376-378 (1984).
25. A. J. Cross, T. J. Crow, I. N. Ferrier, J. A. Johnson, and D. Markakis, Striatal dopamine receptors in Alzheimer-type dementia. Neurosci.Lett. 52:1-6 (1984).
26. K. L. Marek, D. M. Bowen, N. R. Sims, and A. N. Davison, Stimulation of acetylcholine synthesis by blockade of presynaptic muscarinic inhibitory autoreceptors: observations in rat and human brain preparations and comparison with the effect of choline. Life Sci. 30:1517-1524 (1982).
27. M. N. Rossor, L. L. Iversen, G. P. Reynolds, C. Q. Mountjoy, and M. Roth, Neurochemical characteristics of early and late onset types of Alzheimer's disease. Brit.Med.J. 288:961-964 (1984).
28. C. G. Gottfries, R. Adolfsson, S. M. Aquilonius, A. Carlsson, S. A. Eckernas, A. Nordberg, L. Oreland, L. Svennerholm, A. Wiberg, and B. Winblad, Biochemical changes in dementia disorders of Alzheimer type (AD/SDAT). Neurobiol.Aging. 4:261-271 (1984).
29. D. M. Bowen, P. White, J. A. Spillane, M. J. Goodhardt, G. Curzon, P. Iwangoff, W. Meier-Ruge, and A. N. Davison, Accelerated ageing or selective neuronal loss as an important cause of dementia ? Lancet i:11-14 (1979).
30. A. J. Cross, T. J. Crow, J. A. Johnson, E. K. Perry, R. H. Perry, G. Blessed, and B. E. Tomlinson, Studies on neurotransmitter receptor systems in neocortex and hippocampus in senile dementia of the Alzheimer-type. J.Neurol.Sci. 64:109-117 (1984).
31. G. P. Reynolds, L. Arnold, M. N. Rossor, L. L. Iversen, C. Q. Mountjoy, and M. Roth, Reduced binding of [^{3}H] ketanserin to cortical 5-HT$_2$ receptors in senile dementia of the Alzheimer type. Neurosci.Lett. 44:47-51 (1984).
32. G. K. Wilcock, M. M. Esiri, D. M. Bowen, and C. C. T. Smith, Alzheimer's disease: correlation of cortical choline acetyltransferase activity with the severity of dementia and histological abnormalities. J.Neurol.Sci. 57:407-417 (1982).
33. R. C. A. Pearson, M. V. Sofroniew, A. C. Cuello, T. P. S. Powell, F. Eckenskein, M. M. Esiri, and G. K. Wilcock, Persistence of cholinergic neurons in the basal nucleus in a brain with senile dementia of the Alzheimer's type demonstrated by immunohistochemical staining for choline acetyltransferase. Brain Res. 289:375-379 (1983).
34. D. N. Middlemiss, and J. R. Fozard, 8-Hydroxy-2-(di-n-propylamino) tetralin discriminates between subtypes of the 5-HT, recognition site. Eur.J.Pharmacol. 90:151-153 (1983).
35. J. H. Morrison, R. Benoit, P. J. Magistretti, and F. E. Bloom, Immunohistochemical distribution of pro-somatostatin-related peptides in cerebral cortex. Brain Res. 262:344-351 (1983).
36. J. H. Morrison, J. S. Rogers, S. Scherr, R. Benoit, and F. E. Bloom, Somatostatin immunoreactivity in neuritic plaques of Alzheimer's patients. Nature 314:90-92 (1985).

BRAIN TOPOCHEMISTRY OF CHOLINERGIC AND MONOAMINERGIC PARAMETERS IN ALZHEIMER'S DISEASE

B. Winblad*, R. Adolfsson, A. Nordberg and P. Nyberg

Department of Geriatric Medicine*, Psychiatry and Pathology, University of Umeå, S-901 87 Umeå and Department of Pharmacology, University of Uppsala, S-751 24 Uppsala, Sweden

INTRODUCTION

Dementia may be defined as a progressive deterioration of intellectual and emotional functions, the commonest causes being the primary degenerative disorders and AD and SDAT. AD/SDAT is characterized histopathologically by the presence of numerous senile plaques and neurofibrillary tangles throughout cortical grey matter. Neurochemically, reductions of brain choline acetyltransferase and acetylcholine esterase have been noted (Perry et al 1977, Davies 1979, Rossor et al 1982). Results regarding reductions of catecholaminergic transmitters in AD/SDAT are less extensive, but lower mean concentrations of dopamine (DA) and noradrenaline (NA) have been observed in some brain areas (Adolfsson et al 1979, Gottfries et al 1983).

The aim of of the present study was to map the anterior to posterior distribution of DA, NA and cholinergic markers in nucleus caudatus, putamen, globus pallidus and hippocampus from postmortem human control brains and AD/SDAT brains.

MATERIAL

A total of 10 brains were analysed, four of which were clinically and histopathologically verified Alzheimer cases (Table 1). The mean age for these cases was 70.8±3.5 years (SEM) and the mean postmortem delay was 29.8±14.9 hours. The duration of the dementing condition varied between 4 and 12 years and immediate causes of death were bronchopneumonia (two cases), incarcerated hernia (one case) and myocardial infarction (one case). For the control subjects, mean age was 64.7±4.8 years and the corresponding values for death-autopsy time were 19.8± 5.5 hours. According to records, all control patients were mentally intact, and histopathology (performed on five of the cases) revealed no signs of dementia. The causes of death were myocardial infarction (four cases) and ruptured aortic aneurysm (two cases). The brain regions analysed included the basal ganglia (nucleus caudatus, putamen, globus pallidus) and hippocampus.

TABLE 1

Clinical and histopathological data on the AD/SDAT patients

Case no symbol (1)	Sex Age	Here-dity (2)	Duration of illness/hospi-talization (yrs)	Long term medi-cation	Medication final month	Cause of death	Time death-autopsy (hs)	Plaques/ tangles (3)
1 ☆	F,76	2/5	12/5	Antispychotics	Morphine	Bronchopneumonia	30	2/1-2
2 □	M,61	3/8	12/3	Antipsychotics, Anticholinergics	Antipsychotics Anticholiner-gics	Myocardial in-farction	24	3/2
3 △	M,76	0/5	6/1	Antipsychotics	Morphine	Bronchopneumonia	59	3/2
4 ■	F,70	0/3	4/2	Antipsychotics	-	Incarcerated hernia	6	2/1

(1) Case symbols used in figures
(2) Number of affected siblings/total number of siblings
(3) Number of senile plaques (Neurofibrillary tangles in sections from frontal cortex and right hippocampus)
Scale: 0, 1, 2, 3 (12)

METHODS

At autopsy, a central block containing the subcortical grey matter and the intact left hippocampus was wrapped in air-tight plastic and immediately frozen. The sectioning procedure, performed in the frozen state, yielded coronal slices 3 mm in thickness. Samples were removed using a scalpel and returned to the freezer. The basal ganglia samples were taken from the right hemisphere. Cutting slices of a determined thickness inevitably means that sometimes equivalens anatomical landmarks appear on different slices in different brains. To ensure as correct an anterior to posterior gradient as possible (and to facilitate graphic presentation) the slice values were moved so that the anatomical landmarks were coincident in all brains (see figures).

Catecholamines

The estimation of DA and NA was performed as follows: weighed tissue samples were put into vials containing 400 µl 0.1 M perchloric acid and appropriate amounts of dihydroxybenzylamine (internal standard). After alumina adsorption and desorption, reversed-phase high performance liquid chromatography with electrochemical detection was used for the determination of the amines. The mobile phase was an acetate--citrate buffer and the column was a 25 cm C18 Nucleosil R. Wilcoxon's rank sum test was used to calculate the significance.

Assay of choline acetyltransferase (ChAT) activity

The brain slices were homogenized in 100 volumes of 1% Triton X-100 in saline and 0.2 mM EDTA and centrifuged at 1000 g for 10 min. An aliquot of the supernatant was incubated with labelled 140 mM 14C-acetyl-CoA (SA 50 Ci/mmol, NEN, U.K.) according to a radioenzymatic method.

Assay of muscarine-like binding sites

Tritium labelled quinuclidinyl benzilate (L, 3H-QNB; SA 43 Ci/mmol); 0.2 nM; the Radiochemical Center, Amersham, U.K.) was incubated with an aliquot of a P2 fraction (0.1-0.2 mg) in a 50 mM NaHPO buffer (pH 7.4) at 25 C for 60 min. After incubation the samples were chilled on ice, centrifuged in a Beckman microfuge. The radioactivity bound to the pellet was quantified. In parallell experiments 10 mM atropine was included in the incubation media for estimation on unspecific binding.

RESULTS

Catecholaminergic data

The biochemical results are shown in Figure 1 and in Table 2. In general, NA concentrations were lowered in the striatal nuclei of the AD/SDAT brains compared with the control brains (significant in slice 5 of caudatus, in slice 7 and 9 of putamen and in slice 9 of globus pallidus, see figure 1 and table 2). In the control brains, an upward concentration gradient for NA towards the more posterior slices of both nucleus caudatus and putamen is clearly implied. Thus, for nucleus caudatus: slice 1 had significantly lower concentrations than slice 7 ($p<0.05$); slice 3 lower than slice 7 ($p<0.01$), 9 ($p<0.05$) and 11 ($p<0.05$). In putamen, slice 3 (most anterior slice) had significantly lower concentrations than slice 9 ($p<0.05$) and 11 ($p<0.05$). In the AD/SDAT brains no such intranuclear variations in NA content could be detected statistically. Hippocampal NA levels in the control brains

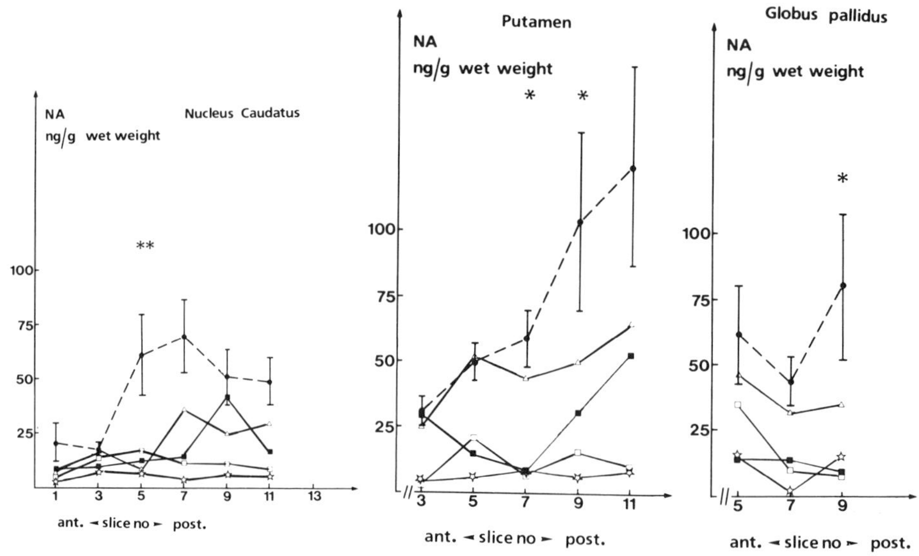

Fig. 1 Noradrenaline concentrations in right nucleus caudatus, right putamen and right globus pallidus. Significance levels are between controls (n=6) and AD/SDAT cases (n=4); *=p<0.05, **=p<0.01. Control values are mean ± SEM (dashed line). AD/SDAT cases are shown individually.

did not differ significantly from those in the AD/SDAT brains (table 2).

Table 2

Whole nuclei concentrations of DA and NA. Values are in ng/g wet weights and are given as mean SEM. Number of control brains=6, and of AD/SDAT brains=4.

Brain Regions	Control brains		AD/SDAT brains	
	DA	NA	DA	NA
Nucleus Caudatus	1454±342	45±12	1238±343	16±6*
Putamen	2745±548	74±17	2593±767	22±8*
Globus Pallidus	243±107	62±19	278± 81	18±7*
Hippocampus	6± 2	17± 5	6± 1	14±7

* Significantly lower than controls, p<0.05

Values for DA were similar in the control group and the AD/SDAT group (Table 2). Significant intranuclear gradients of this transmitter were not seen either in the control group or in the AD/SDAT group (data not shown here).

Cholinergic data

Results are discussed from putamen (Figure 2) and from caudate nucleus and hippocampus (data not shown). It is evident that in the individual Alzheimer case there is no parallel change in NA-content and ChAT activity except in case 1 where there are pronounced decreases in both NA-concentration and ChAT activity in all three regions. The clinical history of the patients reveals a different duration of the disease.

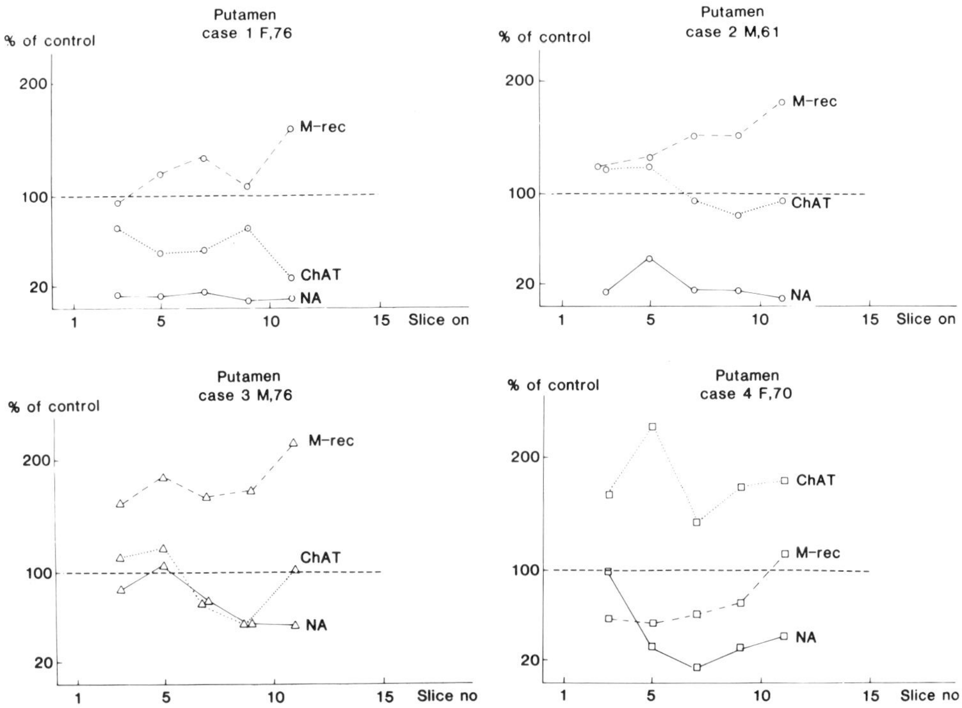

Fig 2. Noradrenaline (NA) concentration cholineacetyltransferase (ChAT) activity and muscarinic receptor (M-rec) in putamen from 4 Alzheimer patients.

Case 4 died after a rather short duration of an incarcerated hernia. In this case only the NA concentration was decreased in all three brain regions. Concerning the muscarinic receptors, all cases (except this case 4) showed an increased number of binding sites in caudate nucleus and putamen as compared to controls. In hippocampus no obvious changes were observed. Intranuclear gradients were observed both for ChAT and muscarinic receptors.

CONCLUSIONS

By demonstrating reduced NA concentrations in the basal ganglia of AD/SDAT brains, this study is in line with earlier reports indicating disturbances in the noradrenergic systems in these disorders. The number of patients is small. However, with a short duration of the disease it seems that the NA changes might preceede the cholinergic changes. With a long duration of the disease there seems to be parallel changes in the noradrenergic and cholinergic systems. In AD/SDAT (caudate nucleus and putamen) an upregulation of muscarinic binding sites was observed in all cases, except for the case with the shortest duration of the disease.

ACKNOWLEDGEMENTS

This study was supported by grants from the Swedish Medical Research Council, King Gustaf V and Queen Victoria's Foundation, Karl-Oskar Hansson's, Loo and Hans Osterman's, Gun och Bertil Stohne's, Fred och Ingrid Thuring's Foundations.

REFERENCES

Adolfsson R., Gottfries C.G., Roos B.E. and Winblad B. Changes in the brain catecholamines in patients with dementia of Alzheimer type. Brit J. Psychiat. 135(1979)216-223.

Davies P. Neurotransmitter-related enzymes in senile dementia of Alzheimer type. Brain Res. 171(1979)319-327.

Gottfries C.G., Adolfsson R., Aquilonius S.M., Carlsson A., Eckernäs S.Å., Nordberg A., Oreland L., Svennerholm L., Wiberg Å. and Winblad B. Biochemical changes in dementia disorders of Alzheimer type (AD/S-DAT). Neurobiol. Aging 4(1983)261-271.

Nordberg A., Larsson C., Adolfsson R., Alafuzoff I., and Winblad B. Muscarinic receptor compensation in hippocampus of Alzheimer patients. J. Neural Transm. 56(1983)13-19.

Perry E.K., Tomlinson B.E., Blessed G., Perry R.H. and Tomlinson B.E. Neurotransmitter enzyme abnormalities in senile dementia. J. Neurol. Sci. 34(1977)247-265.

Rossor M.N., Garrett N.J., Johnson A.L., Mountjoy C.Q. and Roth M. A postmortem study of the cholinergic and GABA systems in senile dementia. Brain 105(1982)313-330.

THE "AUTOCANNIBALISM" OF CHOLINE-CONTAINING MEMBRANE PHOSPHOLIPIDS IN THE PATHOGENESIS OF ALZHEIMER'S DISEASE

Richard J. Wurtman, and Jan K. Blusztajn
Department of Applied Biological Sciences
M.I.T., Cambridge, MA, USA and
Jean-Claude Maire
Pharmacology Department, Université de Genève, Suisse

Brains of patients with Alzheimer's disease exhibit an abundance of possible clues as to the etiology of the disease and the pathophysiologic processes causing its signs and symptoms.(1) These include characteristic aggregations of abnormal proteins in neurons (neurofibrillary tangles) and extracellular spaces (plaques; amyloid); concentrations of a potentially neurotoxic environmental contaminant, aluminum, within affected neurons; and an abnormal aggregate, amyloid, which may itself constitute an infectious particle ("prions"). Additional clues as to the etiology and pathogenesis of Alzheimer's disease may also be provided by the patient's family history - which sometimes reveals a strong genetic component to the disease - or by data, obtained using scanning devices, which show major reductions in brain blood flow and in oxygen and energy consumption.

All of these abnormal findings have spawned research programs designed to test their contributions to the clinical findings of Alzheimer's disease. However, none has affected the conduct of research nearly so much as observations suggesting that Alzheimer's disease preferentially affects particular populations of neurons, distinguishable based on the neurotransmitter that they produce and release. An overwhelming consensus now exists among investigators that a) certain acetylcholine-releasing brain neurons, the septal neurons projecting to the hippocampus and basal forebrain neurons innervating the cerebral cortices, are invariably decimated in Alzheimer's disease;(2-4) b) other neurons (for example, serotonin-releasing neurons in the raphe nucleus; noradrenergic neurons of the locus coeruleus; cortical somatostatin-releasing neurons) are also often afflicted but to a lesser extent; and, c) most neuronal populations are unaffected in the disease. If one or more groups of neurons are invariably damaged in Alzheimer's disease, then examination of their biochemical peculiarities may yield insights as to the disease's etiology or to the pathogenetic process that ultimately cause the neurons to die. Moreover, if the deficient neurotransmitter can be implicated in the abnormal behaviors typical of the disease - like acetylcholine in memory loss, or norepinephrine in the impaired ability to sustain attention, or serotonin in disturbances of mood or in aggressiveness - then drugs which substitute for the deficient transmitter or which increase its availability in synapses might be useful in treating the disease.

This article focusses on the first of these hopes, that is, on the possibility that a particular biochemical property unique to cholinergic neurons underlies their special vulnerability in Alzheimer's disease. This property has to do with the ways that cholinergic neurons metabolize choline: All cells in the body incorporate free choline into phospholipid molecules (which, by the way, constitute the majority of all lipids present in neuronal membranes,[5] like phosphatidylcholine (PC), sphingomyelin, and the 1-acetylcholine glycerophospholipids. However, cholinergic cells use choline for an additional purpose, i.e., both as a constituent of membrane phospholipids and as the precursor for acetylcholine, the neurotransmitter that they release into their synapses. (Indeed, when a cholinergic neuron is physiologically active, the rate at which it synthesizes and releases acetylcholine depends upon its choline levels).[6] We propose that their need to obtain choline for acetylcholine synthesis may sometimes cause cholinergic neurons to destroy their membranes, particularly when the neurons are firing frequently or when free choline is in relatively short supply: they may cannibalize the choline stored in the phospholipid "reservoir," thus altering membrane composition (and, presumably, function) and even blocking the production of new membranes.[6]

Our hypothesis begs the question of the etiology of the Alzheimer's disease, focusing instead on why cholinergic neurons are more likely than others to be damaged by the etiologic factor: It applies equally well whether the etiologic factor is present only in diseased cells or is distributed throughout the brain. The factor itself that presumably causes a choline deficiency might be a decrease in choline's production (by de novo synthesis); a decrease in its uptake from the synaptic cleft and extracellular space; or an excessive utilization of choline to form a particular phospholipid. Choline uptake might be impaired if the delivery of oxygen or glucose to the nerve terminals is deficient, perhaps secondary to a diffusion block caused by the perivascular amyloidosis that is characteristic of Alzheimer's disease.[7] Alternatively, the hypothetical choline deficiency might simply result from its overuse for acetylcholine synthesis, as might happen if the firing frequency of vulnerable neurons is persistently enhanced, or if the presynaptic storage of acetylcholine is impaired. Once cholinergic terminals begin to deteriorate and to release less of the transmitter, it seems likely that surviving, "healthy" terminals might start to release <u>more</u> acetylcholine -- because the firing frequencies of their neurons will increase or because release is no longer subject to presynaptic inhibition. Increased acetylcholine synthesis might also be expected to increase the demand for its precursor, choline, within "healthy" terminals, a process which might ultimately lead to "autocannibalism" in these terminals as well.

The choline obtained by "autocannibalism" could derive from the general metabolic "pool" of choline phospholipids, or perhaps from a pool specifically mobilized for that purpose. Membrane phospholipids like PC are compartmented in three ways: by their subcellular localization [for example, synaptic vesicles <u>vs.</u> plasma membranes]; by their fatty acid composition; and by their mode of synthesis [methylation of phosphatidylethanolamine <u>vs.</u> incorporation of pre-existing choline via the CDP-choline or base-exchange pathways]. Excessive destruction of membrane PC might lead to changes in membrane composition (for example, in the ratios of PC to other phospholipids, or to proteins) or to a loss in total membrane surface. Either alteration could affect the neuron's functional properties and even its viability. Such changes would be most likely to occur in nerve terminals, the neuronal structures that are specialized for neurotransmitter synthesis and release, initially damaging them and only later affecting cell bodies.

The "autocannibalism" hypothesis of the pathogenesis of Alzheimer's disease is not presently supported by an overwhelming body of clinical or experimental evidence; however, it is consistent with a number of observations:

1. It is the terminals of cholinergic neurons, in the cerebral cortex, and not the perikarya, in the basal forebrain, which apparently degenerate first in Alzheimer's disease.(8,9) This is consistent with the fact that most of the neurons' acetylcholine is formed in the pre-synaptic terminals.

2. Only long-axon cholinergic neurons are affected by the disease process: the short-axon interneurons in the striatum are spared. Perhaps the short-axon neurons can more easily resynthesize their membranes because choline phospholipids are more readily available to them through axoplasmic transport.(10,11) This transport would occur over a considerably shorter distance than that separating cholinergic perikarya in the nucleus basalis or septum from terminals in the frontoparietal cortex or hippocampus.

3. Choline is synthesized in brain neurons, de novo, by a multienzymatic pathway; the terminal steps in this pathway, catalyzed by phosphatidyl-ethanolamine N-methyltransferase (PeMT), involve the stepwise methylation of phosphatidylethanolamine (PE) to PC, using S-adenosylmethionine (SAM) as methyl donor. This newly formed PC is hydrolyzed to free choline by a number of phospholipases and other hydrolases. We found that free choline constituted 23% of the total PC synthesized by synaptosomal PeMT (from ^{3}H-methyl-SAM) during a 30-min incubation period. Furthermore, the enrichment of the free choline pool with newly formed [^{3}H]-choline was 50-fold greater than that of the PC pool by newly formed [^{3}H]-PC.(12) Thus, the relatively small amount of PC synthesized in nerve terminals de novo may have a considerably faster turnover than the bulk of synaptosomal PC, possibly because this PC preferentially provides free choline for acetylcholine synthesis.

4. To determine whether an endogenous choline source (perhaps PC) in brain tissue can support acetylcholine synthesis in the absence of free choline, we measured acetylcholine release from rat striatal slices superfused with or without choline.(13) In the absence of free choline, acetylcholine was released spontaneously at a rate of 7.5 $\pm$ 1.3 pmol/mg protein/min (mean $\pm$ S.D.). Electrical field stimulation (15Hz for 30 min) accelerated this release (25.6 $\pm$ 5.9 pmol/mg protein/min), and addition of choline (20 uM) to the superfusate significantly enhanced both the spontaneous (22.7 $\pm$ 5.7 pmol/mg protein/min) and the electrically evoked (37.4 $\pm$ 6.7 pmol/mg protein/min) release of the transmitter. Although the amount of acetylcholine in the tissue did not depend on extracellular choline concentration in this concentration range, the choline contents of the slices did increase as choline levels in the superfusate were raised. In the absence of exogenous choline, the combined efflux of free choline plus acetylcholine into the superfusate was 75 pmol/mg protein/min; the decrease in free choline plus acetylcholine within the tissue, however, was only 16 pmol/mg protein/min. Thus, an endogenous pool of bound choline must have provided additional free choline for acetylcholine synthesis, and to maintain tissue choline and acetylcholine levels. The only known compounds whose pool sizes would be sufficient for this purpose are the choline-containing phospholipids. Apparently, the choline liberated from striatal phospholipids must first enter the extracellular space and then be transported into cholinergic neurons by the high-affinity choline uptake system: addition of hemicholinium-3 (which blocks this uptake process) to the superfusate suppressed electrically evoked acetylcholine release and decreased striatal acetylcholine levels, even when compared with acetylcholine release from, and levels in, tissues that had been incubated without free choline.

Choline efflux from the isolated, perfused chicken heart was found to be enhanced by cholinesterase inhibitors or by muscarinic cholinergic agonists, and blocked by muscarinic antagonists.(14) This choline apparently also originates from the hydrolysis of tissue phospholipids. The rate at which this hydrolysis occurs apparently is modulated by cholinergic activity.

5. Stimulation of the preganglionic trunk of the cat's superior cervical ganglion for 20 min at 20, 4 or 1 Hz decreased the number of synaptic vesicles in cholinergic nerve terminals by 75, 54 or 56%, respectively,[15] without altering ganglionic acetylcholine contents.[16] This finding was interpreted as suggesting that the choline phospholipids in vesicular membranes were the source of the choline for acetylcholine synthesis. When, in a similar experiment, the cat's superior cervical ganglion was stimulated for a shorter period, PC levels and the number of synaptic vesicles in presynaptic terminals did not fall: however, if the ganglion was also exposed to hemicholinium-3, the number of synaptic vesicles decreased after stimulation to 18% of control, while ganglionic PC levels fell to 69% of control.[17] (Other phospholipids were not affected.) These observations indicate that when adequate extracellular choline is not available (after inhibition of its uptake by hemicholinium-3) vesicular PC is used to supply choline for acetylcholine synthesis.

No information is available concerning the possibility that neuronal choline-phospholipids provide choline for acetylcholine synthesis in human brain, nor that this process is pathologically accelerated in Alzheimer's disease. Conceivably, brain regions rich in diseased cholinergic terminals might exhibit reductions in the ratio of PC to other phospholipids. However, a reduction would not occur if, for example, the terminal's failure to sustain adequate PC levels caused it simply to stop producing PC-containing membranes -- a possibility that appears compatible with the preferential loss of cholinergic terminals over perikarya in Alzheimer's disease.

The hypothesized ability of the choline-phospholipids in cholinergic terminals to serve both as a structural component and as a reservoir for an important molecule of lower molecular weight (free choline) is not, of course, unique: circulating albumin both contributes to the maintenance of colloid osmotic pressure and provides free amino acids when protein consumption is inadequate; bone is both a structural unit and a vast reservoir for calcium. Protein malnutrition can cause edema when too much albumin is broken down to provide free amino acids; calcium malnutrition can cause osteomalacia and bone breakage when bone is demineralized to provide the blood with free calcium. If our hypothesis concerning the reservoir functions of neuronal choline-phospholipids is correct, then consumption of supplemental choline -- as such or as dietary PC (lecithin) -- might serve an important nutritional function in patients with Alzheimer's disease, providing their diseased cholinergic neurons with some protection against "autocannibalism" of their choline- containing membrane.

REFERENCES

1. Wurtman, R.J. Alzheimer's disease. Scientific American, 252:62-75, 1985.
2. Perry, E.K., Tomlinson, B.E., Blessed, G., Bergman, K., Gibson, P.H., and Perry, R.H. Correlation of cholinergic abnormalities with senile plaques and mental test scores in senile dementia. Brit. J. Med., 2:1458-1459 (1978).
3. Bowen, D.M., Benton, J.S., Spillane, J.A., Smith, C.C.T., and Allen, S.J. Choline acetyltransferase activity and histopathology of frontal neocortex biopsies of demented patients. J. Neurol. Sci., 57:191-202 (1982).
4. Wilcock, G.K., Esiri, M.M., Bowen, D.M., and Smith, C.C.T. Alzheimer's disease: correlation of cortical choline acetyltransferase activity with the severity of dementia and histological abnormalities. J. Neurol. Sci., 57:407-417 (1982).

5. Ansell, G.B. Phospholipids and the nervous system. In: "Form and Function of Phospholipids," G.B. Ansell, J.N. Hawthorne, and R.M.C. Dawson,eds. Elsevier, Amsterdam (1973)
6. Blusztajn, J.K. and Wurtman, R.J. Choline and cholinergic neurons. Science, 221:614-620 (1983).
7. Mandybur, T.I. The incidence of cerebral amyloid angiopathy in Alzheimer's disease. Neurology (Minneap.), 25:120-126 (1975).
8. Perry, R.H., Candy, J.M., Perry, E.K., Irving, D., Blessed, G., Fairbairn, A.F., and Tomlinson, B.E. Extensive loss of choline acetyltransferase activity is not reflected by neuronal loss in the nucleus of Meynert in Alzheimer's disease. Neuroscience Letters, 33:311-315 (1985).
9. Pearson, R.C.A., Sofroniew, M.V., Cuello, A.C. Powell, T.P.S., Eckenstein, S., Esiri, M.M., Wilcock, G.K. Persistence of cholinergic neurons in the basal nucleus in a brain with senile dementia of the Alzheimer's type demonstrated by immunohistochemical staining for choline acetyltransferase. Brain Research, 289:375-379 (1983).
10. Abe, T., Haga, T., Kurokawa, M. Rapid transport of phosphatidylcholine occurring simultaneously with protein transport in the frog sciatic nerve. Biochem. J., 136:731-740 (1973).
11. Droz, B., Brunetti, M., DiGiambernadino, L., Koenig, H.L., Porcellati, G. Axonal transport of phosphoglycerides to cholinergic synapses. In: "Cholinergic Mechanisms," G. Pepeu, ed., Plenum Press, New York (1981)
12. Blusztajn, J.K. and Wurtman, R.J. Choline biosynthesis by a preparation enriched in synaptosomes from rat brain. Nature, 290:417-418 (1981)
13. Maire, J.-C., Tacconi, M.T., Wurtman, R.J. Source of choline for the release of choline and acetylcholine from brain slices. Soc. Neurosci., 9:283.8, abstract (1983).
14. Corradetti, R., Lindmar, R., Loffelholz, K. Mobilization of cellular choline by stimulation of muscarinic receptors in isolated chicken heart and rat cortex in vivo. J. Pharmacol. Exp. Ther., 226:826-832 (1983).
15. Birks, R.I. The relationship of transmitter release and storage to the fine structure in a sympathetic ganglion. J. Neurocytol., 3:133-160 (1974).
16. Birks, R.I. and MacIntosh, F.C. Acetylcholine metabolism of a sympathetic ganglion. Can. J. Biochem. Physiol., 39:787-827 (1961).
17. Parducz, A., Kiss, Z., Joo, F. Changes of the phosphatidylcholine content and the number of synaptic vesicles in relation to neurohumoral transmission in sympathetic ganglia. Experientia, 32:1520-1521.

TROPHIC FACTORS AND NEUROLOGIC DISEASE

Stanley H. Appel, Yasuko Tomozawa, and
Robert Bostwick

Department of Neurology
Baylor College of Medicine
Houston, Texas

INTRODUCTION

The causes of some of the most common and devastating diseases of the human nervous system remain unknown. Prominent on this list are amyotrophic lateral sclerosis (ALS), parkinsonism, and Alzheimer's disease. Each of these conditions is presently considered to be a degenerative disorder of unknown origin. In each, there may be a variable clinical expression reflecting different etiologies in different patients. A specific inherited metabolic disorder may account for a small percentage of cases, while immunological, viral, or other etiologies may be responsible for the remainder.

Our own thesis is that in ALS, parkinsonism, and Alzheimer's disease, there is a common denominator. We propose that the clinical deficit may be explained by the lack or functional deficiency of specific neurotrophic hormones elaborated or stored in the synaptic target of the affected neurons and acting in a retrograde fashion (Appel, 1981). Thus, ALS, Parkinson's disease, and Alzheimer's disease would be analogous to thyroid disease or other endocrinopathies. For example, genetically induced alterations either in hormone or its receptor would present with a functional deficiency. Furthermore, the presence of antibodies against either the hormone or its receptor on the innervating cell may interfere with hormone action and present as ALS, parkinsonism, or Alzheimer's disease, depending upon the specific neurotrophic hormones and specific systems involved. Thus, any process which interferes with neurotrophic hormone metabolism, release, interaction with receptor, second messenger effects, internalization of the hormone, or interaction with key intracellular constituents would give rise to the network dysfunction noted in these disorders. Any effort to correct the deficit, including tissue transplantation, which did not take account of the functional hormonal alterations of the target cell or the persistence of antibodies against the hormone or its receptor, would be unsuccessful.

TROPHIC FACTORS

Recent studies in developmental neurobiology have demonstrated the importance of target cells for the survival, growth, and differentiation of innervating neurons. The discovery of nerve growth factor was the first major step in the molecular analysis of nervous system development (Levi-Montalcini and Hamburger, 1951), and suggested that the effect of the target might be mediated by diffusible molecules (Cohen, 1960). NGF can be isolated as an active 26,500-dalton component containing two identical polypeptide chains (Cohen, 1960; Levi-Montalcini and Angeletti, 1968; Thoenen and Barde, 1980; Yanker and Shooter, 1982; Bradshaw, 1983). NGF can reverse naturally-occurring as well as experimentally-induced cell death in sympathetic and sensory neurons in vivo. Anti-NGF antibodies can block the development of the sympathetic nervous system in vivo (Levi-Montalcini, 1982). Thus, competition for a limited supply of NGF may determine which neurons live and which die during development. Furthermore, NGF may be required for neuronal maintenance in adulthood (Levi-Montalcini and Angeletti, 1968; Thoenen and Barde, 1980; Yanker and Shooter, 1982; Bradshaw, 1983).

The existence of naturally-occurring cell death in most populations of vertebrate neurons (Oppenheim, 1981) and the early realization that only a few neuronal systems are sensitive to NGF led to speculation that NGF may be only one of a family of trophic agents. The search for new factors that regulate neuronal growth and development has employed in vitro assays similar to those used for NGF. A wide range of activities that stimulate neuronal growth and development have been noted with target tissue extracts and cell-conditioned media. However, the significance of such studies is still unclear since most results have been obtained with impure components and may be dependent on unknown features of the assay. Only complete purification of the trophic factors will permit unambiguous identification. A new factor that stimulates survival of sensory neurons in culture has been purified to homogeneity from pig brain (Barde et al, 1982). The molecule has a molecular weight of 12,300 daltons, an isoelectric point of greater than 10.1, and a specific activity estimated to be 0.4 mg/ml/units. It migrates as a single band on SDS gel electrophoresis. Its effect is additive to that of NGF, and it is not blocked by anti-serum to NGF.

Partially purified factors have been documented to have effects on neuronal survival, neurite extension, substrate adhesion, and neurotransmitter specification. NGF clearly has more than one kind of stimulatory activity, but the degree of multiple activities in other trophic factors is unclear because of the impurity of the preparations employed. Chick ciliary ganglion has been a useful preparation for identifying neuronal survival factors, and such activity has been found in extracts prepared from embryotic eye tissue (Adler et al, 1979), chick heart (Nishi and Berg, 1979), and in CNS wounds in developing and young adult rats (Nietro-Sampedro et al, 1982). Further purification of the eye extract demonstrates activity in the 20,000-dalton component as determined by gel filtration (Varon et al, 1983). A similar molecular weight factor has been found in another laboratory to stimulate neuronal growth with no effects on levels of choline acetyltransferase (CAT) (Nishi and Berg, 1981). Whether these are identical or merely similar factors is unclear, but they are clearly distinct from the pig brain factor. Similar ambiguities surround our understanding of neurite extension factors, substrate adhesion and neurite promoting factors and differentiation and development factors (reviewed by Berg, 1984). Different trophic acitivities with different specificities and functions clearly exist in different target tissues. Whether a single factor can have diverse activities, or diverse factors can have a single activity must await purification and characterization of the specific factors.

TROPHIC FACTORS IN THE NEUROMUSCULAR SYSTEM

In our own laboratories, our initial efforts have focused on the motor unit and the extent to which muscle-derived factors can influence the survival, neurite outgrowth and cholinergic activity of spinal motor neurons in vitro. Co-culture of skeletal myotubes with spinal cord cells enhances neuron survival, promotes outgrowth of neurites, and increases the activity of choline acetyltransferase (Giller et al, 1977). Media conditioned with myotubes can reproduce some of the effects of co-culturing, thereby suggesting the existence of diffusible trophic factors (Dribin and Barrett, 1980; Brooks et al, 1980). Furthermore, soluble extracts of rat skeletal muscle increase neurite outgrowth and cholinergic activity of dissociated spinal neurons in culture (Smith and Appel, 1983). The question of how many different motor neurotrophic agents exist is presently unresolved. In our own studies, we have separated one morphological factor and two cholinergic factors with differing properties. The isolation and characterization of such growth factors should help us begin to understand how motor neurons can control and, in turn, be controlled by the supply of such factors. Furthermore, investigations of the relevant genes may lead to other motor neuron growth factors presently not detectable by our in vitro assays. The availability of purified neurotrophic factors from muscle would enable us to determine whether deficiencies in such factors are present in ALS, and whether antibodies against either the motor neurotrophic factors or their receptors on presynaptic terminals participate in the disease process.

PARKINSON'S DISEASE AND TROPHIC FACTORS

A similar strategy of defining striatal trophic factors and determining their relevance for substantia nigra neuronal survival, growth, differentiation, and maintenance has been adopted in our approaches to Parkinson's disease.

Parkinson's disease is a disorder of older individuals with a mean age of onset of 67. It is characterized by tremor, bradykinesia, and rigidity as well as the loss of postural reflexes. The primary pathological abnormality appears to be a loss of neurons in the substantia nigra. Pathologically, eosinophilic inclusions termed Lewy bodies are present in nigral neurons. In cases of postencephalitic parkinsonism, neurofibrillary alterations are noted in nigral neurons. The loss of nigral cells leads to marked impairment in the nigrostriatal pathway, and diminution in the dopaminergic synaptic input to the caudate and putamen. Of importance is the fact that no diminution is noted in the dopaminergic receptors within the striatum. Thus, the presynaptic neuron is impaired and the postsynaptic neuron is intact.

Extending the hypothesis of retrograde neurotrophic factors to Parkinson's disease suggests the absence or impairment of neurotrophic factors normally supplied by the striatum to nigral neurons. With the failure of neurotrophic factors, nigral cells would gradually die.

Furthermore, if the major cause of the difficulty were antibodies directed against striatal trophic factors or their receptors on presynaptic terminals, then transplantation of fetal substantia nigral cells would be unlikely to have any beneficial effect unless the antibodies themselves could be eliminated.

The question of whether soluble trophic factors are present in the nigrostriatal system has not been previously documented. The dopaminergic nigrostriatal pathway has been extensively studied with respect to anatomic relations, developmental neurogenesis, and biochemistry (Specht et al, 1981). Prochiantz et al demonstrated that the dissociated mesenchephalic dopaminergic neurons from embryonic mouse will grow and differentiate in vitro, with development being enhanced when mesencephalic cells are grown in the presence of striatal target cells (Prochiantz et al, 1979). Subsequent experiments from the same laboratories demonstrated that striatal membranes from 2- and 3-week-old animals and not soluble components specifically stimulate the development of dopaminergic neurons (Prochiantz et al, 1981).

Our own laboratory has examined the effects of soluble striatal extracts on substantia nigra neurons as a means of monitoring and purifying specific neurotrophic factors. Both explant and dissociation cultures are obtained from 14-day-old rat embryos at a time when the mesencephalic dopaminergic neurons are postmitotic, and have extended to striatal targets. The dopaminergic activity is monitored by H^3 dopamine uptake in the presence and absence of specific inhibitors. Our data have confirmed the enhancing effects of striatal membrane fractions on neurite extension, and dopaminergic activity. However, soluble factors are even more potent and are additive to the membrane constituents. These soluble factors have a molecular weight of less than 2,000 daltons and are inactivated by proteolytic enzymes. They enhance 1) the survival of dopaminergic neurons in culture, (2) neurite outgrowth and density, (3) the uptake of H^3 dopamine, and (4) the appearance of positive histofluorescence for catecholamines. Other tissues, such as skeletal muscle and liver, as well as cerebellum, do not have a similar effect on dopaminergic activity of mesencephalic cultures. These same soluble fractions from the striatum have no effect on cholinergic activity of cultured ventral spinal cord neurons. Purification of these factors should enable us to determine their potential relevance to Parkinson's disease.

ALZHEIMER'S DISEASE AND TROPHIC FACTORS

Our approach to Alzheimer's disease has involved a strategy similar to that adopted in our investigations of the neuromuscular and the nigrostriatal systems, namely to establish the existence of trophic factors which act in a retrograde manner in a system known to be compromised in Alzheimer's disease. The specific network we have studied is the septo-hippocampal cholinergic pathway.

Alzheimer's disease is a disorder of the later decades of life characterized by diffuse deterioration of mental functions primarily in thought and memory and secondarily in feeling and conduct. The diagnosis depends upon ruling out secondary causes of loss of memory and impaired cognitive function such as depression, multiple infarcts, intracranial mass lesions, infections or toxic and metabolic disorders. However, even when such secondary causes are ruled out, the clinical manifestations of the remaining patients do not comprise a discrete homogeneous entity. As a result, it is difficult to understand how any single process could cause such devastation and leave so few clues.

The brains of patients with Alzheimer's disease and senile dementia of the Alzheimer's type are characterized by a profusion of senile plaques, neurofibrillary tangles, granulovacuolar degeneration, and Hirano bodies. No single one of these features is specific for Alzheimer's disease, but their presence is vastly increased in Alzheimer's disease as compared with age-matched controls. In senile dementia as well as in Alzheimer's disease, there is a more significant loss of neurons than in age-matched controls. In addition, there is compromise of neurons in the nucleus basalis of Meynert (Whitehouse et al, 1982) as well in the diagonal band of Broca, and in the medial septal nucleus, all of which represent a basal forebrain cholinergic system with widespread projections to the amygdala, hippocampus, and cortex.

In patients with presenile Alzheimer's disease as well as senile dementia of the Alzheimer's type, there is a several-fold accentuation of neuronal loss in the same areas noted in normal brains from age-matched controls. In the case of the amygdala, the neuronal loss of Alzheimer's disease occurs in areas that fail to show age-related cell losses. The density of neurofibrillary tangles varies from region to region. Such tangles are present in lowest density in the primary cortices, with increasing density in the primary and secondary association cortices, and highest density in the multi-modal association area, which is reciprocally related to the limbic cortex and the hippocampal complex.

The impaired cortical projections from subcortical nuclei such as nucleus basalis and locus ceruleus together with impaired cortical-cortical association systems appear responsible for the profound deficits in cognitive function that are characteristic of Alzheimer's disease.

Biochemical changes are quite marked in the brains of patients with Alzheimer's disease and appear to result from the loss of these subcortical projections to the cortex and hippocampus. A reduction in choline acetyltransferase, acetyl cholinesterase, and the synthesis of acetylcholine were among the first reproducible changes noted (Davies, 1976). This observation was then followed by the demonstration of neuronal loss in the nucleus basalis of Meynert (Whitehouse et al, 1982). Of interest is the fact that cholinergic receptors in cortex and hippocampus are normal. Thus, the primary defect appears to be one of presynaptic neurons, with relative sparing of the postsynaptic cell.

Transmitter depletion is not confined to acetylcholine or the enzymes that synthesize or degrade acetylcholine. A diminution in serotonin uptake has been noted in biopsied cerebral cortex (Bowen, 1983). Approximately 70% depletion was noted with relatively little change in imipramine binding or indoleamines by comparison (Bowen, 1983). In certain Alzheimer's patients, especially those with extrapyramidal signs and substantia nigra cell loss, concentrations of dopamine and dopamine metabolites may be decreased. A significant reduction of the concentration of norepinephrine in senile dementia was reported by Adolfsson et al (1979), and a 40% reduction of dopamine-beta-hydroxylase activity was found in the cerebral cortex of patients with SDAT. Both of these observations may relate to the loss of about 80% of locus ceruleus neurons in younger patients with Alzheimer's disease (Bonderaff, 1982).

The many neurotransmitter alterations in Alzheimer's disease have raised doubt about the primacy of the cholinergic changes. Nevertheless, the ability of inhibitors of the cholinergic network to impair performance in healthy young adults (Drachman, 1983) and the depletion of acetylcholine synthesis in early cases of Alzheimer's disease (Bowen, 1983) certainly attest to the importance of the cholinergic changes. Evidence supporting the importance of other neurotransmitters is far less compelling. For example, the hallmark of Alzheimer's disease, namely impairment of memory, is not a characteristic feature of manipulation of dopaminergic, noradrenergic, serotonergic, or GABAergic systems. However, it is of interest that manipulation of the noradrenergic system does have an effect on long-term potentiation, a hippocampal synaptic model of memory (Hopkins and Johnston, 1984). Thus, any theory attempting to explain Alzheimer's disease will have to explain why several of these subcortical projection systems are involved.

Neuropeptides have also been extensively examined in Alzheimer's disease. Of all the neuropeptides examined to date, only somatostatin appears to undergo significant change in Alzheimer's disease (Davies et al 1980). Unlike neurotransmitters such as acetylcholine, serotonin, dopamine, and norepinephrine, which are largely derived from neurons projecting from subcortical nuclei, somatostatin is unaffected by lesions in the subcortical areas. Thus, somatostatin is present in intrinsic cortical and hippocampal neurons. None of the other peptides present in large numbers of cortical and hippocampal neurons such as cholecystokinin or vasoactive intestinal peptide are altered in Alzheimer's disease. Of considerable interest are the recent observations that somatostatin immunoreactivity is present in neuritic plaques of Alzheimer's patients (Morrison et al 1985) and neuronal tangles are present in somatostatin neurons (Roberts et al, 1985). These observations suggest that, at the very least, both acetylcholine and somatostatin-containing nerve terminals participate in plaque formation. Such findings suggest that plaques may occur at cortical or hippocampal sites where inputs from subcortical nuclei containing acetylcholine, norepinephrine, serotonin, or dopamine may converge with inputs from intrinsic cortical or hippocampal neurons containing somatostatin. The tangles would then be most marked in the neurons which project to such sites.

NEUROTROPHIC EFFECTS IN THE SEPTAL-HIPPOCAMPAL SYSTEM

Although several neuronal networks appear to be compromised in Alzheimer's disease, our own efforts have focused on establishing the existence of trophic factors in only one of these, namely the cholinergic septo-hippocampal pathway. Our investigations have employed cultured medial septal tissue as an assay for morphological and cholinergic-enhancing effects of hippocampal extracts. Explants of medial septal tissues are obtained from the brains of 16-day-old embryonic albino Sprague-Dawley rats. Explants are grown either in Sato's defined media or in heat-inactivated horse serum. In defined media, hippocampal membranes are required to demonstrate that soluble hippocampal extracts can enhance cholinergic activity. However, heat-inactivated horse serum can substitute for the membrane constituents. In the presence of serum, the addition of hippocampal supernatant results in a substantial increase in the length and density of neuritic outgrowth after 3 days in vitro. Within the same period, there is an enhancement of acetylcholine synthesis as well as choline acetyltransferase activity, which continues for at least eight days, by which time a three- to four-fold enhancement is noted (Ojika and Appel, 1984). Other tissues, such as cerebellum, spinal cord, muscle, liver, and kidney, do not contain soluble factors with similar enhancing effects. Furthermore, nerve growth factor cannot reproduce the effects of hippocampal extract nor can antibodies to nerve growth factor alter the cholinergic enhancement of hippocampal extract. The supernatant activity resides primarily in peptide fractions of less than 2,000 daltons. Neither cholecystokinin, vasoactive intestinal peptide, nor somatostatin have any effects on the morphologic or cholinergic activities of cultured medial septal neurons.

DISCUSSION

The etiology of both Parkinson's disease and Alzheimer's disease are unknown. Although clinical manifestations of both conditions are seen with aging, the pathological expression of both disorders is much more marked than what is normally seen in the brain of any aged individual. Thus, these two disorders are not simply an acceleration of aging, but reflect specific disease processes. Nevertheless, one cannot exclude the possibility that both normal aging and these two degenerative diseases of the nervous system are reflections of a common denominator. The gradual alteration in cholinergic, dopaminergic, noradrenergic, and possibly even serotonergic projections with aging may give rise to the gradual dysfunction in motor and cognitive function noted with aging. The common denominator could be the gradual age-related loss of specific trophic factors.

However, diseases such as parkinsonism or Alzheimer's cannot be due to the same age-related depletion. In Parkinson's disease there may be an accentuation of age-related retrograde trophic factor loss, either through toxic factors, immunological attack against the neurotrophic factors or their receptors, or other mechanisms. The common denominator would be a diminution in retrograde trophic function, but the process would be accentuated by specific attack on striatal dopaminergic factors or their receptors on nigral terminals. Depending upon the nature of the specific etiological factor (e.g. autoimmunity or toxins), different clinical syndromes may result (e.g., post-encephalitic parkinsonism, idiopathic parkinsonism).

Similar impairment in retrograde trophic effects could explain the gradual depletion of cholinergic activity in normal aging. A marked accentuation of this process could result in senile dementia of the Alzheimer's type. A number of disease processes, including antibodies directed against cells containing cholinergic neurotrophic factor or against cells containing trophic factor receptors as well as toxins, viruses, or other agents would apply in different cases. Similarly, in younger patients with Alzheimer's disease, impairment in the retrograde trophic effects may be present in several systems, including dopaminergic, noradrenergic, serotonergic, as well as cholinergic networks.

The impairment of several neurotransmitter systems has suggested that the primary lesion may be subcortical, and that the cortical and hippocampal pathology may result from transsynaptic degeneration caused by the loss of the afferent input. However, with this explanation it would be difficult to understand the loss of somatostatin immunoactivity in intrinsic cortical or hippocampal neurons. Conversely, lesions of the cortex or hippocampus at sites where somatostatin-containing neurons converge with projections from subcortical cholinergic, noradrenergic, serotonergic, or dopaminergic neurons may result in retrograde degeneration of these afferent projections.

The key question is whether the cortical or the subcortical changes are primary. Our own thesis is that the cortical and hippocampal changes are primary, and that the subcortical changes are secondary. Alterations in the cortical or hippocampal supply of neurotrophic factors could impair the normal retrograde trophic action on afferents projections from subcortical nuclei. The secondary degenerative changes could then lead to widespread dysfunction. The common denominator would be the loss of specific neurotrophic factors. Whether a single factor could regulate the different subcortical projectives in a retrograde fashion or whether several factors are required (i.e., cholinergic, noradrenergic, dopaminergic, and serotonergic trophic factors) is presently unclear. What is clear already is that trophic peptides with dopaminergic or cholinergic enhancing activities do exist. Finally, the pathological process which initiates the retrograde changes is undefined. If the analogy with the endocrinopathies is valid then multiple etiologies could account for trophic factor alterations. The most prominent would be an autoimmune process which compromised either the source of the neurotrophic factors or their interaction with receptors on afferent projections.

Acknowledgement: Supported in part by grants from the Harkins Foundation Fund for Alzheimer's Research, the Tex Collins Fund for ALS Research, and the Robert J. and Helen C. Kleberg Foundation.

REFERENCES

Adler, R., Landa, R.B., Manthorpe, M. and Varon, S., 1979, Cholinergic neurotrophic factors: Intraocular distribution of trophic activity for ciliary neurons, Science, 204:1434-1436.

Appel, S.H., 1981, A unifying hypothesis for the cause of amyotrophic lateral sclerosis, parkinsonism and Alzheimer's disease, Ann. Neurol., 10:499-505.

Barde, Y.A., Edgar, D., and Thoenen, H., 1982, Purification of a new neurotrophic factor from mammalian brain, EMBO J., 1:549-553.

Berg, D.K., 1984, New neuronal growth factors, Ann. Rev. Neurosci., 7:149-170.

Bondareff, W., Mountjoy, C.Q., Roth, M., 1982, Loss of neurons of origin of the adrenergic projection to cerebral cortex (nucleus locus ceruleus) in senile dementia, Neurology 32:164-168.

Bowen, D.M., 1983, Biochemical assessment of neurotransmitter and metabolic dysfunction and cerebral atrophy in Alzheimer's disease, Katzman, R., (ed), Banbury Report 15, Biological Aspects of Alzheimer's Disease, Coldspring Harbor, NY, pp. 219.

Bradshaw, R.A., 1983, What cloned genes can tell us about nerve growth factor, Nature, 303:751.

Brookes, N., Burt, D.R., Goldberg, A.H. and Bierkamp (1980), Influence of muscle-conditoned medium on cholinergic modification in spinal cord cell cultures, Brain Res., 186:474-479

Cohen, S., 1960, Purification of a nerve-growth promoting protein from the mouse salivary gland and its neurocytotoxic antiserum, Proc. Natl. Acad. Sci. USA, 302-311.

Davies, P., Katzman, R., Terry, R.D., 1980, Reduced somatostatin-like immunoreactivity in cerebral cortex from cases of Alzheimer's disease and Alzheimer's senile dementia, Nature, 288:279

Davies, P., and Maloney, A.J.F., 1976, Selective loss of central central cholinergic neurons in Alzheimer's disease, Lancet 2:1403.

Dribin, L.B. and Barrett, J.N., 1980, Conditioned medium enhances neuritic outgrowth from rat spinal explants, Dev. Biol., 74:184

Giller, E.L., Jr., Schrier, B.K., Shainberg, A., Fisk, H.R., and Nelson, P.B., 1977, Choline acetyltransferase activity of spinal cord cell cultures increased by co-culture with muscle and by muscle-conditioned medium, J. Cell Biology, 74:16

Hopkins, W.F., Johnston, D., 1984, Frequency-dependent noradrenergic modulation of long-term potentiation in the hippocampus, Science, 226:350-352.

Levi-Montalcini, R., 1982, Developmental neurobiology and the natural history of nerve growth factor, Ann. Rev. Neurosci., 5:341-362.

Levi-Montalcini, R., and Angeletti, P.U., 1968, Nerve growth factor, Physiol. Rev., 48:534-569.

Levi-Montalalcini, R., and Hamburger, V., 1951, Selective growth stimulating effects of mouse sarcoma on the sensory-sympathetic nervous system of the chick embryo, J. Exp. Zool., 116:321-361.

Morrison, J. H., Rogers, J., Scherr, S., Benoit, R., and Bloom, F. E., 1985, Somatostatin immunoreactivity in neuritic plaques of Alzheimer's patients, Nature, 314:90-92

Nieto-Sampedro, M., Lewis, E.R., Cotman, C.W., Manthorpe, M., Skaper, S.D., Barbin, G., Longo, F.M., and Varon, S., 1982, Brain injury causes a time-dependent increase in neuronotrophic activity at the lesion site, Science, 217:860-861.

Nishi, R., and Berg, D.K., 1979, Survival and development of ciliary ganglion neurones grown alone in cell culture, Nature, 277:232-234.

Nishi, R., and Berg, D., 1981, Two components from eye tissue that differentially stimulate the growth and development of ciliary ganglion neurons in cell culture, J. Neuroscience 1:505-513.

Ojika, K., Appel, S. H., 1984, Neurotrophic effects of hippocampal extracts on medial septal nucleus in vitro, PNAS, 81:2567-2571.

Oppenheim, R.W., 1981, Neuronal cell death and some related regressive phenomena during neurogenesis: A selective historical review and progress report, in: "Studies in Developmental Neurobiology," W.M. Cohen, ed., Oxford University, New York.

Price, D.L., Struble, R.G., Clark, A.W., Coyle, J.T., Delon, M.R., 1982, Alzeimer's disease and senile dementia: Loss of neurons in the basal forebrain, Science 215:1237

Prochiantz, A., di Porzio, U., Kato, A., Berger, B., and Glowinski, J., 1979, In vitro maturation of mesencephalic dopaminergic neurons from mouse embryos is enhanced in presence of their striatal target cells, Proc. Natl. Acad. Sci. USA, 76:5387-5391.

Prochiantz, A., Daguet, M-C, Herbert A., Glowinski, J., 1981, Specific stimulation of in vitro maturation of mesencephalic dopaminergic neurons by striatal membranes, Nature, 293:570-572.

Roberts, G. W., Crow, T. J., and Polak, J.M., 1985, Location of neuronal tangles in somatostatin neurones in Alzheimer's disease, Nature, 314:92-94

Smith, R.G. and Appel, S.H., 1983, Extracts of skeletal muscle increase neurite outgrowth and cholinergic activity of fetal fat spinal motor neurons, Science, 219:1079-1081.
Specht, L.A., Pickel, V.M., Joh, T.H. and Reis, D.J., 1981, Light microscopic immunocytochemical localization of tyrosine-hydroxylase in prenatal rat brain: I Early ontogeny, Comp. Neurol., 199:233-253.
Specht, L.A., Pickel, V.M., Joh, T.H. and Reis, D.J., 1981, Light microscopic immunocytochemical localization of tyrosine-hydroxylase in prenatal rat brain: II Late ontogeny, Comp. Neurol., 199:255-276.
Theonen, H., and Barde, Y., 1980, Physiology of nerve growth factors, Physiol. 60:1284.
Varon, S., Manthorpe, M., Longo, F.M., and Williams, L.R., 1983, in: "Nerve, Organ, and Tissue Regeneration: Research Perspective," F.J. Siel, ed., Academic Press, New York.
Yanker, B.A. and Shooter, E.M., 1982, The biology and mechanism of action of nerve growth factor, Ann. Rev. Biochem., 51:845-868.

NEURONAL LOSS AND NEUROTRANSMITTER RECEPTOR ALTERATIONS IN ALZHEIMER'S DISEASE

Peter J. Whitehouse

Neuropathology Laboratory, Departments of Neurology and Neuroscience, The Johns Hopkins University School of Medicine, 600 North Wolfe Street, Baltimore, MD 21205 USA

INTRODUCTION

Alzheimer's disease (AD) is characterized by degeneration of neurons in several neurotransmitter-specific systems (Price et al., in press; Whitehouse et al., in press b). Alterations in telencephalic presynaptic cholinergic markers, such as choline acetyltransferase (ChAT), have been most closely linked to the severity of clinically apparent dementia and to the density of senile plaques and neurofibrillary tangles (Blessed et al., 1968; Wilcock et al., 1982). The anatomical basis for the presynaptic cholinergic dysfunction in amygdala, hippocampus, and neocortex appears to be loss of neurons in the basal forebrain cholinergic system (Ch1-4 system) (Whitehouse et al., 1981; Whitehouse et al., 1982; Arendt et al., 1983; Candy et al., 1983; Tagliavini and Pilleri, 1983). This system is composed of neurons in the medial septum (Ch1), diagonal band of Broca (Ch2), and the nucleus basalis of Meynert (nbM) (Ch4) (Hedreen et al., 1983; Mesulam et al., 1983). A role for acetylcholine in dementia is supported by animal experiments in which anticholinergic drugs and anatomical lesions of the Ch1-4 system have been shown to produce memory dysfunction (Deutsch, 1971; Aigner et al., 1984; Olton et al., 1984). In this paper, I will review: our recent clinical studies of neuronal loss in this system in AD and related disorders; evidence for neuronal loss in other neural systems; studies of neurotransmitter receptor alterations in AD; and recent characterizations of cholinergic receptor alterations.

CH1-4 SYSTEM IN ALZHEIMER'S DISEASE AND RELATED DISORDERS

Our original reports (Whitehouse et al., 1981; Whitehouse et al., 1982) of neuronal loss occurring in the nbM (Ch4) in AD has been supported by several other groups (Arendt et al., 1983; Candy et al., 1983; Tagliavini and Pilleri, 1983). We have recently completed a study which confirms this finding in a larger sample of patients and which includes assessment of neurons in all components of the Ch1-4 system (Whitehouse et al., 1984a). Using our atlas of normal Ch1-4 anatomy (Hedreen et al., 1983), we selected five standard regions of the Ch1-4 system and counted neurons in 50 patients with AD, 10 patients with other dementias, and 20 age-matched controls. Statistically significant neuronal loss (54-76%) occurred throughout the entire extent of the Ch1-4 system in AD cases. At every level assessed, neuronal loss was more severe in younger (<70 years of age at death) AD cases than in older cases. To date, we have found no evidence of severe neuronal loss in brainstem cholinergic nuclei (Ch5-6) in AD (Mesulam et al., 1983; Zweig et al., submitted for presentation).

Although neuronal loss in the Ch1-4 system appears to be a consistent feature of AD, it is not specific for this condition. Dysfunction in this system also occurs in Parkinson's disease (Whitehouse et al., 1983a; Nakano and Hirano, 1984), Down's snydrome (Price et al., 1982; Casanova et al., in press b), dementia pugilistica (Uhl et al., 1983; Whitehouse et al., in press c), and several other rarer forms of dementia. Ch1-4 neuronal loss does not occur in all dementias, however, as we have also shown this system is intact in Huntington's disease (Clark et al., 1983b) and corticostriatospinal degeneration (Clark et al., 1983a). Whether neuronal dysfunction occurs in the Ch1-4 system in Pick's disease is controversial (Pilleri, 1966; Uhl et al., 1983).

The relationship between neuronal dysfunction in the Ch1-4 system and the formation of senile plaques and neurofibrillary tangles has been studied in several laboratories (Struble et al., 1982; Price et al., in press). We have shown that some senile plaques demonstrate acetylcholinesterase (AChE) activity (Struble et al., 1982) and ChAT-like immunoreactivity (Kitt et al., 1984b). Several other neurotransmitter system markers (including somatostatin, tyrosine hydroxylase, and substance P-like immunoreactivity [Struble et al., 1984; Powers et al., in press]) have also been shown to occur in senile plaques, emphasizing that AD is a multisystem disorder. Neurofibrillary tangles occur in high density in the Ch1-4 system, as well as in other affected brainstem and telencephalic neurons (Hirano and Zimmerman, 1962; Ishii, 1966; Price et al., in press).

OTHER NEUROTRANSMITTER SYSTEMS IN ALZHEIMER'S DISEASE

In AD, neuronal loss occurs in several telencephalic and brainstem regions. Neuronal loss in neocortex and hippocampus occurs consistently (Shefer, 1972; Colon, 1973; Ball, 1977; Terry et al., 1981; Hyman et al., 1984). We have not been able to confirm (Casanova et al., in press a) the specific pattern of hippocampal pathology noted by Hyman et al. (1984) which they claim results in disconnection of hippocampus from other regions of brain. The amygdala also demonstrates considerable neuronal loss and senile plaque formation, particularly in corticomedial nuclear groups (Hooper and Vogel, 1976; Corsellis, 1978; Herzog and Kemper, 1980).

In brainstem, reductions in neuronal density occurs in the noradrenergic locus coeruleus (Forno, 1978; Bondareff et al., 1982) and serotonergic raphe nuclei (Curcio and Kemper, 1984). Whether severe cell loss in these nuclei occurs in all cases or only in certain subtypes (Bondareff et al., 1982) is currently being studied.

CHOLINERGIC RECEPTORS IN ALZHEIMER'S DISEASE

Although reductions in presynaptic cholinergic markers and loss of neurons in the Ch1-4 system appear to be a consistent feature of AD, the nature of cholinergic neurotransmitter receptor alterations in this condition remains unclear. Using the drug ligands [^{3}H] quinuclidinyl benzilate (QNB) (Bowen et al., 1978; Davies and Verth, 1978), [^{3}H] N-methyl scopolamine (Perry et al., 1977), and [^{3}H] atropine (White et al., 1977), early studies showed no significant alterations in muscarinic cholinergic receptor density in frontal, parietal, and temporal cortices in hippocampus in AD when compared to controls. Recently, however, Rinne et al. (1984), using [^{3}H] QNB, showed a significant reduction of muscarinic receptors in the amygdala, nucleus accumbens, and hippocampus in brains of patients with AD. Reduction in hippocampal [^{3}H] QNB binding was also found by Reisine et al. (1978). Mash and Potter (1983) have recently claimed that muscarinic receptor densities are decreased in the cortex of patients with AD. They report that the loss primarily involves the M2 receptor, a subtype of muscarinic receptor characterized by high affinity for muscarinic agonists (such as carbachol) and low affinity for the antagonist pirenzepine (Hammer et al., 1980). Lesions of Ch4 neurons in rats produce a decrease in density of cortical M2 high-affinity agonist receptor which correlates with the magnitude of reduction in ChAT activity (McKinney and Coyle, 1982; Mash and Potter, 1983). However, Caulfied et al. (1983), using [^{3}H] pirenzepine to define M1 and M2 subtypes, found no difference in binding between AD and control subjects.

Although the existence of subtypes of muscarinic cholinergic receptors appears to be established, the terminology used to describe these subtypes needs to be clarified. The original distinction between M1 and M2 muscarinic receptors was made on the basis of affinity of the receptor for a novel muscarinic antagonist, pirenzepine. M1 receptors were defined as having high affinity for pirenzepine, whereas M2 had low affinity. Recently, however, the affinity of receptors for agonists has also been used to define subtypes (Whitehouse et al., 1981; Mash and Potter, 1983). Anatomical distributions of high-affinity agonists and low-affinity pirenzepine muscarinic subtypes are similar (Mash and Potter, 1983). In man, high-affinity agonists and low-affinity pirenzepine receptors appear to occur in areas enriched in cholinergic neurons such as the ventral horn of the spinal cord (Whitehouse et al., 1983b) and the Ch1-4 system (Whitehouse et al., 1984b). High-affinity pirenzepine and low-affinity agonist receptors predominate in cortex and other areas of telencephalon (Whitehouse et al., in press d). However, relationships between the subtypes of receptors defined by antagonist binding and agonist-binding affinities need to be studied further.

We have recently reported two studies of muscarinic cholinergic receptor subtypes in AD using *in vitro* receptor autoradiography (Young and Kuhar, 1979; Kuhar, 1985; Whitehouse, in press). The autoradiographic technique allows mapping neurotransmitter receptors with a higher degree of anatomical resolution than previously possible using homogenate techniques. [^{3}H] ligands are incubated with tissue sections rather than tissue homogenates to determine the pattern of binding to tissue. Preincubation, incubation, and wash conditions are chosen to maximize specific binding and to minimize the effects of endogenous ligands. The autoradiograph is produced by juxtaposing the labeled tissue to a piece of tritium-sensitive film or to an emulsion-coated coverslip.

In our first study, we mapped the distribution of high-affinity and low-affinity agonist muscarinic cholinergic subtypes in the amygdala in patients with AD and in age-matched controls (Whitehouse et al., 1984c). Although some reduction of total muscarinic cholinergic receptor density occurred in the amygdala, the greatest reduction in receptor density occurred in the high-affinity agonist subtype of muscarinic receptor in the basolateral and basomedial nuclei which receive dense innervation from the Ch1-4 system (Kitt et al., 1984a). This finding supports the claim that this high-affinity agonist subtype receptor may be the presynaptic muscarinic cholinergic receptor and is selectively affected in AD (Mash and Potter, 1983).

In a subsequent autoradiographic study of muscarinic cholinergic receptor subtypes in patients with AD, we also demonstrated that the density of high-affinity agonist presynaptic cholinergic subtype was selectively reduced in frontal cortex (Whitehouse et al., in press a). In this study, we also examined high- and low-affinity antagonist receptor subtypes using [^{3}H] pirenzepine to map the M1 receptors. We found no differences in M1 or M2 antagonist subtypes of receptors in AD when compared to age-matched controls.

Although a selective loss of the high-affinity agonist presynaptic muscarinic cholinergic receptor appears to occur in AD, some authors have reported evidence suggesting an up-regulation of total muscarinic cholinergic receptor binding, perhaps related to a compensatory denervation supersensitivity. London and Waller (in press) have reported finding increased QNB binding in several regions of cortex from patients with AD. In addition, a negative correlation between ChAT activity and muscarinic receptor densities has been taken as evidence for receptor up-regulation in the face of presynaptic dysfunction (Nordberg et al., 1983).

Although muscarinic cholinergic receptors are the predominant cholinergic receptor type in the central nervous system, some central cholinergic receptors have nicotinic pharmacological and physiological characteristics (Segal, 1978; Morley et al., 1979). Davies and Feisullin (1981) demonstrated a reduced density of alpha-bungarotoxin binding sites in the temporal cortices of patients with AD, although this finding has not been confirmed in an autoradiographic study (Lang and Henke, 1983). Alpha-bungarotoxin is not a good ligand to label nicotinic cholinergic receptor subtypes in the central nervous system, however, since it demonstrates different pharmacological properties in brain than at the neuromuscular junction (Morley et al., 1979). Recently, a novel method for labeling nicotinic cholinergic receptors in the central nervous system has been described using [^{3}H] acetylcholine with a selective displacer (atropine) to block binding of [^{3}H] acetylcholine to muscarinic sites (Schwartz et al., 1982). We have recently examined the density of muscarinic and nicotinic cholinergic receptors using [^{3}H] acetylcholine and [^{3}H] QNB in three regions of cortex from patients with AD and age-matched controls. We found no statistically significant alterations in [^{3}H] QNB or [^{3}H] acetylcholine muscarinic binding sites, although there was a trend for the AD cases to have somewhat higher concentrations of muscarinic cholinergic receptors. We did, however, find statistically significant reductions of nicotinic cholinergic receptors in all three cortical regions studied in the left hemisphere and also in right frontal cortex. Reductions in nicotinic cholinergic receptors showed the same anatomical distribution as reductions in ChAT activity measured in aliquots of the same cortical homogenates. In animal experiments, nicotinic cholinergic binding sites defined using [^{3}H] acetylcholine were shown to be unaffected by lesions in the cholinergic basal forebrain (Schwartz et al., 1984), suggesting that these nicotinic receptors may be located postsynaptically.

OTHER NEUROTRANSMITTER RECEPTOR CHANGES IN ALZHEIMER'S DISEASE

Subtypes of both serotonin and noradrenergic receptors have been studied in the brains of patients with AD. Alterations in these receptors bear an unclear relationship to dysfunction of neurons in the raphe nucleus and locus coeruleus. Serotonin receptors in the central nervous system have been classified into several types: S-1 receptors have a high affinity for serotonin; S-2 receptors have a lower affinity for serotonin but a higher affinity for the dopamine antagonist spiperone. Lysergic acid diethylamide (LSD) binds to both receptor types. Bowen et al.

(1983a) demonstrated a significant reduction in [^{3}H] LSD binding in temporal cortices and in [^{3}H] serotonin binding in frontal cortices of patients with AD. Cross et al. (1984b), using [^{3}H] LSD binding displaced by serotonin and spiperone, found a marked reduction of both S-1 and S-2 receptors in frontal and temporal cortices and hippocampus. In a more recent study using [^{3}H] serotonin and [^{3}H] ketanserin, Cross et al. (1984a) reported a reduction of S-1 receptors in the amygdala, hippocampus, and temporal cortex and a more extensive reduction of S-2 receptors in frontal, temporal, and cingulate cortices and amygdala. In this study, a greater reduction of [^{3}H] serotonin binding was found in AD patients with a younger age of onset consistent with other studies which reported more extensive dysfunction in monoaminergic cell groups in younger patients (Bondareff et al., 1982).

To date, the few postmortem studies of noradrenergic receptor densities in brains of patients with AD have not shown any significant alterations as compared to controls. Bowen et al. (1983b), measuring [^{3}H] dihydroalprenol (DHA) binding, found no significant changes in ß-adrenergic receptors in frontal and temporal cortices. In another study, Cross et al. (1984b), measuring [^{3}H]-WB4101, [^{3}H]-Rauwolscine, and [^{3}H] DHA binding, found no changes in alpha 1, alpha 2, and ß-receptor densities, respectively, in hippocampus and occipital cortex.

In some studies, presynaptic markers for GABAergic neurons, such as the activity of glutamic acid decarboxylase, have been found to be reduced in patients with AD (Bowen et al., 1974; Perry et al., 1977). Using [^{3}H] GABA, Reisine et al. (1978) reported a marked reduction in GABA receptors in the caudate nucleus and frontal cortex but found no significant difference in the putamen and hippocampus in AD. In two other studies, however, [^{3}H] muscimol binding was found to be unaltered in temporal and occipital cortices (Bowen et al., 1979; Bowen et al., 1983b). Muscimol is a GABA agonist which binds to a subpopulation of high-affinity GABA receptors.

Dopaminergic receptor density measured by [^{3}H] spiroperidol was found to be reduced in the caudate nucleus in AD but unaltered in the frontal cortex, hippocampus, and putamen (Reisine et al., 1978). Opiate receptor densities, using [^{3}H] naloxone, were also found to be unchanged in the temporal lobe of patients with AD (Bowen et al., 1979).

CONCLUSION

Dysfunction in the basal forebrain cholinergic system is a consistent feature of AD and related disorders. In AD, attempts at therapy designed to enhance cholinergic dysfunction have met with limited success. These attempts have usually employed either precursor loading strategies with lethicin or choline or anticholinesterase inhibitors, such as physostigmine. Part of the explanation for failure of these cholinergic therapies undoubtedly lies in AD being a disorder which affects multiple neurotransmitter systems. Nevertheless, improved understanding of cholinergic neurotransmitter receptor alterations in AD may permit the development of more effective therapies to enhance cholinergic function. For example, if presynaptic high-affinity agonist muscarinic subtypes of receptors are inhibitory, selective M1 postsynaptic agonists or M2 antagonists may be more effective in improving memory function. Finally, the possibility of drugs active at central nicotinic sites should be considered, since nicotinic receptors also appear to be affected in this condition.

ACKNOWLEDGEMENTS

The contributions of the following individuals for the ideas and work reported in this paper are gratefully acknowledged: Drs. Manuel F. Casanova, Linda C. Cork, Joseph T. Coyle, John C. Hedreen, Kenneth J. Kellar, Cheryl A. Kitt, Michael J. Kuhar, Andrea M. Martino, Richard E. Powers, Donald L. Price, Robert G. Struble, and Richard M. Zweig. The assistance of Mrs. Carla R. Jordon in preparation of the manuscript is greatly appreciated.

REFERANCES

Aigner, T., Mitchell, S., Aggleton, J., DeLong, M., Struble, R., Price, D., and Mishkin, M., 1984, Effects of scopolamine and physostigmine on recognition memory in monkeys after ibotenic acid injections into the area of the nucleus basalis of Meynert, in: "Alzheimer's Disease: Advances in Basic Research and Therapies. Proceedings of the Third Meeting of the International Study Group on the Treatment of Memory Disorders Associated with Aging," R. J. Wurtman, S. H. Corkin, and J. H. Growdon, eds., Zurich, p. 429.

Arendt, T., Bigl, V., Arendt, A., and Tennstedt, A., 1983, Loss of neurons in the nucleus basalis of Meynert in Alzheimer's disease, paralysis agitans, and Korsakoff's disease, Acta Neuropathol., 61:101-108.

Ball, M. J., 1977, Neuronal loss, neurofibrillary tangles and granulovacuolar degeneration in the hippocampus with ageing and dementia. A qualitative study, Acta Neuropathol., 37:111-118.

Blessed, G., Tomlinson, B. E., and Roth, M., 1968, The association between quantitative measures of dementia and of senile change in the cerebral grey matter of elderly subjects, Br. J. Psychiatry, 114:797-811.

Bondareff, W., Mountjoy, C. Q., and Roth, M., 1982, Loss of neurons or origin of the adrenergic projection to cerebral cortex (nucleus locus ceruleus) in senile dementia, Neurology, 32:164-168.

Bowen, D. M., and Davison, A. N., 1978, Changes in brain lysosomal activity, neurotransmitter-related enzymes, and other proteins in senile dementia, in: "Alzheimer's Disease: Senile Dementia and Related Disorders" (Aging, Vol. 7), R. Katzman, R. D. Terry, and K. L. Bick, eds., Raven Press, New York, pp. 421-424.

Bowen, D. M., Allen, S. J., Benton, J. S., Goodhardt, M. J., Haan, E. A., Palmer, A. M., Sims, N. R., Smith, C. C. T., Spillane, J. A., Esiri, M. M., Neary, D., Snowdon, J. S., Wilcock, G. K., and Davison, A. N., 1983a, Biochemical assessment of serotonergic and cholinergic dysfunction and cerebral atrophy in Alzheimer's disease, J. Neurochem., 41:266-272.

Bowen, D. M., Davison, A. N., and Sims, N. R., 1983b, The cholinergic system in the ageing brain and dementia, in: "Aging of the Brain" (Aging, Vol. 22), D. Samuel, S. Algeri, S. Gershon, V. E. Grimm, and G. Toffano, eds., Raven Press, New York, pp. 183-190.

Bowen, D. M., Flack, R. H. A., White, P., Smith, C. B., and Davison, A. N., 1974, Brain-decarboxylase activities as indices of pathological change in senile dementia, Lancet, __:1247-1249.

Bowen, D. M., Spillane, J. A., Curzon, G., Meier-Ruge, W., White, P., Goodhardt, M. J., Iwangoff, P., and Davison, A. N., 1979, Accelerated ageing or selective neuronal loss as an important cause of dementia?, Lancet, 1:11-14.

Candy, J. M., Perry, R. H., Perry, E. K., Irving, D., Blessed, G., Fairbairn, A. F., and Tomlinson, B. E., 1983, Pathological changes in the nucleus of Meynert in Alzheimer's and Parkinson's diseases, J. Neurol. Sci., 59:277-289.

Casanova, M. F., Struble, R. G., Glaser, E. M., Powers, R. E., Whitehouse, P. J., Tagamets, M., and Price, D. L., in press a, Distribution of plaques and tangles in the hippocampi of patients with Alzheimer's disease, Neurology.

Casanova, M. F., Walker, L. C., Whitehouse, P. J., and Price, D. L., in press b, Abnormalities of the nucleus basalis in Down's syndrome, Ann. Neurol.

Caulfield, M. P., Higgins, G. A., and Straughan, D. W., 1983, Central administration of the muscarinic receptor subtype -- selective antagonist pirenzepine selectively impairs passive avoidance learning in the mouse, J. Pharm. Pharmacol., 35:131-132.

Clark, A. W., Lehmann, J., Whitehouse, P. J., Struble, R. G., Coyle, J. T., and Price, D. L., 1983a, Cortico-striato-spinal degeneration (CSSD) mimicking Alzheimer's disease (AD): studies of the nucleus basalis of Meynert (nbM) and cortical choline acetyltransferase (CAT), J. Neuropathol. Exp. Neurol., 42:334.

Clark, A. W., Parhad, I. M., Folstein, S. E., Whitehouse, P. J., Hedreen, J. C., Price, D. L., and Chase, G. A., 1983b, The nucleus basalis in Huntington's disease, Neurology, 33:1262-1267.

Colon, E. J., 1973, The cerebral cortex in presenil dementia. A quantitative analysis, Acta Neuropathol., 23:281-290.

Corsellis, J. A. N., 1978, Posttraumatic dementia, in: "Alzheimer's Disease: Senile Dementia and Related Disorders" (Aging, Vol. 7), R. Katzman, R. D. Terry, and K. L. Bick, eds., Raven Press, New York, pp. 125-133.

Cross, A. J., Crow, T. J., Ferrier, I. N., Johnson, J. A., Bloom, S. R., and Corsellis, J. A. N., 1984a, Serotonin receptor changes in dementia of the Alzheimer type, J. Neurochem., 43:1574-1581.

Cross, A. J., Crow, T. J., Johnson, J. A., Perry, E. K., Perry, R. H., Blessed, G., and Tomlinson, B. E., 1984b, Studies on neurotransmitter receptor systems in neocortex and hippocampus in senile dementia of the Alzheimer-type, J. Neurol. Sci., 64:109-117.

Curcio, C. A., and Kemper, T., 1984, Nucleus raphe dorsalis in dementia of the Alzheimer type: neurofibrillary changes and neuronal packing density, J. Neuropathol. Exp. Neurol., 43:359-368.

Davies, P., and Feisullin, S., 1981, Postmortem stability of alpha-bungarotoxin binding sites in mouse and human brain, Brain Res., 216:449-454.

Davies, P., and Verth, A. H., 1978, Regional distribution of muscarinic acetylcholine receptor in normal and Alzheimer's-type dementia brains, Brain Res., 138:385-392.

Deutsch, J. A., 1971, The cholinergic synapse and the site of memory, Science, 174:788-794.

Forno, L. S., 1978, The locus caeruleus in Alzheimer's disease, J. Neuropathol. Exp. Neurol., 37:614.

Hammer, R., Berrie, C. P., Birdsall, N. J. M., Burgen, A. S. V., and Hulme, E. C., 1980, Pirenzepine distinguishes between different subclasses of muscarinic receptors, Nature, 283:90-92.

Hedreen, J. C., Bacon, S. J., Cork, L. C., Kitt, C. A., Crawford, G. D., Salvaterra, P. M., and Price, D. L., 1983, Immunocytochemical identification of cholinergic neurons in the monkey central nervous system using monoclonal antibodies against choline acetyltransferase, Neurosci. Lett., 43:173-177.

Herzog, A. G., and Kemper, T. L., 1980, Amygdaloid changes in aging and dementia, Arch. Neurol., 37:625-629.

Hirano, A., and Zimmerman, H. M., 1962, Alzheimer's neurofibrillary changes. A topographic study, Arch. Neurol., 7:227-242.

Hooper, M. W., and Vogel, F. S., 1976, The limbic system in Alzheimer's disease. A neuropathologic investigation, Am. J. Pathol., 85:1-20.

Hyman, B. T., Van Hoesen, G. W., Damasio, A. R., and Barnes, C. L., 1984, Alzheimer's disease: cell-specific pathology isolates the hippocampal formation, Science, 225:1168-1170.

Ishii, T., 1966, Distribution of Alzheimer's neurofibrillary changes in the brain stem and hypothalamus of senile dementia, Acta Neuropathol., 6:181-187.

Kitt, C. A., Mobley, W. C., Struble, R. G., Cork, L. C., Hedreen, J. C., Wainer, B. H., and Price, D. L., 1984a, Evidence for cholinergic processes in neuritic plaques of aged primates, Neurology, 34:121.

Kitt, C. A., Price, D. L., Struble, R. G., Cork, L. C., Wainer, B. H., Becher, M. W., and Mobley, W. C., 1984b, Evidence for cholinergic neurites in senile plaques, Science, 226:1443-1445.

Kuhar, M. J., 1985, Receptor localization with the microscope, in: "Neurotransmitter Receptor Binding", 2nd edition, H. I. Yamamura, S. J. Enna, and M. J. Kuhar, eds., Raven Press, New York, pp. 153-176.

Lang, W., and Henke, H., 1983, Cholinergic receptor binding and autoradiography in brains of non-neurological and senile dementia of Alzheimer-type patients, Brain Res., 267:271-280.

London, E. D., and Waller, S. B., in press, Relations between choline acetyltransferase and muscarinic binding in aging and Alzheimer's disease, in: "Dynamics of Cholinergic Function," I. Hanin, ed., Plenum Press, New York.

Mash, D. S., and Potter, L. T., 1983, Changes in M1 and M2 muscarine receptors in Alzheimer's disease and aging, and with lesions of cholinergic neurons in animals, Soc. Neurosci. Abstr., 9:582.

McKinney, M., and Coyle, J. T., 1982, Regulation of neocortical muscarinic receptors: effects of drug treatment and lesions, J. Neurosci., 2:97-105.

Mesulam, M-M., Mufson, E. J., Levey, A. I., and Wainer, B. H., 1983, Cholinergic innervation of cortex by the basal forebrain: cytochemistry and cortical connections of the septal area, diagonal band nuclei, nucleus basalis (substantia innominata), and hypothalamus in the rhesus monkey, J. Comp. Neurol., 214:170-197.

Morley, B. J., Kemp, G. E., and Salvaterra, P., 1979, Alpha-bungarotoxin binding sites in the CNS, Life Sci., 24:859-872.

Nakano, I., and Hirano, A., 1984, Parkinson's disease: neuron loss in the nucleus basalis without concomitant Alzheimer's disease, Ann. Neurol., 15:415-418.

Nordberg, A., Larsson, C., Adolfsson, R., Alafuzoff, I., and Winblad, B., 1983, Muscarinic receptor compensation in hippocampus of Alzheimer patients, J. Neural Transm., 56:13-19.

Olton, D. S., Hepler, D., Wenk, G., Lehman, J., and Coyle, J., 1984, Lesions of the nucleus basalis magnocellularis and medial septal area in rats produce similar memory impairments, in: "Alzheimer's Disease: Advances in Basic Research and Therapies. Proceedings of the Third Meeting of the International Study Group on the Treatment of Memory Disorders Associated with Aging," R. J. Wurtman, S. H. Corkin, and J. H. Growdon, eds., Zurich, pp. 461.

Perry, E. K., Gibson, P. H., Blessed, G., Perry, R. H., and Tomlinson, B. E., 1977, Neurotransmitter enzyme abnormalities in senile dementia, J. Neurol. Sci., 34:247-265.

Pilleri, G., 1966, The Kluver-Bucy syndrome in man. A clinico-anatomical contribution to the function of the medial temporal lobe structures, Psychiatr. Neurol., 152:65-103.

Powers, R. E., Struble, R. G., Casanova, M. F., Kitt, C. A., O'Connor, D. T., and Price, D. L., in press, Immunocytochemical localization of putative neurotransmitter substances in human hippocampus, J. Neuropathol. Exp. Neurol.

Price, D. L., Whitehouse, P. J., and Struble, R. G., in press, Cellular pathology in Alzheimer's and Parkinson's diseases, Trends Neurosci.

Price, D. L., Whitehouse, P. J., Struble, R. G., Coyle, J. T., Clark, A. W., DeLong, M. R., Cork, L. C., and Hedreen, J. C., 1982, Alzheimer's disease and Down's syndrome, Ann. N. Y. Acad. Sci., 396:145-164.

Reisine, T. D., Yamamura, H. I., Bird, E. D., Spokes, E., and Enna, S. J., 1978, Pre- and postsynaptic neurochemical alterations in Alzheimer's disease, Brain Res., 159:477-481.

Rinne, J. O., Rinne, J. K., Laakso, K., Paijarvi, -.-., and Rinne, U. K., 1984, Reduction in muscarinic receptor binding in limbic areas of Alzheimer brain, J. Neurol. Neurosurg. Psychiatry, 47:651-653.

Schwartz, R. D., Lehmann, J., and Kellar, K. J., 1984, Presynaptic nicotinic cholinergic receptors labeled by [^{3}H]acetylcholine on catecholamine and serotonin axons in brain, J. Neurochem., 42:1495-1498.

Schwartz, R. D., McGee, R., Jr., and Kellar, K. J., 1982, Nicotinic cholinergic receptors labeled by [^{3}H]acetylcholine in rat brain, Mol. Pharmacol., 22:56-62.

Segal, M., 1978, The acetylcholine receptor in the rat hippocampus: nicotinic, muscarinic or both?, Neuropharmacology, 17:619-623.

Shefer, V. F., 1972, Absolute number of neurons and thickness of the cerebral cortex during aging, senile and vascular dementia, and Pick's and Alzheimer's diseases, Zh. Neuropatol. Psikhiatr., 72:1024-1029.

Struble, R. G., Cork, L. C., Whitehouse, P. J., and Price, D. L., 1982, Cholinergic innervation in neuritic plaques, Science, 216:413-415.

Struble, R. G., Kitt, C. A., Walker, L. C., Cork, L. C., and Price, D. L., 1984, Somatostatinergic neurites in senile plaques of aged non-human primates, Brain Res., 324:394-396.

Tagliavini, F., and Pilleri, G., 1983, Neuronal counts in basal nucleus of Meynert in Alzheimer disease and in simple senile dementia, Lancet, 1:469-470.

Terry, R. D., Peck, A., DeTeresa, R., Schechter, R., and Horoupian, D. S., 1981, Some morphometric aspects of the brain in senile dementia of the Alzheimer type, Ann. Neurol., 10:184-192.

Uhl, G. R., Hilt, D. C., Hedreen, J. C., Whitehouse, P. J., and Price, D. L., 1983, Pick's disease (lobar sclerosis): depletion of neurons in the nucleus basalis of Meynert, Neurology, 33:1470-1473.

Uhl, G. R., McKinney, M., Hedreen, J. C., White, C. L., III, Coyle, J. T., Whitehouse, P. J., and Price, D. L., 1982, Dementia pugilistica: loss of basal forebrain cholinergic neurons and cortical cholinergic markers, Ann. Neurol., 12:99.

Unnerstall, J. R., Kuhar, M. J., Niehoff, D. L., and Palacios, J. M., 1981, Benzodiazepine receptors are coupled to a subpopulation of gamma-aminobutyric acid (GABA) receptors: evidence from a quantitative autoradiographic study, J. Pharmacol. Exp. Ther., 218:797-804.

White, P., Goodhardt, M. J., Keet, J. P., Hiley, C. R., Carrasco, L. H., Williams, I. E. I., and Bowen, D. M., 1977, Neocortical cholinergic neurons in elderly people, Lancet, 1:668-670.

Whitehouse, P. J., in press, Receptor autoradiography: applications in neuropathology, Trends Neurosci.

Whitehouse, P. J., Hedreen, J. C., Clark, A. W., Zweig, R. M., Jones, B. E., Terry, R. D., Antuono, P. G., Coyle, J. T., Davies, P. F., and Price, D. L., 1984a, Clinical and neurochemical correlates of neuronal loss in the cholinergic basal forebrain system in Alzheimer's disease, Soc. Neurosci. Abstr., 10:290.

Whitehouse, P. J., Hedreen, J. C., White, C. L., III, and Price, D. L., 1983a, Basal forebrain neurons in the dementia of Parkinson disease, Ann. Neurol., 13:243-248.

Whitehouse, P. J., Jones, B. E., Kopajtic, T. A., Price, D. L., and Kuhar, M. J., 1984b, Receptors in the nucleus basalis of primates: an *in vitro* autoradiographic study, Ann. Neurol., 16:118.

Whitehouse, P. J., Kopajtic, T., Jones, B. E., Kuhar, M. J., and Price, D. L., in press a, An in vitro receptor autoradiographic study of muscarinic cholinergic receptor subtypes in the amygdala and neocortex of patients with Alzheimer's disease, Neurology.

Whitehouse, P. J., Price, D. L., Clark, A. W., Coyle, J. T., and DeLong, M. R., 1981, Alzheimer disease: evidence for selective loss of cholinergic neurons in the nucleus basalis, Ann. Neurol., 10:122-126.

Whitehouse, P. J., Price, D. L., Struble, R. G., Clark, A. W., Coyle, J. T., and DeLong, M. R., 1982, Alzheimer's disease and senile dementia: loss of neurons in the basal forebrain, Science, 215:1237-1239.

Whitehouse, P. J., Rajagopalan, R., Kitt, C. A., Jones, B. E., Niehoff, D. L., Kuhar, M. J., and Price, D. L., 1984c, Muscarinic cholinergic receptors in the amygdala in Alzheimer's disease, Neurology, 34:121.

Whitehouse, P. J., Struble, R. G., Hedreen, J. C., Clark, A. W., and Price, D. L., in press b, Alzheimer's disease and related dementias: selective involvement of specific neuronal systems, C.R.C. Press.

Whitehouse, P. J., Struble, R. G., Uhl, G. R., and Price, D. L., in press c, Dementia: bridging brain and behavior, in: "Proceedings of the Norman Rockwell Conference on Alzheimer's Disease," J. T. Hutton, and A. D. Kenny, eds., Alan R. Liss, Inc., New York.

Whitehouse, P. J., Trifiletti, R. R., Jones, B. E., Folstein, S., Price, D. L., Snyder, S. H., and Kuhar, M. J., in press d, Neurotransmitter receptor alterations in Huntington's disease: autoradiographic and homogenate studies with special reference to benzodiazepine receptor complexes, Ann. Neurol.

Whitehouse, P. J., Wamsley, J. K., Zarbin, M. A., Price, D. L., Tourtellotte, W. W., and Kuhar, M. J., 1983b, Amyotrophic lateral sclerosis: alterations in neurotransmitter receptors, Ann. Neurol., 14:8-16.

Wilcock, G. K., Esiri, M. M., Bowen, D. M., and Smith, C. C. T., 1982, Alzheimer's disease. Correlation of cortical choline acetyltransferase activity with the severity of dementia and histological abnormalities, J. Neurol. Sci., 57:407-417.

Young, W. S., III, and Kuhar, M. J., 1979, Autoradiography of opiate and benzodiazepine receptors: in vitro labeling of tissue sections, Fed. Proc., 38:687.

Zweig, R. M., Whitehouse, P. J., Casanova, M. F., Walker, L. C., Jankel, W. R., and Price, D. L., 1985, Loss of putative cholinergic neurons of the pedunculopontine nucleus in progressive supranuclear palsy. Submitted for presentation at the 1985 meeting of the American Neurological Association.

BRAIN NICOTINIC AND MUSCARINIC RECEPTORS IN NORMAL AGING AND DEMENTIA

Agneta Nordberg and Bengt Winblad*

Department of Pharmacology
University of Uppsala
Box 591
S-751 23 Uppsala, and

*Department of Geriatric Medicine
University of Umea
S-901 87 Umea
Sweden

INTRODUCTION

The cholinergic receptors are classically divided into two kinds, namely the nicotinic acetylcholine receptor and the muscarinic acetylcholine receptor. The existence of these receptor types in the peripheral nervous system is well established. This is true also for the muscarinic receptors in the CNS. Attempts to study and characterize nicotinic receptors in brain have been initiated recently. Data on muscarinic receptors in the literature indicate similarities between rodent and human brain concerning number of binding sites and sub-populations (Birdsall et al., 1978; Nordberg and Winblad, 1981; Unden et al., 1983; Garrey et al., 1984). A comparison between fresh surgical and frozen autopsy samples (Unden et al, 1983) showed no difference in binding data, while Whitehouse et al. (1984), using a rat model of the human autopsy process, observed a significant decrease (18%) in Bmax after 48 h at room temperature. The muscarinic receptors seem to be more stable post mortem than the activity of choline acetyltransferase (ChAT) (Perry and Perry, 1980).

Four different nicotinic ligands have been used hitherto to characterize nicotinic receptors in the brain, namely α-bungarotoxin (Btx) (Morley and Kemp, 1981), tubocurarine (TC) (Larsson and Nordberg, 1980), nicotine (NIC) (Larsson and Nordberg, 1985) and acetylcholine (ACh) (Schwartz et al., 1982). The findings indicate a complex pattern of subpopulations of nicotinic binding sites (Larsson and Nordberg, 1985). Few reports on nicotinic receptors in human brain are available. In these studies the ligands Btx (Volpe et al., 1979; Davies and Feisullin, 1981; Nordberg et al., 1982 a, b; Lang and Henke, 1983), tubocurarine (Nordberg and Winblad, 1981 ; Nordberg et al., 1982 a, b), nicotine (Nordberg et al., 1985 a) and ACh (Larsson et al., 1985) have been used. In table 1 a comparison is made between the binding of nicotinic ligands to different brain regions of mouse and human brain obtained in our laboratory. As can be noticed a general lower number of binding sites was obtained for

^{3}H-nicotine and ^{3}H-ACh (in the presence of atropine) in human than in mouse brain. For ^{3}H-tubocurarine and ^{3}H-Btx the differences were less pronounced. Davies and Feisullin (1981) reported a 25-30% lower content of Btx sites in human cortex than in mouse brain. This is in agreement with our findings in the hippocampus (table 1). It is possible that some of the differences noted between species might be due to the postmortem delay. While in rodent brain a regional distribution of ^{3}H-nicotine binding sites was found with the highest content of ^{3}H-nicotine in the cerebral cortex (Larsson and Nordberg, 1985), the ^{3}H-nicotine binding in human brain is more even (table 1).

Table 1. Specific binding of ^{3}H-ACh (10nM), ^{3}H-NIC (20nM), ^{3}H-Btx (1.5nM) and ^{3}H-TC (3nM) to cortex and hippocampus of mouse and human brain.

	CORTEX pmol/g protein		HIPPOCAMPUS pmol/g protein			CAUDATE NUCLEUS pmol/g protein
	^{3}H-ACh	^{3}H-NIC	^{3}H-NIC	^{3}H-Btx	^{3}H-TC	^{3}H-NIC
MOUSE	16±1	110±23	41±7	9.6±0.3	90±9	68±10
	(n=5)	(n=5)	(n=5)	(n=3)	(n=3)	(n=5)
HUMAN	3.1±0.5	15±5	21±3	7.0±1.0	147±10	27±4
	(n=4)	(n=5)	(n=15)	(n=10)	(n=10)	(n=5)

Mv ± SE
n = number of individuals
Data from Larsson and Nordberg, 1985
Larsson et al, 1985
Nordberg et al., 1982 a
Nordberg et al., 1985 a, b

CHOLINERGIC RECEPTORS IN HUMAN BRAIN DURING NURMAL AGING

The muscarinic receptors have been reported to be both decreased and unchanged in number with age (table 2). In most studies the material were obtained from individuals over 50 years, excluding younger individuals. As seen in figure 1 a significant decrease in number of muscarinic receptors with age was found when hippocampus from 44 individuals (0-100 years) were analysed. In the hippocampus, a similar decrease with age was found from the nicotinic receptors (^{3}H-tubocurarine binding): no change in ^{3}H-Btx binding and a significant increase in ^{3}H-NIC binding with age could be demonstrated (see table 3). For the nicotinic receptors these findings might indicate different age influence on nicotine receptor subpopulations.

Although thalamus is a main link for different neurotransmitter pathways projecting to and from cortex, little is known about the cholinergic pathways to the thalamus. From immunochemical studies thalamus appears to receive afferents from the reticular formation while no intrinsic cholinergic cells have been detected (Cuello and Sofroniew, 1984). Due to these facts normal and pathological aging processes might affect thalamus in a way different to other structures. When looking at the influence of age (60-90 years) on muscarinic and nicotinic receptors in the thalamus (fig. 2) we obtained a picture different from that seen

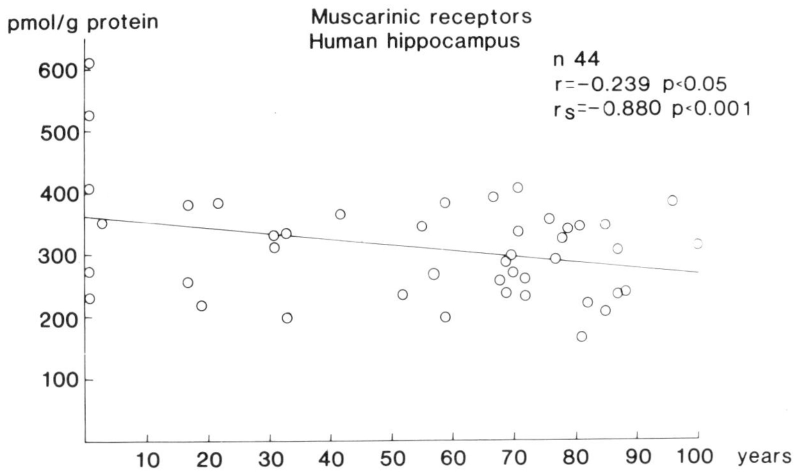

Fig. 1. Number of muscarinic binding sites (^{3}H-QNB) in human hippocampus from 44 controls (age span 0-100 years) with no psychiatric or neurological disease. The linear regression coefficient (r) and Spearman rank correlation coefficient (r_s) indicate a significant decrease in ^{3}H-QNB sites with age.

in the hippocampus. Thus, the number of nicotinic binding sites (^{3}H-Btx) decreased with age while that of muscarinic (^{3}H-QNB) binding sites significantly increased (fig. 2). The natural cell loss with age must in the case of the muscarinic receptors in the thalamus be well compensated by an upregulation of the receptors on target cells.

CHOLINERGIC RECEPTORS IN HUMAN BRAIN IN ALZHEIMER'S DISEASE AND MULTI-INFARCT DEMENTIA

A consistent finding in the literature concerning senile dementia of Alzheimer type (SDAT) has been a significant decrease in choline acetyltransferase (ChAT) activity in brain (for review see Bartus et al., 1982). The reported loss varies considerably between research groups, which might be due to different selection criteria for the patients. As seen in table 2 the loss in ChAT activity does not appear to be mirrored by losses in postsynaptic muscarinic and nicotinic receptor binding sites. As Alzheimer's Disease is a primary degenerative disorder it is surprising that the number of cholinergic binding sites is unchanged. An explanation put forward to this is an ongoing receptor-compensation (Nordberg et al., 1983). When studying the influence of age on different cholinergic receptors we observed (see above) different significant effects, for example a significant decrease of ^{3}H-QNB binding in the hippocampus but a significant increase in the thalamus. These age effects are not so obvious in Alzheimer's disease and are lost in multi-infarct dementia (MID). These data are schematically summarized in table 3.

Table 2. Cholinergic receptors in human brain at normal aging and different dementia conditions.

1. MUSCARINIC RECEPTORS

A. Normal aging	age	change	reference
Frontal cortex	65-93 ys	decrease	White et al., 1977
19 brain regions	46-79 ys	no change	Davies and Verth, 1978
Cerebral cortex	61-92 ys	decrease	Perry, 1980
Hippocampus	0-87 ys	decrease	Nordberg et al., 1982a
Temporal lobe, caudate nucleus	50-90 ys	no change	Allen et al., 1983
B. SDAT			
Cerebral cortex caudate nucleus	71.7±3.9 ys	no change	Perry et al., 1977
19 regions	53-75 ys	no change	Davies and Verth, 1978
Caudate nucleus putamen, frontal cortex	59-79 ys	no change	Reisine et al., 1978
Hippocampus		decrease	
Temporal lobe	71-89 ys	no change	Bowen et al., 1979
Temporal cortex		no change	Perry, 1980
Hippocampus	67-85 ys	no change	Nordberg et al., 1980
Hippocampus (autoradiography)	82±6 ys	no change	Palacios, 1982
Frontal cortex Temporal cortex Hippocampus gyrus cinguli (autoradio-graphy)	62-93 ys	no change 3/7 diffuse labelling throughout cortex	Lang & Henke, 1983
Hippocampus	76-93 ys	receptor compensation	Nordberg et al., 1983
Hippocampus Amygdala Accumbens	79±1 ys	decrease	Rinne et al., 1984
Caudate nucleus Putamen Pallidum Frontal cortex		no change	
5 regions	76-100 ys	no change	Jenni-Eiermann et al., 1984
Cortex		increase	London and Waller (personal communication)
Frontal cortex	56-89 ys	6/11 decrease	Wood et al., 1983

C. MID			
Cerebral cortex	74±2.3 ys	no change	Perry et al., 1977
Caudate nucleus			
Frontal cortex	83±9 ys	no change	White et al., 1977
Hippocampus	67-90 ys	decrease	Nordberg et al., 1982a
Temporal lobe	81-102 ys	decrease	Jenni-Eiermann et al.,1984
D. Pick's disease			
Temporal lobe	63; 68 ys	decrease	White et al., 1977
Cortex		decrease	Yates et al., 1980
Frontal cortex	61-83 ys	no change	Wood et al., 1983
Alcohol dementia			
Hippocampus Caudate nucleus	52.8±4.3	decrease no change	Nordberg et al., 1980
4 regions		no change	Antuono et al., 1980
Hippocampus	29-58 ys 59-68 ys	no change decrease	Nordberg et al., 1982b
Parkinson dementia			
Frontal cortex	73±2 ys	increase	Dubois et al., 1983
2. NICOTINIC RECEPTORS			
A. Normal aging			
Tubocurarine			
Hippocampus	57-87 ys	decrease	Nordberg et al., 1982a
B. SDAT			
α-bungarotoxin			
Midtemporal gyrus	49-96 ys	decrease	Davies and Feisullin, 1981
Frontal cortex		no change	
Hippocampus	65-85 ys	no change	Nordberg et al., 1982a
4 regions (autoradiography)	62-93 ys	no change	Lang and Henke, 1983
Tubocurarine			
Hippocampus	65-85 ys	no change	Nordberg et al., 1982a
C. MID			
α-bungarotoxin, tubocurarine			
Hippocampus	65-85 ys	no change	Nordberg et al., 1982a
D. Alcohol dementia			
α-bungarotoxin, tubocurarine			
Hippocampus	29-68 ys	no change	Nordberg et al., 1982b

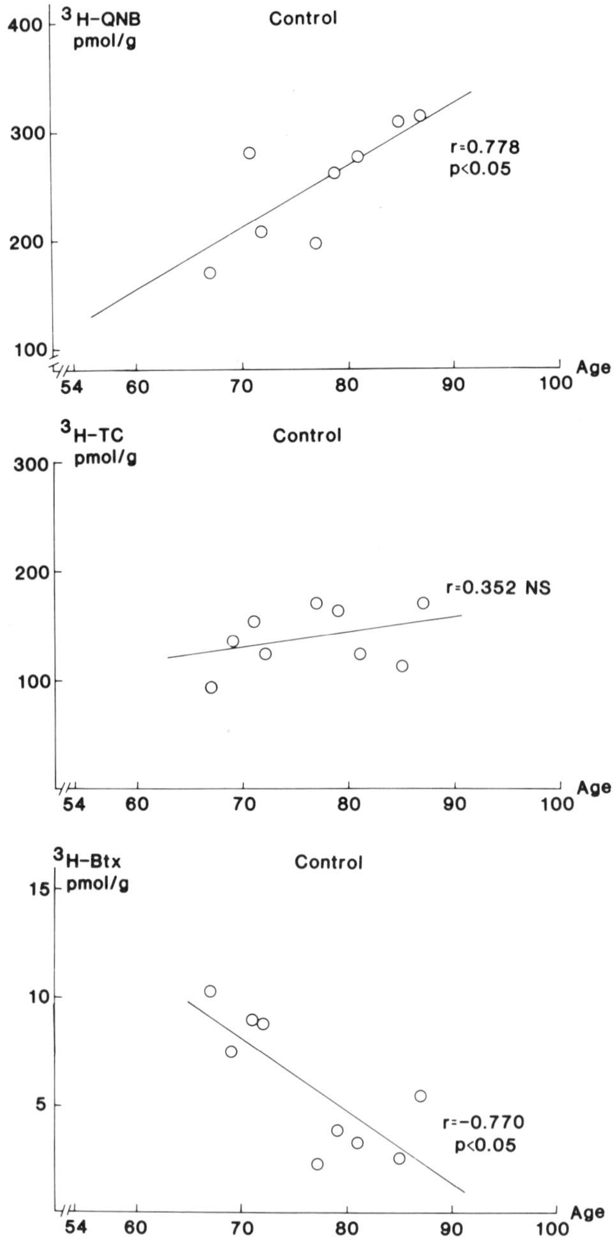

Fig. 2. Number of muscarinic (^{3}H-QNB) and nicotinic (^{3}H-Btx) binding sites in human thalamus from 9 controls (age span 65-90 years) with no psychiatric or neurological disease. Linear regression coefficients (r) indicate a significant positive regression line for ^{3}H-QNB, but a significant negative regression line for ^{3}H-Btx.

Table 3. Change in ^{3}H-QNB, ^{3}H-Btx, ^{3}H-Tubocurarine, ^{3}H-Nicotine binding with age in normal aging, SDAT and MID.

	THALAMUS			HIPPOCAMPUS			
	^{3}H-QNB	^{3}H-TC	^{3}H-Btx	^{3}H-QNB	^{3}H-TC	^{3}H-Btx	^{3}H-NIC
Control	↑*	→	↓*	↓*	↓*	→	↑*
SDAT	↓	→	↓	↓	→	→	
MID	→	→	→	→	→	→	

* $p < 0.05$

The clinical differentiation of multi-infarct dementia from Alzheimer's Disease is easily made in typical cases but is difficult and often impossible in other cases unless there is a typical history with cerebrovascular incidents (Kohlmeyer, 1982). One explanation for this might be that 15-25% of demented patients show clinical signs of both multi-infarct dementia and Alzheimer's disease (Hutton, 1980; Reisberg and Ferris, 1982). As seen in table 4 we found a marked decrease in ChAT activity in the hippocampus both in Alzheimer's disease and multi-infarct dementia. No significant change in ChAT activity was observed in the thalamus. In multi-infarct dementia (MID) there was a significant decrease in number of muscarinic binding sites in the hippocampus (table 5). A similar decrease was observed by Eiermann et al (1984) in the temporal

Table 4. Choline acetyltransferase activity (ChAT) in the hippocampus and thalamus of control, SDAT and MID brains.

	HIPPOCAMPUS nkatal/g tissue	THALAMUS nkatal/g tissue
Control	1.55±0.10 n=11	1.50±0.26 n=9
SDAT	0.74±0.12*** n=9	1.49±0.34 n=9
MID	0.81±0.13*** n=12	1.07±0.26 n=13

*** $p < 0.001$ compared with control

n = number of individuals

Mv ± SE

Table 5. Muscarinic (^{3}H-QNB) and nicotinic (^{3}H-TC, ^{3}H-Btx) binding sites in the hippocampus and thalamus of control, SDAT and MID brains.

Brain region	HIPPOCAMPUS			THALAMUS		
Ligand	^{3}H-QNB	^{3}H-TC	^{3}H-Btx	^{3}H-QNB	^{3}H-TC	^{3}H-Btx
Control	305±18 n=13	145±11 n=9	7.8±1.0 n=9	243±16 n=10	136±9 n=10	5.9±1.0 n=9
SDAT	294±13 n=8	154±9 n=8	8.8±0.8 n=8	251±20 n=8	151±15 n=8	9.2±1.1* n=8
MID	252±13* n=13	155±20 n=13	7.3±0.5 n=13	226±10 n=13	164±12 n=13	8.1±0.9 n=13

* $p < 0.05$ compared with control

n = number of individuals

Mv ± SE

cortex (table 2). No change has been reported in other cortical areas by Perry et al. (1977), White et al. (1977). The different findings are probably due to difficulties in obtaining uniform histopathological diagnosis in this type of vascular dementia (Alafuzoff et al., 1985).

Most biochemical studies have been done on homogenates from whole brain regions. This method overlooks the possibility of an internuclear regional variation. To avoid this obstacle we have looked at the

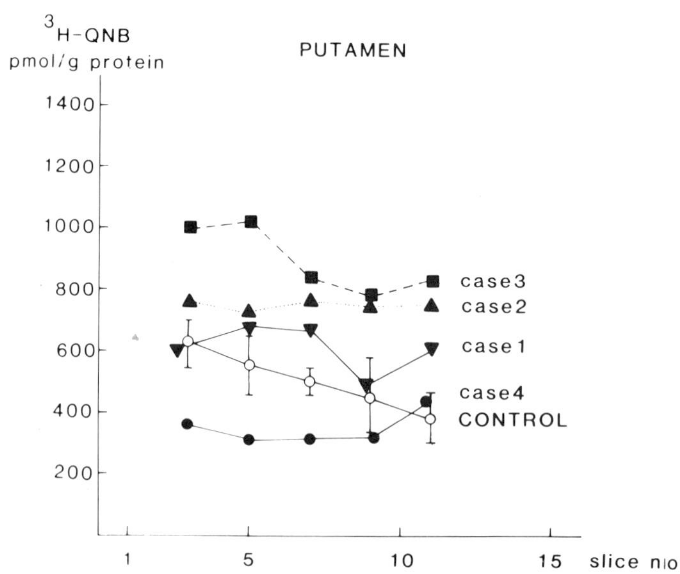

Fig. 3. Anterio-posterior topochemical distribution of muscarinic (^{3}H-QNB) binding sites in human putamen from control (n=5) and Alzheimer (case 1-4) brains. For the controls mean value ±SE are given. For the Alzheimer cases each point represents an individual value.

topochemical localization of the muscarinic receptors in different brain regions. It is evident from figure 3 that in three out of four Alzheimer cases there is an increased number of muscarinic binding sites in the whole anterio-posterior direction of the putamen. The patient (case 4) showing no receptor compensation died after a short duration of Alzheimer's disease of an incarcerated hernia.

To get a deeper understanding at neuronal level of the underlying mechanism for Alzheimer's disease, we have developed a method to dissect brain tissue with short post-mortem delay, freeze it in sucrose to -70°C and keep its functional integrity. After preloading with labelled choline both a spontaneous and potassium (35mM) induced release of radioactivity can be observed from frontal cortical slices of both control and Alzheimer brains.

CHOLINERGIC RECEPTORS IN HUMAN BRAIN IN OTHER DEMENTIA DISORDERS

Research on rare dementia conditions have been performed on a few cases, making the conclusions of our studies less secure (table 2). In Pick's disease decrease or unchanged number of muscarinic receptors were obtained (table 2).

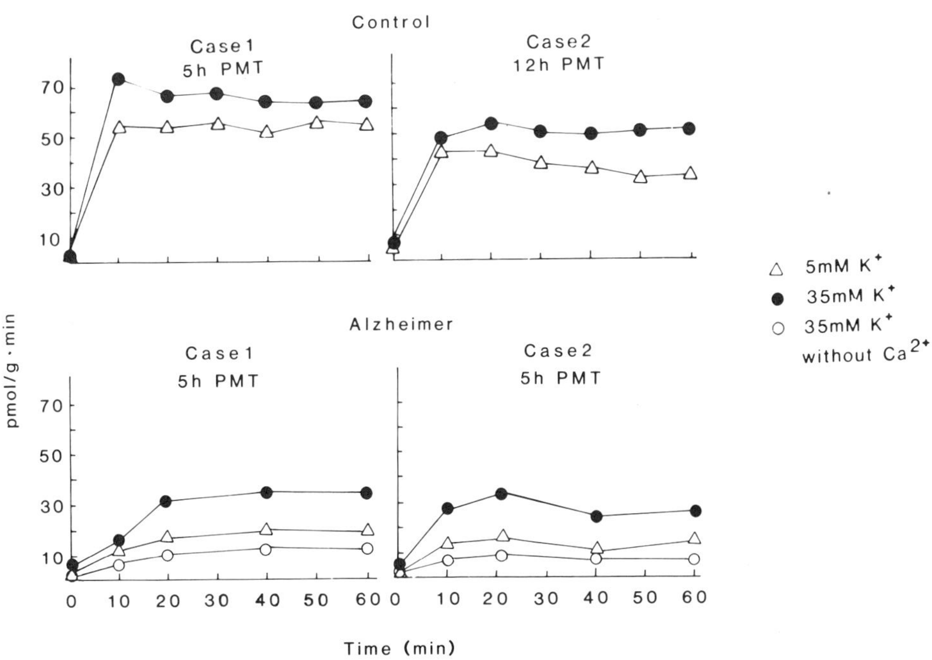

Fig. 4. Release of ^{3}H from human frontal cortex slices of control and Alzheimer brains obtained 5-12 h post mortem. The cortical slices were preincubated with $6x10^{-6}$ M ^{3}H-choline for 30 mins and spontaneous (5mM K^+) as well as stimulated release (35mM K^+) were followed (Nilsson et al., unpublished observations).

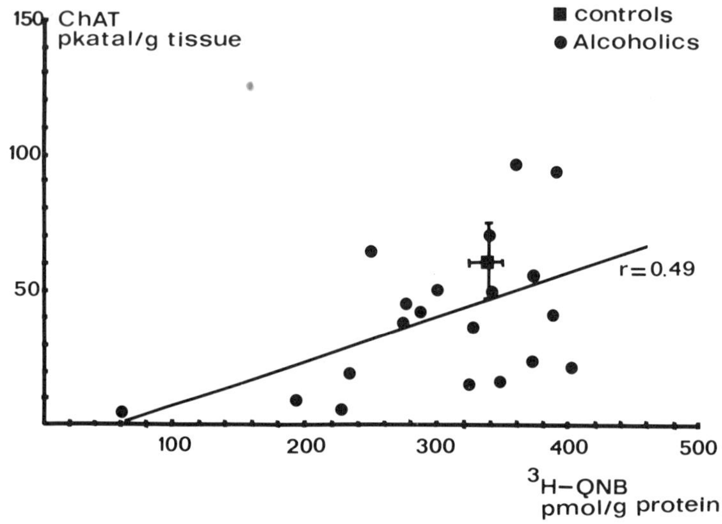

Fig. 5. Correlation between number of muscarinic (^{3}H-QNB) binding sites and ChAT activity in hippocampus of chronic alcoholics (29-64 years). Each point represents an individual value. Mean values of the age-matched control group is given with relevant standard errors.

In chronic alcoholism a decrease in number of muscarinic receptors is observed in the hippocampus of older age groups while in the younger age groups the receptors seem to be less affected (Nordberg 1982b, table 2). This might be due to an additive effect of the normal aging process and the toxic effect of a prolonged alcohol abuse. As seen in figure 5 a positive correlation between ChAT activity and number of muscarinic binding sites is obtained when data for the hippocampus chronic alcoholics (29-64 years) are plotted. Both chronic alcoholics and Alzheimer patients have memory disturbances. The cholinergic system has been linked to the memory function making a biochemical comparison between these two dementia conditions of interest. In contrast to the finding in chronic alcoholism the correlation between ChAT activity and muscarinic receptors in the hippocampus is negative in Alzheimer's disease (Nordberg et al., 1983). In multi-infarct dementia there was a decrease in both ChAT activity and muscarinic receptors but a significant correlation was not obtained. Thus the biochemical findings seem to be more comparable in multi-infarct dementia and chronic alcoholism. A plausible explanation at the synaptic level is that in Alzheimer's disease there is more selective presynaptic change with the possibility of receptor compensation at the more intact post-synaptic part of the neuron. The normal aging process and the pathological mechanisms involved in ethanol abuse and multi-infarct dementia seem to cause a more unselective damage of the brain neurons, i.e. both pre- and post-synaptically.

The prevalence for dementia is increased in Parkinson's disease. Dubois et al. (1983) observed in cortical tissue from demented Parkinson patients an increased number of muscarinic binding sites while no

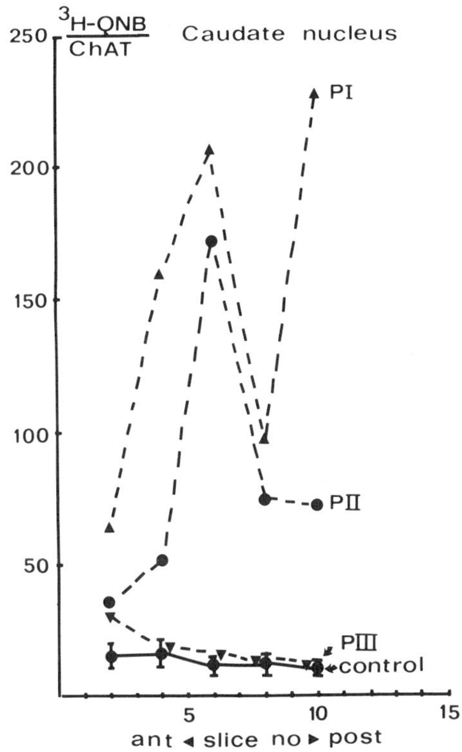

Fig. 6. Anterio-posterior distribution of the ratio of muscarinic (^{3}H-QNB) binding sites/ChAT activity in the caudate nucleus of three Parkinson patients (PI-III) and six controls. For the Parkinson cases each point indicates an individual value and for the controls mean values ±SE are given.

significant increase was found in non-demented Parkinson patients. When looking on topochemical distribution in the basal ganglia of three Parkinson patients we found a similar upregulation in two out ot three individuals (fig. 6). These two patients (P1, P2) had a marked reduced ChAT activity and a long disease duration (12-16 years) combined with severe dementia (5 years) in one of them (P2) while the patient (P3) showing no change in these cholinergic markers (ChAT, ^{3}H-QNB) had a short history of Parkinson's disease (2 years). Consequently the duration of Parkinson's disease might be of great importance for the biochemical disturbances of the cholinergic system.

Acknowledgement. The financial support by the Swedish Medical Research Council, the Swedish Tobacco Company and the Osterman's foundation is highly acknowledged.

REFERENCES

Alafuzoff, E., Adolfsson, R., Grundki-Iqbal, I. and Winblad, B., 1985, Perivascular deposits of serum proteins in cerebral cortex in vascular dementia, Acta neuropathol. (Berlin), (in press).

Allen, S.J., Benton, J.S., Goodhardt, M.J., Haan, E.A., Sims, N.R., Smith, C.C.T., Spillane, J.A., Bowen, D.M., and Davison, A.N., 1983, Biochemical evidence of selective nerve cell changes in the normal ageing human and rat brain, J. Neurochem., 41:256.

Antuono, P., Sorbi, S., Bracco, L., Fusco, T., and Amaducci, L., 1980, A discrete sampling technique in senile dementia of the Alzheimer type and alcoholic dementia: study of the cholinergic system, in: "Aging of the Brain and Dementia," Aging vol. 13, L. Amaducci, A.N. Davison, P. Antuono, eds., Raven Press, New York.

Bartus, R.T., Dean, R.L., Beer, B., and Lippa, A.S., 1982, The cholinergic hypothesis of geriatric memory dysfunction, Science 217:408.

Birdsall, N.J.M., Burgen, A.S.V., and Hulme, E.C., 1978, Multiple classes of muscarinic receptor binding sites in the brain, in: "Advances in Pharmacology and Therapeutics, vol. 1 Receptors," J. Jacob, ed., Pergamon Press, Oxford, New York.

Bowen, D.M., Spillane, J.A., Curzon, G., Meier-Ruge, W., White, P., Goodhardt, M.J., Iwangoff, P., and Davison, A.N., 1979, Accelerated ageing or selective neuronal loss as an important cause of dementia?, Lancet, I:11.

Cuello, A.C., and Sofroniew, M.V., 1984, The anatomy of the CNS cholinergic neurons, TINS, 7:74.

Davies, P., and Feisullin, S., 1981, Postmortem stability of α-bungarotoxin binding sites in mouse and human brain, Brain Res., 216:449.

Davies, P., and Verth, A., 1978, Regional distribution of muscarinic acetylcholine receptor in normal and Alzheimer's type dementia brains, Brain Res., 138:385.

Dubois, B., Ruberg, M., Javoy-Agid, F., Plosha, A., and Agid, Y., 1983, A subcortical - cortical cholinergic system is affected in Parkinson's disease, Brain Res., 288:213.

Garvey, J.M., Rossor, M., and Iversen, L.L., 1984, Evidence for multiple muscarinic receptor subtypes in human brain, J. Neurochem., 43:299.

Hutton, J.T., 1980, Clinical nosology of the dementing illnesses, in: "Advances in Neurogerontology," G.J. Maletta, F.J. Pirozzolo, eds., Praegen, New York.

Jenni-Eiermann, S., von Hahn, H.P., Honegger, C.G., and Ulrich, J., 1984, Studies on neurotransmitter binding in senile dementia, Gerontology, 30:350.

Kohlmeyer, K., 1982, (Multiinfarct-)dementia versus primary degenerative (Alzheimer's) dementia: A study of r-CBF and computed tomography (CT), in: "The Aging Brain," S.Hoyer, ed., Springer-Verlag, Berlin, Heidelberg, New York.

Lang, H., and Henke, H., 1983, Cholinergic receptor binding and autoradiography in brains of non-neurological and senile dementia of Alzheimer-type patients, Brain Res., 267:271.

Larsson, C., Lundberg, P-Å., Nordberg, A., Halén, A., and Adem, A., 1985, In vitro binding of ^{3}H-acetylcholine to nicotine-like receptors in human and rodent brain, Acta Physiol. Scand., (submitted).

Larsson, C., and Nordberg, A., 1985, Comparative analysis of nicotine-like receptor - ligand interactions in rodent brain homogenate, J. Neurochem., (in press).

Larsson, C., and Nordberg, A., 1980, Studies of nicotine-like binding sites in brain, in: "Neurotransmitters and Their Receptors," V.Z. Littauer, Y. Dudai, J. Silman, V.I. Vogel, eds., John Wiley & Sons Ltd.

Morley, B.J., and Kemp, G.E., 1981, Characterization of putative nicotinic acetylcholine receptor in mammalian brain, Brain Res. Rev., 3:81.

Nordberg, A., Adolfsson, R., Aquilonius, S-M., Marklund, S., Oreland, L., and Winblad, B., 1980, Brain enzymes and acetylcholine receptors in dementia of Alzheimer type and chronic alcohol abuse, in: "Aging in the Brain and Dementia," Aging vol. 13, L. Amaducci, A.N. Davison, P. Antuono, eds., Raven Press, New York.

Nordberg, A., Adolfsson, R., Marcusson, J., and Winblad, B., 1982a, Cholinergic receptors in the hippocampus in normal aging and dementia of Alzheimer type, in: The Aging Brain: "Cellular and Molecular Mechanisms of Aging in the Nervous System," Aging vol. 20, E. Giacobini, G. Filogamo, G. Giacobini, A. Vernadakis, eds., Raven Press, New York.

Nordberg, A., Larsson, C., Adolfsson, R., Alafuzoff, I., and Winblad, B., 1983, Muscarinic receptor compensation in hippocampus of Alzheimer patients, J. Neural. Transmission, 56:13.

Nordberg, A., Larsson, C., Perdahl, E., and Winblad, B., 1982b, Cholinergic activity in hippocampus in chronic alcoholism, Drug and Alcohol Dependence, 10:333.

Nordberg, A., Marcusson, J., and Winblad, B., 1985a, ^{3}H-QNB binding in human hippocampus - selective increase of ^{3}H-nicotine sites with age. To be submitted.

Nordberg, A., Nyberg, P., and Winblad, B., 1985b, Topochemical distribution of choline acetyltransferase activity, muscarinic and nicotinic receptors in Parkinson brains. To be submitted.

Nordberg, A., and Winblad, B., 1981, Cholinergic receptors in human hippocampus - regional distribution and variance with age, Life Sci., 29:1937.

Palacios, J.M., 1982, Autoradiographic localization of muscarinic cholinergic receptors in the hippocampus of patients with senile dementia, Brain Res., 243:173.

Perry, E., 1980, The cholinergic system in old age and Alzheimer's disease, Age and Aging, 9:1.

Perry, E.K., and Perry, R.H., 1980, The cholinergic system in Alzheimer's disease, in: "Biochemistry of Dementia," P.H. Roberts, ed., John Wiley & Sons Ltd.

Perry, E.K., Perry, R., Blessed, G., and Tomlinson, B., 1977, Necropsy evidence of central cholinergic deficits in senile dementia, Lancet, I:189.

Perry, E.K., Perry, R.H., Gibson, P., Blessed, G., and Tomlinson, B.E., 1977, A cholinergic connection between normal aging and senile dementia in the human hippocampus, Neuroscience Letters, 6:85.

Reisberg, B., and Ferris, S.H., 1982, Diagnosis and assessment of the older patient, Hosp. Com. Psychiat., 33:104.

Reisine, T.D., Yamamura, H.I., Bird, E.D., Spokes, E., and Enna, S.J., 1978, Pre- and postsynaptic neurochemical alterations in Alzheimer's disease, Brain Res., 159:477.

Rinne, J.O., Rinne, J.K., Laakso, K., Paljärvi, L., and Rinne, V.K., 1984, Reduction in muscarinic receptor binding in limbic areas of Alzheimer brain, J. Neurol. Neurosurg, Psychiat., 47:651.

Schwartz, R.D., McGee, R., and Kellar, K.J., 1982, Nicotinic cholinergic receptors labelled by ^{3}H-acetylcholine in rat brain, Mol. Pharmacol., 22:56.

Undén, A., Meyerson, B., Winblad, B., Sachs, C. and Bartfai, T., 1983, Postmortem changes in binding to the muscarinic receptor from human cerebral cortex, J. Neurochem., 41:102.

Volpe, B., Francis, A., Gazzaniga, M.S., and Schechter, N., 1979, Regional concentration of putative nicotinic - cholinergic receptor sites in human brain, Exp. Neurol., 66:737.

White, P., Goodhardt, M.J., Keet, J.P., Hiley, C.R., Carrasco, L.H., and Williams, I.E.I., 1977, Neocortical cholinergic neurons in elderly people, Lancet, I:668.

Whitehouse, P.J., Lynch, D., and Kuhar, M.J., 1984, Effects of postmortem delay and temperature on neurotransmitter receptor binding in a rat model of the human autopsy process, J. Neurochem., 43:553.

Wood, P.L., Etienne, P., Lal, S., Nair, N.P.V., Finlayson, M.H., Gauthier, S., Palo, J., Haltia, M., Paetau, A., and Bird, E.D., 1983, A post-mortem comparison of the cortical cholinergic system in Alzheimer's disease and Pick's disease, J. Neurol. Sci., 62:211.

Yates, C.M., Simpson, J., Maloney, A.F.J., and Gordon, A., 1980, Neurochemical observations in a case of Pick's disease, J. Neurol. Sci., 48:257.

EXAMINATION OF CHOLINERGIC AND NEUROPEPTIDE RECEPTOR ALTERATIONS IN SENILE DEMENTIA OF THE ALZHEIMER's TYPE (SDAT)

K. Gulya[1], M. Watson[1], T.W. Vickroy[1], W.R. Roeske[1], R. Perry[2], E. Perry[2], S.P. Duckles[1] and H.I. Yamamura[1]

[1]Depts. of Pharmacology and Internal Medicine, University of Arizona, Tucson, Arizona, and [2]Dept. of Neuropathology Newcastle General Hospital, Newcastle upon Tyne, England

INTRODUCTION

Senile dementia of the Alzheimer's type (SDAT) is a progressive cerebral neurodegeneration which is known to affect approximately 5% of the population over age 65 in every industrialized country. SDAT patients show correlative changes in various physiological, morphological, biochemical and clinical parameters. In recent years, a number of biochemical studies have attempted to define neurochemical changes which occur during SDAT. The characteristics of a number of neurotransmitter systems have been investigated (Terry and Davies, 1980) and changes in the number of receptors (Reisine et al., 1978), transmitter synthesizing enzyme activities (Perry et al., 1978) and transmitter levels (Richter et al., 1980) have already been demonstrated. Since changes in the cholinergic and some neuropeptide transmitter systems (Rossor et al., 1982; Davies et al., 1982) have been reported in brain tissue of patients with this disorder, we decided to simultaneously characterize biochemical markers for the cholinergic system (choline acetyltransferase (CAT, EC 2.3.1.6), muscarinic acetylcholine receptor (mAChR) and to investigate the possible changes in the somatostatin, delta and mu opiate receptor systems.

MATERIALS AND METHODS

Twenty two clinically well-documented cases were selected for this study. Deaths were from a variety of causes that were thought not to have any neurological complications aside from SDAT in diagnosed patients. Brain samples (12) of SDAT and age-matched control (10) patients between 69 and 90 years (Table 1) were studied. Following a post mortem delay (Table 1) during which bodies were maintained at 4°C, samples (150 - 200 mg) were taken out from the hippocampal gyrus, the cingulate and parietal cortices and stored at -70°C until biochemical analyses could be carried out.

Brain tissues were dissected into grey and white matter and the grey matter was homogenized in 50 vols of ice-cold 10 mM Na/K buffer (pH 7.4 at 4°C) with a Polytron homogenizer. CAT activity was determined in this homogenate (see below). Subsequently, the homogenate was centrifuged at 18,000 g for 15 min and the pellet was resuspended in the same buffer to 100 vols, and a portion was saved for the determination of somatostatin and opiate receptor binding sites. The other portion was centrifuged again as above. The resulting pellet was rehomogenized in 100 vols of fresh, ice-cold Na/K buffer and used for the determination of $[^3H](+)CD$, $[^3H]PZ$ and $[^3H](-)QNB$ binding sites according to the method of Vickroy et al, 1984, Watson et al, 1983, and Yamamura and Snyder, 1974, respectively. Approximately 0.75 mg, 0.25 mg or 0.05 mg protein in a final volume of 2 ml of 10 mM Na/K buffer (pH 7.4 at 25°C) was incubated with 6.8 nM $[^3H](+)CD$, 10 nM $[^3H]PZ$ or 0.25 nM $[^3H](-)QNB$ in the absence or presence of 1 uM atropine at 25°C, respectively. After one hour ($[^3H]PZ$) or two hours (in the case of $[^3H](+)CD$ and $[^3H]QNB$) of incubation, the reaction was stopped with rapid vacuum filtration of the incubation mixture through Whatman GF/B filters which were pretreated with 0.1% polyethylenimine. The filters were washed 4 times with 3 ml of 10 mM Na/K buffer (pH 7.4) at 4°C and then placed in vials to dry overnight. Scintillation fluid was added and following a minimum six hours for extraction, the radioactivity was determined in a liquid scintillation counter.

For the neuropeptide receptor binding studies, the homogenate was centrifuged at 19,000 g for 10 min and the resulting pellet was resuspended in 50 mM Tris-HCl buffer (pH 7.4 at 4°C) containing 5 mM $MgCl_2$, 2 mg/ml bovine serum albumin (BSA) (RIA grade, Sigma, St. Louis, MO) and 20 ug/ml bacitracin and centrifuged again at 19,000 g for 10 min. The pellet was resuspended in the same buffer (pH 7.4 at 25°C) and a portion (approximately 0.15 mg protein) was incubated with $[^{125}I]$CGP 23,996 (0.5 nM) for 90 min. in 50 mM Tris-HCl buffer (pH 7.4 at 25°C, the same as above). For the determination of delta and mu opiate receptor binding capacity, 1 nM of $[^3H]$(2-D-penicillamine, 5-D-penicillamine)enkephalin ($[^3H]$DPDPE) or $[^3H]$naloxone was used in the same manner (90 min at 25°C) in the absence or presence of 1 uM met-enkephalin or naltrexone, respectively. The incubation was stopped by rapid vacuum filtration of the mixture as stated above, and the radioactivity was counted as above.

CAT enzyme activity was assayed from the original homogenate. The phosphate buffered (pH 7.4 at 37°C and 0°C, respectively) incubation medium contained in final concentrations; 0.2 mM ^{14}C-acetyl coenzyme A, 300 mM NaCl, 20 mM choline chloride, 1 mM EDTA and 0.15 mM eserine sulfate. After incubation (15 min at 37°C and 0°C for the blank) the tubes were transferred to scintillation vials and the contents were washed out with 3 ml 50 mM sodium phosphate buffer (pH 7.4 at 4°C). The $[^{14}C]$ACh formed was extracted with the acetonitrile-tetraphenylborona-te-toluene scintillation cocktail for direct measurement.

Protein was assayed by the method of Lowry et al. (1951) using BSA as standard.

$[^3H]PZ$ (84 Ci/mmoles), $[^3H](-)QNB$ (33 Ci/mmoles), $[^3H](+)CD$ (38.1 Ci/mmoles) and $[^{14}C]$acetyl-coenzyme A (51.9 Ci/mmoles) were purchased from New England Nuclear. $[^3H]$DPDPE (40 Ci/mmoles) was custom synthesized by Amersham. $[^{125}I]$CGP 23,996 was radioiodinated by the method of Czernik and Petrack (1983). All other chemicals were obtained from commercial sources.

RESULTS

All SDAT patients showed histological changes that are known to be associated with SDAT. The senile plaque number (Table 1) is significantly higher (Student's t-test, $p<0.001$) in SDAT patients as compared with those from controls. CAT activity decreased in all SDAT

TABLE 1. Characteristics of Control and SDAT Groups

	Control	SDAT
Sex	6 males 4 females	2 males 10 females
Age (years)	81 ± 8	78 ± 6
Post-Mortem Delay (hours)	21 ± 7	33 ± 14
Mean Plaque Number	2 ± 3	36 ± 19*

± S.E.M. * $p < 0.001$

brain areas examined (Table 2). The largest decrease was found in the cingulate cortex where only 36% of the control CAT activity was detected. We found no significant changes in the number of binding sites for three muscarinic ligands (Table 3). Table 4 shows the density of somatostatin binding sites in our samples. [^{125}I]CGP 23,996 binding sites were unformly decreased ($p < 0.05$, Student's t-test) by 45.9 - 48.5% of the control value in all brain areas examined. Our preliminary results show an unchanged opiate receptor system in SDAT as compared to the age-matched controls (data not shown).

DISCUSSION

Senile plaques are present in SDAT brains and the density of these plaques in the cortex and hippocampus correlates with the severity of the neurological defects found in SDAT patients (Blessed et al., 1968). In our SDAT samples the average number of senile plaques was 36 indicating that the disease had reached an advanced stage. The average post mortem delay to autopsy differed in the two groups, although nonsignficantly, being 33 h in the SDAT group and 21 h in the control one.

The activity of the enzyme CAT is reported to be decreased in SDAT (Perry et al., 1978; Reisine et al., 1978). We also found the enzyme that synthesizes acetylcholine, is significantly reduced (by 52 - 64%) in all brain areas examined as compared to age-matched controls. This degree of decrease of CAT activity is in good agreement with previous reports. Reisine et al. (1978) reported a 60 - 80% reduction of CAT activity in the caudate nucleus, putamen, frontal cortex and hippocampus. Perry et al. (1978) reported a similar decrease in four cortical lobes of SDAT patients. Rossor et al. (1980) found a significant fall in CAT activity in several cortical areas and in posterior hippocampus, although there was no significant reduction in CAT activity in basal ganglia areas. The loss of this substantial amount of CAT activity observed in SDAT probably due to the damage of the terminals of the cholinergic afferents arising from the basal forebrain nuclei rather than intrinsic cortical cholinergic neurons (Rossor et al., 1982; Coyle et al., 1983). Kitt et al. (1984) presented the first direct evidence that some of the neurites in senile plaques were of cholinergic nature and that they originated in part from neurons in the basal forebrain. Thus, it is understandable that the severely damaged

TABLE 2. CAT Activity in Three Regions of Human Brain

Brain Region		CAT activity[a]	
Hippocampal	C	3.1 ± 0.4	(6)
Gyrus	SDAT	1.5 ± 0.4*	(6)
Parietal	C	3.2 ± 0.4	(6)
Cortex	SDAT	1.0 ± 0.4*	(6)
Cingulate	C	4.4 ± 0.5	(6)
Cortex	SDAT	1.6 ± 0.5*	(6)

[a]expressed as nmoles ^{14}C-ACh formed/mg prot/h

All values are expressed as mean ± S.E.M. *$p < 0.05$, Student's t-test. The number of separate experiments is in brackets.

TABLE 3. Muscarinic Ligand Binding in Three Regions of Human Brain

Brain Region		$[^3H](+)CD$[a] bound		$[^3H]PZ$ bound		$[^3H](-)QNB$ bound	
Hippocampal	C	12 ± 1	(6)	296 ± 30	(6)	272 ± 57	(4)
Gyrus	SDAT	16 ± 2	(6)	222 ± 28	(6)	226 ± 29	(4)
Parietal	C	14 ± 3	(6)	257 ± 24	(6)	221 ± 7	(4)
Cortex	SDAT	15 ± 3	(6)	199 ± 44	(6)	231 ± 53	(4)
Cingulate	C	11 ± 2	(6)	261 ± 83	(6)	249 ± 64	(3)
Cortex	SDAT	12 ± 2	(6)	304 ± 50	(6)	263 ± 46	(3)

[a]specific binding expressed as fmoles/mg protein

TABLE 4. Somatostatin Binding in Three Regions of Human Brain

Brain Region		^{125}I-CGP 23,996[a]	
Hippocampal	C	17.1 ± 2.1	(6)
Gyrus	SDAT	8.3 ± 1.7*	(5)
Parietal	C	20.3 ± 6.9	(6)
Cortex	SDAT	9.3 ± 2.2*	(4)
Cingulate	C	23.5 ± 4.3	(5)
Cortex	SDAT	11.1 ± 0.8*	(5)

[a]Values are expressed as mean ± S.E.M. (fmoles/mg protein)

The number of separate experiments is in brackets.

*$p < 0.05$, Student's t-test

forebrain cholinergic system appears to be related to this dramatic decrease of CAT, a selective marker for cholinergic neurons.

During the past few years several groups have studied post mortem SDAT tissues for neurotransmitter receptor alterations. Most of these investigations have been focused on muscarinic cholinergic receptors with the majority of reports based upon [^{3}H]QNB binding. Reisine et al. (1978; 1980) demonstrated a significant reduction in specific [^{3}H]QNB binding sites in the hippocampus with no changes in the caudate nucleus, putamen or frontal cortex. No change in the receptor affinity for [^{3}H]QNB was evident in other studies (Davies and Verth (1978)). Recently however, Nordberg et al. (1983) have reported that while significant differences between SDAT and control patients in the number of hippocampal [^{3}H]QNB binding sites were not evident, there was a significant negative correlation between CAT activity and the number of muscarinic receptors in the SDAT group but not in the controls. In the present study, we found a consistent but nonsignificant increase in the number of sites labeled by [^{3}H](+)CD, a muscarinic agonist. The greatest increase (127.7% of the control value) was found in the hippocampal gyrus, where muscarinic antagonists [^{3}H]PZ and [^{3}H](-)QNB were found to be decreased (75% and 83% of the control values, respectively). However, there were no significant differences between cortices of SDAT and control tissues in [^{3}H]antagonist binding.

The reason for the apparently normal levels of mAChR in the parietal and cingulate cortices could be that cholinergic fibers to the cortical areas do not carry a significant proportion of receptors (presynaptic localization) or that the loss of these receptors by degenerating (cholinergic) neurons is compensated by other, possibly cholinoceptive neurons. There is another complication which must be considered. Garvey et al. (1984) have reported evidence for multiple muscarinic receptor subtypes in human brain. There is a possibility that unique subclasses may be differentially or preferentially affected in SDAT. This could possibly explain the slightly increasing trend of ^{3}H(+)CD binding in our assay. Under the assay conditions used here [^{3}H](+)CD binds only to the highest affinity state of receptors. Thus, the observed increase in [^{3}H](+)CD binding could reflect an increased receptor sensitivity which occurs to compensate against reduced Ach levels. Similar phenomena have been observed in the periphery (denervation hypersensitivity) and could be the basis for receptor compensation to diminished presynaptic cholinergic activity in this disease (Nordberg et al., 1983).

It was shown previously that somatostatin immunoreactivity is reduced in the temporal cortex (Rossor et al., 1980) and in different parts of the cerebral cortex (Davies et al., 1980; Davies and Terry, 1981) of SDAT patients. We found a significant decrease in the density of somatostatin receptors (45.9 - 48.5% of the control value) in SDAT which was almost identical in the three areas examined. Interestingly, these reductions are similar to those that were found in CAT activity. However, it would appear that these parallel decreases are attributable to a coincidental reduction rather than co-localization of these neurotransmitter systems since no current evidence supports the neuronal colocalization of these neurotransmitters (McKinney et al., 1982; Vincent et al., 1983).

There has been no previous reports concerning the status of opiate receptors in SDAT (Bowen et al., 1979), although Messing et al. (1980,1981) and Roth (1983) reported decreased opiate receptor concentrations in several parts of aged rat brain. Our preliminary results show an unchanged opiate receptor system in SDAT as compared to the age-matched controls indicating that there is no additional delta and mu opiate receptor loss in this disease.

ACKNOWLEDGEMENT

Supported in part by USPHS grants. S.D.D. is an established investigator of the American Heart Association. W.R.R. and H.I.Y. are recipients of a RCDA and RSDA from the NIH.

REFERENCES

BLESSED, G., TOMLINSON, B.E. and ROTH, M.: The association between quantitative measures of dementia and of senile change in the cerebral grey matter of elderly subjects. Br. J. Psych., 114, 797-811, (1968).

BOWEN, D.M., SPILLANE, J.A., CURZON, G., MEIER-RUGE, W., WHITE, P., GOODHARDT, M.J., IWANGOFF, P. and DAVIDSON, A.N.: Accelerated ageing or selective neuronal loss as an important cause of dementia? Lancet, 1, 11-14, 1979.

COYLE, J.T., PRICE, D.L. and DELONG, M.R.: Alzheimer's disease: a disorder of cholinergic innervation. Science, 219, 1184-1190, 1983.

CZERNIK, A.J. and PETRACK, B.: Somatostatin receptor binding in rat cerebral cortex. J. Biol. Chem., 258, 5525-5530, 1983.

DAVIES, P. and VERTH, A.H.: Regional distribution of muscarinic acetylcholine receptor in normal and Alzheimer's-type dementia brains. Brain Res., 138, 385-392, 1978.

DAVIES, P., KATZMAN, R. and TERRY, R.D.: Reduced somatostatin-like immunoreactivity in cerebral cortex from cases of Alzheimer disease and Alzheimer senile dementia. Nature, 288, 279-280, 1980.

DAVIES, P. and TERRY, R.: Cortical somatostatin-like immunoreactivity in cases of Alzheimer's disease and senile dementia of the Alzheimer type. Neurobiol. of Aging, 2, 9-14, 1981.

DAVIES, P., KATZ, D.A. and CRYSTAL, H.A.: Choline acetyltransferase, somatostatin, and substance P in selected cases of Alzheimer's disease, Alzheimer's disease: A report of progress. (Aging, Vol. 19), ed. S. Corkin et al., Raven Press, New York, 1982.

GARVEY, J.M., ROSSOR, M. and IVERSEN, L.L.: Evidence for multiple muscarinic receptor subtypes in human brain. J. Neurochem. 43, 299-302, 1984.

KITT, C.A., PRICE, D.L., STRUBLE, R.G., CORK, L.C., WAINER, B.H., BECHER, M.W. and MOBLEY, W.C.: Evidence for cholinergic neurites in senile plaques. Science, 226, 1443-1445, 1984.

LOWRY, O.H., ROSEBROUGH, N.J., FARR, A.L., and RANDALL, R.J.: Protein measurement with the folin phenol reagent. J. Biol. Chem. 193:265-275, 1951.

MCKINNEY, M., DAVIES, P. and COYLE, J.T.: Somatostatin is not co-localized in cholinergic neurons innervating the rat cerebral cortex - hippocampal formation. Brain Res., 243, 169-172, 1982.

MESSING, R.B., VASQUEZ, B.J., SPIEHLER, V.R., MARTINEZ, J.L., JENSEN, R.A., RIGTER, H. and MCGAUGH, J.L.: ^{3}H-dihydromorphine binding in brain regions of young and aged rats. Life Sci., 26, 921-927, 1980.

MESSING, R.B., VASQUEZ, B.J., SAMANIEGO, B., JENSEN, R.A., MARTINEZ, J.L. and MCGAUGH, J.L.: Alterations in dihydromorphine binding in cerebral hemispheres of aged male rats. J. Neurochem. 36, 784-790, 1981.

NORDBERG, A., LARSSON, C., ADOLFSSON, R., ALAFUZOFF, I. and WINBLAD, B.: Muscarinic receptor compensation in hippocampus of Alzheimer patients. J. Neural. Transmission, 56, 13-19, 1983.

PERRY, E.K., TOMLINSON, B.E., BLESSED, G., BERGMAN, K., GIBSON, P.H. and PERRY, R.H.: Correlation of cholinergic abnormalities with senile plaques and mental test scores in senile dementia. Br. Med. J., 2, 1457-1459, 1978.

REISINE, T.D., YAMAMURA, H.I., BIRD, E.D., SPOKES, E. and ENNA, S.J.: Pre- and postsynaptic neurochemical alterations in Alzheimer's disease. Brain Res., 159, 477-481, 1978.

REISINE, T.D., PEDIGO, N.W., MEINERS, B., IQBAL, K. and YAMAMURA, H.I.: Alzheimer's disease: studies on neurochemical alterations in the brain. Aging of the Brain and Dementia (Aging, Vol. 13), ed. L. Amaducci et al., Raven Press, New York, 1980.

RICHTER, J.A., PERRY, E. and TOMLINSON, B.E.: Acetylcholine and choline levels in post-mortem human brain tissue: preliminary observations in Alzheimer's disease. Life Sci., 26, 1683-1689, 1980.

ROSSOR, M., FAHRENKRUG, J., EMSON, P., MOUNTJOY, C., IVERSEN, L. and ROTH, M.: Reduced cortical choline acetyltransferase activity in senile dementia of Alzheimer's type is not accompanied by changes in vasoactive intestinal polypeptide. Brain Res, 201, 249-253, 1980.

ROSSOR, M.N., EMSON, P.C., IVERSEN, L.L., MOUNTJOY, C.Q., ROTH, M., FAHRENKRUG, J. and REHFELD, J.F.: Neuropeptides and neurotransmitters in cerebral cortex in Alzheimer's disease. Alzheimer's disease: A report of progress. (Aging, Vol. 19), ed. S. Corkin et al., Raven Press, New York, 1982.

ROSSOR, M.N., SVENDSEN, C., HUNT, S.P., MOUNTJOY, C.Q., ROTH, M. and IVERSEN, L.L.: The substantia innominata in Alzheimer's disease: an histochemical and biochemical study of cholinergic marker enzymes. Neurosci. Lett., 28, 217-222, 1982.

ROTH, G.S.: Brain dopaminergic and opiate receptors and responsiveness during aging. Aging Brain and Ergot Alkaloids (Aging, Vol. 23), ed. A. Agnoli et al., Raven Press, New York, 1983.

TERRY, R.D. and DAVIES, P.: Dementia of the Alzheimer type. Ann. Rev. Neurosci., 3, 77-95, 1980.

VICKROY, T.W., ROESKE, W.R. and YAMAMURA, H.I.: Pharmacological differences between the high-affinity muscarinic agonist binding states of the rat heart and cerebral cortex labeled with (+)-^{3}H cismethyldioxolane. J. Pharm. Exp. Ther., 229, 747-755, 1984.

VINCENT, S.R., STAINES, W.A. and FIBIGER, H.C.: Histochemical demonstration of separate populations of somatostatin and cholinergic neurons in the rat striatum. Neurosci. Lett., 35, 111-114, 1983.

WATSON, M., YAMAMURA, H.I. and ROESKE, W.R.: A unique regulatory profile and regional distribution of [^{3}H]pirenzepine binding in the rat provide evidence for distinct M_1 and M_2 muscarinic receptor subtypes. Life Sci., 32, 3001-3011, 1983.

YAMAMURA, H.I. and SNYDER, S.H.: Muscarinic cholinergic receptor binding in rat brain. Proc. Natl. Acad. Sci., U.S.A., 71, 1725-1729, 1974.

QUANTITATIVE AUTORADIOGRAPHY AND HISTOCHEMISTRY IN THE HUMAN BRAIN POST MORTEM

Anat Biegon and Marilyn Wolff

Isotope Department
The Weizmann Institute of Science
Rehovot, Israel

INTRODUCTION

The cholinergic system has been repeatedly implicated in diseases involving loss of memory and cognitive function.[1] It is also evident that disease or aging may affect some discrete nuclei in the brain and spare others.[1] In the following pages we will describe the adaptation of two classical morphological methods - histochemistry and autoradiography - for quantitative measurement of cholinergic elements in the human brain post mortem. This new methodology will make it feasible to perform quantitative but anatomically discrete comparisons between normal brains and brains of patients with senile dementia and related diseases.

METHODOLOGY AND RESULTS

A. Quantitative Histochemistry of the Enzyme Acetylcholine esterase (ACHE)

Brains were collected at autopsy, sliced in 2 cm coronal slices and frozen in powdered dry ice. Storage was at -70°C. Thin (40 μ) sections were cut at -20°C in a Bright croyotome and thaw-mounted onto gelatin coated glass plates, dried on a warm (30°C) surface, kept at -20°C overnight and then used or stored again at -70°C.

The histochemical staining method consisted of small modifications of the method of Koelle.[2] (Fig. 1).

Standard preparation: cerebellum from 4 rats was collected fresh, rinsed and mashed to a paste-like consistency. The homogeneous paste was divided into 6 glass test tubes. Increasing amounts of a purified ACHE preparation in a constant volume of buffer were added to the tubes, mixed well and the excess buffer was removed by lyophilization. The paste was mixed again with a wooden stick, centrifuged at a low (1000 x g) speed and frozen on powdered dry ice. The frozen paste samples were then transferred to a cryostat and cut to the same (40 μ) thickness as the brains. Alternate sections were taken for protein determination and for a biochemical ACHE assay using tritiated acetyl choline. The sections from the brain-mash standards were thaw-mounted onto gelatin coated glass slides and taken through the same histochemical procedure as the human brain sections. The stained sections and standards were then analyzed using a computerized, video-camera based image analysis system. A standard curve was constructed by the computer using the optical density

I. 2 hours incubation at 37°C in:
   50 mM Acetate buffer, pH 5.0
   10 mM Glycine
   2 mM Copper Sulphate
   1.15 gr/li Acetylthiocholine Iodide
   60 mg/li Ethopropazine (pseudo-choline blocker)

II. 4 washes in double distilled water, room temperature

III. 1 min in 1.25% Na_2S; pH 7.5

IV. 4 washes in double distilled water

V. 1 min in $AgNO_3$

VI. 2 washes in double distilled water

VII. Overnight fixation in 10% formalin

Fig. 1. Histochemistry of ACHE.

and the calculated enzyme content in ng/mg protein, so that densities derived from experimental sections were printed out in the same units. As expected, very high levels of ACHE activity were found in the caudate and putamen, and relatively low levels in the cortex (Fig. 2). A partial list of areas analyzed by the image analyzer is given in Table 1.

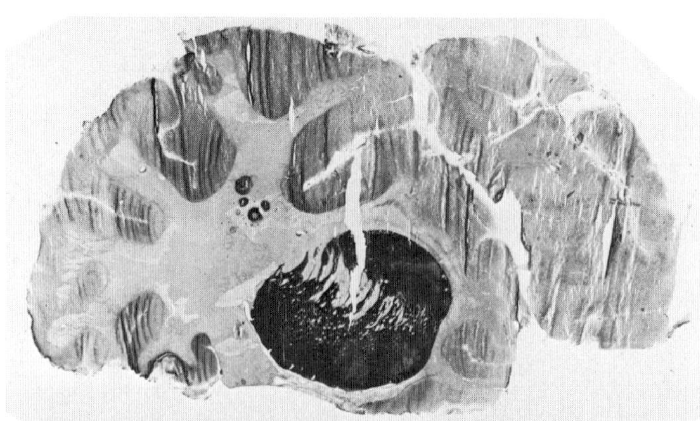

Fig. 2. Photograph of section from the anterior basal ganglia stained for ACHE.

B. Quantitative Autoradiography of cholinergic Muscarinic Receptors

Brain sections prepared exactly as for histochemistry, were labeled *in vitro* with tritiated QNB, a selective muscarinic ligand, following previously published procedures for rat brain.[3] Each section was covered with 10 ml of ^{3}H-QNB, 1 nM, for 2 hours at room temperature, washed for 5 min at 4°C, dipped in ice-cold double distilled water (to remove buffer salts) and finally dried and exposed to ^{3}H-LKB ultrafilm for 3 to 4 weeks, alongside with brain mash standards containing known amounts of radioactivity.[4]

The computerized image analysis system was used to measure the density of labeling over various regions and convert it to fm/mg protein via the standard curve. Table 1 summarizes the density of muscarinic receptors over areas similar to those in which ACHE content was analyzed. A detailed description of muscarinic receptors in the human hippocampus has been published earlier.[5]

Table 1. Regional Distribution of ACHE and Muscarinic Receptors in the Human Brain Post Mortem

Region	ACHE Content, ng/mg Protein	^{3}H-QNB Specifically Bound, pm/mg Protein	
Basal Ganglia:			
Caudate	42.3±1.7	10.1 ±2.4 (Lateral)	
Putamen	43.2±1.8	4.4 ±1.5	
Globus Pallidus:			
Lateral	20.7±0.7	0.49±0.06	
Medial	25.0±0.5	0.7 ±0.02	
Claustrum:	7.6±2.1	0.6 ±0.15	
Cortex:			
Frontal Superior	11.2±1.5	5.8±0.8 (s)	3.2±0.4 (i)
Frontal Medius	11.5±2.2	4.5±0.4 (s)	2.8±0.2 (i)
Frontal Inferior	11.7±3.2	3.8±0.3 (s)	2.5±0.2 (i)
Cingulate	9.0±2.1	7.4±1.2 (s)	3.4±0.5 (i)
Temporal Superior	8.5±1.1	5.3±1.1 (s)	2.6±0.5 (i)
Insula	10.9±3.0	3.7±0.3 (s)	2.4±0.3 (i)
Hippocampus:			
CA1	14.0±1.0	2.3	
Dentate Gyrus	17.5±1.8	3.0 ±0.3	

Results are means ± S.E.M. of 2-6 determinations on sections collected from six drug and neuropathology free individuals. s = superficial layers; i = inner layers.

DISCUSSION

In the present work, we have shown that qualitative histochemical methods can be made quantitative through the use of appropriate standards. In conjunction with quantitative autoradiography, these two methods allow a thorough analysis of anatomically localized changes in several elements of a given neurotransmitter system.

In the cholinergic system in the human brain post mortem, both elements (ACHE and muscarinic receptors) have been previously shown to be surprisingly stable post mortem.[6] Thus, we believe that the values we report on brains with a post-mortem delay no longer than 40 hours, are quite close to what is found in vivo.

The lack of correlation, in our hand, between ACHE content and post mortem delay also argues in this direction.

As others have reported using different methodologies[7] there is only a poor correlation between ACHE content and muscarinic receptor distribution. The most obvious difference is in the cortex, where muscarinic receptors are almost as dense as in the striatum while ACHE content is extremely low compared to the striatum.

However, the methods and results we describe here may now serve to study this matter, and the possible changes in the cholinergic system due to aging and disease in an accurate, quantitative manner.

REFERENCES

1. Bowen, D.M., Davison, A.N. and Sims, N.R. (1983). The cholinergic system in aging brain and dementia. In: Aging of the Brain, Samuel et al., ed. Raven Press, N.Y., p. 183-195.
2. Koelle, G.B. (1954). The histochemical localization of cholinesterase in the central nervous system of the rat. J. Comp. Neurol. 100, 211-235.
3. Rainbow, T.C., Bleisch, W.V., Biegon, A. and McEwen, B.S. (1982). Quantitative densitometry of neurotransmitter receptors. J. Neuroscience Methods 5, 127-138.
4. Rainbow, T.C., Biegon, A. and Berck, D.J. (1984). Quantitative receptor autoradiography with tritium labeled ligands: comparison of biochemical and densitometric measurements. J. Neuroscience Methods 11, 231-241.
5. Biegon, A., Rainbow, T.C., Mann, J.J. and McEwen, B.S. (1982). Neurotransmitter receptor sites in human hippocampus: a quantitative autoradiographic study. Brain Res. 247, 379-382.
6. Hardy, J.A. and Dodd, P.R. (1983). Metabolic and functional studies on post mortem human brain. Neurochemistry International 5, 253-266.
7. Greenfield, S. (1984). Acetylcholinesterase may have novel functions in the brain. TINS 10, 364-368.

INCREASED VASOPRESSIN PRODUCTION IN SENESCENCE AND DEMENTIA DUE TO KIDNEY CHANGES

R. Ravid, D.F. Swaab, E. Fliers and J.E. Hoogendijk

Netherlands Institute for Brain Research, Meibergdreef 33

1105 AZ Amsterdam ZO, the Netherlands

ABSTRACT

Vasopressin (VP) is involved as a neurotransmitter in a number of central functions that are frequently disturbed during aging and dementia. Therefore, this peptide has been used in clinical trials as a 'substitution therapy' for the degenerating peptidergic neurons, aimed at improving cognitive functions in aged and demented individuals with unequivocal results. In order to investigate whether the VP systems indeed show the claimed degenerative changes during aging and dementia, we focused in the first place on the Supra Optic Nucleus (SON) and the Para Ventricular Nucleus (PVN). VP cells were identified by means of immunocytochemistry in a series of 32 formalin-fixed human hypothalami, including 4 patients with senile dementia of the Alzheimer type (SDAT). In the SON and PVN, VP cell and nucleolar size was determined by means of a digitizer device, as parameter for peptide synthesizing activity. VP cell size and nucleolar size increased beyond 80 years of age, both in the PVN and in the SON. In SDAT patients these measures fell within the range for their age group. Instead of degenerative changes, these results show an activation of the vasopressinergic system, in senescence and in SDAT patients, similar to earlier observations in the aged rat and in accordance with a rise in human neurophysin and VP levels reported recently. The cause for these changes might be in the kidney.

Immunocytochemical staining of VP binding sites in the renal tubuli was strongly diminished in kidneys of old (25 and 34 months) as compared to young (3 and 5 months) Wistar and Brown-Norway rats. Urine production did not significantly increase in old age and the activation of the vasopressin neurons thus seems to be a secondary mechanism to compensate for loss of VP receptors in the old kidney.

VASOPRESSIN, AGING AND DEMENTIA

Advanced age is associated with a decreased ability of the organism to adapt to changes in its environment, and at a more fundamental level, with a decreased capacity of certain tissues to adapt their physiological responses to changes in neuronal or hormonal environment. This reduced adaptive capacity may be based upon deficiencies in neurotransmitters and neurohormones. Neuropeptides are the largest and most variable class of neurotransmitters (for review see Swaab, 1982). In the last few years, the changes in neuropeptide-containing neurons were studied in our group, in rat and human brain, and in patients with senile dementia of the Alzheimer type (SDAT). In the first place, the morphological basis for central effects of neuropeptides was described with special emphasis on vasopressin, which is known to be a neurohormone with many central effects (cf. De Wied, 1983). For a long time this peptide has been known to be produced in the Supra Optic Nucleus (SON) and Para Ventricular Nucleus (PVN), transported to the neurohypophysis and released as a neurohormone into the bloodstream.

The observations of De Wied et al. (1983) on vasopressin effects on 'memory' and the reports of Legros et al., (1980) on decreased plasma levels of the vasopressin precursor molecule Neurophysin in normal subjects between the ages of 55 and 60, were a strong stimulus for the hypothesis that a degeneration of vasopressin neurons at older age would be a basis of memory impairment. This idea was reinforced by the observations of Legros et al. (1980), who reported that administration of vasopressin by nasal spray to healthy volunteers of 50-65 years of age, improved performance in psychometric tests. Later trials in aged and demented patients were no longer unequivocal, however (for review see Jolles, 1983).

SON, PVN AND SUPRACHIASMATIC NUCLEUS (SCN) CHANGES DURING AGING AND DEMENTIA

Consequently, the question was studied whether indeed the vasopressin neuron was degenerating in senescence and dementia in the rat and human brain. Combining immunocytochemical (ICC) investigations with morphometric techniques for localization of vasopressin and measuring changes in peptide production, revealed that vasopressin neurons in some brain areas indeed degenerate during aging, and even more pronouncedly in dementia (i.e., in the SCN). A marked decrease in the SCN volume, VP cell number (fig. 1) and total SCN cell number was found in 80-100 year-old patients as compared with the youngest age group (Swaab et al., 1984; Swaab et al., 1985b). However, other vasopressin neurons, viz., the SON and PVN, were found to be activated in senescence and dementia, and to maintain an increased level of neurosecretion in these conditions (Fliers and Swaab, 1983; Swaab et al., 1984; Swaab et al., 1985a,b; Fliers et al., 1985). Cell size of immunocytochemically identified VP cells was measured as a parameter for peptide production in these areas (Swaab et al., 1984; Fliers et al., 1985). A significant increase was observed in the size of VP cell profiles, beyond the age of 80 (Swaab et al., 1984; Swaab et al., 1985). In brains from patients with SDAT, this morphometric parameter was within the range of their respective age group. Assuming that the well-known relation between neurosecretory cell size and peptide-synthesizing activity (cf. Fliers et al., 1985) also holds for the aging brain, the observed increase in VP cell size after 80 years of age may imply an increased activity of these cells. This interpretation is strengthened by recent nucleolar measurements (Hoogendijk et al., 1985), which show identical results (fig. 2). Our morphometric observations are in good agreement with the decreased blood levels of neurophysins (Legros, 1975) and increased peripheral levels of VP (Frolkis et al., 1982; Kirkland et al., 1984). Legros et al. (1980) reported also a secondary increase in immunoreactive neurophysin blood levels after the age of 70. A similar activation of VP production and release was found in aged Wistar rats (Fliers and Swaab, 1983).

AGE-RELATED CHANGES IN RENAL VP BINDING SITES

Immunocytochemical staining of VP binding sites in the rat kidney has given a possible explanation for the activation of the neurosecretory function of the vasopressin neurons. This procedure revealed a significant diminution of VP binding sites in the aged kidney (Ravid et al., 1985; Swaab et al., 1985b; Swaab et al., 1985c). The staining of renal tubuli in young and old Wistar and Brown-Norway rats was confined to medullary and cortical portions of collecting ducts and an occasional staining in the distal convoluted tubes only after preincubation of the kidney sections with VP, which enhanced the staining. In young kidneys (3 and 5 months) a very intense staining of medullary collecting ducts was observed and a marked staining of cortical collecting ducts and distal convoluted tubes. In old kidneys (25 and 34 months) only occasional and weak staining of medullary collecting ducts was observed (fig. 3). This diminution in VP binding sites in the old kidney is in accord with the impaired urinary concentrating ability (Bengele et al., 1981) and reduced c-AMP generation of the old kidney (Beck and Yu, 1982). In addition, 24 hr VP excretion was found to be increased in the 25-month-old animals compared to the 3-month-old rats (Swaab et al., 1985b). Bengele et al. (1981) reported that the ability to conserve water in the kidney diminishes with age, and the same decrease was observed in senescent human subjects (Rowe et al., 1976). The maximum urinary concentrating ability is decreased in old subjects after VP administration and after water deprivation (Rowe et al., 1976), which suggests that the impairment is due to a decrease in renal response to VP. Bengele et al. (1981) found that the critical step for decrease in concentrating ability of old kidneys was significant impairment of water permeability across the epithelium of collecting ducts, even when normal circulating levels of VP were maintained.

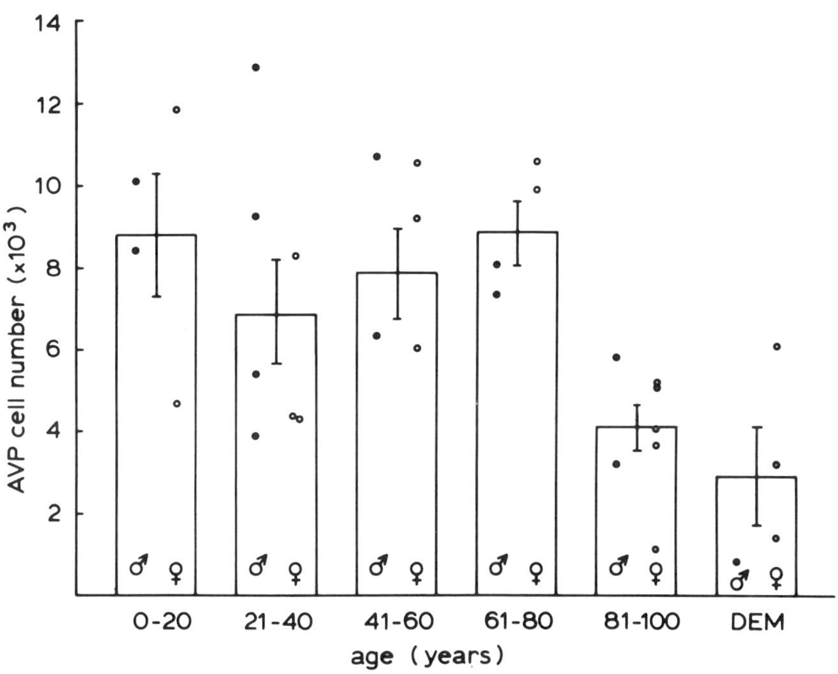

Fig. 1 - Suprachiasmatic nucleus vasopressin (AVP) cell number. Note the decrease in cell number in the oldest age group (81-100 years) and the strong decrease in the demented patients, in spite of their relatively young mean age (76 years). The vertical lines denote the SEM. (This figure is reproduced by permission from the paper: The suprachiasmatic nucleus of the human brain in relation to sex, age and dementia, Brain Research, 1985, in press).

These findings are in line with the increased activity of the vasopressin neurosecretory neuron and the enhanced VP blood levels in the old rat as described earlier (Fliers and Swaab, 1983). Urine production does not decrease at old age and the VP neuron activation in senescent rats thus seems to compensate for loss of VP receptors in the old kidney.

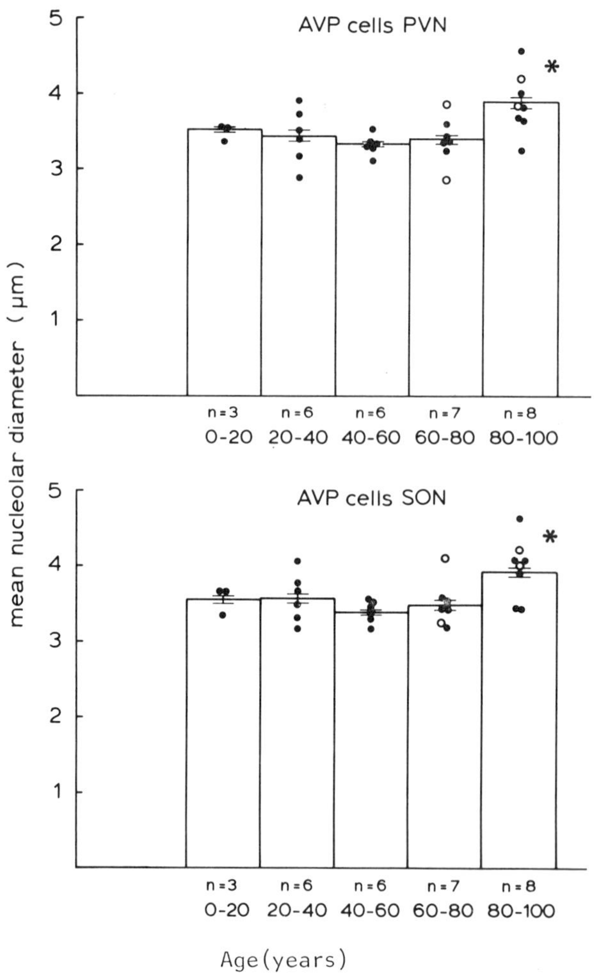

Fig. 2 - Mean nucleolar diameter of vasopressin (VP) cells in the Paraventricular Nucleus (PVN) and Supraoptic Nucleus (SON) as a function of age. There is a significant effect of age on mean nucleolar diameter of AVP cells. Values in the 80-100 year-old group are higher than the 20-80 year-old groups in the PVN and the 40-80 year-old groups in the SON, as indicated by the asterisk. Bars indicate mean values per two decades, vertical lines indicate SEM, n representing the number of brains examined in each age group. Open circles represent values from SDAT patients. (This figure is reproduced by permission from the paper: Activation of the vasopressin neurons of the human supraoptic and paraventricular nucleus in senescence and senile dementia, by Hoogendijk, J.E., Fliers, E., Swaab, D.F. and Verwer, R.W.H., J. of Neurol. Sci., 1985, in press).

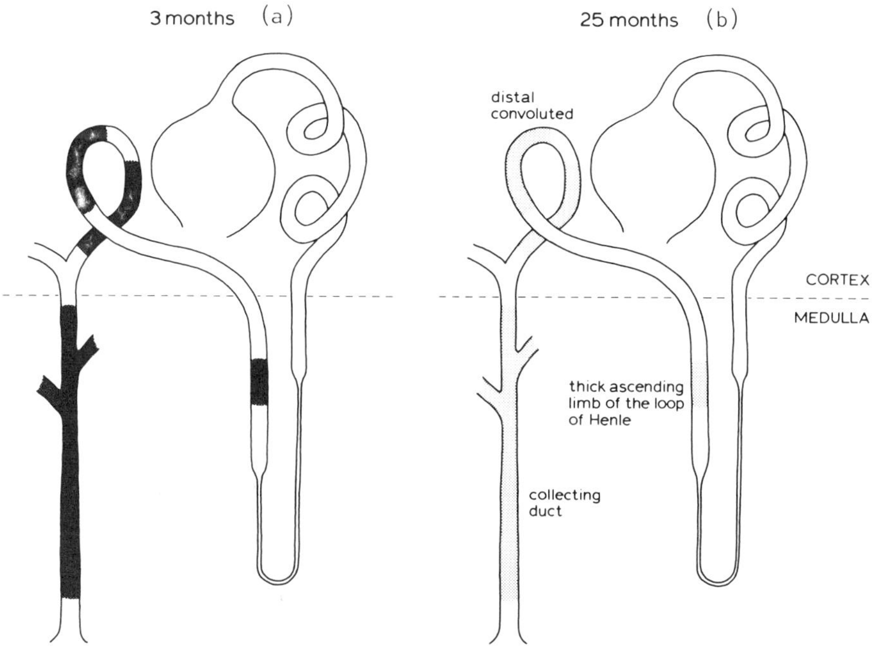

Fig. 3 - Schematic illustration of VP binding, revealed by an immunocytochemical staining method, in the kidney of Wistar rats of 3(a) and 25(b) months of age. The very intense staining of medullary collecting ducts is indicated in (a) and the weak and occasional staining of the same tubes in (b). This difference becomes most obvious when the kidney sections are incubated with 600 nM VP prior to staining with anti-VP antibody.

CONCLUSIONS

VP seems to act as a neurohormone when released from the neurohypophysis and as a neurotransmitter when released within the brain. It appears that neurosecretory VP neurons in the SON and PVN are activated in senescence, while patients with senile dementia of the Alzheimer type (SDAT) follow this curve in accordance with their age. In the SCN, on the other hand, a clear decrease in the amount of VP neurons was observed in SDAT. Depending on the area studied, the VP neuron is thus either activated or degenerated, and therefore little specific benefit might be derived from a general way of administration of exogenous VP during aging and dementia. Thus, our findings might explain the negative results of clinical trials involving VP administration to these patient groups (cf. Jolles, 1983). In addition, one should take into consideration that the primary cause of the VP neurosecretory activation seems to lie in the diminished VP binding in the kidney. Our findings also emphasize that SDAT can neither be regarded as merely a 'general degenerative process' of the brain, since VP cells in the SON and PVN are activated, nor as a 'cholinergic disease', in view of the clear changes in the SCN of VP-containing cells and the other SCN cells. These findings do not rule out beneficial effects of peptides during aging and dementia as a result of other, e.g., metabolic or trophic effects of neuropeptides or their analogues.

REFERENCES

Beck, N. and Yu, B.P., 1982, Effect of aging on urinary concentrating mechanism and vasopressin-dependent cAMP in rats, Am. J. Physiol., 243: F121-F125.

Bengele, H.H., Mathias, R.S., Perkins, J.H. and Alexander, E.A., 1981, Urinary concentrating defect in the aged rat, Am. J. Physiol., 240: F147-F150.

De Wied, D., 1983, Central actions of neurohypophyseal hormones. In: The Neurohypophysis: Structure, Function and Control, Progress in Brain Research, Vol. 60, B.A. Cross and G. Leng, Eds., Elsevier, Amsterdam.

Fliers, E. and Swaab, D.F., 1983, Activation of vasopressinergic and oxytocinergic neurons during aging in the Wistar rat. Peptides, 4: 165-170.

Fliers, E., Swaab, D.F., Pool, Chr.W. and Verwer, R.W.H., 1985, The vasopressin and oxytocin neurons in the human supraoptic and paraventricular nucleus; changes with aging and senile dementia, Brain Research, in press.

Frolkis, V.V., Golovchenko, S.F., Medved, V.I. and Frolkis, R.A., 1982, Vasopressin and cardiovascular system in aging, Gerontol., 28: 290-302.

Hoogendijk, J.E., Fliers, E., Swaab, D.F. and Verwer, R.W.H., 1985, Activation of vasopressin neurons in the human supraoptic and paraventricular nucleus in senescence and senile dementia, J. of Neurol. Sci., in press.

Jolles, J., 1983, Vasopressin-like peptides and the treatment of memory disorders in man, In: The Neurohypophysis: Structure, Function and Control, Progress in Brain Research, Vol. 60, Cross, B.A. and Leng, G., Eds., Elsevier, Amsterdam, 169-182.

Kirkland, J., Lye, M., Goddard, C., Vargas, E. and Davies, I., 1984, Arginine vasopressin in dehydrated elderly patients. Clin. Endocrinol., 20: 451-456,

Legros, J.J., 1975, Radioimmunoassay of human neurophysins: contribution to the understanding of the physiopathology of neurohypophyseal function. Ann. N.Y. Acad. Sci. 248: 281-303

Legros, J.J., Gilot, P., Schmitz, S., Bruwier, M., Mantanus, H., and Timsit-Berthier, M., 1980, Neurohypophyseal peptides and cognitive function: a clinical approach, In: Progress in Psychoneuroendocrinology, Brambilla, F., Racagni, G. and De Wied, D., Eds., Elsevier/North Holland Biomedical Press, 325-337.

Ravid, R., Swaab, D.F. and Pool, Chr.W., 1985, Immunocytochemical localization of vasopressin binding sites in the rat kidney. J. Endocrinol., in press.

Rowe, J.W., Shock, N.W. and De Fronzo, R.A., 1976, The influence of age on the renal response to water deprivation in man. Nephron, 17: 270-278.

Swaab, D.F., 1982, Neuropeptides. Their distribution and function in the brain. In: Chemical Transmission in the Brain. Progress in Brain Research, Vol. 55, Buijs, R.M., Pévet, P., and Swaab, D.F., Eds., Elsevier, Amsterdam, 97-122.

Swaab, D.F., Fliers, E. and Fisser, B., 1984, The vasopressin containing neuron in the human brain. Changes during aging and senile dementia. Proc. EURAGE Workshop 'Aging of the Brain and Senile Dementia: The Inventory of EEC Potentialities', D.L. Knook et al. Eds., Eurage, 71-78.

Swaab, D.F., Fliers, E. and Partiman, T.S., 1985a, The suprachiasmatic nucleus of the human brain in relation to sex, age and dementia, Brain Research, in press.

Swaab, D.F., Fliers, E. and Ravid, R., 1985b, The vasopressin neuron in the aging humand and rat brain. In: Proceedings of the conference: 'Comparative Aspects of Opioid and Related Neuropeptides', Sunny, U.S.A., in press.

Swaab, D.F., Fliers, E. and Van Gool, W.A., 1985c, Immunocytochemical localization of neuropeptides in the human brain; its consequences for therapeutic strategies in aging and dementia. In: Progress in Brain Research, in press.

Acknowledgements

We gratefully acknowledge the V.D. Houten Fund for supporting this research, The Dutch Gerentology Foundation for supporting the participation in the 30th Oholo Conference and Peter V. Niewkoop, G.U.D. Meulen and H. Stoffels for preparing the manuscript for publication.

CLINICAL HETEROGENEITY IN PATIENTS WITH DEMENTIA OF THE ALZHEIMER TYPE

Richard Mayeux and Yaakov Stern

Columbia University, College of Physicians and Surgeons
Neurological Institute, 710 West 168th Street, New York
New York 10032, USA

Clinical criteria for the diagnosis of dementia of the Alzheimer type (DAT) vary considerably in the current literature (1-4). Most investigators develop uniform criteria in order to be certain of homogeneity within a given cohort of patients for research purposes. Restricted criteria can lead to refinement in diagnosis, particularly when supported by careful postmortem verification (4-6). In view of this, several investigations are currently in progress to develop both qualitative and quantitative clinical and diagnostic measures for use in DAT.

The definite diagnosis of Alzheimer's disease requires postmortem confirmation, but in practice rigid clinical criteria can improve the pre-morbid diagnosis to nearly 90% (1). Such criteria may exclude atypical but recognized variations of DAT, and may not adequately reflect the range of severity of the disease. For example, patients with parietal lobe syndrome (7) or aphasia resulting from DAT can be excluded by current criteria.

Biochemical and pathological correlates of Alzheimer's disease vary with age at onset, family history of dementia, and the presence of myo-clonus (8). However, these clinical features have not been shown to be predictive of severity or other aspects of the disease. Myoclonus (9-11), and extrapyramidal signs (12-14) such as rigidity, simian posture, and bradykinesia have been observed in patients with DAT and autopsy verified Alzheimer's disease, and do not represent an exclusionary criteria in most studies. These motor manifestations suggest some degree of heterogeneity in the diagnosis of DAT. We investigated the possibility that patients with these motor manifestations or other unique clinical features might represent subgroups of DAT that would progress at different rates. Our hypothesis was that this heterogeneity would have important prognostic implications.

METHODS

Subjects

We reviewed the records of 138 patients who met our research criteria for DAT. These included: 1) intellectual impairment for at least 6 months; 2) objective evidence of dementia on neuropsychological testing; and 3) the diagnostic criteria from the Diagnostic and Statistical Manual of Mental Disorders, Third edition (DSM-III) (15).

We excluded patients with any of the following: 1) affective disorder within one year of onset of dementia; 2) history or signs of Parkinson's disease prior to onset of dementia; 3) history of stroke or a Hachinski Ischemic score >5 (16); 4) history of cancer, cardiac, hepatic, pulmonary, or renal disease or anoxia; 5) seizures prior to onset of dementia. Computed tomography and EEG excluded focal lesions and periodicity. Other possible causes of dementia were excluded by the appropriate studies.

Procedure

Neurological assessment included history of the present illness, review of past medical and neurological histories, and family history, all obtained from a family member or patient advocate. The neurological examination included a modified version of the Columbia University Parkinson's disease rating scale (17), and the Columbia University dyskinesia rating scale. Ability to perform functional activities of daily life were rated and scored on the Blessed Dementia Rating Scale (18) (BDRS).

Neurospychological assessment included a modified version of the Mini-Mental State Examination (mMMS, 19-20). Aphasic, mute, and uncooperative patients were so designated. Psychiatric assessment included a semi-structured interview to derive symptoms of depression and psychosis using guidelines from the DSM-III (15) and the Brief Psychiatric Rating Scale (21). These excluded patients with affective disorder and schizophrenia.

In order to investigate the prognostic utility of clinical symptoms, a subset of the patients were included in a longitudinal analysis. We reviewed the records and later evaluations of 62 of the original 138 patients. These were subjects followed exclusively at this institution. We chose to include only those subjects evaluated on at least two occasions at least 6 months apart for this analysis.

Data Entry and Statistical Analysis

All information was entered into a data base. Historical and demographic information was collected at the initial evaluation. All neurological and psychiatric information derived from each visit was entered and dated appropriately. Data collected from the first visit of the 138 patients was used to isolate clinical factors that might differentiate patient performance on the mMMS or the BDRS. These factors were then used to predict decline in intellectual performance and functional capacity in the longitudinal analysis of data for the 62 patients. Differences in the progression of mMMS and BDRS scores in patients with distinguishing features were investigated to test the hypothesis that certain motor manifestations might segregate subgroups.

RESULTS

Initial Assessment

The mean age of the patients was 68.9 (± 9.7). The mMMS and BDRS scores varied widely, yet correlated ($r=-0.54$, $p<.001$) and were related to symptom duration ($r=-0.23$ & 0.2 respectively, $p<.01$). mMMS also correlated with education $r=0.34$, $p<.001$). Surprisingly age and age at onset did not related to mMMS or BDRS scores.

Thirty-six (25.9%) of the patients had extrapyramidal signs considered unrelated to the use of psychotropic medications. Twelve additional patients had extrapyramidal signs deemed secondary to medications. Rigidity and bradykinesia were most frequently observed, and tremor was rare. As a group, patients with extrapyramidal signs did not differ from the others in terms of age, age at onset, or duration of symptoms. However, mMMS scores were significantly lower and BDRS scores higher in both groups (sporadic and drug-induced).

Twelve (11.5%) of the patients had myoclonus. These patients did not differ from others with regard to age, education, or duration of symptoms, but were younger at age of onset. Myoclonus and extrapyramidal signs coexisted in 5 patients. mMMS scores were significantly lower and BDRS scores higher in patients with myoclonus with or without extrapyramidal signs.

Longitudinal Analysis

By definition, these 62 patients had been re-examined at least 6 months after the initial evaluation. Most had more than one subsequent visit over a period spanning 4 years. In comparison to the original cohort this group was slightly younger (66.7 $\pm$ 9.3) and had lower BDRS scores.

We found evidence of four distinct groups: 1) typical DAT (n=16); 2) DAT with extrapyramidal signs (n=14) or drug-induced extrapyramidal signs (n=16); 3) DAT with myoclonus (n=9); and 4) DAT-benign (n=7). Patients were classified into subgroups if they displayed signs noted above at any time during the follow-up.

Patients with extrapyramidal signs or myoclonus at their initial visit had significantly lower mean mMMS and higher mean BDRS scores as a group at the last evaluation point ($p<.01$ for both measures). They also experienced a more rapid change in these measures over time compared to the typical DAT patient. Patients with drug-induced extrapyramidal signs deteriorated even more rapidly. In contrast, 7 of the 23 patients with typical DAT appeared to remain relatively stable over the time period and were subclassified as DAT-benign. mMMS and BDRS scores for the "benign" patients were significantly better than in the rest of the cohort at the final visit ($p<.001$).

Other factors were also evaluated for their value in predicting the clinical course of DAT. Family history and age at onset did not differentiate patients over the period of study. However, patients with evidence of thought disorder such as organic delusions or hallucinations (15) also deteriorated more rapidly over the time period (mMMS, $p<.01$; BDRS, $p<.05$).

DISCUSSION

We found clinical evidence to support the existence of 4 unique subgroups of DAT: extrapyramidal (sporadic and drug-induced), myoclonic, benign, and typical. However, a study of this type is difficult to interpret without postmortem verification of the diagnosis of DAT in each patient and within each subgroup. To date, four patients from the longitudinal study have died and Alzheimer's disease has been confirmed in all. However, given the clinical criteria we have chosen and the experience of other investigators who have used similar criteria, we expect our diagnostic accuracy to be about 90%.

The observation of myoclonus, extrapyramidal signs, and minimal progression in patients with DAT and postmortem confirmed Alzheimer's disease is not new (3,9-14), but the relationship of these signs to the course of DAT has not been critically examined.

Pearce (12) originally described extrapyramidal signs in patients suspected of having Alzheimer's disease. No pathological confirmation of diagnosis was ever reported, and the impact on the course was never described. A recent retrospective review of the records of patients found to have Alzheimer's disease at postmortem revealed clinical evidence of parkinsonism (14). More detailed examination of the brains also indicated the presence of Lewy bodies and degenerative changes within the substantia nigra in that study, and Perl et al (23) have made similar observations. Investigators have suggested that some patients have both Alzheimer's and Parkinson's disease (24-27). Demented parkinsonians are alleged to have increased neurofibrillary tangles and neuritic plaques, and cell loss in the basal forebrain cholinergic complex at postmortem examination (28). Biochemical changes in the cerebral cortex (29-30) and the clinical manifestations of dementia in Parkinson's disease (31) are remarkably similar to those observed in Alzheimer's disease.

Patients in this investigation with DAT and extrapyramidal signs probably do not have Parkinson's disease. Extrapyramidal signs were subtle and would not warrant that diagnosis. These signs never antedated the onset of dementia. We consider this subgroup to represent a more severe form of DAT, but its pathological and biochemical correlates remain to be determined. This group was further distinguished by psychosis occurring more frequently than in other subgroups; family history of dementia was also more prevalent. Unfortunately, drug-induced extrapyramidal signs were associated with an even more rapid deterioration.

Bird et al (8), found that the presence of myoclonus in patients with DAT was the best predictor of the amount of choline acetyltransferase activity found at postmortem. Myoclonus has been considered to occur late in Alzheimer's disease and to be associated with a more rapid evolution (9,10). We did not find a difference in duration of illness in our patients, but they were younger at the onset of the disease and the progression of symptoms was significantly more rapid. Two patients in this subgroup have had postmortem examinations confirming the diagnosis of Alzheimer's disease. In one, reported earlier (11), dementia, mutism and myoclonus began simultaneously and progressed to death within a 2 year period. Mutism and coincident muscular rigidity was noted in our groups and also described by Jacob (9).

The "benign" group is unusual. Over a four year period the progression of dementia was minimal. This group, distinct from Kral's description of "benign senescent forgetfulness" (32), met criteria for DAT but continues to function quite well compared to other patients. This could represent a milder form of the disease, such as the "simple" dementia (33). Perhaps a more likely explanation is that the rate of deterioration is simply slower than that seen in more typical DAT. Berg et al (34) also found that some patients progressed very little during a one year follow up study; this could be predicted by the initial neuropsychological test performance. One patient in our "benign" group deteriorated rapidly after seven years. This was associated with the onset of severe delusions. The "benign" group was not segregated by age, age at onset, or any other factor except progression of illness. Longitudinal studies should help to clarify the pathogenesis of this form of DAT.

The majority of our patients had no clinical manifestations other than dementia. This more typical form of DAT progressed as expected over the follow up period. In the few patients with initial high mMMS and preserved BDRS scores the eventual rate of deterioration was similar to that observed in other patients within the "typical" subgroup.

Data presented here imply that DAT may be a more heterogeneous disorder than previously considered, despite the use of relatively restricted criteria. We have demonstrated that consideration of certain motor manifestations and psychiatric features may aid in determining the prognosis in DAT. However, we have not addressed the pathological or biochemical issues raised by these observations. Future studies of this cohort will be essential to substantiate our conclusions.

ACKNOWLEDGMENTS

Support for this investigation was provided by the Charles S. Robertson Memorial Gift for research in Alzheimer's disease and grants from the National Institutes of Health (AG-02802 & RR-00645).

REFERENCES

1. Eisendorfer C, Cohen D: Diagnostic criteria for primary neuronal degeneration of the Alzheimer type. J Fam Pract 1980;2:553-7.
2. Hughes CP, Berg L, Danziger WL, Coben LA, Martin RD: A new clinical scale for the staging of dementia. Brit J Psychiat 1982; 140:566-72.
3. Berg L, Hughes CP, Coben LA, Danziger WL, Martin RL, Knesevich J: Mild senile dementia of the Alzheimer type: Research diagnostic criteria,recruitment and description of a study population. J Neurol Neurosurg Psychiat 1982;45:962-8.
4. Todorov AB, Go RCP, Constantinidis J, Elston RC: Specificity of the clinical diagnosis of dementia. J Neurol Sci 1975;26:81-98.
5. Ron MA, Toone BK, Graralda ME, Lishman WA: Diagnostic Accuracy in presenile dementia. Brit J Psychiat 1979: 161-8.
6. Sulka R, Matti H, Paetan A, Wikstom J, Palo J: Accuracy of clinical diagnosis in primary degenerative dementia: Correlation with neuropathological findings. J Neurol Neurosurg Psychiat 1983;46:9-13.
7. Crystal HA, Horoupian DS, Katzman R, Jotkowitz S: Biopsy-proven Alzheimer disease presenting as a right parietal lobe syndrome. Ann Neurol 1982; 12:186-8.
8. Bird TD, Stranahan S, Sumi M, Raskind M: Alzheimer's disease and choline acetyltransferase activity in brain tissue from clinical and pathological subgroups. Ann Neurol 1983;14:284-93.
9. Jacob H: Muscular twitching in Alzheimer's disease. In: Wolstenholme GEW, O'Conner M, eds. Alzheimer's disease and related conditions. London: Churchill. 1970: 75-93.
10. Faden AL, Townsend JJ: Myoclonus in Alzheimer's disease. Arch Neurol 1976; 33:278-80.
11. Mayeux R, Hunter S, Fahn S: More on myoclonus in Alzheimer's disease. Ann Neurol 1980;8:200.
12. Pearce J: The extrapyramidal disorder of Alzheimer's disease. Europ Neurol 1974; 12:94-103.
13. Molsa PK, Martilla R, Rinne UK: Extrapyramidal signs in Alzheimer's disease. Neurology 1984; 34:1114-6.
14. Leverenz J, Sumi SM: Prevalence of Parkinson's disease in patients with Alzheimer's disease. Neurology 1984; 34:101.

15. American Psychiatric Association, Diagnostic and Statistical Manual of Mental Disorders, Third Edition, Washington, D.C. 1980, pp.205-24.
16. Hachinski VC, Iliff LD, Zhilka E, duBoulay GHD, McAllister VC, Marshall J, Russell RWR, Symon L: Cerebral blood flow in dementia. Arch Neurol 1975;32: 632-7.
17. Lesser RP, Fahn S, Snider SR, Cote LJ, Isgreen WP, Barrett RE: Analysis for the clinical problems in parkinsonism and the complications of long-term levodopa therapy. Neurology 1979;29: 1253-60.
18. Blessed G, Tomlinson BE, Roth M: The association between quantitative measures of dementia and of senile changes in the cerebral grey matter of elderly subjects. Brit J Psychiat 1968;225:797-811.
19. Folstein MF, Folstein SE, McHugh PR: "Mini-Mental State" a practical method for grading the cognitive state of patients for the clinician. J Psychiatr Res 1975; 12:189-98.
20. Mayeux R, Stern Y, Rosen J, Leventhal J: Depression, intellectual impairment and Parkinson's disease. Neurology 1981;31:645-50.
21. Overall JE, Groham DR: The Brief Psychiatric Rating Scale. Psychol Rep 1962;10:799-812.
22. Rosenblum WI, Ghatak NR: Lewy bodies in the presence of Alzheimer's disease. Arch Neurol 1979:36:170-1.
23. Perl DP, Pendlebury WW, Bird ED: Detailed neuropathological evaluation of banked brain specimens submitted with a clinical diagnosis of Alzheimer's disease. In: Wurtman RJ, Corkin SH, Growdon JH, eds. Alzheimer's Disease: Advances in Basic Research and Therapies. Center for Brain Sciences and Metabolism Charitable Trust: Zurich, 1984:463.
24. Alvord EC: The pathology of parkinsonism: etiologic, pathogenetic and pronostic implications. Trans Am Neurol Assoc 1965;90:167-8.
25. Alvord EC, Forno LS, Kusske JA, Kauffman RJ, Rhodes JS, Goetowski CR: The pathology of parkinsonism: A comparison of degeneration in the cerebral; cortex and brain stem. Adv Neurol 1975;5:175-93.
26. Hakim AM, Mathieson G: Dementia in Parkinson disease: A neuropathologic study. Neurology 1979;29:1209-14.
27. Boller F, Mizutani T, Roessmann V, Gambetti P: Parkinson disease, dementia, and Alzheimer disease: Clinicopathological correlations. Ann Neurol 1980;1:329-35.
28. Whitehouse P, Hedreen JC, White C, DeLong M, Price DL: Basal forebrain neurons in the dementia of Parkinson's disease. Ann Neurol 1983;13:243-8.
29. Ruberg M, Ploska A, Javoy-Agid F, Agid Y: Muscarinic binding and choline acetyltransferase activity in parkinsonian subjects with reference to dementia. Brain Res 1982;232:129-33.
30. Perry RH, Tomlinson BE, Candy JM, Blessed G, Foster JF, Blaxham CA, Perry E: Cortical cholinergic deficit in mentally impaired parkinsonian patients. Lancet 1983; 309:789-90.
31. Mayeux R, Stern Y, Rosen J, Benson DF: Is subcortical dementia a recognizable clinical entity? Ann Neurol 1983;14:278-83.
32. Kral VA: Benign Senescent forgetfulness. In: Katzman R, Terry RD, Bick KL, eds. Alzheimer's disease: Senile dementia and related disorders. New York: Raven Press, 1978:47-51.
33. Tagliavini F, Pilleri G: Neuronal counts in basal nucleus of Meynert in Alzheimer disease and in simple senile dementia. Lancet 1983;1:469-70.
34. Berg L, Danziger WL, Storandt M, Coben LA, Gado M, Hughes CP, Knesevich JW, Botwinick J: Predictive features in mild senile dementia of the Alzheimer type. Neurology 1984;34:563-9.

PATTERNS OF COGNITIVE IMPAIRMENT IN PATIENTS WITH ALZHEIMER'S DISEASE AND PARKINSON'S DISEASE: ARE THEY SIMILAR OR DIFFERENT?

Bracha Mildworf, Mordechai Globus and Eldad Melamed

Laboratory for Cerebrovascular Research, Department of Neurology, Hadassah University Hospital, Jerusalem, Israel

INTRODUCTION

Cognitive impairment is the hallmark of Alzheimer's disease (AD) and is caused by pathological and biochemical changes in the brain. There is a correlation between the number of senile plaques and neurofibrillary tangles and extent of cholinergic neuronal degeneration and the severity of AD dementia[1,2]. In Parkinson's disease (PD) the main feature is a movement disorder which may be accompanied by cognitive impairment[3,4,5,6]. The causes for the dementia in PD are undetermined[6]. It may be due to superimposed AD in PD patients[7,8]. This view is supported by similarities in pattern of the cognitive impairment in AD and PD patients reported by some but not all investigators[7,8]. In addition, there is a high prevalence of "Alzheimer-like" changes[9], and degeneration of neuronal perikaria in the nucleus basalis of Meynert and of the innominato-cortical cholinergic neurons in PD brains[10,11,12]. However, some authors suggest that the characteristics of the dementia in PD are different from those of AD and are of "subcortical" origin[13,14]. Also, in some demented PD patients, there was no evidence for senile plaques and neurofibrillary tangles post-mortem[15]. The latter raises the possibility that the cognitive impairment in Ad an PD are not identical and may be caused by different mechanisms. To gain more information on this controversial issue we have now examined whether the pattern of cognitive dysfunction is similar or different in AD and PD patients.

METHODS

Subjects: This study included 96 PD patients (age range 38-80, mean 65 years), 23 AD patients (age range 45-86, mean 66 years) and 41 age-matched normal controls (age range 48-80, mean 65 years), matched for level of education. All subjects underwent a detailed neuropsychological evaluation.

Neuropsychological test battery: All tests were performed in a quiet, well-illuminated room, without time limitation and the motor component was reduced to exclude possible effect of bradykinesia on the results in all tests. The neuropsychological battery included the following tests: specific cognitive functions:

A. Minimental test[16] . B. A set of tests for specific cognitive functions: 1. Memory: Short-term visual memory was tested using the Benton test[17] short term verbal memory was assessed using the Super-Span test[18] and long term memory was evaluated using questions relating to important events from the past. 2. Language: The following components were included: auditory comprehension, verbal expression, object naming, abstraction, reading and writing. Fluency was assessed by categorial naming and the F.A.S. test[19]. 3. Hooper test: To mainly test visual-spatial perception, and perceptual organization[20]. 4. Drawing: The subject had to draw from memory a clock and a house. Afterwards he had to copy a three-dimensional house and a clock[19]. The abilities required include constructional skills, visual-spatial perception, perceptual organization, visual copying and spatial memory. 5. Block design: Subjects arrange blocks manually to match a design displayed in a test booklet[21]. Abilities required include constructional skills, visual-spatial perception, spatial orientation and information processing. 6. Trail-making test: The test used was a version of the trail-making B[22]. Subjects draw lines to interconnect, as rapidly as possible, a sequence of ascending numbers and letters, alternating between the two sequences. Abilities required include visual-spatial perception, visuo-motor coordination and the concept of set shifting. 7. Paced Auditory Serial Additon Test (PASAT): This test examines the ability of simple calculation by the addition of numbers heard during three-trails. In each trial a different time interval was given between the numbers, ranging from 2.5 to 1.5 seconds[18].

RESULTS

In normal subjects (age range 48-80), advancing age did not affect cognitive functions except for some mild decrease in attention (r=0.40; p= 0.008) and in recent memory (r=0.46; p= 0.002) in the elderly subjects (Figure 1)

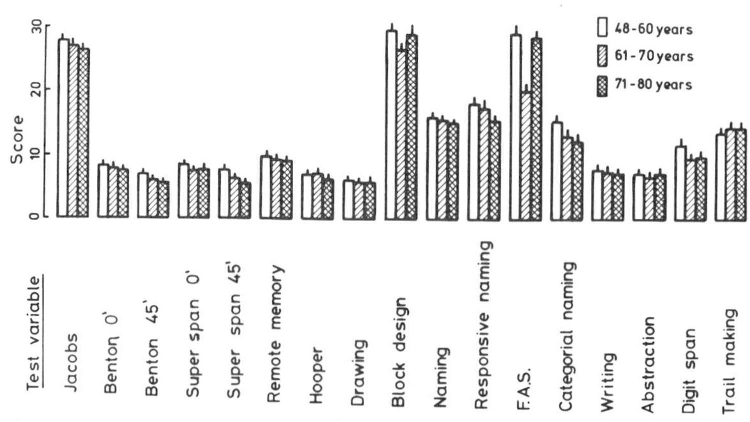

Figure 1: Cognitive functions in various age groups of normal control subjects (age-range 48-80 years) Advancing age did not affect cognitive functions except for some mild decrease in attention, recent memory, and categorial naming.

AD patients showed impaired performance in all tests (Figure 2).

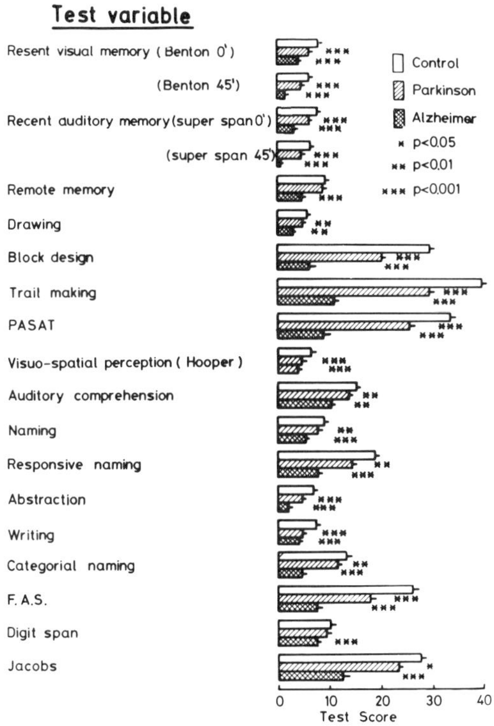

Figure 2: Cognitive functions in controls, parkinsonian patients and Alzheimer's patients.

Transformation of data to z-scores showed that verbal memory, remote memory, naming, abstraction and shifting and maintaining a task, were particularly impaired (Figure 3).

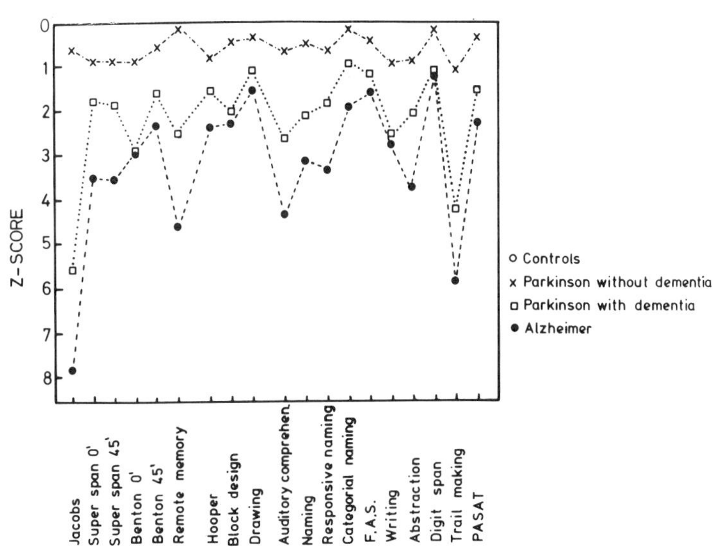

Figure 3: Pattern of cognitive functions in Alzheimer patients, Parkinsonians with dementia (minimental test < 21), and in Parkinsonians without dementia (minimental test > 21).

As a whole group, PD patients were different from both age-matched controls and AD patients. They displayed poorer performance on most tests as compared with controls. Remote memory and attention were, however, preserved (Figure 2). PD patients performed better than AD patients in all tests (Figure 2).

PD patients were divided into two subgroups according to their performance on the minimental test (Jacobs). The first group (66%) included patients without dementia, (minimental > 21) and the second (34%) patients with dementia (minimental < 21). The first group did not differ from the controls on most of the tests except for specific dysfunctions in recent memory, visuo-spatial organization, and shifting and maintaining a task (Figure 3). The demented subgroup exhibited a global deterioration in all tests as compared with controls. Pattern was similar to that of AD patients except for recent verbal memory, remote memory, abstraction and categorial naming, which were relatively preserved (Figure 3).

DISCUSSION

There are conflicting views concerning the effects of normal aging on cognition[23]. Our study suggests that there is almost no deterioration in the intelectual functions during advancing age except for a mild decrease in attention, recent memory and categorial naming. Our AD patients were markedly impaired in all neuropsychological tests as compared with age-matched normal control subjects. They also performed worse than PD patients in all tests. Among the various tests, verbal memory, remote memory, naming and abstraction were relatively more impaired whereas attention drawing and fluency were relatively less abnormal. As a whole group, our PD patients showed cognitive impairment in all tests (except for attention and remote memory) as compared with normal age-matched subjects. They performed better than the AD group on all tests. Similar results were reported by Gainotti et al[24].

Based on the minimental test, two subgroups of PD patients can be identified i.e. demented and non-demented. The non-demented PD subjects showed impairment only in recent memory, visual-spatial perception and shifting and maintaining a task. Such pattern of cognitive impairment is compatible with that described by several authors in subcortical dementia[14,25,26]. The demented PD patients showed a global cognitive deterioration. However, when pattern of their performance is compared with that of the AD subjects, they were relatively better on verbal recent memory, remote memory, naming and abstraction. It seems therefore that the dementia in PD is not entirely identical to that of AD. There are other indices for such a discrepancy[27,28,30]. For instance, the regional cerebral blood flow is reduced in both AD[28] and PD[29]. However, there is a correlation between the extent of flow reduction and the severity of the dementia only in AD but not in PD[30,31]. Likewise, there is a correlation between the severity of dementia to central atrophy in PD[32] and to cortical atrophy in AD. All these do not rule out the possibility that the dementia in PD is due to superimposed AD of lesser severity, or that AD occurs only in some, but not all PD patients. Clarification of this controversial issue can be acheived only by development of more sensitive and specific neuropsychological tests and by combined post-mortem studies.

ACKNOWLEDGEMENT

Supported, in part, by the Lena P. Harvey Endowment Fund for Neurological Research.

REFERENCES

1. G. Blessed, B.E. Tomilson, M. Roth, The association between quantitative measures of dementia and senile change in the cerebral grey matter of elderly subjects. Brit. J. Psychiat. 114:797 (1968).
2. P.J. Whitehouse, D.L. Price, R.G. Struble, A.W. Glark, J.T. Coyle, Alzheimer's disease and senile dementia-loss of neurons in the basal forebrain. Science 218:1237 (1982).
3. M. Pollock and R.W. Hornabrook, The prevalence, natural history and dementia of Parkinson's disease. Brain 89:429 (1966).
4. A. Liberman, M. Dziatolowski, M. Kupersmith et al. Dementia in Parkinson disease. Ann. Neurol. 6:355 (1979)
5. F.J. Pirozzolo, E.C. Hansch, J.A. Mortimer, D.D. Webster, M.A. Kuskowski, Dementia in Parkinson disease: a neuropsychological analysis. Brain & Cognition 1:71 (1982)
6. R. Mayeux and Y. Stern, Intellectual dysfunction and dementia in Parkinson disease in: The Dementia, R. Mayeux and W.G. Rosen, eds. Raven Press, New York (1983) pp 211-227.
7. F. Boller, T. Mizutani, U. Roessman, P. Gambetti, Parkinson disease, dementia and alzheimer disease: clinicopathological correlation. Ann. Neurol. 7: 329 (1980)
8. S. Corkin, J.H. Growdon, M.J. Nissen, Comparison of the dementia in Parkinson disease and Alzheimer disease: VII the International Symposium on Parkinson disease. Frankfurt,1982.
9. A.M. Hakim and G. Mathieson, Dementia in Parkinson disease: A neuropathologic study. Neurology 29:1209 (1979)
10. J.M. Candy, R.H. Perry, E.K. Perry, et al. Pathological changes in the nucleus of Meynery in Alzheimer's and Parkinson's disease. J. Neurol. Sci. 59:277 (1983).
11. M. Ruberg, A. Ploska, F.J. Agid, Y. Agid, Muscarinic binding and choline acetyltransferase activity in parkinsonian subjects, with reference to dementia. Brain Res. 232:129 (1982).
12. P.J. Whitehouse, J.C. Hedreen, C.L. White, D.L. Price, Basal forebrain neurons in the dementia of Parkinson disease.Ann. Neurol.13:243 (1983).
13. M.L. Albert, Subcortical dementia. In: R. Katzman, R.D. Terry, K.L. Bick, eds. Alzheimer disease: senile dementia and related disorders (Aging, Vol. 7). New York, Raven Press, (1978) pp 173-80.
14. F. Boller, D. Passafune, N.C. Keefe, K. Rogers, L. Morrow, Y. Kim, Visuospatial impariments in Parkinson's disease. Arch. Neurol. 41: 485, (1984).
15. I. Nakano and A. Hirano, Parkinson's disease: neuron loss in the nucleus basalis without concomitant Alzheimer's disease. Ann. Neurol. 15:415 (1984).
16. J.W. Jacobs, M.R. Bernhard, A. Delgado, J. Strain, Screening for organic mential syndromes in the medically ill. Ann. Int. Med.86: 40 (1977).
17. A.L. Benton, A multiple choice type of visual retention test. Arch of Neurol. Psych. 64:699 (1950).
18. D. Gronivall, P. Wrightson, Delayed recovery of intellectual functions after minor head injuries. Lancet 2:605 (1974).
19. H. Goodglass, E. Kaplan, The assessment of aphasia and related disord disorders. Philadelphia, Lea & Febiger (1972).
20. H.E. Hooper, The Hooper visual organization test manual, California: Western Psychological Services (1958).
21. D. Wechsler, The measurement and appraisal of adult intelligence. Baltimore, Williams & Wilkins (1958).
22. R.M. Reitan, T.J. Boll, Intellectual and cognitive functions in Parkinson's disease. J. Cons. Clin. Psycho. 37:364, (1971).

23. N.A. Kramer and L. F. Jarvik, Assessment of intellectual changes in the elderly, in: Psychiatric symptoms and cognitive loss in the the elderly. Washington D.C. (1979) pp. 221-271.
24. G. Gainotti, C. Caetragirone, C. Masullo , G. Micelli, Pattern of neuropsychological impairment in various diagnostic groups of dementia in:Aging of the brain and dementia. Amaduci (ed), (1980) pp. 131-244.
25. F. Bowen, Behavioral alteration in patients with basal ganglia lesions (ed.) M.D. Yahr, The Basal Ganglia, Raven Press, N.Y. (1976).
26. R. Mayeux, Y. Stern, J. Rosen, D.F. Benson, Subcortical dementia: A recognizable clinical entity. Trans. Am. Neurol. Assoc. 106:313 (1981).
27. E.E. Alvord, L.S. Forno, J.A. Kusske, et al. The pathology of parkinsonism: A comparison of degeneration in cerebral cortex and brain stem. Advances in Neurology, 5:1175 (1974).
28. W.D. Obrist, E. Chivian, S. Cronquist, D.H. Ingvar, Regional cerebral blood flow in senile and presenile dementia. Neurology 20:315,(1970).
29. S. Lavy, E. Melamed, S. Bentin et al. , rCBF in patients with Pakrinson's disease. Arch. Neurology 36:344 (1979).
30. M. Globus, B. Mildworf, E. Globus, rCBF changes in Parkinson's disease correlation with dementia, Neurology, in press(1985).
31. R. Portin, R. Rainink and U.K. Rinne, Dementia and brain atrophy in Parkinsonism. Paper presented at the VII th International Symposium on Parkinson Disease. Frankfurt (1982).
32. E. Melamed, M. Globus and B. Mildworf, Non invasive measurements and regional cerebral blood flow in man: effect of normal aging and dementia. in: Alzheimer's disease: Advances in Basic research and therapies, ed: R.J. Wurtman, S.H. Corkin and J.H. Growdon, in press, (1985).

RISK FACTORS IN ALZHEIMER'S DISEASE

Barclay, LL, Kheyfets, S, Zemcov, A, Blass, and JP, McDowell, FH

The Burke Rehabilitation Center
Cornell University Medical Center
White Plains, New York, U.S.A.

ABSTRACT

The role of specific risk factors for Alzheimer's disease (AD) is undefined. We compared medical histories in 259 patients with clinically diagnosed AD with those in cognitively intact patients (CI;n=36). The two groups were comparable in age (mean±SEM 73.3±0.6 in AD, 70.9 ±2.1 in CI), race (>95% white), and socioeconomic status, although they differed in male:female ratio (1:2 in AD; 1.6:1 in CI). Stroke was more common in CI (11.1% vs 1.5%, p=.006), presumably because demented patients with stroke tend to be diagnosed as multi-infarct dementia rather than AD. Family history for dementia was positive in 35.9% of AD patients, but only 5.6% of CI patients (p<0.001). Family history of other genetic disorders was more often positive in AD than in CI, but these differences were not statistically significant (thyroid disease in 1.5% vs 0%; Down's in 0.8% vs 0%, and congenital malformations in 1.2% vs 0%). Other factors previously implicated in AD were not significantly more common in AD than in CI (head trauma in 4.2% vs 8.3%; peptic ulcers (presumably with aluminum-containing antacid use) in 5.8% vs 8.3%, alcoholism in 0.7% vs 0%, job-related toxic exposures in 1.5% vs 0%, and thyroid disease in 2.3% vs 0%). There were also no significant differences in prevalence of cancer; lung, biliary, or gastrointestinal disease; or arthritis. These data suggest that genetic factors are more important than environmental ones in the pathogenesis of AD, although case-control studies of large numbers of subjects are needed to determine if small differences in exposure to environmental factors are statistically significant.

INTRODUCTION

Risk factors for Alzheimer's disease (AD) are undefined, although both genetic and environmental factors have been implicated. Familial aggregation in AD has been well-described (1,2,3), and life-table analysis used to adjust for competing risks in an aging population suggests that the 90-year lifetime incidence of dementia approaches 50% in siblings and children of agraphic probands with AD (4). Genetic predisposition to AD is also suggested by an excess of Down's syndrome and immunoproliferative disorders in relatives of patients with AD (2,5,6), although these findings have not been confirmed by other studies (7).

Environmental risk factors for AD are well-documented. Thyroid disease (3,8), organic solvents (9,10), aluminum (11,12), head trauma (8), and herpes zoster infection (8), have all been proposed,, but the evidence is far from compelling. Determining genetic and environmental risk factors for AD might elucidate the pathogenesis of this disorder, might identify groups at high risk to develop AD, and might even lead to avoidance of environmental exposures that might trigger the disease. We therefore compared the prevalence of familial traits and environmental exposures in patients with AD and in cognitively intact controls.

METHODS

Patient Evaluation: All patients were seen and followed in an outpatient dementia clinic, described in detail elsewhere (13), and had a complete medical, neurological, psychiatric, and laboratory evaluation including head CTT and EEG. Patient data were entered in a computerized data base (13). Patients and their relatives and/or caretaker were questioned carefully as to medical and family history, and detailed pedigrees were obtained whenever possible. Psychometric rating scales included the mental status quotient (MSQ) measuring recent memory and orientation (14), the modified Hachinski ischemic score measuring the likelihood of ischemic dementia (15), and the Haycox scale measuring behavioral impairment (16).

Diagnostic Criteria: Patients with treatable cases of dementia were excluded. Patients with Alzheimer's disease (AD;n=259) had a duration of illness of at least 6 months, mental status quotient score (MSQ) (14), $\leq$ 7/10, and no superimposed delirium, and met consensus criteria for "probable Alzheimer's disease" (17). Cognitively intact subjects (n=36) were also referred to our clinic, but had no cognitive or behavioral evidence of dementia on thorough evaluation, and had MSQ $\geq$ 9/10.

Statistical Analysis: Statistical significance of differences between groups was determined using chi-square, with Yates correction for sample size <5, or unpaired t-test.

RESULTS

Patients with AD were similar to controls in age (mean$\pm$SEM 73.3$\pm$0.6 vs 70.9$\pm$2.1 and racial composition (>95% white). Male:female ratio was 1:2 in AD and 1.6:1 in controls. Modified Hachinski score measuring vascular markers was higher in controls (3.6$\pm$0.5 vs 1.5$\pm$0.1; P<0.001), presumably because demented patients with prominent markers for vascular disease tend to be diagnosed as multi-infarct dementia or as mixed dementia rather than as AD. As expected, MSQ was significantly higher in controls (9.5$\pm$0.2 vs 3.0$\pm$0.2; P<0.001) and Haycox behavioral impairment score was significantly lower (1.3$\pm$0.0 vs 15.8$\pm$0.6, P<0.001).

Past medical history of stroke was significantly more common in controls than in patients with AD (11.1% vs 1.5%, P=0.006), presumably because demented patients with stroke tend to be diagnosed as multi-infarct dementia. Past medical history of other neurological disorders, including brain tumor, Parkinson's disease, amyotrophic lateral sclerosis, meningitis, poliomyelitis, epilepsy, Guillain-Barre, myasthenia gravis, and Bell's palsy, was not significantly different in the two groups. Past history of head trauma was present in 4.2% of patients with AD and in 9.1% of controls.

Past or present history of depression was significantly higher in patients with AD (13.9% vs 2.8%, P<0.05). Prevalence of other psychiatric disorders was not significantly different in the two groups; neither was prevalence of cardiovascular, immunoproliferative, respiratory, gastrointestinal, endocrine, orthopedic, rheumatic, urological, or gynecological disorders. History of thyroid disease was present in 2.3% of patients with AD and in no controls, but this difference was not statistically significant. Peptic ulcer disease, which might be associated with increased exposure to aluminum-containing materials, did not differ in prevalence in the two groups (5.8% in AD and 8.3% in controls). History of job-related toxic exposure was present in 4 patients with AD (1.5%) and in no controls (not significant). History of herpes zoster infection was positive in no patients with AD and in one control (2.8% not significant).

Family history of dementia was present in 35.9% of patients with AD, but in only 5.6% of controls (P<0.001). The 259 patients with AD and their families reported on 2458 relativs, and 129 of these (5.3%) were thought to be demented. In AD, 65/259 patients (25.1%) had one demented relative, 21 (8.1%) had two, 6 (2.3%) had three, and 1 (0.4%) had four demented relatives. Female relatives were demented twice as often as male relatives. (Table 1).

Family history of stroke, Parkinson's disease, brain tumor, and amyotrophic lateral sclerosis was not significantly different in AD versus controls; nor was family history of cardiovascular or pulmonary disease cancer, thyroid dysfunction, or peptic ulcer. Family history of psychiatric disturbances, Down's syndrome, and congenital malformations was more common in AD than in controls, although these differences were not statistically significant (Table 2).

Table 1: Composition of Demented Relatives in Alzheimer's Disease

FEMALE		MALE	
Mother	38 (29.5%)	Father	22 (17.1%)
Sister	32 (24.8%)	Brother	16 (12.4%)
Maternal aunt	8 (6.2%)	Maternal uncle	3 (2.3%)
Maternal grandmother	4 (3.1%)	Paternal uncle	1 (0.7%)
Paternal grandmother	1 (0.7%)	Paternal grandfather	1 (0.7%)
Maternal greatgrandmother	1 (0.7%)	First cousin	1 (0.7%)
		Distant cousin	1 (0.7%)
TOTAL	84/129 (65/1%)	TOTAL	45/129 (34.9%)

Table 2: Family History of Other Disorders

(N.B. # Pts. = # of patients with a positive family history
relatives = total # of affected relatives)

	Alzheimer's Disease		Controls	
	#Pts.	#Relatives	#Pts.	#Relatives
	(n =36)	(n= 2458)	(n=36)	(n=351)
Psychiatric				
Depression	27 (10.4%)	41 (1.7%)	4 (11.1%)	4 (1.1%)
Alcoholism	23 (8.9%)	27 (1.1%)	1 (2.8%)	1 (0.2%)
Other Psychiatric	16 (6.2%)	20 (0.8%)	0 (0.0%)	0 (0.0%)
Suicide or Behavioral Disturbance	13 (5.0%)	13 (0.5%)	0 (0.0%)	0 (0.0%)
Genetic				
Down's Syndrome	2 (0.7%)	2 (0.1%)	0 (0.0%)	0 (0.0%)
Cognenital Malformation	3 (1.2%)	3 (0.1%)	0 (0.0%)	0 (0.0%)

CONCLUSIONS

Family history for dementia was positive in 35.9% of patients with AD, but in only 5.6% of controls (P<0.001), even though all patients and families were questioned thoroughly regarding family history. Since AD is a disorder of late adult life, with many genetically predisposed individuals dying before the disease could be expressed, the true prevalence may approach 50%, suggesting a dominant pattern of inheritance. The male:female ratio of 1:2 in both probands and affected relatives raises the possibility of a sex-linked dominant gene.

Family history of other genetic disorders was more often positive in AD than in controls, but these differences were not statistically significant (thyroid disease in 1.5% vs 0%; Down's syndrome in 0.8% vs 0%, and congenital malformations in 1.2% vs 0%). Similarly, family history of other psychiatric disorders was more often positive in AD. The gene or genes predisposing to AD may also predispose to other diseases, and more extensive genetic studies of this type may uncover genetic linkages that may ultimately lead to discoveery of an abnormal gene product in AD.

Other factors previously implicated in AD were not significantly more common than in controls (head trauma in 4.2% vs 8.3%); peptic ulcers (presumably with aluminum-containing antacid use) in 5.8% vs 8.3% alcoholism in 0.8% vs 0%, job-related toxic exposure in 1.5% vs 0.9%, and thyrod disease in 2.3% vs 0%).

Genetic factors seem to be more important than environmental ones in the pathogenesis of Alzheimer's disease, although case-control studies of large numbers of subjects are needed to determine if small differences in exposure to environmental factors are statistically significant.

REFERENCES

1. Larsson T, Sjogren T, Jacobson G: Senile dementia: a clinical, sociomedical, and genetic study. Acta Psychiatr. Scand (suppl.) 39: Supl. 167 (1963).

2. Heston LL, Mostri AR, Anderson VE, White J: Dementia of the Alzheimer type: clinical genetics, natural history and associated conditions. Arch. Gen. Psychiat. 38: 1085-1090 (1981).

3. Heyman A, Wilkinson WE, Hurwitz BJ, Schmechel D, Sigmon AH, Weinberg T, Helms MJ, Swift M: Alzheimer's disease: genetic aspects and associated clinical disorders. Ann. Neurol. 14: 507-515 (1983).

4. Chase GA, Folstein MF, Breitner JCS, Beaty TH, Self SG: The use of life tables and survival analysis in testing genetic hypotheses, with an application to Alzheimer's disease. Am J. Epidemiol. 17: 590-597 (1983).

5. Heston LL. Mostri AR: The genetics of Alzheimer's disease: associations with hematologic malignancy and Down syndrome. Arch. Gen. Psychiat. 34: 976-981 (1977).

6. Heston LL: Alzheimer;s disease, trisomy 21 and myeloproliferative disorders. Associations suggesting a genetic diathesis. Science 196: 322-323 (1977).

7. Whalley LJ, Carothers AD, Collyer S, DeMey R, Frackiewicz: A study of familial factors in Alzheimer's disease. Brit. J. Psychiat. 140: 249-256 (1982).

8. Heyman A. Wilkinson WE, Stafford JA, Helms MJ, Sigmon AH, Weinberg T: Alzheimer's disease: a study of epidemiological aspects. Ann. Neurol. 15: 335-341 (1984).

9. Mikkel S: A cohort study of disability, pension, and death among workers with special regard to disabling presenile dementia as an occupational disease. Scand. J. Soc. Med. Suppl 16: 34-43 (1980).

10. Olsen J, Sabaroe S: A case reference study of neuropsychiatric disorders among workers exposed to solvents in the Danish wood and furniture industry. Scand. J. Soc. Med. Suppl 16: 44-49 (1980).

11. Crapper DR, Kushman SS, Quittkat S: Aluminum, neurofibrillary degeneration and Alzheimer's disease. Brain 99: 67-80 (1976).

12. Trapp GA, Miner GD, Zimmerman RL, Mastri AR, Heston LL: Aluminum levels in brain in Alzheimer's disease. Biol. Psychiat. 13: 709-718 (1978).

13. Zemcov A, Barclay LL, Brush D, Blass JP: Computerized data base for evaluation and follow-up of demented outpatients. J. Amer. Geriat. Soc. 32: 801-842 (1984),

14. Kahn RL, Goldfarb AI, Pollack MK, Peck A; Brief objective measures for the determination of mental status in the aged. Am. J. Psych. 117:326-329 (1960).

15. Rosen WG, Terry RD, Fuld PA, Katzman R, Peck A: Pathological Verification of ischemic score in differentiation of dementias. Ann. Neurol. 7:486-488 (1980).

16. Haycox JA: A simple reliable clinical behavioral scale for assessing demented patients. J. Clin. Psychiat. 45:23-24, (1984).

17. McKahnn G, Drachman D, Folstein M, Katzman R, Price D, Stadlan EM: Clinical diagnosis of Alzheimer's disease. Neurol 34: 939-944 (1984).

ENHANCING COMMUNICATION FOR THE DEMENTED PATIENT AND HIS FAMILY

A. J. Rosin, L. Abramowitz, J. Diamond, S. Beitz,
S. Hirsch, and S. Rifkin

Shaare Zedek Medical Center, Jerusalem; National Insurance Institute, Israel

INTRODUCTION

The cognitive impairment and personality change in a demented individual engender a situation in which he is unable to cope or come to terms with the norms of society or family life. In the absence of therapeutic means of altering the dementing process, a useful and practical approach in the long-term management of the behavioural problem is to change the environment. This well-known principle of milieu therapy was applied to cognitively impaired people who were living at home by the establishment of a number of therapeutically orientated clubs in community centers in Jerusalem. Implicit in the model to be described in this paper are the ramifications which we consider to be an integral part of the project - the family support groups, group meetings with the children of the patients, the medical coverage, the team meetings of the staff, the case conferences, and the educational programs on problems of old age which have stemmed from the initiation of the project.

AIMS AND METHODS Each club has aimed at becoming a regular social setting in which the patient could feel that he belongs, and in which his acceptance is enhanced by personal contact, and he can realize his potential by programmed activity. Referral of subjects has been from social workers in the community, from the hospital geriatric department, from families, and from volunteers working with old people. Residents of institutions are not admitted as yet. The majority of those accepted suffer from dementia of Alzheimer's type, or that associated with strokes. Parkinsonism, depression and other conditions associated with cognitive disability are other causes of referral, but patients with psychotic states are generally sent back to mental hospital clinics. The reasons for accepting a patient have been to stimulate him out of apathy, and to induce some more purposive activity other than the inevitable repetitive questions and annoyance that the relative has to tolerate. Another major reason is to give the relative or care-giver a few hours free of the responsibility of looking after the patient. Selection of patients is made after a home visit by the group leader, who documents and discusses the goals of treatment with the executive.

Four clubs, each comprising up to 15 members have been opened in different districts in Jerusalem in the last 4 years, located in community centers or day centers for the elderly. Transport is provided in order to assure safe arrival and return of the patient, to stimulate him to come and also to note any change in his health condition, and to relieve the relative from the chore of taking him and bringing him back. The drivers, often volunteers, build up an acquaintance with the patient, and the journey thereby becomes part of the club activity.[1]

PROGRAM The basis and aims of the program are:

1. To promote communication by verbal and non-verbal means.
2. To enchance participation, counter apathy and stimulate wakefulness through various types of physical and occupational activity.
3. To enhance orientation to the immediate group environment and to current events through conversation and activity.
4. Goal-directed activity to bring out expression of identity and induce a sense of achievement.

The following summary illustrates some of these principles.

REALITY ORIENTATION Introducing and naming members of the group, hand shaking and holding, and imparting information on date, significant calendar events and personal happenings connected to the group - all these procedures are aimed at establishing identity and developing participation within the group.

ANECDOTES AND TALKS This part consists of simple stories with a strong cultural association, and the members are encourage to contribute. For example, former rabbinical scholars may express some familiar themes, and those who can sing may perform folk songs or synagogue music. As each activity is completed, the leader explains what has been said, and correct reactions by the patients are rewarded and acknowledged.

PHYSIOTHERAPY AND GROUP EXERCISES This popular activity by its very dynamics induces participation by even the most passive members. Exercises include limb movement, breathing and relaxation techniques, the use of sticks and balls, and goal directed movement, and by maintaining a gentle pace the physiotherapist is able to involve the groups for up to 45 minutes.

DANCE THERAPY The aim is communication on an emotional level through movement, gesture and rhythm. With patients who are confused, intellectually cut off, or isolated, the language of body movement and pantomime can be meaningfully applied to achieve participation and a feeling of belonging. The music selected in relation to the varied cultural backgrounds, played in demanding rhythms attuned to folk dance, waltz or tango has a very persuasive appeal, and can evoke spontaneity in a demented patient to dance in rhythmic steps, or lead others in a dance line.

The activity, lasting for 30-45 minutes in a group setting, starts with the participants seated in a circle, after each is greeted individually by the therapist. Melodious or stirring tunes are played, according to the wakefulness of the group, and movements are practised of the major joints in time to the music. With hands joined and contact established among the members of the group they are led to standing and then moving in a circle, with the tempo of the rhythm as a constant signal to further activity. This may be in the form of step dancing in couples, in small circles, or in line formation, while the therapist passes around, encouraging and gaining response from every member of the group. Even those who are unable to stand receive attention, e.g. by hand swinging or by the others dancing around them. Gradually, the quiet that started is converted into a rhythmic moving group of active people. At the end, they all retire to their places, relax with deep breathing exercises, and so the music, sound and movement decline to a halt.

OCCUPATIONAL SKILLS AND CRAFT ACTIVITY The accent of this part of the program is on enhancing self-worth of the patient, and talking <u>to</u> him rather than about him. The effort demanded from the patient is tailored to his ability, but perhaps more important than the type of work done is the sense of fulfilment experienced by him when he describes his work before the group. Allowing the patient to comment or criticize his own or other people's work is another means of expression of self-identity in front of his peers. While choosing the subjects for the patient to work on, the therapist evokes other sensory memories - visual, auditory, tactile or smell - by story-telling around the objects to be painted or modelled. Many subjects are selected from nature or the immediate environment. The concern with which these demented people undertake their painting is reflected in the pride they evince by seeing it as their own possession, and often by taking it home. The crafts activity encourages verbal communication among the group, and also co-operation between members in the actual tasks, and the ensuing emotional uplift is a frequent concomitant of the 60-75 minutes activity.

SPOUSE GROUPS The caregiver, usually the spouse, is not only the pillar of the therapeutic team, but also one who requires treatment.[2] Because we saw the bewilderment and perplexity as well as the loneliness of those spouses, we set up regular sessions specially with them once fortnightly on a semi-obligatory basis, with the group leader as moderator.[3,4] It became clear that talks by experts or specialist counselling did not answer their real need. The groups often evolve from an initial state of polite restraint to the ability to engage in ventilation and exposure of personal conflict, indecision and tragedy. The leader, who has to know the personal situation of each participant, plays a guiding role by putting before them situations and suggestions of coping with them. The group itself then analyzes the problems which are raised in the light of their own conflicts.

Among the important topics that have emerged has been the gross imbalance in these people's lives due to the caring role, which can bring them to the point of being unable to "let go", in order to care a little for themselves.[5] The group has also dealt with suggested help for the physical problems of lifting and toiletting, of insomnia, and of feeding, but discussion usually focusses on the emotional overtones implicit in dealing with these problems. In trying to put some order into a life disrupted by a demented partner, the group leader orientates them to the essential tasks of a care-giver - to attend to the physical needs of the patient; to try and lighten the emotional burden on himself; to strike a proper and positive relationship between the care-giver, his family and his immediate society.

In addition to the rather close and intimate meetings of the spouse group, a get-together is arranged every few months for the children of the patients. The purpose is to maintain a wider contact with families, albeit on a more superficial level, and to allow public discussion of their management difficulties and personal adaptive problems. Discussion often brings to light deficiencies in community services or suggestions for an answer to needs such as counselling, medical supervision, and admission of the patient to care in an institution in order to give the care-giver a holiday, or short periods of relief.

ACTIVITY OF THE CLUBS Table 1 summarizes the diagnoses and the turnover of the participants in the 4 clubs during 12 months of 1983-84. The figures illustrate the high morbidity of this population, accounting for the relatively rapid turnover, thus allowing acceptance of new patients without a long waiting time. The criteria of suitability for the club permitted certain people to be accepted whose physical disability was more dominant than the cognitive disorder. The discrepancy in intellectual range was more than compensated for by the very fact that they could take part in some organized social activity.

Table 1: DYNAMICS OF 4 TREATMENT CENTERS

June 1983-June 1984

Total referrals - 157

Average number in each club - 15

Dropped Out		Main Diagnoses	
Not suitable	25	Dementia	79
Unwilling	36	Post-stroke	42
Died	14	Parkinsonism	13
Became ill	12	Depression	10
Entered nursing home	17	Brain tumor	3
		Isolation	5

50 patients continued attendance

Inevitably, some of the demented patients are eventually admitted for long-term care in an institution. The clubs are purported to be a practical means of delaying this irrevocable step of separation from the family, and discussion on this theme with the families and among the team occupies much time and thought. Sometimes an indecisive tendency by the family towards admission to a nursing home may be reversed by demonstrating the positive behavior patterns that emerge in the club setting. The importance of correlating the observations of the club leaders with the family attitudes has led us to delegate one of the staff, who is a social worker, to deal only with casework with problem families, or more properly, problem situations.

STAFFING Each group or club is staffed by a leader, usually a trained social worker, and an assistant, and if possible a volunteer to assist disabled patients. The clubs meet 3 or 4 times weekly for about 3½ hours, and comprise up to 15 participants. Special therapists work on a basis of 1-2 hours per club every 1-2 weeks - physiotherapist, art and creative therapist, dance therapist and music therapist. Case conferences with all the staff members take place with each club every 2-3 months, chaired by the physician to the organization, when progress and problems of all the participants are raised, and decisions are made regarding the usefulness of the project to the patient and his family.

"Journal clubs" are held every month for the staff, including the director, co-ordinator and executive members, during which a paper is discussed, new ideas are exchanged, and administrative information is passed on.

A steering committee consisting of representatives of the Municipality and various public bodies, meets every 3 months to monitor progress, and to supervise policy, administration and finance.

EVALUATION OF THE PROJECT What impact has all this activity had on the patients and their families? A preliminary investigation through semi-structured interviews was carried out on 46 families by the Research Department of the National Insurance Institute of Israel in regard to the possible contribution made by the clubs. The club leaders were also interviewed on how they saw the reaction and behavior of the patients within the clubs. The degree of dependency and disability among the patients was marked - 74% needed a lot of help in bathing, 35% could not dress themselves at all and only 33% were able to prepare a cup of tea for themselves. There was a correlation between physical and mental impairment - 20% showed both to a highly significant degree, and over 40% had severe difficulty with remembering names and events of the day before. Thus of the 46 care-givers, 27 pointed to the physical strain of caring for the patient as the main problem, and 16 suffered from tension and depression. Thirty of the care-givers (60%) were motivated to send the patient to the clubs in order that they could mix with people. The group leaders saw the chief indication for attendance as rehabilitation and social integration in approximately three-quarters of the group.

The main contribution of the clubs in the opinion of the relatives was in the improvement of the patients' spirits, a greater interest in doing things inside the house, and some increased orientation outside the home. These comments, however, only applied to between 20-25% of the participants, and mainly concerning those with less cognitive or physical impairment, who could therefore benefit more from the club atmosphere. Fifty percent of the care-givers stated that for themselves, the main benefit was that they had more free time, and another 33% commented on the emotional relief and on the knowledge that some treatment was being given to their sick relative. Altogether, the care-givers saw the clubs as of positive benefit to themselves and the patients, although their judgement was necessarily a subjective one. However, we saw this subjective opinion as important because the actual handling of the patient was largely dependent on how the relative care-giver felt and these feelings can be a dominant influence on his long-term care.[6]

DISCUSSION The increasing public awareness of what Alzheimer and other dementias are has resulted in more obvious efforts to investigate, alleviate or cure the disease.[7] These efforts are reflected in grants and support for scientific and medical research at the basic and clinical level. However, one of the problems handicapping the support of community programs is that dementia is an organic disease of which the manifestations are for the most part behavioral and communicative, and the long-term management of the these disorders is in the field of the social services. The latter are often unwilling to deal with problems based on disease; the health authorities may contend that the home-based patient with dementia is not sick in the physical or even psychiatric sense, and therefore may not be under their jurisdiction.

As with many aspects of rehabilitation, the chronic management of dementia demands a multi-disciplinary team that is well co-ordinated. Delegation of staff duties will result in bringing fresh aspects of treatment into the patient's life, e.g. awareness of natural surroundings and expressing it in painting, increased sensitivity of body movement and gesture as an expression of identity.

The model presented in this paper is more than a club to fill in old people's time at a low intellectual level. As it has developed, the roles of each party have been more clearly defined. The patient is often given a role, a situation of which he was previously bereft because of the dementia and the consequent isolation.[8] Along with his role and tasks come a resurgence of identity and some self-respect. The spouse, who is often overwhelmed by the enormous new responsibilities facing her, the difficulty of coping with a unique and unpleasant situation and the constant state of "on-call", may find her task undefinable. The support engendered not only by the interest taken in her spouse but by the attention focussed on her by the group leader serves to allow her to see her own life in a more real perspective.[4] Through the spouse groups, she should become able to undergo the role of caring and of grieving in correct proportions, and to come to terms emotionally with a situation whose demands are often not requited with satisfaction or achievement. The group leader who has to inject a spirit of activity into the sessions has sometimes difficulty in completing all the items on the program - a welcome contrast to the emptiness which time inflicts on demented persons. In addition, she becomes an authority to whom patients, families and others can turn, and may become the arbiter of decisions such as keeping the patient at home or sending him into an institution. Her role is also educational to the family, to other members of the public and to herself. Thus, the organization as a whole takes on an educational character which varies from "showing the way" to other bodies on how to cope with the dementia situation, to actual course instruction for old people or for relatives in management techniques.[7]

Evaluation of this kind of project is difficult because of the unlikelihood of improvement in the cognitive impairment. One measurement is the amount of activity carried out by the patient in the club as compared with the home setting. Most cases show an increase, but this is hardly a valid comparison since the nature of the circumstances is so different. Nevertheless, the fact of the patient's activity and participation do add quality to a life that often lacks any program. Similarly, although many relatives express appreciation for the service, our pilot survey found only 39% who felt a significant lightening of the burden in terms of free time, and 28% who experienced emotional relief. This could be because as long as the patient is alive, whether at home, in a club or in a nursing home, the relative lives in constant anxiety and strain, and requires the support that only a specialized agency such as the club can give her.

Because of the tensions and frustrations which arise round the demented individual, it is important that a professional and social community of interest be maintained among the staff. We have found the educational features, case conferences and presentation of professional papers as essential secondary features to the main purpose of the organization. In this way the group becomes a focus of professional interest, activity and pressure within the community, so that its outreach can encompass more and more of those who need their services.

REFERENCES

1. T. Arie, Day care in geriatric psychiatry 1978, *Age and Ageing* 8(suppt): 87 (1979).
2. N. L. Mace, and P. V. Rabins, The 36 hour day, Johns Hopkins University Press, Baltimore (1981).
3. A. Fengler, and N. Goodrich, Wives of elderly disabled men: the hidden patients, *The Gerontologist* 19:175 (1979).
4. L. W. Lazarus, B. Stafford, K. Cooper, B. Cohler, and M. Dysken, A pilot study of an Alzheimer patients' relatives group, *The Gerontologist* 21:353 (1981).

   J. Fuller, E. Ward, A. Evans, K. Massam, and A. Gardner, Dementia: supportive groups for relatives, *British Medical Journal* 1:1684 (1979).

6. B. Isaacs, Geriatric patients: Do their families care? British Medical Journal 4:282 (1981).
7. Report of the Royal College of Physicians by the College Committee on Geriatrics: Organic mental impairment in the elderly, Journal of Royal College of Physicians 15:141 (1981).
8. P. Ernst, B. Biran, R. Safford, and H. Kleinhauz, Isolation and chronic brain syndrome, The Gerontologist 18:468 (1978).

REACTION TIMES IN TASKS OF VARYING DEGREES OF COMPLEXITY,

AN INDICATION OF THE DEGREE AND THE EVOLUTION OF MENTAL DETERIORATION:

A PRELIMINARY STUDY

Tony Waegemans

Leuven, Belgium

The present text describes the initial results obtained with a new measurement apparatus. In an open study, the influence of suloctidil on reaction times of elderly patients with slight to moderate mental deterioration was determined. The study was designed to test a number of working hypotheses in preparation for a controlled, double-blind study (currently in progress).

Previous studies indicate that it is possible to measurably influence mental deterioration with suloctidil primarily during its initial stages. Therefore, the target group was recruited from various rest homes for the elderly. The presence of mental deterioration was established by means of a psychiatric examination.

Method. In total, 52 subjects were selected of whom 40 participated in the complete protocol. The drop-outs were due to intervening illness or death. For six months, the subjects were given suloctidil in its commercial form (donated by Continental Pharma, Belgium). The reaction times were measured before treatment and after two, four, and six months of treatment. The protocol provided for the exclusion of mentally confused patients, or patients with mental dysfunction not associated with psycho-organic causes, and of subjects with diabetes. Other products that would influence mental functioning were not permitted, and other medication was maintained as stable as possible. The recording of the reaction times took place for each subject at the same time of day in order to eliminate diurnal variations. In addition to the evaluation of reaction times, a simplified form of the SCAG scale was administered, and medical data pertinent to cerebral and vascular diseases were recorded.

The apparatus. In view of the objectives of this study, appropriate measurement apparatus were developed and constructed. A specially constructed microcomputer (around a Z80 microprocessor) with the capability of controlling external signals for acoustical and visual stimuli was used. The apparatus had to satisfy a number of requirements.

1. In order to obtain a sufficiently large group of elderly subjects who met the rather stringent selection criteria, the study had to be performed in several institutions and thus the apparatus had to be portable.

2. Simplicity of operation was achieved by building in a high degree of automation in the test. The microcomputer stores the measurements in a permanent memory that can be read and processed by a more powerfull computer. This excludes human reading and writing errors and allows the administrator to concentrate more on the test and the subjects. This simplicity makes it possible for the nursing staff to administer the test, which gives the advantage of familiarity with the patients.

3. Splitting the reaction time into the time between stimulus and beginning of execution (premotoric or central time) and the time needed for the execution of the movement (motoric time) was achieved by the use of contact plates.

4. The complete reaction-time measurement consisted of three tasks of increasing difficulty. The first task is reacting as quickly as possible to an acoustic signal. In the second task, a choice has to be made, the task being to touch the signal area under one of the two lamps that randomly lights up. In the third task, a dissociation is made between signal and target: the subject is instructed to touch the signal area under the lamp that does NOT light up. The hypothesis is that this third degree of difficulty would permit a better discrimination of subjects with a psycho-organic syndrome because more cerebral processes are involved, some of which are described as specifically disturbed by mental deterioration. There is a strong tendency among demented patients to return to a previous task (retroactive interference). In addition the motility of the gaze is limited.

The learning effect

In a rest home for healthy elderly people, fifteen subjects were selected who were mentally alert and manifested a minimum of mental deterioration. Should no learning effect occur with these subjects, a fortiori none would occur with subjects with mental deterioration, who have a decreased learning capacity. These fifteen subjects were tested with the same protocol with the exception of the treatment with suloctidil.

The results indicate that there is a slight, but statistically insignificant, slowing of the simple central times over the six month period, with the more complex central times and the motoric times remaining practically unchanged. When the measurements taken at two, four and six months are considered with respect to the first measurement, the correlations remain very high, which indicates a large degree of stability in the subject's performance. This high re-test reliability confirms the conclusion that reaction time is an indication of the speed of performance of an individual that is stable and repeatable in time.

The SCAG as an independent criterion for mental deterioration

From the complete Idiopathic Cerebral Dysfunction Scale (IDSC or SCAG scale) of 18 items, 10 were selected that seemed good indications of mental deterioration. In the processing of the research results, the scale serves as an independent criterion for the seriousness of the mental deterioration. The intercorrelations of the 10 items on the correlation matrix are very high.

The selected SCAG items were: confusion, impairment of mental alertness, of recent memory, of orientation, of self-care, indifference of surroundings, fatigue, emotional lability,irritability, and hostility.

From the factor matrix of principal factors only two factors emerge. (Factor 1: Organic psychosyndroms, factor 2: demented behaviour).

Reaction times as a measure for the seriousness of mental deterioration

In this study, a measurement of speed of reaction is used as a means of estimating mental deterioration and to demonstrate the influence of suloctidil on these deterioration processes. Important is here the question of whether the measured slowing is indeed an indication of aging and of pathological aging. It can be shown by the demonstration of relations between the research data that reaction time does actually fulfill these conditions. (see table)

Table : Correlations of the times registered at the first administration (before treatment), with global Scag score age.

		global Scag score		age	
C1	central simple RT	.39	p=.002	.27	p=.037
M1	motoric simple RT	.445	p=.0007	-	
T1	total simple RT	.438	p=.0008	-	
C2	central choice RT	.59	p=.00002	.29	p=.024
M2	motoric choice RT	.52	p=.0001	-	
T2	total choice RT	.622	$p<.00001$	.27	p=.036
C3	central complex RT	.557	p=.00004	-	
M3	motoric complex RT	.518	p=.0001	.26	p=.05
T3	total complex RT	.611	p=.00002	.29	p=.027

There appears to be a weak though significant relationship between slower reaction times and advanced age. The literature would lead one to expect a stronger relationship here. Thus, it may be supposed that other, non-age related factors influence the reaction times. Since there is, in the research group, no correlation between the SCAG score and age, it may be assumed that the strong SCAG-reaction time correlation causes the age-reaction time relationship to disappear. It is also clear from the table that the correlation with the SCAG scores for the complex times is greater than for the simple reaction times. This is a confirmation of the hypothesis that mental deterioration can be more clearly revealed by the building in of increasing complexity into the measurement method.

When taking the 10 SCAG items separately, there is a recurring association with the reaction times, an association that is almost always larger with the more complex reaction times.

In the selection, use was also made of a list of signs that could indicate the presence of beginning dementia. These indications of the presence of mental deterioration also manifest a high degree of association with the various reaction times. The association of these clinical signs with the SCAG score constitutes an additional indication that they both describe the same phenomenon of mental deterioration.

The last indication for the relationship between reaction times and mental deterioration comes from the clinical judgment criterion. After recording the SCAG score, the attending physician indicated on a 4-point scale his judgment on the presence or absence of mental deterioration. This global clinical judgment also correlates rather high with slower reaction times, and particularly with the complex reaction times. The correlation of this clinical judgment with the global SCAG score is extremely high, namely .92. This may be interpreted as justifying the use of the SCAG scale as an indication of the degree of mental deterioration.

One may conclude from the above that reaction time is a reliable indication for the degree of mental deterioration and that the division into more complex tasks increases its reliability considerably.

Evolution of the reaction times with suloctidil treatment

The following figure gives the decrease observed in the central (pre-motoric) reaction times after treatment with suloctidil for two, four, and six months. This improvement is not yet complete after two months. After four months, the complex reaction times reach a plateau, the difference between four and six months not being statistically significant. For the simple reaction times, the improvement still continues after four months.

In the motoric times, no appreciable evolution was observed. Owing to this, it is clear that the total reaction times, which are the sum of the central and motoric times, follow the curve of the central reaction time.

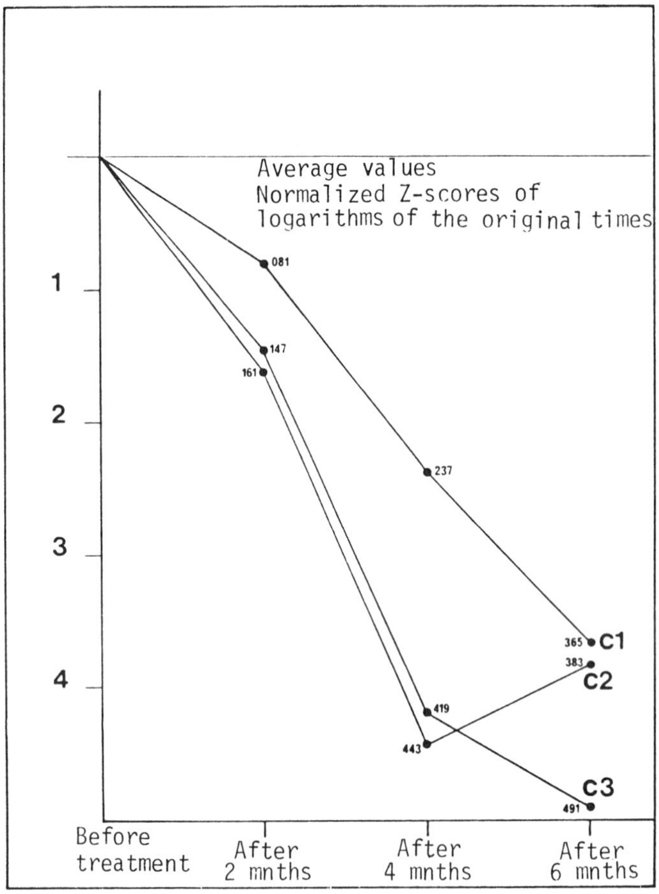

Figure: C1 being simple, C2 being choice, and C3 being complex central RT

One may conclude that the cerebral processes of perception, information processing, and decision making are more efficient and thus more rapid after treatment. Very important here is the observation that the more cerebral processes involved in the execution of an activity, the greater the relative gain in efficiency. There is thus a broader influencing of not only one, but several cerebral processes, the favorable effects of which are cumulative. From the nature of the test design, the influenced functions must be sought among attention, concentration, and mental alertness.

SUMMARY

The objective of this open study was to test a number of hypotheses.

1. The reaction-time measurement apparatus developed for this study can be used with slightly to moderately demented patients in rest homes. Its acceptability by elderly patients is high. The apparatus can be reliably operated by the nursing staff of the rest house.

2. Reaction times as measured with the apparatus have good retest reliability and are a good indication of the speed of performance, which is stable and reproducible. There is no learning effect with repeated measurements.

3. Slow reaction times are an expression of mental deterioration. The more complex reaction-time tasks correlate stronger with mental deterioration than do simple reaction times. The reaction time may be considered a quantitative measure of mental deterioration and can thus be used to follow its evolution. Changes under treatment can be more clearly seen when the total reaction time is taken apart in its two components, the changes taking place only in the central part of the reaction-time task. The large resolution capacity of the apparatus also makes it possible to discriminate small changes. This makes the test a useful tool in the geriatric clinic.

4. The reaction times manifest a strong relationship with cerebrovascular pathology. A strong vascular factor in the etiology of mental deterioration in the research group may be assumed.

5. By means of reaction times, the improvement that occurs in patients with mental deterioration when treated with suloctidil can be measured unambiguously. This implies that the improvement in alertness, decision-making capacity, and flexibility of adaptation is sufficiently large to be demonstrated by reaction-time measurements.

CONCLUSION

This open study demonstrates that an evolution in the process of mental deterioration can be reliably evaluated by means of reaction-time measurements. The division of the total reaction time into its premotoric (central) and motoric components and, in the same test design, the variation of the degree of complexity in the tasks to be executed appear to be valuable techniques. Further, it is shown that the reaction time (and thus the underlying mental deterioration) can be favorably influenced by suloctidil. Since the improvement occurs in the premotoric component and since this improvement is greater when more cerebral processes are mobilized, it is postulated that this increase of speed indicates more efficient functioning of attention and concentration, a higher degree of mental alertness, more efficient information processing and decision making, and increased flexibility in changing to new tasks.

AN INTRANOSOLOGICAL CLASSIFICATION OF ALZHEIMER'S DISEASE AS A MULTI-STAGE DEMENTING PROCESS - THE BASIS FOR INDIVIDUALIZED THERAPEUTIC STRATEGIES (a developmental-semiological approach)

Meinhardt S. Tropper and Jacob Wagner

Neuropsychiatric Department, Zamenhof Multi-Disciplinary Central Out-Patient Clinic, Tel-Aviv and Mental Health Services and Geriatric Center, Rishon Le-Zion, Israel

Key words. Alzheimer's Disease. Dementia of Alzheimer Type. Classification of dementing processes. Developmental approaches (stages) of dementing processes. Semiology of dementing processes. Diagnostical bases for individualized therapeutic strategies in Alzheimer's diseases.

Those working in the field of psychiatry of old age are confronted with growing difficulties in choosing proper therapeutic strategies for Alzheimer's disease patients. The evaluation of the efficacy of interventional strategies on pathognomonic clinical manifestations belonging to different stages of Alzheimer's disease remains an intriguing issue of theoretical and practical importance. By overcoming this challenge it will be possible to answer the following three questions: (a) what are the typical stages along the temporal trajectory of Alzheimer's disease; (b) are there any reliable ways of intervention, e.g. functional rehabilitation according to the stages concept of Alzheimer's disease; (c) what are the reasons for different progressions of Alzheimer's disease; and whether there are strategies to delay this process by keeping patients on a definite functional level.

Studying the current literature concerning the Dementia of Alzheimer Type (DAT), we have encountered a series of classifications each one from different viewpoints (Hasegawa and Karasawa, 1975; Verwoerdt, 1976; Lishman, 1978; Reisberg and Ferris, 1982).

With feeling of deep appreciation for our distinguished colleagues, mentioned above, and many others not mentioned here, we would like to add to their valuable contributions, some of our observations. The emphasis in our work was put on the search of such an intranosological classification of DAT, which could serve as a basis for individualized therapeutic strategies. This interventional oriented approach is based on three principles. The first, a developmental one (Brainerd, 1978), is a concept of stages, phases and levels of functioning applied by us to DAT (Tropper, 1983). This approach designates a period, which is characterized by qualitative changes that differentiates each of them from the adjacent stages and constitutes one step in a progression.

The second, the semiological (from the greek word semiotikon), is the concept of course, signs and symptoms and their diagnostic importance, mechanisms of their appearance and correlations.

The third, the taxonomic concept (Russel, Neuringer and Goldstein, 1970) concerns brain damage and the polythetic system of classification.

Based on these principles we turn to our data base. This is a sample of 467 patients, who were under our observation during the last six years (1979-1985). The patients (age range 54-86, mean age 70+0.4) underwent thorough geropsychiatric, geropsychological, neuropsychological assessments, as well as general physical examinations, EEG, CTscan, biochemical, endocrinological, immunological investigations. The patients were followed up every 3-5 months during the observation period. Parallel to this sample of patients we followed up a group of demented patients (N=115), whose anamnestical clinical and paraclinical data proved that they fitted into the diagnostical category of Multi-infarct dementia (according to DSM-11).

As to the main sample of 467 patients, the results of manifold clinical and paraclinical investigations, especially the follow up course of the disease show that they fit into the diagnostic criteria (DSM-11) of primary degenerative dementia of early or late onset, with a symptomatology very close to the clinical picture of DAT.

We would like to emphasize that all patients involved in this study were thoroughly investigated from different aspects, as age of onset, kind of presenting symptoms, appearance of new symptoms and signs along the axis of time, peculiarities of the transformation of symptoms and syndromes. Our special interest was devoted to the issue of brain-behavior relationship along the course of DAT, to the yet preserved functions and abilities, which could serve as the basis for target oriented individualized therapeutic strategies (Tropper, 1984).

In this light, the most intriguing issue was the selection of the typical pathognomic symptoms and signs for each of the clinical stages, through which our patients pass along their via dolorosa of this cruel disease. The succession of stages along the trajectory of time is a very complex process. The sequence of segments along the temporal axis was characterized by typical changes, e.g. symptoms and syndromes relative to the adjacent ones. And here we turn to one of the most interesting issues - the peculiarities of the brain-behavior relationship along the whole stretch of time starting from the insiduous and often undetected onset till the tragic final stage of DAT.

We approach the DAT patient independently of age, sex, educational and cultural background according to our hypothesis (Tropper, 1983) concerning the model of cognitive intactness of the normal human being. This model, postulating a "structural formula of cognitive intactness"

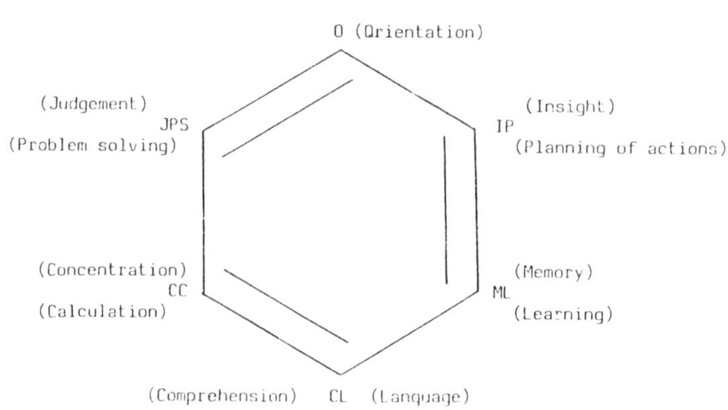

Fig. 1 The "Structural Formula" of Cognitive Intactness

includes the main cognitive functions, as orientation, language, comprehension, concentration, calculation, memory, judgement and problem solving (Fig. 1).

According to our main task, the search for individualized therapeutic strategies in DAT, we tried to follow up the qualitative and quantitative changes of the above mentioned components of cognitive intactness along the course of the disease. Based on the dynamics of changes we assume the existence of the following intranosological classification of DAT, which includes 5 stages. These stages are:

Stage I	-	the stage of increased cognitive difficulties
Stage II	-	the stage of overt memory-cognitive-language difficulties
Stage III	-	the stage of manifested memory-orientation-language-affective-confusional disorders
Stage IV	-	the stage of deep behavioral defects ("psychosocial breakdown")
Stage V	-	the stage of final cognitive deterioration ("the cognitive dead but physically alive patient")

Each of these five stages is characterized by a wide range of clinical behavioral, psychological, neuropsychological symptoms and signs. However, for practical purposes we have chosen 10 principal symptoms which according to their frequency and significance among the patients of our sample appear to be pathognomonic for this or that respective stage.

The following (Table 1) is the detailed description of the principal symptoms of stage I:

Table 1 - STAGE I

Of "increased" cognitive difficulties 10 principal symptoms (in percents of patients sample)	
- Difficulties in finding the proper names	84
- Forgetfulness for placement of objects	81
- Difficulties in planning complex actions	72
- Difficulties in remembering appointments	64
- Decrease in energy, "cerebral asthenia"	63
- Difficulties in work capacity or in house work	62
- Difficulties in understanding logical-grammatical structures	62
- Attentional difficulties	61
- Difficulties in understanding of wits and lessening of sense of humour	58
- Hypochondriazation	52

We would like to mention some points concerning this first, so often overlooked and underdiagnosed stage of DAT. In this stage as well as in Stage II the thorough undertaken neurological examination often fails to supply us with pathognomonic signs. In this stage the neurological signs were as follows: slowed pupil reactions 25 percent, decrease of vibration perception-27 percent, diminished Achilles reflexes-32 percent, unequal tendon reflexes-34 percent. These neurological signs, the search of which should be undertaken in each case, are neither significant nor pathognomic for this stage, and consequently of low diagnostic value. However, the modern neuropsychological thoroughly performed assessment and its proper interpretation emanating from the taxonomic and "functional system" approaches, could enormously contribute to early diagnostics of this stage (Tropper and Wagner, 1983). The peculiarities of Stage II are presented in Table 2.

Table 2 - STAGE II

Of "obvious" memory-cognitive-language disorders
10 principal symptoms (in percents of patients sample)

Symptom	%
- Obvious forgetfulness	91
- Loss of insight, of interpretation of sensory defects and metamemory	86
- Decrease in capitalizing appropriate cues in memory strategies and organization	85
- Anxiety during psychological testing and social demands	72
- Disorders in clearly expressing of thoughts	69
- Difficulties in reading of anagrams	63
- Difficulties in understanding metaphors	61
- Expressed mood swings	58
- Mild expressed and evaluated only by special testing language disorders	57
- Appearance of prefrontal abnormal reflexes	54

In this table we point out two systems and signs. The first is defined by us as "expressed mood swings". This is a pre-depressive stage, which resembles a mild or moderate neurotic reaction. In more than half of these patients referred to us, it appears that though they are not always aware of the losses, they feel, however, as if "they are on the top of an iceberg in the middle of the ocean and loosing ground". (Assael and Tropper, 1981). The other system is the appearance of prefrontal abnormal reflexes and frontal lobe disfunctions. The peculiarities of Stage III are illustrated in Table 3.

Table 3- STAGE III

Of "manifested" mnestic-orientation-language-affective-confusional disorders;10 principal symptoms(in percents of patients sample)

Symptom	%
- Facial recognition disorders	82
- Topographic memory disorders	80
- Restlessness and psychomotor agitation	67
- Aggression and hostility	63
- Paranoid mood (Wahnstimmung)and the hiding possession symptom	60
- Inability to detect own errors	58
- Inability to perform arithmetical operations	58
- Disorders in verbal fluency	57
- Manifested social withdrawal	55
- Disorders in narrative speech	51

Here we point to two most pathognomonic symptoms, the appearance of prosopagnosia and topographic memory disorders. Both represent usually those alarm symptoms which have urged prompt referring of patients to the gero-psychiatrist, and not to the general practioner. Apart from these symptoms we paid special attention to the phenomenon of "paranoid mood" (or "Wahnstimmung", according to the German authors). This state of mind is of transient character along the course of DAT and is often erroneously coined as paranoid reaction, when indeed it represents a segment in the chain of pathognomonic psychopathological symptoms.

The detailed description of Stage IV, main symptomatology, is presented in Table 4. We have not included in this table the increased frequency of prefrontal abnormal reflexes, which appeared for the first time in Stage III. However, in this stage, the snout, suck and grasp reflexes were found in 73 percent of the patients.

We have not included in this table the increased frequency of prefrontal abnormal reflexes, which appeared for the first time in Stage III. However, in this stage, the snout, suck and grasp reflexes were found in 73 percent of the patients.

Table 4 - STAGE IV

Of "deep behavioural defects" (psychosocial breakdown) based on cognitive deterioration; 10 principal symptoms (in percents of patients sample)	
- Deep spatial disorientation	92
- Significant language deterioration (omission of words, incomplete sentences, verbal iteration stable intrusions of coherent kind)	89
- Confabulations	86
- Misidentifications	85
- Total lack of critical attitudes	85
- Total helplessness	84
- Hypersexuality (verbal and in activities)	66
- Disturbances of the diurnal rhythm	64
- Delusional behaviour	53
- Diogenes-like syndrome	32

Stage V - the stage of final cognitive deterioration ("the cognitive dead, but physically alive patient") is characterized by total agnosia, dyspraxia, spatial disorientation, very high percentage of abnormal frontal reflexes, significant aphasia, loss of diurnal rhythm, incontinence, almost total abolition of alpha waves and prominent theta and delta activities on the EEG. Now we turn to the psychogeriatric intervention of DAT patients - the most important subject for us physicians.

Based on the development-semiological approach and starting from the assumption that DAT represents a multi-stage dementing process, we have carried out during the reported observation period, some therapeutic trials. In the light of our topic the main conclusions of these therapeutic strategies will be discussed here briefly.

In a trial with a representative of the Nootropic class of drugs (Piracetam-UCB, resp. 1-acetamide-2-pyrrolidone acetate) we have treated 94 patients, among them 63 suffering from DAT (Tropper, Wagner, Manulescu and Glinternik, 1981). Every patient was given 2.4 g Piracetam daily for 40 consecutive days. The results were statistically processed. Although the therapeutic results concerning the whole (N=63) group, were not significant, however, by dividing the symptoms according to stages, a definite tendency in amelioration was achieved, and this predominantly in the Stages I, and II, and partly in Stage III. We have followed up these symptoms, according to the stages.

In Stage I, temporary improvement was achieved among 64 percent of the patients. However, in respect of some symptoms, the results varied: in attentional difficulties-70 percent; in difficulties in work capacity or housework-68 percent; in forgetfulness of finding proper names-56 percent. Among patients in Stage II improvement was achieved in 53 percent. However, in some symptoms, the results were the following: in expressed mood swings-68 percent; in interpretation of sensory defects and meta-memory-64 percent; in obvious forgetfulness-54 percent. Among patients in Stage III, temporary improvement was achieved only in 35 percent. However, in disorders of verbal fluency-54 percent; in coping with social withdrawal-63 percent. Among patients belonging to Stage IV, the improvement rate was very low-18 percent and this predominantly in one sense, the disturbances of the diurnal rhythm. In Stage V, we have not seen any improvement.

In our trials (Tropper and Wagner, 1982) with Lecithin, for comparison, the total improvement rate was 59 percent. However, according to our approach, the improvement reached-68 percent in Stage I; 64 percent in Stage II and 58 percent in Stage III. Piracetam appeared to be of value in the recovery from states of apathy, in coping with attentional difficulties, in improving alertness and interests. Even in memory disorders in Stage I (31 percent), Stage II (29 percent) piracetam proved to be of some value in improving the patient's abilities in categorization of items presented in the frame of memory tasks, in promoting patients to choose more attributes and retrieval cues. We have also undertaken a comparative interventional trial (Tropper and Wagner, 1984). In this cross-over study the efficacy of piracetam (as a representative of Nootropics) was compared with the efficacy of lecithin (a cholinergic substance) administered in a daily dose of 3.6 g daily during 42 days. Assessments and reassessments by a developed geriatric neuropsychological battery (Tropper, 1984) were undertaken four times during this trial of two years duration. This study shows a clear-cut relationship between the therapeutic results and the clinical stage of DAT. Verbal fluency was accelerated by lecithin administration, while paracetam appeared to be more valuable in improving attention, alertness and interest.

Similar to current literature, we have undertaken also non-drug interventional trials in DAT patients belonging to different stages (Tropper and Wagner, 1984). Two strategies were followed: One was the application of various individual memory-cognitive functions training and enhancing techniques, the others were the classroom memory-cognitive functional rehabilitation sessions conducted by us. These 40 minute bi-weekly sessions were accompanied by slide demonstrations and intensive exercises performed by the patients on the blackboard. Results show that memory-cognitive functions training and classroom sessions are beneficial.

In Stages I and II, these interventional strategies are (a) promoting the patients to capitalize organizational strategies and cues facilitating the act of remembering; (b) helping to accelerate the ecphoric ability of items excepted from long-term memory to the working memory; (c) promoting the use of spatial and temporal cues in the structurization of semantic and episodic memory and (d) allowing to sift out redundancy in the material presented for memorization and recall during the sessions.

With Stage III patients, these non-drug strategies appear to be helpful in improving motivation, in provoking a positive competition and creativity in the classroom, in forcing the patients out of social isolation, in raising their interest in their surroundings.

Our results with drugs and non-drug interventional methods are in line with the results obtained by many of our colleagues in different countries in their reports on various therapeutic approaches to DAT. However, the peculiarity of our work are the encouraging results (the amelioration rate in Stages I, II and partly III) achieved in DAT, seen and treated as a multi-stage process. The proposed developmental-semiological approach can help us to understand better the so often encountered negative results in DAT therapeutic trials.

Conclusions

1. According to our experience, Alzheimer's disease (Dementia of Alzheimer Type) can be interpreted as a multi-stage process, and this approach represents the basis of our individualized therapeutic strategies.

2. The concept of co-existence of impaired and concomitantly preserved abilities and functions in different stages of DAT heralds the prospects of uninterrupted search for individualized therapeutic strategies in DAT patients.

3. Drug and no-drug interventional therapeutic strategies used by us as well as by other specialists, might delay the progression of DAT and contribute to the patient's functional rehabilitation and management.

REFERENCES

Assael, M. and Tropper, M., 1981, Depressions: an affective trigger of organicity or vice versa., in XII. Intern. Congress of Gerontology, Abst. vol. 2,32 Hamburg.

Brainerd, C.J., 1978, The stage question in cognitive development theory, Behav. Brain Sci. 1: 173-213.

Hasagawa, K. and Karasawa., 1975, The epidemiological study of senile psychoorganic syndromes, in: X. Intern. Congress of Gerontology, Abst. vol. 2,95 Jerusalem.

Lishman, W.D., 1978, Organic Psychiatry, Blackwell Scient. Public., Oxford, London.

Reisberg, B. and Ferris, S.H., 1982, Diagnosis and assessment of the older patient, Hospit. & Community Psychiatry, 33: 2, 104.

Russel, W.W., Neuringer, C. and Goldstein, G., 1970, Assessment of brain damage: a neuropsychological approach, Wiley, New York.

Tropper, M., 1978, Memory control in geropsychiatric rehabilitation, in: XI. Intern. Congress of Gerontology, Abst. vol. 1,151 Tokyo.

Tropper, M., Wagner, J., Manulescu, J. & Glinternik, S., Piracetam as a possible mnemotropic and congniactive drug in geriatric psychiatry, in: XII Intern. Congress of Geronotology, Abst. vol. 2, 258, Hamburg.

Tropper, M. and Wagner, J. 1982, Nootropic drugs in short-term memory rehabilitation, in: 13. Collegium Intern. Psychopharmacol., Abst. vol. 2, 725 Jerusalem.

Tropper, M., 1983, Dementias as multi-stage processes (conceptual semiological approaches), in: VII. World Congress of Psychiatry, Abst. vol. 1, S859, 192, Vienna.

Tropper, M. and Wagner, J., 1983, Neuropsychological approaches in Geropsychiatry, Abst. vol. P396, 519, Vienna.

Tropper, M. 1984, Neuropsychology and Psychogeriatrics (new dimensions in assessment, intervention and functional rehabilitation of elderly patients), in: 1st. Intern. Workshop of the Intern. Psychogeriatric Association, 1, 2, Cologne.

Tropper, M. and Wagner, J., 1984, Nootropic vs Cholinergic drugs in memory-cognitive functional rehabilitation, Isr. J. Med. Sci. 20, 287.

Verwoerdt, A., 1976, Clinical Geropsychiatry, Williams & Wilkins, Co. Baltimore.

THE EPIDEMIOLOGY OF ALZHEIMER'S TYPE PRESENILE DEMENTIA IN ISRAEL

Therese Treves, Nelly Zilber, Amos D. Korczyn, Esther Kahana, Yaffa Leibowitz, Milton Alter, and Bruce S. Schoenberg

Sackler School of Medicine, Tel Aviv University and Hadassah University Hospital, Jerusalem, Israel; INSERM Villejuif, France, Temple University Medical School Philadelphia, Pa. and National Institutes of Health Bethesda, MD., U.S.A.

INTRODUCTION

Population studies of dementia can determine data concerning frequency, clinical patterns and risk factors of the disorder, and thus shed light on the pathophysiology. For example, in Alzheimer disease, if epidemiologic features of dementia with early and later onset are found similar, the likelihood will be strengthened that they represent one disease process.

Israel offers special advantages for epidemiologic studies. The population comprises several distinct ethnic groups. Medical care in this country has a high standard and is readily available, usually at no cost. Moreover, the availability of accurate demographic data and the existence of a nation-wide, centralized register of neurologic disease based on patients discharged from hospital (Israel National Neurologic Disease Register) make a study of dementia of early onset in Israel particularly attractive.

METHODS AND PATIENTS

All cases of dementia with onset of disease between the years 1974 through 1978 were included. Sources for information were: Israeli National Neurology Disease Register (1), patients' records from general and psychiatric hospitals, and from institutions for the chronically ill as well as death certificates for the years 1974-1983. The long ascertained period was used to assure that individuals diagnosed after 1978 but with onset between 1974 and 1978 would be identified. A large number of diagnoses was so screened that patients with dementia who may have been listed under different diagnostic labels could be included.

Patients were accepted only if the onset of their disease occurred before or through age 60.

Table 1: Inclusion and Exclusion Criteria for Patients

Inclusion	-	Jewish patients, discharged from hospitals 1974-1983. Slowly progressive mental deterioration. Age at onset 60 years or lower. Onset years 1974-1978.
Exclusion	-	Focal neurologic signs. History of stroke(s). Alcoholism. Other causes of dementia. Pseudodementia.

Onset of dementia was considered to have occurred during the year when the patient or a knowlegeable observer (e.g. spouse) noted the first change in mental function consistent with the diagnosis of dementia.

Patients were accepted as having presenile dementia of the Alzheimer type (PDAT) according to strict clinical diagnostic criteria as follows: if there was proven progressive deterioration in at least three of the following functions: attention, memory, orientation, cognition (learning, calculation, comprehension, abstraction) and behavior (at work and socially.).

Clinical records were reviewed independently by two neurologists. If they disagreed, a third senior neurologist would certify the diagnosis so that for all cases accepted, there was consensus between two neurologists concerning the diagnosis of PDAT. Other criteria used for inclusion or exclusion of patients are detailed in Table 1.

Sex- and age-adjusted incidence rates of PDAT in the Israeli population were calculated by taking the total Jewish population as the standard (indirect adjustments). Demographic data for the calculation of incidence rates were obtained from official publications.

Probability of survival of the patients was calculated by the life-table method and compared to the expected survival in the general population of Israel of the same age and sex using life tables of the National Insurance Institute.

RESULTS

Seventy-one cases were finally accepted as suffering from PDAT; 30 as definite, 18 as probable (because of incomplete data to permit absolute exclusion of either other causes of dementia or mild focal neurological signs), and 23 as possible (where other disorders, such as renal failure were present but seemed insufficient to explain the dementia and the clinical course). Computerized tomograms and/or pneumoencephalograms were available in 56 of the 71 patients and in no instance was there evidence of another disease which could account for the dementia. In 48 cases, there was evidence of cerebral atrophy or ventricular enlargement which are compatible with PDAT. An electro-encephalogram was available in 61 cases. It was read as normal in 29 and diffusely slow in another 24. In 3 other cases, bilateral sharp waves were noted with diffuse bilateral theta activity and in five

Table 2. Age specific incidence rates (IR) by region of birth

Age at onset	Europe-America		Africa-Asia		T O T A L*	
	N	IR	N	IR	N	IR
40-44	2	0.8	0	-	2	0.3
45-49	4	0.9	3	1.0	7	0.8
50-54	11	2.5	4	1.6	16	2.2
55-59	28	7.1	5	2.6	36	5.8
60	9	11.5	1	3.1	10	8.7
T O T A L	54	3.5	13	1.2	71	2.4
Age adjust		3.0		1.4		

* Three patients born in Israel and one for whom country of origin is unknown were included only under "Total".

N Number of patients
IR Annual incidence rate per 10^5 population

cases there was bilateral slowing, greater on one side. In no case was the EEG indicative of a seizure disorder or a focal destructive lesion.

The distribution of cases by age at onset of PDAT, and continent of birth are shown in Table 2. The youngest patient was 43 years old at onset.

The average annual incidence rate of PDAT was calculated for the 70 cases with onset of the disease in Israel and was found to be 2.4 per 100,000 population (2.5 in females and 2.2 in males, a difference which was not statistically significant). The age-adjusted incidence rate per 100,000 population per year was 3.0 among European-American born patients and 1.4 among African-Asian born patients. The differences between these two groups is highly significant ($p < 0.004$).

By the end of 1983 a total of 33 patients had died. The median survival time (MST) for the entire group (life-table method) was 8.1 years.

Fig. 1 shows that the survival of the patients is reduced by about 60% when compared to the expected survival in the general population after adjustment for the age and sex distribution of the cases. Patients with onset of dementia after 55 years had a shorter survival time than those with earlier onset even after correction for expected survival, as shown in Fig. 2.

Twelve of the cases died from the usual complications of chronic disease: pneumonia, urosepsis, decubiti; 8 died from cardiovascular disease; 2 from strokes and one each from malnutrition, cancer and hypoglycemic coma. For 8, the cause of death was unknown.

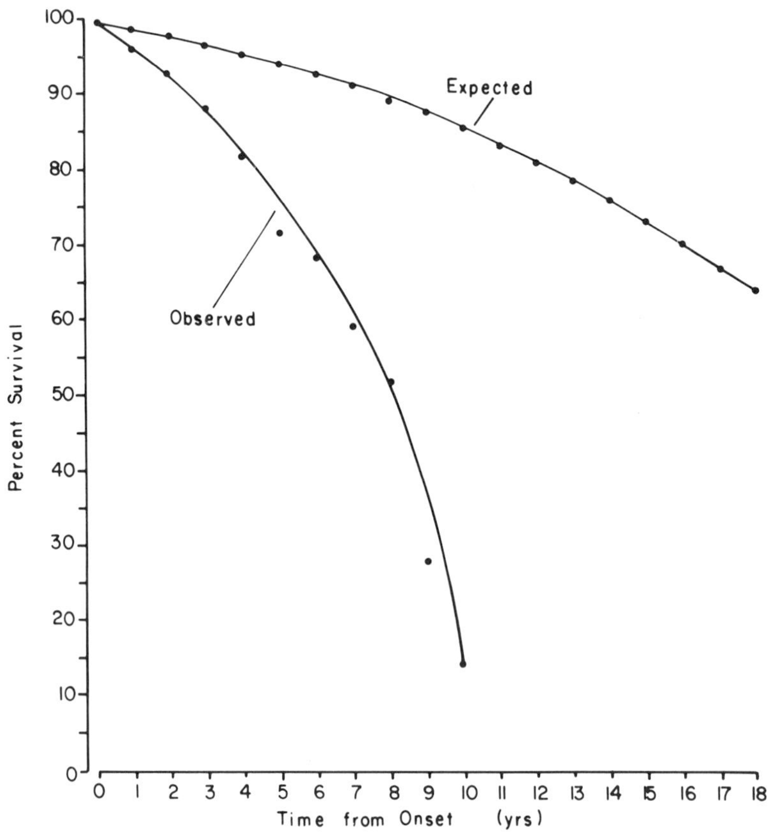

Fig. 1. Survival of patients with presenile dementia of the Alzheimer type as compared to expected survival.

DISCUSSION

The availability, at no cost, of hospital services in Israel assured that patients with dementia, particularly if it started at a young age while the individual was still working, would be admitted for evaluation. To further minimize an ascertainment bias due to delayed referral, every case with a diagnosis of dementia, either of the senile or presenile type, born from 1913 onward was reviewed and records were screened through 1983. Thus, although data included in this report represent minimal incidence figures for PDAT, they cannot be far below the actual frequencies.

The unexpected finding of a significantly lower incidence of PDAT among Jews born in Africa or Asia could be due to an artifact, for example, if this ethnic group would tend to care for PDAT cases at home to a greater extent, or if the family would fail to recognize the dementing process because of the patient's background and education level. When diagnosed,those patients would then be expected to be at a more advanced stage, to be older and to have a shorter life expectancy. As this was not found in our material, we conclude that the lower incidence of PDAT in African-Asians may, in fact, be real. Moreover patients with advanced dementia and urinary incontinence would be referred to the hospital for evaluation in this age group before admission to a nursing home and, as we screened through 1983, we will ascertain them in this stage. In the

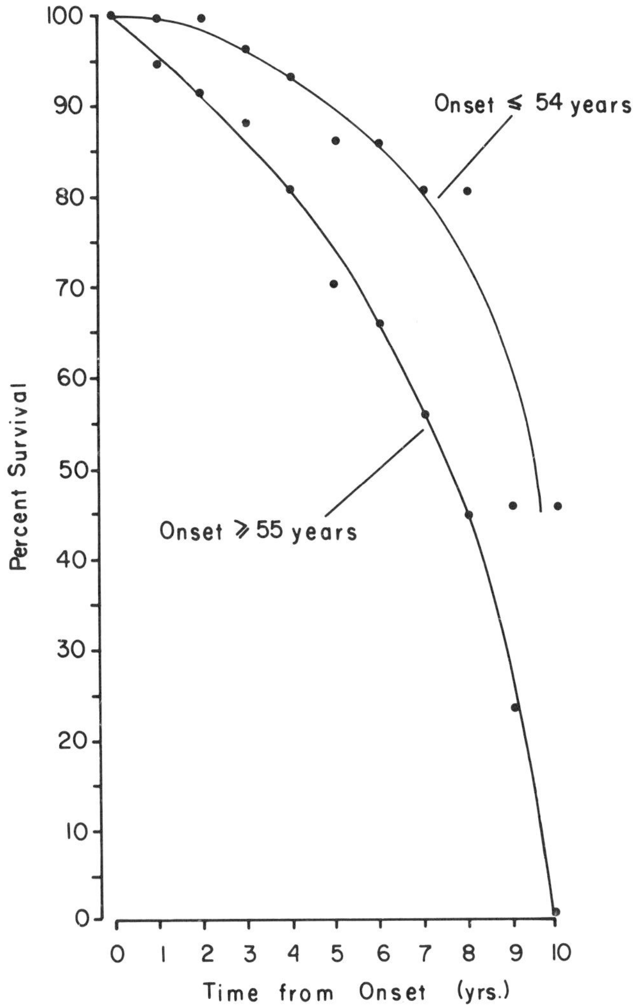

Fig. 2. Effect of age at onset on survival of patients with presenile dementia of the Alzheimer type.

United States ethnic difference in rates of dementia were not observed when blacks were compared to whites in a county of rural Mississippi (2).

Previous epidemiological studies of Alzheimer's disease stressed the relatively high female preponderance (3,4). In Israel, the female to male ratio was only 1.14. However, while a large female excess was found in the senile group, both Molsa, Marttila and Rinne (5) and Sulkava (6) found female to male ratio similar to ours in presenile patients. The reason for the higher prevalence of dementia of the Alzheimer type among older women as compared to older men is unknown at present.

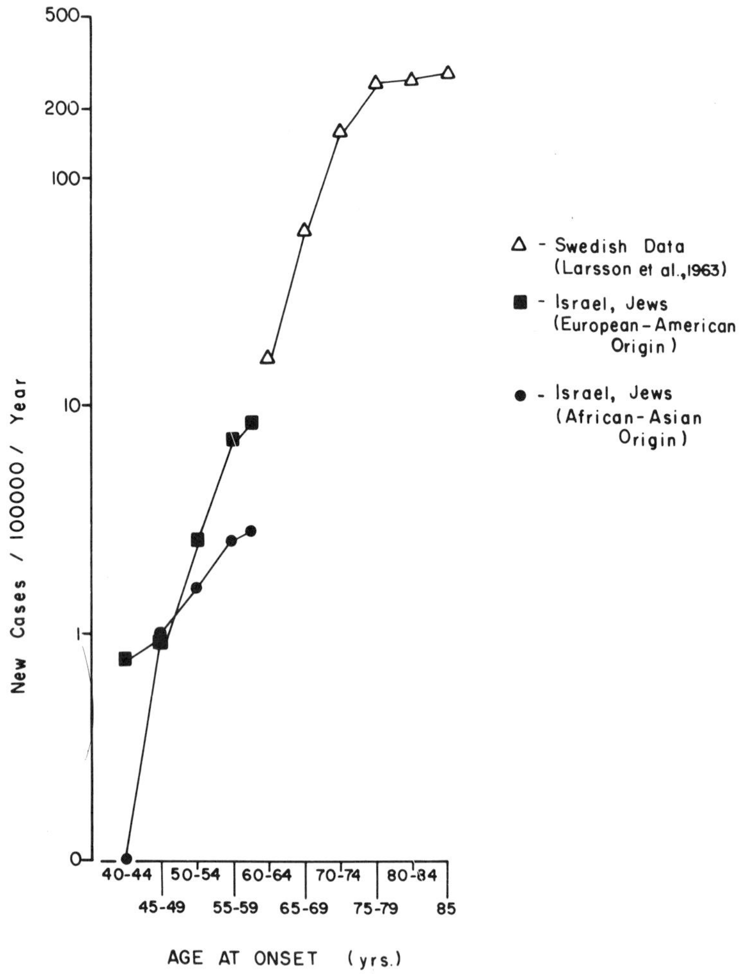

Fig. 3 Incidence of presenile dementia of the Alzheimer type in Israel, for the two ethnic groups, as compared to data from Sweden.

Poor prognosis of Alzheimer disease was particularly stressed by Go, Todorov, Elston et al (7), Goodman (3) and Katzman (8). In the present series, the mean survival time was 8.1 years, corresponding to a reduction of life expectancy by about 60%. As shown in Fig. 2, the reduction in survival was dependent on the age of the patient at the onset of the disease. The mean survival time (corrected for expected life expectancy), was longer for patients with onset of dementia before age 55 as compared to those with older age of onset. A similar age effect was noted by other authors (6,9) in senile dementia of the Alzheimer type (SDAT), although this is not a universal finding (7,10,11).

The disease in European-American born patients was not more "malignant" than in those born in Africa-Asia. The similar mean survival time in the two ethnic groups in Israel, despite their difference in incidence, suggests that the pathologic process is similar.

The curve of the incidence rate of presenile dementia by age for European-American born Jews appears to be continuous with that obtained by Larsson, Sjogren and Jacobson in Sweden for a different Caucasian group with SDAT (12) (Fig. 3). This is consistent with the hypothesis that the disease in these two populations reflects a single nosologic entity (13). Interestingly, the slope of the curve for incidence rate of PDAT by age among Jews from Europe-America differs from the slope for African-Asian Jews (Fig. 3). The difference may represent the effect of environmental factors, though genetic differences may also contribute since the two Jewish ethnic groups have lived apart for centuries. If bias in social behavior toward demented individuals can be excluded and the difference in frequency of dementia proves to be real, then the relationship of genetic and environmental factors to dementia in different groups should be studied further in Israel.

REFERENCES

1. E. Kahana, Y. Leibowitz, B. S. Schoenberg, and M. Alter, Israeli National Disease Register, Neuroepidemiology 1:239 (1982).
2. B. S. Schoenberg, D. W. Anderson, and A. F. Haerer, Prevalence and clinical features of dementia in a biracial US population: Neuroepidemiological study of a county in rural Mississippi, Ann Neurol. 10:72 (1981).
3. L. Goodman, Alzheimer's disease. A clinico-pathologic analysis of twenty-three cases with a theory on pathogensis, J. Nerv. Ment. Dis. 127:97 (1953).
4. E. H. Liston, The clinical phenomenology of presenile dementia. A critical review of the literature, J. Nerv. Ment. Dis. 167 329 (1979).
5. P. K. Molsa, R. J. Marttila, U. K. Rinne, Epidemiology of dementia in a Finnish population, Acta Neurol. Scand. 65:541 (1982).
6. R. Sulkava, Alzheimer's disease and senile dementia of Alzheimer type. A comparative study, Acta Neurol. Scand. 65:636 (1982).
7. R. C. P. Go, A. B. Todorov, R. C. Elston, and J. Constantinidis, The malignancy of dementias, Ann Neurol. 3:559 (1978).
8. R. Katzman, The prevalence and malignancy of Alzheimer disease, Arch. Neurol. 33:217 (1976).
9. J. Constantinidis, Is Alzheimer's disease: a major form of senile dementia. Clinical, anatomical and genetic data, in: "Alzheimer's Disease: Senile Dementia and Related Disorders, " R. Katzman, R. D. Terry, and K. L. Bick, eds., Raven Press, New York (1978).
10. D. W. K. Kay, Outcome and cause of death in mental disorders of old age: a long-term follow-up of functional and organic psychoses, J. Ment. Sci. 102:249 (1955).
11. B. Seltzer, and I. Sherwin, A comparison of clinical features in early- and late-onset primary degenerative dementia, Arch. Neurol. 40:143 (1983).
12. T. Larsson, T. Sjogren, and G. Jacobson, Senile dementia: A clinical, socio-medical and genetic study. Acta Psychiat. Scand. 39: Suppl 167, 1-259 (1963).
13. E. M. Gruenberg, Epidemiology of senile dementia, in: "Advances in Neurology," vol. 19, B. S. Schoenberg, ed., Raven Press, New York (1978).

DEMENTIA IN PARKINSON DISEASE

Amos D. Korczyn

Tel Aviv University Sackler School of Medicine
Ramat Aviv, Israel

INTRODUCTION

The possibility that Parkinson disease is associated with dementia has been negated by neurologists for several decades. However, the story is more complex. It should be recalled that predating levodopa therapy, patients could not be formally tested because of bradykinesia and speech difficulties, and this would be a problem particularly in more advanced cases. If cognitive functioning was impaired, this was ascribed to "bradyphrenia" (1), presumably implying a normal mental state, but "slow thinking" as a manifestation of the disease, paralleling bradykinesia. If a patient was frankly disoriented, it would be difficult to be sure to what extent this was a manifestation of drug-induced confusion (2). Other factors could account for pseudodementia, such as social isolation and depression. Finally, if dementia could not be denied it could always be ascribed to a chance association with "senility" or "cerebral arteriosclerosis". With the introduction of modern drug therapy, however, many of the above factors could be ruled out as contributing to the dementia, or at least could be accounted for. Surprisingly, however, the impression emerged that cognitive changes are common in Parkinson disease.

Prevalence data of dementia in Parkinson disease vary (3-5), probably reflecting the population studied as much as the criteria used for diagnosing dementia.

Two factors were immediately thought of as possibly accounting for the high prevalence of dementia in Parkinson disease. The first was that the introduction of dopaminergic agonists has increased the longevity of the patients, thus enabling them to develop and exhibit changes. Indeed, while prior to the levodopa era Parkinsonian patients had a markedly reduced life expectancy, this was practically normalized by drugs. It was suggested that with this increased life expectancy patients now could develop SDAT changes, or that such changes were there all the time, but their expression was suppressed by the motor impairment, and uncovered when levodopa was given. However, although prevalence data on dementia in Parkinson disease vary, they are definitely higher than expected for the general population. Therefore, increased life expectancy or improved motor control alone could not explain the frequent dementia.

The second hypothesis which was suggested as possibly accounting for the high frequency of dementia is that these changes may be related to the drug therapy rather than to the disease (4). Since levodopa is hardly used for indications other than Parkinson disease, and since advanced cases of non-treated Parkinsonism are not available (or cannot be tested), this theory was hard to disprove.

The recognition that extrapyramidal features commonly accompanied Alzheimer disease only added to the confusion since some patients would be hard to classify: Are they suffering from Parkinson disease with marked dementia, or from Alzheimer disease with marked Parkinsonism, or from chance co-occurrence of the two conditions? Phrased differently, are Parkinson disease and Alzheimer disease two extreme points on a continuum? Indeed, Appel has recently suggested (6) that both diseases result from impaired neurotrophic influences. If this is true, it would not be surprising that neurotrophic failure may include more than a single neuronal population.

It could be expected that histological data would solve the question, but they have not. Neurofibrillary tangles as well as senile plaques, the hallmark of Alzheimer disease, are rather frequent in the brains of parkinsonian patients (7,8). It is unclear, however, to what extent these histological changes reflect, or parallel, the cognitive decline in Parkinsonism as they do in SDAT (9).

Changes in the nucleus basalis of Meynert (nbM), which are central to the cholinergic deficit of Alzheimer disease, were also described in Parkinson disease (10-12) although they may not be identical in the two diseases (13). However, the analogy is also limited since nbM changes can also occur in presumably non-demented patients with Parkinson disease (11). It could, perhaps, be argued that nbM lesions predate the classical cortical changes and that the degeneration of nbM neurons may actually lead to delayed cortical senile plaque formation together with clinical evidence of dementia.

On another level, detailed neuropsychological testing in patients with Parkinson disease suggested that the dementia may have certain characteristics, possibly grouping it with other forms of "subcortical" dementia (14). This view is difficult to reconcile with the anatomical cortical changes detailed above, which are similar in Alzheimer disease and in Parkinson disease.

Thus, several questions arise. Are the cognitive changes an integral part of Parkinson disease? Are they related to drug therapy? Does the mental change reflect "subcortical" or "cortical" dementia, and - if the latter is the case - are they identical, clinically and pathologically, with changes of Alzheimer disease? We have recently initiated a prospective study of Parkinsonian patients with a special emphasis on their cognitive deterioration and some biologic correlates. The present report will give some of our preliminary results.

One way to try and approach the problem of the dementia in Parkinson disease was to see whether there are EEG alterations in this condition. Normal aging is accompanied by EEG changes, particularly slowing of the alpha rhythm. This shift towards the slow end of the alpha frequency spectrum is associated with anterior temporal theta and delta wave foci, which have been reported in 30-40°/o of healthy people over the age of 50 years (15). The EEG changes associated with Alzheimer disease consist of accentuation of the features seen in normal aging (16).

Previous EEG studies on patients with Parkinson disease have shown that although in the majority the EEG is unaffected, the prevalence of abnormalities is greater than in a normal population (17). However, these studies failed to distinguish between demented and non-demented Parkinsonian patients.

EXPERIMENTAL METHODS

We have studied 119 consecutive patients with Parkinson disease diagnosed by the conventional clinical criteria of this disease. Other diseases were excluded by family and personal history, neurological examination, CT scans and routine laboratory tests. All patients were on an optimal dose of dopa derivatives and anticholinergics.

EEG recording consisted of 30 min: tracing performed in an 8- or 18-channel Grass machine using the standard 10/20 system of electrode placement, and utilizing scalp-to-scalp and referential montages. Recording was done during wakefulness, 3-minute hyperventilation and photic stimulation. All patients were instructed to have their meal before their EEG.

EEG analyses were done blindly by a qualified electroencephalographer who had no information concerning the mental or motor status of the patient. The average frequency of the dominant occipital rhythm was measured in several points of the record. In addition we evaluated overall disturbances, accentuation of theta and delta rhythms, fluctuations in alertness and paroxysmal activity. EEG recordings were classified as either *normal* or *abnormal*. *Normal* background activity was adjusted for age, *8 Hz* and above for age 45-70, 7.5 Hz and above for age 70-85. Intermittent bitemporal delta slowing was considered as essentially normal for patients above the age of 50. The EEG was considered *abnormal* if the occipital rhythm was below the values indicated above. Variable degree of local and generalized slowing (excluding intermittent bitemporal slowing above age 50), as well as paroxysmal epileptiform activity were also considered.

The motor function of the patients was evaluated according to the classification of Hoehn and Yahr (18).

The mental status was evaluated in all groups of patients by a short questionnaire. The questionnaire included 22 items of attention, memory, learning ability, calculation, naming, comprehension, visuo-spatial skill, reading, writing and abstraction. The test was previously performed by 400 controls and 80 demented patients and was found to be valid for our Hebrew-speaking population. Our previous analysis demonstrated that a score of 85% or above indicated a "normal" mental status, while a cut point of 62% was used to separate definitely demented patients. An overlap between normal and demented subjects exists for scores between 62 and 85. Accordingly, we have divided our Parkinsonian patients into 3 subgroups:

A. Patients with "normal" scores (85%).
B. Patients with mild dementia - scores 62-85%.
C. Patients with moderate to severe dementia - scores below 62.

RESULTS AND DISCUSSION

EEG abnormalities consisted mainly of slowing of the background rhythm, and essentially identical results were obtained if all abnormalities were considered or if abnormalities other than slowing were excluded. In the total group, abnormal records were common (68%) and occurred increasingly more frequently with advanced age (Table 1). However, a closer look at the results indicates that slowing was more common in the elderly Parkinsonian patients because they were more likely to be demented. In separate subgroups (non demented, mildly demented and markedly demented), age did not affect the frequency of abnormal records. Marked and statistically significant differences were observed between the groups, with a prevalence of abnormalities corresponding to the degree of dementia (Table 1). On the other hand, EEG abnormalies were also related to motor disability.

Table 1. Correlation between dementia score, Parkinsonian stage and EEG findings

Mental State		Parkinsonian stages I + II	III	IV	Total
	Normal	8.3°/o (24)	25°/o (16)	33°/o (3)	15.6°/o (43)
	Mild dementia	40°/o (10)	31°/o (19)	67°/o (3)	37.5°/o (32)
	Severe dementia	25°/o (16)	47°/o (19)	89°/o (9)	45.7°/o (44)
	Total	19.2°/o (50)	37.7°/o (54)	73.3°/o (15)	33.6°/o (119)

The figures denote percentage of abnormal records. (Number of cases in brackets).

Our results therefore demonstrated an interaction, both the mental state and the degree of movement impairment being correlated with EEG abnormalities. The fact that in our study dementia correlated with slowing of the dominant alpha frequency is compatible with the view that parkinsonian dementia is akin to Alzheimer disease. On the other hand, the association between motor disability and EEG changes seems surprising and may suggest a dopaminergic effect on the EEG. There is meager data on the influence of subcortical structures on the EEG. It should be stressed, however, that data are not available correlating EEG slowing with dementia score in Alzheimer disease. It is therefore unknown whether such a correlation exists, and which other factors also influence the EEG changes in SDAT.

In addition we have made CT studies on our patients. Using horizontal cuts, we have measured several anatomical parameters and correlated them with the degree of dementia. Previously, Sroka et al. (19) examined CT scans of demented and non-demented parkinsonian patients; they found <u>all</u> demented patients to have abnormal CT scans. The frequency of similar changes in the non-demented group was much lower (50°/o), in fact very similar to that of a control group (44°/o). The demented cases had primarily sulcal enlargement but also ventricular dilatation. We have measured the width of the frontal horns of the lateral ventricles, the septo-caudate and intercaudate distances, the width of the third ventricle, the cortical sulcus score and the number of sulci seen on the uppermost cuts. As in the study of Sroka et al. (19) all these factors correlated significantly with age, and several with the Parkinsonian score. Our results show a considerable overlap between the demented and non-demented group. The only parameters which correlated with the degree of dementia were the intercaudate distance and the width of the third ventricle. These results are particularly interesting since de Leon and his colleagues reported that among linear ventricular measures, the width of the third cerebral ventricle was the best correlate of cognitive decline (20). In this respect, then, Parkinson dementia parallels Alzheimer's dementia.

Since both EEG and CT studies support the association of subcortical changes with dementia, it is interesting to recall that Mortimer et al. (21) found a correlation between the motor impairment and the degree of cognitive decline.

The clinical features of parkinsonian patients with or without dementia were also compared, and the results are detailed in Table 2. This Table shows that patients with dementia are slightly (and non-significantly) older than the non-demented and Parkinson disease was diagnosed in them at a more advanced age than those without dementia. The duration of the disease is but slightly longer in the demented. These results are on the whole similar to those of Lieberman et al. (5) although these workers found a shorter duration of parkinsonism in the demented group, implying a more aggressive form of disease. It is, of course, well known that confusion and dementia tend to appear late in the course of the disease. On the other hand, there is also a considerable number of patients who do not develop cognitive changes even after many years. However, since the mean age of the groups does not differ significantly, this may be due to selective high mortality of more advanced, demented cases. We are currently investigating this hypothesis.

In our study, we have excluded patients with stroke, when the latter was diagnosed either by history, clinical findings or CT. The results show a slightly higher percentage of patients with coronary or peripheral artery disease among demented parkinsonians. However, this probably reflects their more advanced age rather than implying a vascular etiology to their dementia.

Table 2. Clinical Characteristics of Demented or Non Demented Parkinsonian Patients

	MENTAL STATE		
	Normal	Mild dementia	Marked dementia
No. of cases	36	25	35
Mean age (years)	67.2	70.4	71.4
Age at diagnosis of Parkinson disease (years)	62.5	65.3	65.1
Mean duration of Parkinsonism (years)	4.8	5.0	6.2
Mean duration of levodopa therapy (years)	3.9	4.2	4.0
Vascular background	66°/o	70°/o	72°/o
Smoking	39°/o	42°/o	17°/o
On-off	25°/o	37°/o	22°/o

In summary, our data confirm the high prevalence of dementia among patients with Parkinson disease. It is our belief that dementia is one of the protean manifestations of Parkinson disease, together with hyperkinesis, rigidity, tremor and loss of postural reflexes. The demented patients are somewhat older than the non-demented but the duration of treatment with dopaminergic drugs is similar. It is therefore unlikely that these agents play an important role in the development of the dementia. Similarly, a vascular cause is unlikely. Demented parkinsonian patients are similar to patients with SDAT in manifesting EEG abnormalities (primarily slowing of the alpha activity). On CT, they show ventricular dilatation, again similar to the finding in Alzheimer disease. This striking parallelism between Parkinson dementia and Alzheimer disease is intriguing and is an important field of future research.

REFERENCES

1. R. Hassler, Zur pathologieschen Anatomie der Paralysis Agitans und des postenzephalitischen Parkinsonismus, J. Psychol. Neurol. 48:390 (1938).
2. A. D. Korczyn, and M. D. Yahr, Psychiatric side effecrs of antiparkinson drugs, in: Geriatric Psychopharmacology, K. Nandy, ed. Elsevier, Amsterdam (1979).
3. R. H. S. Mindham, S. W. A. Ahmed, and C. G. Clough, A controlled study of dementia in Parkinson's disease, J. Neurol. Neurosurg. Psychiat. 45:969 (1982).
4. P. R. Sweet, F. H. McDowell, J. S. Feigenson, A. W. Loranger, and H. Goodell, Mental symptoms in Parkinson's disease during chronic treatment with levodopa, Neurology 26:305 (1976).
5. A. Lieberman, M. Dziatolowski, M. Kupersmith, M. Serby, A. Goodgold, J. Korein, and M. Goldstein, Dementia in Parkinson disease, Ann. Neurol. 6:355 (1979).
6. S. H. Appel, A unifying hypothesis for the cause of amyotrophic lateral sclerosis, parkinsonism and Alzheimer disease, Ann. Neurol. 10:499 (1981).
7. F. Boller, T. Mizutani, U. Roessmann, and P. Gambetti, Parkinson disease, dementia and Alzheimer disease: Clinicopathological correlations, Ann. Neurol. 7:329 (1980).
8. A.H. Hakim and G. Mathieson, Dementia in Parkinson disease: A neuropathologic study, Neurology 29:1209 (1979).
9. E. K. Perry, B. E. Tomlinson, G. Blessed, K. Bergmann, P. H. Gibson, and R. H. Perry, Correlation of central cholinergic abnormalities with senile plaques and mental test scores in senile dementia, Br. Med. J. 2:1457 (1978).
10. P. J. Whitehouse, J. C. Hedreen, C. L. White, and D. L. Price, Basal forebrain neurons in the dementia of Parkinson disease, Ann. Neurol. 13:243 (1983).
11. I. Nakano, and A. Hirano, Parkinson disease: Neuron loss in the nucleus basalis without concomitant Alzheimer's disease, Ann. Neurol. 15:415 (1984).
12. F. Tagliavini, G. Pilleri, C. Bouras, and J. Constantinidis, The basal nucleus of Meynert in idiopathic Parkinson's disease, Acta Neurol. Scand. 69:20 (1984).
13. J. M. Candy, R. H. Perry, E. K. Perry, D. Irving, G. Blessed, A. F. Fairbeirn, and B.E. Tomlinson, Pathological Changes in nucleus of Meynert in Alzheimer's and Parkinson's diseases, J. Neurol. Sci. 54:272 (1983).

14. M. L. Albert, Subcortical dementia, _in_: Alzheimer's Disease; Senile Dementia and Related Disorders. R. Katzman, R.D. Terry, and K.L. Bick, eds. Raven, New York (1978).
15. J. R. Hughes, The EEG in patients at different ages without organic cerebral disease, _Electroceph. Clin. Neurophysiol_. 42:776 (1977).
16. H. Soininen, V. J. Partanen, and E. L. Helkala, EEG findings in senile dementia and normal aging, _Acta Neurol. Scandinav_. 65:59 (1982).
17. C. L. Yeager, W. W. Alberts, and L. D. Delattre, Effect of sterotaxic surgery upon electroencephalographic status of Parkinsonian patients, _Neurology_ 16:904 (1966).
18. M. M. Hoehn, and M. D. Yahr, Parkinsonism: Onset, progression and mortality, _Neurology_ 17:427 (1967).
19. H. Sroka, T. S. Elizan, M. D. Yahr, A. Burger, and M. R. Mendoza, Organic mental syndrome and confusional states in Parkinson's disease, _Arch. Neurol._ 38:339 (1981).
20. M. J. de Leon, S. H. Ferris, and A. E. George, Computed tomography evaluation of brain-behavior relationship in senile dementia of the Alzheimer type. _Neurobiol. Aging_ 1:69 (1980).
22. J. A. Mortimer, F. J. Pirozzolo, E. C. Hansch, and D. D. Webster, Relationship of motor symptoms to intellectual deficits in Parkinson disease, _Neurology_ 32:133 (1982).

POSSIBLE DOPAMINERGIC BASIS FOR PERCEPTUAL MOTOR DYSFUNCTION

Yaakov Stern, and Richard Mayeux

Neurological Institute, Columbia University College of Physicians and Surgeons, 710 West 168th Street, New York New York 10032, USA

There are at least two different forms of intellectual impairment in patients with Parkinson's disease (PD). Approximately 30% of patients may eventually become demented (1). This dementia is difficult to differentiate from dementia of the Alzheimer type (DAT) (2) and may be associated with similar neuropathologic and neurochemical changes (3,4). In particular, changes in the cholinergic system may be similar (5). The majority of parkinsonians, however, carry on relatively normal lives with unimpaired social and occupational functioning, and meet no recognized criteria for dementia. In these non-demented patients, careful neuropsychological testing often reveals subtle intellectual deficits, most commonly perceptual motor dysfunction (1).

Perceptual motor dysfunction in PD still might be the initial manifestation of developing dementia. If so, it could be attributed to changes in the same cholinergic system implicated in DAT. Alternately, it is possible that this impairment is related to the well established changes in the dopaminergic system in PD. This relation could be present in DAT as well. Changes in non-cholinergic systems have also been described in DAT, but have not been as consistently related to dementia or its severity (6,7). In addition, DAT manifests a wide range of intellectual changes, and perceptual motor dysfunction is common (8). Cholinergic changes in DAT may relate only to particular aspects of intellectual impairment such as poor memory, while changes in other transmitter systems may correlate with other deficits. This chapter will review evidence suggesting that perceptual motor dysfunction in PD is related to changes in the dopaminergic system.

PERCEPTUAL MOTOR DYSFUNCTION IN PD

The most commonly reported intellectual change in non-demented patients with PD is perceptual motor dysfunction. Various tasks have been used to explore this cognitive domain, including puzzle assembly (9,10), tracing (11,12), tracking (13), and drawing (14) tests. These deficits are subtle and typically do not impair patients' functional capacities.

We explored this issue (12) using a test in which patients and controls traced patterns of increasing complexity presented on a vertical transparent screen. Some patterns were presented with missing segments which subjects were required to fill in. Subjects also completed a brief test of intellectual function, and the severity of patients' parkinsonian signs and symptoms were assessed. Patients performed more poorly than controls on complete patterns, and their errors increased more sharply than controls on patterns with missing segments. Patients' errors, but not those of controls, in filling in missing segments were uniquely related to performance on construction tasks. Other aspects of tracing performance correlated with the severity of their parkinsonian symptoms. We noted a similar deficit on a tracing task which made use of only the tactile modality (15). These findings suggest that there is an underlying perceptual motor deficit in PD that affects performance on both tracing and construction tasks.

Flowers (13) used a tracking task, and suggested that patients can not generate movements without immediate feedback to guide them. Marsden (16) also described an inability of parkinsonians to execute motor plans. He stressed that patients' intellectual abilities are unimpaired in the presence of this deficit, and in fact considered it a purely motor impairment. Our studies demonstrated that problems in the control of higher-order movement (such as in the tracing and tracking tasks) correlate with performance on tasks that are generally considered intellectual (such as construction tasks). Further both types of tasks were unrelated to the motor symptoms of PD. We term these deficits "perceptual-motor" since they appear to involve the inability to coordinate the perceptual and motor activities necessary to complete a task (11,12,17).

Performance on tasks that require no motor response would also be affected since the organization and monitoring of responses is also impaired. For example, parkinsonians commonly perform poorly on the Wisconsin Card Sort and Stroop Word-Color Test (18,19). In these tests, behavior must be modulated based on cues that are not actually present. Performance on both of these tasks is disrupted by lesions to specific areas of the frontal lobe (20). Interestingly, these cortical areas project to the basal ganglia, and it is possible that the tasks are affected in PD because of disruption of a cortico-striatal system at the level of the basal ganglia.

PERCEPTUAL MOTOR DYSFUNCTION IN ANIMALS

This concept is supported by behavioral research in animals. Delayed spatial response or spatial alternation tasks can be affected by lesions to either dorsolateral frontal cortex or to anterodorsal head of caudate (21). In the delayed spatial response paradigm, the animal watches food being placed in one of two identical food wells. A delay period follows in which the animal's view of the wells is blocked. The animal then chooses one of the wells. While simpler in many ways than perceptual motor tasks used when testing people, the delayed spatial response task maintains many of the same characteristics. It is not simply a memory test: the animal can solve tasks of similar difficulty that do not have a spatial component, such as visual discrimination tasks. Rather, the animal must operate within a spatial environment with no external guidance. Similarly in the tracing task described above, the patient is required to generate simple movements with no guidance save his past experience.

Manipulation of the dopaminergic system also affects the ability to perform the delayed spatial response task. Depleting dopamine levels with dopaminergic antagonists produces reversible deficits on the task (22).

It is possible, then, that the subtle intellectual deficits seen in PD may be related to changes in the dopaminergic system, particularly the cortico-striatal system where lesions are disruptive of perceptual motor function. If so, they represent a separate entity from the more severe deficits seen in demented patients.

MPTP-INDUCED PARKINSONISM

A unique opportunity to investigate these alternatives presented itself with the recognition of the parkinsonian syndrome induced by 1-methyl-4-phenyl-1,2,3,6-tetrahydropyridine (MPTP) (23). This syndrome has all of the classical motor features of PD, and is responsive to standard dopamine agonist therapy (24). It appears to represent a purely hypodopaminergic condition. Neuropathological changes in primates and in one human case consist primarily of selective destruction of dopaminergic neurons in the pars compacta of the substantia nigra (25-27). The concentration of the major metabolite of dopamine, HVA, is reduced both in cerebrospinal fluid and in brain (25,27,28). Changes in other neurotransmitter levels have also been reported but occurred only in the more acute phase of the syndrome and returned to normal over time.

Patients with MPTP induced parkinsonism represent a unique population in which to explore the underlying basis for intellectual changes in PD. Changes in this group should represent the effects of their hypodopaminergic state and aid in differentiating the effects of dopaminergic and cholinergic changes on intellectual function.

We studied 6 patients with MPTP-induced parkinsonism to assess intellectual function, attention and reaction time (29). Eight people with a similar history of drug abuse participated as age, education and experience matched controls. None of the MPTP patients met criteria for dementia. General intellectual function as assessed by a brief mental status examination was slightly depressed in the MPTP group. In more specific neuropsychological testing, construction, category naming and performance on the Stroop Word-Color test were worse in the MPTP group. Attention, memory, digit span, calculation and overall language performance were comparable in the two groups.

The pattern of intellectual changes seen in the MPTP patients was similar to that reported in idiopathic PD. Both construction and the Stroop Word-Color test can be classified as assessments of perceptual motor abilities. In addition, poor performance on these tests can result from damage to the frontal lobes. Deficient category naming is also associated with damage to this area (20). Further, poor performance on category naming tests has also been reported in idiopathic PD (30). These findings suggest that the pattern of intellectual changes seen in idiopathic PD and in MPTP-induced parkinsonism may be related to changes in the dopaminergic system.

CONCLUSION

This review attempted to develop the concept of perceptual motor dysfunction and to relate it to the loss of dopamine in PD. A neuroanatomic system to mediate perceptual motor function was also suggested. Attributing perceptual motor dysfunction to changes in the dopaminergic system still does not eliminate the possibility that it is an early manifestation of dementia. Longitudinal studies of parkinsonian patients with perceptual motor dysfunction, and additional work relating biochemical and behavioral measures in PD and DAT are necessary to clarify this issue.

ACKNOWLEDGMENTS

Support for this work was provided by grants from the National Institutes of Health (AG-02802) and the Parkinson's Disease Foundation.

REFERENCES

1. Mayeux R, Stern Y. Intellectual dysfunction and dementia in Parkinson's disease. Adv Neurol 1983;38:211-227.
2. Mayeux R, Stern Y, Rosen J, Benson DF. Is "subcortical dementia" a recognizable clinical entity? Ann Neurol 1983;14:278-283.
3. Hakim AM and Mathieson G. Dementia in Parkinson's disease: a neuropathologic study. Neurology, 1979;29:1209-14.
4. Whitehouse P, Hedreen JC, White C, DeLong M, Price DL. Basal forebrain neurons in the dementia of Parkinson's disease. Ann Neurol 1983;13:243-248.
5. Ruberg M, Ploska A, Javoy-Agid F, Agid Y. Muscarinic binding and choline acetyltransferase activity in parkinsonian subjects with reference to dementia. Brain Res 1982;232:129-33.
6. Winblad B, Adolfsson R, Carlsson A, Gottfries CG. Biogenic amines in brains of patients with Alzheimer's disease. Aging 19; 1982:25-33.
7. Adolfsson R, Gottfries CG, Roos BE, Winblad B: Changes in brain catecholamines in patients with dementia of Alzheimer types. Brit J. Psychiat. 1979;135:216-23.
8. Ajuriaguerra J. de, Tissot R. Some aspects of psycho-neurologic disintegration in senile dementia. In: Muller C, Ciompi L (eds.) Senile Dementia. Huber, Switzerland, pp. 69-79.
9. Joubert M and Barbeau A. Akinesia in parkinson's disease. In: Barbeau A. and Brunette J-R (eds.) Progress in Neurogenetics. Excerpta Medica, Amsterdam, 1969, pp. 366-376.
10. Botez MI, Barbeau A. Neuropsychological findings in Parkinson's disease: A comparison between various tests during long-term levodopa therapy. Int J Neurol 1975;10:222-32.
11. Stern Y, Mayeux R, Rosen J. Ilson J. Perceptual motor dysfunction in Parkinson's disease: A deficit in sequential and predictive movement. J Neurol Neurosurg Psychiatry 1983;46:145-51.
12. Stern Y, Mayeux R, Rosen J. Contribution of perceptual motor dysfunction and tracing disturbances in Parkinson's disease. J Neurol Neurosurg Psychiatry 1984;47:983-94.
13. Flowers K. Lack of prediction in the motor behavior of parkinsonism. Brain 1978;101:35-52.
14. Pirozzolo FJ, Hansach EC, Mortimer JA, Webster DD and Kuskowski MA. Dementia in Parkinson's disease: A neuropsychological analysis. Brain cognition 1982;1:71-83.
15. Mayeux R, Tomaino C, Rosen J, Stern Y, Gerstman L. The effects of parkinsonism and aging on tactile-motor skills and perception. Neurology (Abstract), 1983;33:198A.

16. Marsden CD: The mysterious motor function of the basal ganglia: The Robert Wartenberg Lecture. Neurology 1982;32:514-39.
17. Stern Y. Behavior and the basal ganglia. Adv Neurol 1983;38: 195-210.
18. Bowen FP. Behavioral alterations in patients with basal ganglia lesions. In: Yahr MD (ed.) The Basal Ganglia. Raven Press, 1975, pp. 169-80.
19. Lees AJ, Smith E. Cognitive deficits in the early stages of Parkinsons disease. Brain 1983;106:257-70.
20. Lezack M: Neuropsychological assessment. Oxford Press, New York, 1976, pp. 208-211.
21 Divac I. Neostriatum and functions of the prefrontal cortex. Acta Neurobiol Exp 1972;32:461-77.
22. Brozoski TJ, Brown RM, Rosvold HE, Goldman PS. Cognitive deficit caused by regional depletion of dopamine in prefrontal cortex of rhesus monkey. Science 1979;205:929-32.
23. Langston JW, Ballard P, Tefrud JW, Irwin I. Chronic parkinsonism in humans due to a product of mepedrine analogue synthesis. Science 1983;219:979-80.
24. Langston JW, Ballard P. Parkinsonism induced by 1-methyl-4-phenyl-1,2,3,6-tetrahydropyridine (MPTP): Implications for treatment and the pathogenesis of Parkinson's disease. Can J Neurol Sci 1984;11:160-5.
25. Burns RS, Chiveh CC, Markey SP, Ebert MM, Jacobowitz DM, Kopin IJ. A primate model of parkinsonism: Selective destruction of neurons in the pars compacta of the substantia nigra by N-methyl-4-phenyl-1,2,3,6-tetrahydropyridine. Proc Natl Acad Sci. USA, 1983;80:4546-50.
26. Langston JW, Forno LS, Robert CS, Irwin I. Selective nigral toxicity after systematic administration of 1-methyl-4-phenyl-1,2,5,6-tetrahydropyridine (MPTP) in the squirrel monkey. Brain Res. 1984;292:390-4.
27. Davis GC, Williams AC, Markey SP, Ebert MH, Caine ED, Reichert CM, Kopin IJ. Chronic parkinsonism secondary to intravenous injection of mepedrine analogues. Psychiatry Res. 1979;1:249-54.
28. Ballard PA, Langston JW, Tetrud J. Burns Rs. Chemically induced chronic parkinsonism in young adults: Clinical and neuropharmacologic aspects. Neurology (Abstract) 1983;33:90A
29. Stern Y, Langston JW. Intellectual changes in patients with MPTP-induced parkinsonism. Neurology, in press.
30. Matison R, Mayeux R, Rosen J, Fahn S. "Tip-of-the-tongue" phenomenon in Parkinson's disease. Neurology 1982;32:567-70.

DIAGNOSTIC METHODS IN ALZHEIMER'S DISEASE:

MAGNETIC RESONANCE BRAIN IMAGING AND CSF NEUROTRANSMITTER MARKERS

John H. Growdon,[1,2,3] Suzanne Corkin,[2,3]
Ferdinando Buonanno,[1,4] Kenneth Davis,[4]
F. Jacob Huff,[1,2,3] M. Flint Beal,[1,4]
and Carl Kramer,[1,4]

[1]Department of Neurology
Massachusetts General Hospital
Boston, MA

[2]Department of Psychology and [3]Clinical Research Center
Massachusetts Institute of Technology
Cambridge, MA

[4]Department of Neuroradiology
Massachusetts General Hospital
Boston, MA

The clinical diagnosis of Alzheimer's disease (AD) depends upon a history of progressive cognitive impairments, lack of focal neurological signs, and laboratory tests that exclude other known causes of dementia (1,2). A definitive diagnosis of AD depends upon characteristic histopathological features, including abundant senile plaques and neurofibrillary tangles in the cortical neuropil (3,4). Other anatomical features include decreased numbers of neurons in the nucleus basalis of Meynert (5), the brain stem nucleus locus coeruleus (6,7), and the frontal and temporal cortices (8). Frequent neurochemical correlates of AD are decreased choline acetyltransferase (CAT), acetylcholinesterase (AChE), glutamic acid decarboxylase (GAD), and butyrylcholinesterase (BuChE) activities, and decreased somatostatin, norepinephrine, and serotonin levels (9-20). Diagnosis of AD would be enhanced greatly if it were possible to detect any of these pathological or neurochemical changes in patients before death. Without such measures, the clinical diagnosis of AD is confirmed pathologically in only 60-75% of the cases (21,22); in these instances, Parkinson's disease (PD) and vascular disease are the most prevalent unrecognized causes of dementia. This chapter describes our experience with two approaches that may render diagnosis of the dementias more accurate: morphological studies with magnetic resonance imaging (MRI) of the brain and biochemical analyses of neurotransmitter markers in the cerebrospinal fluid (CSF).

MAGNETIC RESONANCE IMAGING IN ALZHEIMER'S DISEASE

Nuclear magnetic resonance techniques have been used for the past 30 years to study the chemical and physical structures of isolated compounds, but the biological applications of magnetic resonance are new and represent a major scientific and technologic advance in medicine. Lauterbur (23) demonstrated the feasibility of imaging biological specimens in 1973. Thereafter, numerous MRI techniques have been reported and applied to the study of various CNS disorders (24,25). The inherent magnetic resonance measures of nuclear spin density, spin-lattice (T_1 relaxation time), and spin-spin (T_2 relaxation time) may be determined spectrometrically on bulk tissue samples, and now by in vivo MRI methods. MRI parameters reflect, and are probably affected by, the metabolic status of the tissue under investigation (26). The underlying principle of MRI is that exposure of atoms with unpaired nuclei to a strong magnetic field and the subsequent application of radiowaves of a particular frequency make the nuclei behave as tiny radiotransmitters by first absorbing and then re-emitting a signal at the same frequency as the one applied (27). Although any atomic nucleus containing an odd number of protons or neutrons is sensitive to MRI study, the proton of the hydrogen atom is the most common one in the human body and therefore the principal nucleus involved in MRI.

MRI brain scans have been performed on a small series of patients with a variety of neu logical disorders, including stroke, hydrocephalus, Huntington's disease (HD), and multiple sclerosis (MS) (28-34); there is only a single preliminary report in AD (35). The study described here determined whether proton MRI brain imaging could detect pathological changes in the brains of patients with AD and patients with multi-infarct dementia (MID), and compared MRI and CT brain scans in these patients.

Methods

The participants in this study were 21 patients with a clinical diagnosis of AD, and 5 patients with MID. Diagnoses were established according to strict clinical criteria (1,2). Among the 21 patients with AD, there were 13 women and 8 men with a mean age of 69 years (range 57-85 years old). Estimates of dementia severity were based upon the Blessed Dementia Scale (36) score, and upon clinical assessment of functional disabilities (1,37). The Blessed scores ranged from 3.5 (mild dementia) to 46.5 (severe dementia) with a mean score of 22.5 for the entire group. The 5 patients with MID included 3 men and 2 women with a mean age of 70 years (range 57-78 years) and a mean Blessed score of 8.5 (range 3.5 to 14.5).

The first 10 patients with AD were examined with the 0.15 tesla Technicare prototype machine; all other patients were examined with the 0.6 tesla Technicare Teslacon. Spatial encoding procedures employed both 3-dimensional projection reconstruction and 2-dimensional Fourrier transform imaging. Three radio frequency pulse sequences were employed: saturation recovery and inversion recovery, both of which give T_1-weighted information, and T_2-weighted Hahn or Carr-Purcell-Meiboom-Gill spin echo. Data reconstruction provided T_1 and T_2 weighted images in coronal, horizontal, and sagittal projections. CT brain scans were obtained with the GE 9800 and Sieman Somatom machines. Comparisons between MRI and CT scans were made on comparable horizontal plane sections. The CT scans were read independently by a neuroradiologist (KD) and the MRI scans by two other members of the magnetic resonance unit (FB & CK). In both instances, a 4-point rating scale (normal, mild, moderate, severe) was used to grade 4 cortical and 4 periventricular white matter regions in each hemisphere, 9 CSF spaces, and 5 subcortical nuclear regions.

Results

MRI brain scans permitted direct imaging of structures of interest in AD, especially the hippocampus-amygdala complex, whereas with CT scans the status of these areas was inferred indirectly from the size of the temporal horns. Furthermore, MRI displayed subcortical white matter thinning associated with cortical atrophy and ventricular enlargement, whereas CT scans suggested thinning only indirectly. For example, we examined an AD patient with visual agnosia and prosopagnosia whose MRI and CT scans showed virtual absence of subcortical white matter in the left temporoparietal region (38). Both techniques revealed greater dilatation of the left posterior horn of the lateral ventricle than of the right, but MRI also displayed abnormal characteristics of the remaining tissue, which possessed prolonged T_1 and T_2 values.

An additional finding of the present study was that MRI scans were superior to CT scans in detecting lesions in white matter, such as small strokes. In our series of 21 cases of suspected AD, 3 had evidence of small infarcts that were detected on MRI images but not on CT scans. Furthermore, lacunes that were seen on CT scans were more clearly displayed with MRI techniques, especially on the T_2-weighted images (Fig. 1). In some cases, the T_2 abnormality exceeded the boundaries of the small cystic component seen by MRI on the inversion recovery pulse sequences or by CT. In another instance, the MRI scan was critical in identifying a case of dementia associated with probable cerebral multiple sclerosis. Although low absorption values were detected in periventricular regions on this patient's CT scan, they were initially felt to be most compatible with transependymal absorption of CSF. The presence, nature, and extent of these lesions were not fully appreciated until an MRI scan was obtained (Fig. 2).

Discussion

The results of this study indicate that MRI brain scans can improve accuracy in the diagnosis of dementia. For example, our observations indicated that MRI was superior to CT in detecting multiple subcortical strokes and unsuspected white matter disease that masqueraded as AD. Because MID is the pathological diagnosis most often confused clinically with AD (22), MRI scans should be included in the evaluation of all patients with dementia. Furthermore, direct assessment of anatomic structures and improved discrimination between gray and white matter with MRI imaging techniques will facilitate research into the pathological substrates of specific behavioral abnormalities in AD.

Although MRI brain scans do not display pathognomonic features of AD, they are superior to CT scans in defining CSF spaces as an indirect measure of brain atrophy. In our study, we found that CSF and brain parenchyma were more clearly distinguished on T_2-weighted MRI than on CT scans. Imprecise estimates of CSF spaces over cerebral cortices based upon CT scans may partly account for the controversy regarding the relationship between brain atrophy and dementia (39). Estimates of ventricular enlargement and widened cortical sulci seen on CT have been examined by a variety of techniques, including linear measurements (39-42), planimetry (43), and visual rank order (40,44), but it is generally believed that volumetric methods correlate more highly with dementia than linear ones (45). Studies relating brain morphology and behavior will be greatly facilitated by MRI techniques in which accurate discrimination between brain parenchyma and CSF will permit calculation of true brain and CSF volumes.

Fig. 1. CT after iodinated contrast and MRI brain scans of a 70-year-old woman with a clinical diagnosis of MID. Bilateral basal ganglia and periventricular lesions were seen on CT scan (upper left) and more clearly seen on the T_1-weighted inversion recovery MRI image (upper right). The lesions appeared more extensive on the T_2-weighted spin-echo images (lower left and right, respectively); periventricular areas of moderately prolonged T_2 were also noted. Pulse repetition times were 1650 ms for one inversion recovery sequence and 2000 ms for the spin-echo study. Inversion time was 450 ms. Echo times were 60 and 120 ms for the T_2 study.

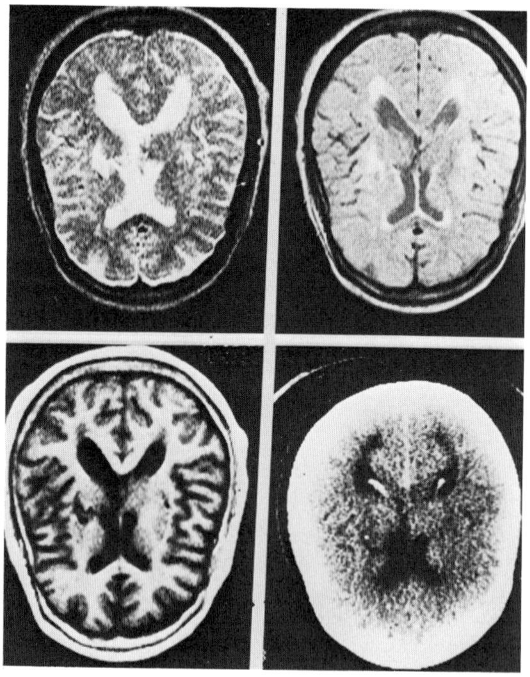

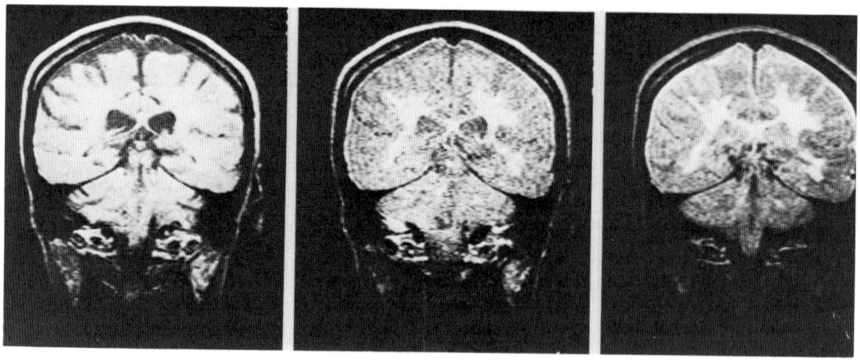

Fig. 2. T_2-weighted images of a 44-year-old woman with dementia. Extensive subcortical white matter lesions and a single left cerebellar lesion were barely detected in the 30 ms echo (left), but were clearly visualized in the 60 ms and 90 ms echos (middle and right). Repetition time was 2000 ms. MRI images helped establish the clinical diagnosis of probable cerebral multiple sclerosis.

CEREBROSPINAL FLUID NEUROTRANSMITTER MARKERS IN ALZHEIMER'S DISEASE

Analysis of CSF neurotransmitter markers has been proposed as a way of separating AD from other neurodegenerative disorders and thereby increasing diagnostic accuracy. This strategy is based upon the expectation that the cholinergic, monoaminergic, and peptidergic abnormalities in the brains of patients with AD (9-20) will be reflected in the CSF.

Cholinergic muscarinic deficits were the initial neurotransmitter abnormalities reported in AD, based upon reports that the activities of CAT and AChE were reduced in brains of patients with AD and the activity of the nonspecific cholinesterase BuChE was increased (9-12). Cell degeneration in the nucleus basalis of Meynert probably accounts for most of the decrease in CAT and AChE activity noted in the cortex (5). Decreases in CAT and AChE activities have been related to the number of senile placques in neocortex and to the number of neurofibrillary tangles in hippocampal neurons, and to the clinical severity of dementia (10,46).

Somatostatin is a 14-amino-acid peptide that is widely distributed in the brain and believed to function as a neurotransmitter or neuromodulator (47,48). Altered brain concentrations of somatostatin-like immunoreactivity (SLI) have been reported in degenerative neurological diseases, including AD and HD. In AD, concentrations of SLI (19,49-51) as well as the number of somatostatin receptors (52) are decreased in cerebral cortex. Cortical concentrations of somatostatin are inversely correlated with neuritic placque counts in the temporal lobes of patients with AD (53), suggesting that decreases in somatostatin levels are possibly related to some of the clinical manifestations of this disorder.

Although not as dramatic as changes in the cholinergic or somatostatinergic systems, reductions in brain monoamines and their metabolite levels greater than those observed in normal aging occur in patients with AD (6,7,16-18,54). Most of the norepinephrine in the mammalian central nervous system is synthesized by neurons within the brainstem nucleus locus coeruleus (55). In AD, noradrenergic cell loss in the locus coeruleus (6,7,16) is common, and many of the remaining neurons contain neurofibrillary tangles (56). As a result, cortical levels of norepinephrine and its metabolite, 3-methoxy, 4-hydroxyphenylethylene glycol (MHPG) are decreased (15,16). Decreased levels of serotonin and its major metabolite, 5-hydroxyindoleacetic acid (5-HIAA), have also been observed in brains examined at autopsy and in brain biopsies from patients with AD (16,17). Serotonergic receptors may also be affected (18).

Methods

The diagnosis of AD and estimates of dementia severity were established according to the same strict clinical criteria (1,2) and rating scales (1,36,37) described for the MRI studies. The diagnosis of PD, HD, and stroke relied upon conventional neurological criteria (57). The clinical characteristics of each patient group are described in the protocols for individual neurotransmitter markers.

Patients who required psychoactive drugs were excluded from the study. All participants consumed a standard 70 gram protein diet during the day prior to lumbar puncture. Patients remained flat in bed for 12 hours prior to lumbar puncture in order to minimize the effects of physical activity. All samples were collected between 9 AM and 11 AM in order to avoid diurnal variations in monoamine metabolite levels. CSF samples were collected from the lumbar subarachnoid space with patients in the supine position. Cell counts and protein and glucose determinations were performed using the first 2 ml of CSF. AChE and BuChE activities and choline level determinations were performed on the second 2 ml sample, monoamine metabolite levels in the 4th through 8th ml aliquot, and somatostatin levels in the 8th through 10th ml aliquot. Choline levels were measured by a radioenzymatic assay (58); cholinesterase activity was determined by a colorometric method using thiocholinester substrates (59). The BuChE inhibitor ethopropazine was used when assaying AChE. Radioimmunoassay of somatostatin was determined by a specific double antibody assay (60) that primarily recognized residue 6-10 of tetradecapeptide somatostatin. Monoamine metabolite levels were measured by high pressure liquid chromatography with electrochemical detection (61).

The data thus obtained were analyzed by analyses of variance and covariance with respect to age, sex, diagnosis, and severity of disease.

Acetylcholine

Subjects. In order to assess cholinergic markers in lumbar CSF, we measured CSF choline levels in 9 patients with AD, in 8 with HD (another neurological degenerative disease associated with decreased CAT activity), and in 14 neurological control subjects. We also measured AChE and BuChE activities in 17 patients with AD and in 6 neurological control subjects. AD subjects in the cholinesterase study had a mean age of 64 years (± 6.9 years) and a mean duration of illness of 4.2 years. The AD group ranged from mildly to severely demented, and the mean Blessed Dementia Scale score was 17.2. The mean age of control subjects did not differ from that of the AD group.

Results. Baseline choline levels were 2.2 ± 0.6 nm/ml in patients with AD; this value did not differ from choline levels measured in control subjects or in patients with HD (62,63). Choline levels increased significantly and to the same extent during choline or lecithin administration in all three groups of subjects. BuChE activity, expressed in volume units, was significantly lower in the CSF of patients with AD than in that of control subjects ($p < .05$), but there was substantial overlap between these groups. Low BuChE activity was related to the degree of dementia severity, memory impairment, and language disorder, whereas low AChE activity was related to impaired visual contrast sensitivity but not to severity of dementia. The ratio of BuChE to AChE activity was decreased in AD and correlated significantly with severity of dementia ($p < 0.05$).

Somatostatin

Subjects. In order to determine the value in the differential diagnosis of dementia of measuring somatostatin levels in CSF, we examined CSF concentrations of SLI in 40 patients with AD, 12 patients with HD, 6 patients with PD, 5 patients with MID, and in 84 nondemented control subjects. The mean age of AD patients was 67 years with a range of 55-78 years; severity of disease ranged from mild to severe. Of the 84 control subjects, 46 were younger and 39 older than 55 years old.

Results. The mean CSF concentration of SLI in patients with AD was 36.9 ± 2.9 pg/ml, and in patients with MID it was 27.7 ± 5.6 pg/ml; levels in both groups were significantly reduced ($p < 0.01$) compared to the mean value of 56.2 ± 2.2 pg/ml in control subjects. Concentrations of SLI in PD and HD did not differ from those of control subjects. A few patients with AD had normal concentrations of CSF SLI with values overlapping those of control subjects and of patients with other degenerative neurological diseases. AD patients with mild dementia had higher concentrations of SLI (41.6 ± 5.5 pg/ml) than did patients with either moderate or severe dementia (33.6 ± 2.8 pg/ml), but the differences were not significant. Six patients with mild dementia and two with moderate dementia had concentrations that fell within the normal range. There was no correlation between age and CSF SLI concentrations.

Monoamines

Subjects. In order to assess the diagnostic value of monoamine metabolite levels in CSF of patients with AD, we measured levels of homovanillic acid (HVA), 5-HIAA, and MHPG, the major brain metabolites of dopamine, serotonin, and norepinephrine, respectively, in patients with AD, and contrasted the results to similar measures in patients with PD who were not demented. CSF was collected from 32 patients with AD and from 33 patients with PD. The mean age of the AD group was 64 years, with a range of 54-79 years, and of the PD group, 57 years, with a range of 32-75 years. All patients had discontinued medications for at least 4 days prior to the lumbar puncture.

Results. Mean HVA levels were 33.1 ± 2.8 ng/ml in patients with AD and 27.1 ± 3.0 ng/ml in patients with PD; this difference was not statistically significant. Levels of 5-HIAA were 19.4 ± 3.5 ng/ml in AD and 18.3 ± 1.8 ng/ml in PD; mean MHPG levels were 7.2 ± 0.3 ng/ml in AD, and 7.4 ± 0.6 ng/ml in PD. None of these differences was statistically significant. The concentrations of all 3 monoamine metabolites increased during probenecid administration (100 mg/kg in 6 divided oral doses over 24 hours), but HVA levels were significantly higher in patients with AD than in patients with PD (151.1 ± 14.4 ng/ml in AD versus 85.1 ± 11.0 ng/ml in PD, $p < .001$). Within the AD group, baseline levels of HVA were lowest in the patients with severe dementia; those with the most severe dementia also had the greatest rise in MHPG levels during probenecid administration.

Discussion

The results of these CSF studies indicate that for the neurotransmitter markers measured here, there were no changes that were unique to AD. Among other possible cholinergic markers, CSF concentrations of CAT activity and acetylcholine (ACh) are too low to measure reliably, although there is a single report that ACh levels were reduced in AD (64). Choline is both the precursor and metabolite of ACh synthesis and degradation. Levels of choline in CSF derive from at least three sources: directly from the blood (65), from the breakdown of endogenous phosphatidylcholine in neuronal membranes (66), and from the choline that is formed intrasynaptically by the hydrolysis of ACh but not taken up into presynaptic terminals (67,68). Choline levels did not distinguish patients with AD from normal subjects or from patients with HD. The status of cholinesterase activity in AD is controversial: Some investigators have found that AChE and BuChE in lumbar CSF from patients with AD did not differ from control subjects (69-72), but others noted low lumbar CSF AChE activity (73,74) or a low ratio of AChE to BuChE activity (75) in AD patients. In ventricular CSF obtained at postmortem examination from histopathologically verified cases of AD, AChE activity was low when expressed per unit volume but not per unit protein (76). Our data differ from these previous reports in that BuChE activity was significantly reduced, although considerable overlap with measures from control subjects limits the value of this observation. Our data also indicate that the ratio of BuChE to AChE is more strongly correlated with cognitive function in AD than is either measurement alone (77).

Our observation that somatostatin levels are decreased in CSF obtained from patients with AD is consistent with most (71,78-81) but not all (82) previous reports. The significance of this finding remains uncertain: It is consistent with a loss of somatostatinergic neurons in the cortex in AD and MID (19,50,51,53), although the contribution of SLI from spinal cord origins may be substantial. The finding that concentrations of CSF SLI in some AD patients overlapped those measured in both normal subjects and in patients with MID indicates that decrements in CSF SLI concentrations lack diagnostic specificity.

Reduced levels of monoamine metabolites in CSF as a reflection of monoamine-containing neuronal atrophy (6,7,56), or decreases in their accumulation during probenecid administration, have been reported in patients with AD by some investigators (83-87) but not all (64,88). Our data indicate that baseline levels of monoamine metabolites in lumbar CSF do not reveal abnormalities that are specific for AD, but that changes in metabolite accumulation during probenecid administration can separate AD from other neurodegenerative disorders. For example, measurement of HVA levels during probenecid administration clearly separated patients with AD from those with PD. Probenecid blocks the transport of acid metabolites across membranes; its administration causes accumulation of HVA, 5-HIAA and, to a lesser extent, MHPG in the CSF and thereby provides an index of the rates at which neurons synthesize and release dopamine, serotonin, and norepinephrine, respectively. The increase in CSF monoamine metabolite levels with probenecid administration is widely used as a test of neuronal function and may be a more sensitive indication of cellular integrity than a single baseline value. In the current study, probenecid administration demonstrated greater dopaminergic functional reserve in AD than in PD, although baseline HVA values did not discriminate these two groups (37).

Our studies indicate that the detection of a distinctive neurotransmitter marker in CSF of patients with AD remains elusive. One way to gain diagnostic specificity may be to construct a composite profile of CSF findings in AD (Table 1) and contrast it with similar profiles in other dementing illnesses. It is possible that a constellation of findings characterizes AD even if a single value does not. Another fruitful new direction in the study of CSF neurotransmitter markers in AD could evolve from longitudinal studies. To date, all reports on neurotransmitter markers in CSF have described cross-sectional studies; no information exists regarding changes during the evolution of dementia. Repeated analysis of markers in the same patient over time, in addition to improving diagnostic accuracy, may provide insights into the neurochemical substrates of the behavioral manifestations of AD. For example, a progressive decline in MHPG levels in an AD patient with depressed mood, or BuChE activity in a patient with prominent memory loss may be highly significant in serially collected CSF samples but be missed entirely if buried in mean values of a large cross-sectional study. If such correlations could be established, different patterns of neurotransmitter change detected in CSF could help explain variations in the clinical manifestations of AD, and possibly guide development of individual drug treatments.

Table 1. Composite profile of neurotransmitter markers in CSF of patients with Alzheimer's disease*

Transmitter system	Finding
Acetylcholine	
Choline level	Normal
AChE activity	Normal or decreased
BuChE activity	Decreased
ACh level	Decreased
Neuropeptides	
Somatostatin level	Decreased or normal
Vasopressin level	Decreased
Dopamine	
HVA level	Decreased or normal
HVA level after probenecid	Normal
Norepinephrine	
MHPG level	Normal or decreased
Serotonin	
5-HIAA level	Normal
Gamma aminobutyric acid	Decreased

*The tabulated CSF profile is based upon findings in the current study and is supplemented by similar data reported by other investigators (37,62,64,69-91).

References

1. Corkin S, Growdon JH, Rasmussen SL: Parental age as a risk factor in Alzheimer's disease. Ann Neurol 13:674-676, 1983.
2. McKhann G, Drachman D, Folstein M, Katzman R, Price D, Stadlan EM: Clinical diagnosis of Alzheimer's disease: Report of the NINCDS-ADRDA Work Group under the auspices of Dept. of Health & Human Services Task Force on Alzheimer's Disease. Neurol 34:940, 1984.
3. Corsellis JAN: Aging and the dementias. In: Greenfield's Neuropathology. Blackwood W, Corsellis JAN (eds). 1976, London, Edward Arnold, pp. 849-902.
4. Terry RD: Structural changes in the dementia of the Alzheimer's type. In: Aging of the Brain and Dementia. Amaducci L, et al (eds). 1980, Raven Press, New York, pp 23-32.
5. Whitehouse PH, Price DL, Coyle JT, DeLong MR: Alzheimer's disease: evidence for selective loss of cholinergic neurons in the nucleus basalis. Ann Neurol 10:122-126, 1981.
6. Mann DMA, Lincoln J, Yates PO et al: Changes in monoamine containing neurons of the human CNS in senile dementia. Brit J Psychiatry 136:533-541, 1980.
7. Bondareff W, Mountjoy CQ, Roth M: Loss of neurons of origin of the adrenergic projection of the cerebral cortex (nucleus locus coeruleus) in

senile dementia. Neurol 32:164-168, 1982.
8. Terry RD, Peck A, DeTheresa R, Schechter R, Horoupian DS: Some morphometric aspects of the brain in senile dementia of the Alzheimer type. Ann Neurol 10:184-192, 1981.
9. Davies P, Maloney AFJ: Selective loss of central cholinergic neurons in Alzheimer's disease. Lancet ii:1403, 1976.
10. Perry EK, Tomlinson BE, Blessed BE, Bergmann K, Gibson PH, Perry RH: Correlation of cholinergic abnormalities with senile plaques and mental scores in senile dementia. Brit Med J 2:1457-1459, 1978.
11. Bowen DM, Sims NR, Benton S, Haan EA, Smith CCT, Neary D et al: Biochemical changes in cortical brain biopsies from demented patients in relation to morphological findings and pathogenesis. In: Alzheimer's Disease: A Report of Progress in Research. Corkin S, Davis KL, Growdon JH et al. (eds). 1982, Raven Press, New York, pp.1-8.
12. Op Den Velde W, Stam FC: Some cerebral proteins and enzyme systems in Alzheimer's presenile and senile dementia. J Amer Geriat Soc 1:12-16, 1976.
13. Rossor MN, Emson PC, Iversen LL, Mountjoy CQ, Roth M, Fahrenkrug J, Rehfeld JF: Neuropeptides and neurotransmitters in cerebral cortex in Alzheimer's disease. In: Alzheimer's Disease: A Report of Progress in Research. Corkin S, Davis KL, Growdon JH et al. (eds). 1982, Raven Press, New York, pp. 15-24.
14. Perry RH, Candy JM, Perry K, Irving D, Blessed G, Fairbain AF, Tomlinson BE: Extensive loss of choline acetyltransferase is not reflected by neuronal loss in the nucleus of Meynert in Alzheimer's disease. Neurosci Lett 33:311-315, 1983.
15. Adolfsson R, Gottfries CG, Roos BE, Winblad B: Changes in the brain catecholamines in patients with dementia of the Alzheimer type. Brit J Psychiatry 135:216-233, 1979.
16. Cross AJ, Crow TJ, Johnson JA, Joseph MH, Perry EK, Perry RH, Blessed G, Tomlinson BE. Monoamine metabolism in senile dementia of the Alzheimer type. J Neurol Sci 60:383-392, 1983.
17. Bowen DM, Allan SJ, Benton JS et al: Biochemical assessment of serotonergic and cholinergic dysfunction and cerebral atrophy in Alzheimer's disease. J Neurochem 41:266-272, 1983.
18. Cross AJ, Crow TJ, Ferrier IN, Johnson JA, Bloom SR, Corsellis JAN: Serotonin receptor changes in dementia of the Alzheimer type. J Neurochem 43:1574-1581, 1984.
19. Davies P, Katzman R, Terry RD: Reduced somatostatin-like immunoreactivity in cerebral cortex from cases of Alzheimer's disease and Alzheimer senile dementia. Nature 228:279-280, 1980.
20. Mountjoy CQ, Rossor MN, Iversen LI, Roth M: Correlation of cortical cholinergic and GABA deficits with quantitative neuropathological findings in senile dementia. Brain 107:507-518, 1984.
21. Terry RD: Aging, senile dementia, and Alzheimer's disease. In: Alzheimer's Disease: Senile Dementia and Related Disorders, Katzman R, Terry RD, Bick KL (eds). New York, Raven Press, 1978, pp. 11-14.
22. Davies P, Katz DA, Crystal HA: Choline acetyltransferase, somatostatin, and substance P in selected cases of Alzheimer's disease. In: Alzheimer's Disease: A Report of Progress in Research, Corkin S, Davis K, Growdon JH et al (eds). 1982, Raven Press, New York, pp. 9-14.
23. Lauterbur PC: Image formation by induced local interactions: examples employing NMR. Nature 242:190-191, 1973.
24. Kaufman L, Crooks, LE, Margulis AR: Nuclear Magnetic Resonance Imaging in Medicine. 1981, Igaku-Shoin, New York.
25. Witcofski RL, Karstaedt N, Aparlain CL: NMR Imaging. 1982, Bowman Gray School of Medicine Press, Winston-Salem.
26. Buonanno FS, Pykett IL, Brady TJ, Pohost GM: Clinical application of nuclear magnetic resonance. Disease-a-Month 29(8), 1983.
27. Kramer CL, Buonanno FS: Physical principles of nuclear magnetic resonance and its application to imaging. In: Head and Spine Imaging,

Gonzalez CF, Grossman CB, Marsden JC (eds). 1985, J Wiley & Sons, New York, pp. 859-887.
28. Doyle FM, Gorew JC, Pennock JM, Bydder GM, Steiner R, Young IR, Burl M, Loq, AH, Gilderdle DH, Bailes DR: Imaging of the brain by nuclear magnetic resonance. Lancet ii:53-57, 1981.
29. Bydder GM, Steinre R, Young IR, Hall AA, Thomas AD, Marshall H, Pallis CA, Legg NJ: Clinical NMR imaging of the brain: 140 cases. Amer J Radiology 139:215-236, 1982.
30. Bailes DR, Young IR, Thomas TJ, Straughan, K, Bydder GM, Steiner RE: NMR imaging of the brain using spin-echo sequences. Clin Radiology 33:395-414, 1982.
31. Lukes SA, Aminoff MJ, Mills C, Normal D, Newton TH: Comparison of nuclear magnetic resonance an computed tomographic findings in patients with extrapyramidal movement disorders. Ann Neurol 12:88, 1982.
32. Buonanno FS, Brady TJ, Pykett IL, et al.: NMR clinical results: Masssachusetts General Hospital. In: Nuclear Magnetic Resonance (NMR) Imaging. Partain CL, James AE, Rollo FD, Price RA (eds). Saunders, Philadelphia, 1983, pp. 207-230.
33. DeWitt LD, Buonanno FS, Kistler JP, Brady TJ, Pykett IL, Goldman MR, Davis KR: Nuclear magnetic resonance imaging in evaluation of clinical stroke syndromes. Ann Neurol 16:535-545, 1984.
34. Lukes SA, Crooks LE, Aminoff MJ, Kaufman L, Panitch HS, Mills C, Norman D: Nuclear magnetic resonance imaging in multiple sclerosis. Ann Neurol 13:592-601, 1983.
35. Besson JAO, Corrigan FM, Foreman EI, Ashcroft GW, Eastwood LM, Smith FW: Differentiating senile dementia of Alzheimer type and multi-infarct dementia by proton NMR imaging. Lancet ii:789, 1983.
36. Blessed G, Tomlinson BE, Roth M: The association between quantitative measures of dementia and of senile change in the cerebral grey matter of elderly subjects. Brit J Psychiat 114:797-811, 1968.
37. Gibson CJ, Logue M, Growdon JH: CSF monoamine metabolite levels in Alzheimer's and Parkinson's disease. Arch Neurol 42:489-495, 1985.
38. Nissen MJ, Corkin S, Buonanno FS, Growdon JH, Wray SH, Bauer J: Spatial contrast sensitivity in Alzheimer's disease: general findings and a case report. Arch Neurol 42:667-671, 1985.
39. Huckman MS, Fox J, Topel J: The validity of criteria for the evaluation of cerebral atrophy by computed tomography. Radiology 116:85-92, 1975.
40. DeLeon MJ, Ferris SH, George AE, Reisberg, B, Kricheff II, Gershon S: Computed tomography evaluations of brain-behavior relationships in senile dementia of the Alzheimer's type. Neurobiol Aging 1:69-79, 1980.
41. Hughes CP, Gado MH: Computed tomography and aging of the brain. Radiology 139:391-396, 1981.
42. Albert M, Naeser MA, Levine HL, Garvey AH: Ventricular size in patients with presenile dementia of the Alzheimer type. Arch Neurol 41:1258-1263, 1984.
43. Roberts MA, Caird FI: Computerized tomography and intellectual impairment in the elderly. J Neurol Neurosurg Psychiat 39:986-989, 1976.
44. Ford CV, Winter J: Computerized axial tomograms and dementia in elderly subjects. J Gerontol 36:164-169, 1980.
45. Gado MH, Hughes CP, Danziger AW, Chi D, Jost G, Berg L: Volumetric measurements of the cerebrospinal fluid spaces in subjects with dementia and in controls. Radiology 144:535-538, 1982.
46. Wilcock GK, Esiri MM, Bowen DM, Smith CCT: Alzheimer's disease: Correlation of cortical choline acetyltransferase activity with the severity of dementia and histological abnormalities. J Neurol Sci 57:407-417, 1982.
47. Bennett-Clark C, Romagno MA, Joseph SA: Distribution of somatostatin in the rat brain: telencephalon and diencephalon. Brain Res 188:473-486, 1980.
48. Delfs J, Robbins R, Connolly JL, Dichter M, Reichlin S: Somatostatin production by rat cerebral neurons in dissociated cell culture. Nature 283:676-677, 1980.

49. Rossor MW, Emson PC, Mountjoy CQ, Roth M, Iversen LL: Reduced amounts of immunoreactive somatostatin in the temporal cortex in senile dementia of Alzheimer's type. Neurosci Lett 20:373-377, 1980.
50. Ferrier IN, Cross AJ, Johnson HA, Roberts GW, Crow TJ, Corsellis JAN, Lee YC, O'Shaughnessy D, Adrian TE, McGregor GP, Baracrese-Hamilton AJ, Bloom SR: Neuropeptides in Alzheimer's type dementia. J Neurol Sci 62:159-170, 1983.
51. Nemoroff CB, Bissette G, Busby WH, Youngblood WW, Rossor M, Roth M, Kizer JS: Regional brain concentrations of neurotensin, thyrotropin releasing hormone and somatostatin in Alzheimer's disease. Neurosci Abstr 9:1052, 1983.
52. Beal MF, Mazurek MF, Tran VT, Chattha G, Bird ED, Martin JB: Reduced numbers of somatostatin receptors in cerebral cortex in Alzheimer's disease. Science 229:289-291, 1985.
53. Perry EK, Blessed G, Tomlinson BE,M Perry RH, Crow TJ, Cross AJ, Dockray GJ, Dimaline R, Arregue A: Neurochemical activities in human temporal lobe related to aging with Alzheimer-type changes. Neurobiol Aging 2:251-256, 1981.
54. Adolfsson R, Gottfries CG, Roos BE et al: Changes in the brain catecholamines in patients with dementia of Alzheimer type. Brit J Psychiat 135:216-223, 1979.
55. Foote SL, Bloom FE, Ashton-Jones G: Nucleus locus coeruleus: new evidence of anatomical and physiological specificity. Physiol Rev 63:844-914, 1983.
56. Ishii T: Distribution of Alzheimer's neurofibrillary changes in the brainstem and hypothalamus of senile dementia. Acta Neurol Path 6:181-187, 1983.
57. Adams RD, Victor M (eds). Principles of Neurology. 1981, McGraw-Hill, New York.
58. Goldberg AM, McCaman RE: The determination of picamole amounts of acetylcholine in mammalian brain. J Neurochem 20:1-8, 1973.
59. Ellman GL, Courtney KD, Andres V, Featherstone RM: A new and rapid colorimetric determination of acetylcholinesterase activity. Biochem Pharmacol 7:88-95, 1961.
60. Arnold MA, Reppert SM, Rorstad OP, Sagar SM, Jeutmann HT, Perlow MJ, Martin JB: Temporal patterns of somatostatin immunoreactivity in the cerebrospinal fluid of the rhesus monkey: effect of environmental lighting. J Neurosci 2:574-580, 1982.
61. Hefti F: A simple, sensitive method for measuring 3,4-dihydroxyphenylacetic acid and homovanillic acid in rat brain tissue using high performance liquid chromatography with electrochemical detection. Life Sci 25:775-782, 1979.
62. Christie JE, Blackburn AM, Glen AIM, Zeisel S, Shering A, Yates CM: Effects of choline lecithin on CSF choline levels and on cognitive function in patients with presenile dementia of the Alzheimer type. In: Nutrition and the Brain, Barbeau A, Growdon JH, Wurtman RJ (eds). Raven Press, New York, pp.377-388, 1979.
63. Growdon JH, Cohen EL, Wurtman RJ: Effects on oral choline administration on serum and CSF choline levels in patients with Huntington's disease. J Neurochem 28:229-231, 1977.
64. Davis KL, Hsieh JY-K, Levy MI, Horvath TB, Davis BM, Mohs, RC: Cerebrospinal fluid acetylcholine, choline, and senile dementia of the Alzheimer type. Psychopharm Bull 18:193-195, 1982.
65. Gardiner JE, Domer FR: Movement of choline between the blood and cerebrospinal fluid in the cat. Arch Int Pharmacodyn Ther 175:482-496, 1968.
66. Schuberth J, Henden DJ: Transport of choline from plasma to cerebrospinal fluid in the rabbit with reference to the origin of choline and to acetylcholine metabolism in brain. Brain Res 84:245-256, 1975.
67. Aquilonius SM, Nystrom B, Schunerth J, Sundwall A: Cerebrospinal fluid

choline in extrapyramidal disorders. J Neurochem 28:229-231, 1972.
68. Jonsson LE, Schuberth J, Sundwall A: Amphetamine effect on the choline concentration of human cerebrospinal fluid. J Neurochem 28:229-231, 1969.
69. Davis PL Neurotransmitter-related enzymes in senile dementia of the Alzheimer type. Brain Res 171:319-327, 1979.
70. Johnson S, Domino EF: Cholinergic enzymatic activity of cerebrospinal fluid in patients with various neurological diseases. Clin Chim Acta 35:421-428, 1971.
71. Wood PL, Etienne P, Lal S, Gauthier S, Cajal S, Nair P: Reduced lumbar CSF somatostatin levels in Alzheimer's disease. Life Sci 31: 2073-2079, 1982.
72. Deutsch SI, Mohs RC, Rothpearl AB, Horvath TB, Davis KL: CSF acetylcholinesterase activity in neuropsychiatric disorders. Bio Psychiat 18:1363-1373, 1983.
73. Soininen H, Halonen T, Riekkinen PJ: Acetylcholinesterase activities in cerebrospinal fluid of patients with senile dementia of Alzheimer type. Acta Neurol Scand 64:217-224, 1981.
74. Tune L, Gucker S, Folstein M, Oshida L, Coyle JT: Cerebrospinal fluid acetylcholinesterase activity in seniile dementia of the Alzheimer type. Ann Neurol 17:46-48, 1985.
75. Arendt T, Bigl V, Walther F, Sonntag M: Decreased ratio of CSF acetylcholinesterase to butyrylcholinesterase activity in Alzheimer's disease. Lancet i:173, 1984.
76. Appleyard ME, Smith AD, Wilcock GK, Esiri MM: Decreased CSF acetylcholinesterase activity in Alzheimer's disease. Lancet i: 452, 1983.
77. Huff FJ, Maire J-C, Growdon JH, Corkin S, Wurtman RJ: CSF cholinesterases in Alzheimer's disease. Neurol (Suppl 1) 35:218, 1985
78. Oram JJ, Edwardson J, Millard PH: Investigation of cerebrospinal fluid neuropeptides in idiopathic senile dementia. Gerontology 27:216-223, 1981.
79. Soininen HS, Jolkonen JT, Reinidainen KJ, Halonen TO, Riekkinen PJ: Reduced cholinesterase activity and somatostatin-like immunoreactivity in the cerebrospinal fluid of patients with dementia of the Alzheimer type. J Neurol Sci 63:167-172, 1984.
80. Francis PT, Bowen DM, Neary D, Palo J, Wikstrom J, Olney N: Somatostatin-like immunoreactivity in lumbar cerebrospinal fluid from neurohistologically examined demented patients. Neurobiol Aging 5:183-186, 1984.
81. Serby M, Richardson SB, Twente S, Siekierski J, Corwin J, Rotrosen J: CSF somatostatin in Alzheimer's disease. Neurobiol Aging 5:187-189, 1984.
82. Thal LJ, Rosenbaum DM, Horowitz SG, Sharpless NS, Waltz JM, Amin IM: Alterations in CSF somatostatin in neurologic disease. Neurol 33(Suppl 2):119, 1983.
83. Gottfries CG, Gottfries E, Roos BE: Homovanillic acid and 5-hydroxyindoleacetic acid in the cerebrospinal fluid related to rated mental and motor impairment in senile and presenile dementia. Acta Psychiat Scand 49:257-263, 1970.
84. Gottfries CG, Roos BE: Acid monoamine metabolites in cerebrospinal fluid patients from patients with presenile dementia (Alzheimer's disease). Acta Psychiat Scand 49:257-263, 1973.
85. Gottfries CG, Kjallquist A, Ponten Y, Roos BE, Sundbarg G: Cerebrospinal fluid pH and monoamine and glucolytic metabolites in Alzheimer's disease. Brit J Psychiat 124:280-287, 1974.
86. Guard O, Renaud B, Chazot G: Metabolisme cerebral de la dopamine et de la serotonine au cours des maladies d'Alzheimer et de Pick. Etude dynamique par le test au probenecide. Encephale 2:293-303, 1976.

87. Raskin MA, Peskind ER, Halter JB, Jimerson DX: Norepinephrine and MHPG levels in CSF and plasma in Alzheimer's disease. Arch Gen Psychiat 41: 343-346, 1984.
88. Mann JJ, Stanley M, Neophytides A, deLeon MJ, Ferris SH, Gershon S. Central amine metabolism in Alzheimer's disease: in vivo relationship to cognitive deficit. Neurobiol Aging 2:57-60, 1981.
89. Beal MF, Growdon JH, Mazurek MF: CSF somatostatin in dementia. Neurol 34(Suppl 1):120, 1984.
90. Mazurek MF, Growdon JH, Beal MF: CSF vasopressin levels reduced in Alzheimer's disease. Neurol 34(Suppl 1):280, 1984.
91. Foster NL, Hare TA, Chase TN: Spinal fluid GABA in Alzheimer's disease. Neurol 33(Suppl 2):68, 1982.

NEUROIMAGING STUDIES OF ALZHEIMER'S DISEASE

M. J. de Leon, A. E. George, S. H. Ferris,
G. Budzilovich and A. P. Wolf

New York University Medical Center
Brookhaven National Laboratories

COMPUTED TOMOGRAPHY (CT) in ALZHEIMER's DISEASE (AD)

To a large extent *in vivo* structural brain studies of Alzheimer's disease (AD) have been restricted to estimates of dilation of the cerebral ventricles and the cortical sulci. While there are consistently reported increases in these areas in normal aging and in AD patients, when compared with age matched normal controls there is considerable overlap. As a result, these estimates are of limited diagnostic value (de Leon and George, 1983).

More recently CT studies of AD have turned to direct assessment of brain parenchyma rather than indirect measures of parenchymal loss (i.e. CSF distributions) and there is growing evidence to suggest that these investigations may be of value. For the most part white matter changes have played a prominent role in these investigations, in part due to relative accessibility of the white matter in the centrum semiovale to measurement and in part due to the limitation of CT to accurately measure tissue adjacent to bone, i.e., cortical gray matter. The results from these studies suggest that CT attenuation values from white matter decrease in AD (Naesser, et al. 1980, Albert, et al., 1984).

Subjective estimates of parenchymal changes have suggested a complex pattern of change. We found that the relationship between gray matter and white matter attenuation was changed such that the visual discrimination of these tissues from each other was reduced in AD. In other words in AD, with increasing disease severity there was a reduced discriminability of these tissues (George, et al., 1981). Hypothetically, such results when taken together suggest that if the white matter attenuation values are decreased in AD then in order for there to also be a discriminability reduction the gray matter may be shrinking or alternatively the attenuation values of the gray matter are also changing possibly to an even greater extent. (The white matter has attenuation values that are lower than those found for the gray matter.)

In the most general of terms the CT literature is not in disagreement with the neuropathological literature. At present there is a marked absence of CT-pathologic correlation studies. As reviewed by Kemper (1984) increases in post-mortem ventricular size, gyral atropy and loss of myelin are often found in AD. Of diagnostic value, increased numbers of neurofibrillary tangles and senile plaques are found in the neocortex of AD patients.

Leukoencephalopathy of Aging

Subjectively, it is frequently observed using CT that focal periventri- zones of decreased white matter density are found in aging populations. More recently, using nuclear magnetic resonance (NMR) these white matter changes have been observed to an even greater extent.

In our recent studies of normal aging and the dementias we carefully examined 340 patients and controls with a standard protocol consisting of medical, neurological, psychiatric, cognitive and CT examinations. From these examinations the following four research groups were determined: young normals ($\bar{X}$ age = 26.4 $\pm$ 5.0, N = 35), old normals (X age = 69.5 $\pm$ 6.5, N = 89), AD (X age = 72.5 $\pm$ 7.5, N = 151) and a group whose dementia was judged to be due to a cascular etiology or multi-infarct dementia (MID) ($\bar{X}$ age = 72.0 $\pm$ 7.6, N = 65).

Table 1 shows the regional distribution of CT periventricular lucencies in 45 AD patients. These data indicate a strong prediliction for the frontal white matter to be involved. The results showing the incidence of leukoencephalopathy (lucency) in the four research groups are found in Table 2. These results show an increased lucency incidence that is age associated among normals and a further increase with the dementias. Furthermore within each of the three geriatric groups there is a significant increase in the lucency incidence with increasing age (see Table 3).

Our hypothesis that groups demonstrating lucencies would be characterized by increased numbers of persons demonstrating hypertension, heart disease, peripheral vascular disease or diabetes was not confirmed. Our findings indicate that only for the normals was hypertension associated with an increased incidence of lucency. We found 57% of our normal lucency subjects to be hypertensive and 24% of those without lucency to be hypertensive. For both AD and MID patients we found nearly equal percentages of hypertensives among lucent as among non-lucent patients. Approximately 23% of the AD patients and approximately 45% of the MID patients were hypertensive. The other medical, neurological and psychiatric parameters did not distinguish between lucent and non-lucent subgroups.

Table 1. Regional Distribution of CT Periventricular Lucencies (N = 45)

	%
Anterior	39
Anterior and Posteriar	32
Posterior	14
Diffuse	16

Table 2. Incidence of CT Leukoencephalopathy

Group	(N)	%
Young Normal	(35)	0
Old Normal	(89)	16
AD	(151)	30
MID	(65)	46

Table 3. Age-Related Incidence of Leukoencephalopathy

Diagnosis	Age Group 55-69 (N)	%	70-85 (N)	%
Old Normal	(44)	7	(45)	24
AD	(40)	18	(102)	35
MID	(23)	30	(42)	55

POSITRON EMISSION TOMOGRAPHY in AD

PET studies of oxidative metabolism in AD have consistently demonstrated significant decreases in AD. These disease related metabolic changes have been reported using 18-F deoxyglucose, a tracer for glucose metabolism (Ferris, et al., 1980, Benson, et al., 1983, de Leon, et al, 1983, Friedland, et al., 1983 and Chase et al., 1984) and oxygen metabolism 15-02 (Frackowiak et al., 1981). Interestingly, the PET determined metabolic changes in AD greatly exceed the CT determined structural changes (de Leon et al., 1983). Furthermore, in comparison to age related structural brain changes, metabolic changes with normal aging are minimal (de Leon et al., 1984).

Utilizing 11-C deoxyglucose (a compound with a 20 min. half-life as compared with the 110 min. of 18-F deoxyglucose), we have recently replicated our FDG findings of generalized metabolic reductions in AD relative to age matched controls. The results consistently indicate that diminutions found with AD are most striking in the middle and inferior temporal gyri and the parietal lobe (angular gyrus region) (see Table 4). Also, in this analysis we studied two lucency groups, normal and AD. Table 4 shows that the two lucency groups are very similar to each other and both demonstrate small regional diminutions as compared with non-lucent normal aged controls.

Table 4. % Change in Glucose (11-CDG) Utilization Relative to Normal Elderly (N = 4)

Region	AD	N(L)	AD(L)
Frontal	-13	-8	-5
Sup. Temp.	-15	-3	+2
Mid. Temp.	-28	-9	-7
Inf. Temp.	-33	-8	-7
Parietal	-27	-9	-6
Occipital	-23	-5	-9

POST-MORTEM

Diffuse periventricular lesions in geriatric populations have been described pathologically as vascular in origin (Goto et al., 1981, Tomonaga et al., 1982). In our studies we examined the brains of 10 patients who clinically had received the diagnosis of AD and who also retained the AD diagnosis at post-mortem. In this group we examined the severity of the CT lucency and examined the specific white matter locations microscopically.

There existed a nearly linear relationship between the ante and post mortem studies of lesion severity. In all cases the postmortem change was on a vascular basis whose severity was correlated with the severity of the CT lesion. Most typically we found hyalinization of arterioles with an associated demyelination of the periventricular white matter.

DISCUSSION

In conclusion, CT studies have not been able to establish definitive criteria for the diagnosis of AD. CT has enabled us however to describe some specific brain changes that may be of value in diagnosing dementias other than AD. To the large list of CT exclusion factors in the diagnosis of AD, we believe that the periventricular lucency should be added.

Our evidence suggests lucencies are commonly found among patients clinically diagnosed as AD. As many as 30% in our series showed this pathological change. NMR study of this group confirms and extends our appreciation of these lesions. PET study reveals that lucency AD patients do not appear metabolically similar to non-lucent AD patients. Rather, the lucency AD patients show smaller regional diminutions of glucose utilization than those found with non-lucent AD. Lucency patients also show specific metabolic diminutions that follow the anatomic locations of the lucencies. In other words, in pure AD there is a marked temporo-parietal reduction of metabolism that is not found in the AD cases with lucency. Pathologically there is clear evidence that these changes are of a vascular nature even in patients with the pathologic diagnosis of AD. It is curious that the AD patients with lucencies do not show the marked metabolic diminutions characteristic of AD. Speculatively, perhaps small lesions presumably of a vascular nature have caused the cognitive loss. Alternatively, perhaps these patients have an early AD that is potentiated by the additional burden of a vascular disease. Only longitudinal and postmortem investigations will illuminate these issues. The potential development of such a subgroup of patients will be of interest in the pharmacologic study of AD and in the investigation of the interaction between vascular and Alzheimer type brain changes.

REFERENCES

Albert, M., 1984, CT density numbers in patients with senile dementia of the Alzheimer's type, Arch Neurol, 41:1264-1269.

Benson, D.F., Kuhl, D.E., Hawkins, R.A., Phelps, M.E., Cummings, J.L. and Tsai, S.Y., 1983, The fluorodeoxyglucose 18F scan in Alzheimer's disease and multi-infarct dementia, Arch Neurol, 40:711-714.

Chase, T.N., Foster, N.L., Fedio, P., Brooks, R., Mansi, L. and Di Chiro, G., 1984, Regional cortical dysfunction in Alzheimer's disease as determined by positron emission tomography, Ann Neurol, 15:S170-S174.

de Leon, M.J. and George, A.E., 1983, Computed tomography in aging and senile dementia of the Alzheimer type in the Dementias, R. Mayeux and W.G. Rosen, eds., Raven Press, New York.

de Leon, M.J., Ferris, S.H., George, A., Reisberg, B., Christman, D.R., Kricheff, I.I. and Wolf, A.P., 1983, Computed tomography and positron emission transaxial tomography evaluations of normal aging and Alzheimer's disease, J Cereb Blood Flow and Metab, 3:391-394.

de Leon, M.J., George, A.E., Ferris, S.H., Christman, D.R., Fowler, J.S., Gentes, C., Brodie, J., Reisberg, B. and Wolf, A.P., 1984, Positron emission tomography and computer assisted tomography assessments of the aging human brain, J Comput Asst Tomogr, 8:88-94.

Ferris, S.H., de Leon, M.J., Wolf, A.P., Farkas, T., Christman, D.R., Reisberg, B., Fowler, J.S., MacGregor, R., Goldman, A., George, A.E., and Rampal, S., 1980, Positron emission tomography in the study of aging and senile dementia, Neurobiol Aging, 1:127-131.

Frackowiak, R.S., Wise, R.J., Gibbs, J.M. and Jones, T., 1981, Regional cerebral oxygen supply and utilization in dementia--a clinical and physiological study with oxygen-15 and positron tomography, Brain, 104:753-778.

Friedland, R.P., Brun, A. and Budinger, T.F., 1985, Pathological and positron emission tomographic correlations in Alzheimer's disease, Lancet, Jan. 26, 228.

George, A.E., de Leon, M.J., Ferris, S.H. and Kricheff, I.I., 1981, Parenchymal CT correlates of Alzheimer's disease: loss of grey-white matter discriminability, Amer J Neuroradiol, 2:205-213.

Goto, K., Ishii, N. and Fukasawa, H., 1981, Diffuse white matter disease in the geriatric population, Neuroradiol, 141:687-695.

Kemper, T., 1984, Neuroanatomical and neuropathological changes in normal aging and in dementia in Clinical Neurology of Aging, M.L. Albert, ed., Oxford Univ. Press, New York.

Naeser, M.A., Gebhardt, C. and Levine, H.L., 1980, Decreased computerized tomography numbers in patients with presenile dementia: detection in patients with otherwise normal scans, Arch Neurol, 37:401-409.

Tomonaga, B.M., Yamanouchi, H., Tohgi, H. and Kameyama, M., 1982, Clinicopathologic study of progressive subcortical vascular encephalopathy (Binswanger type) in the elderly, J Am Geriat Soc, 30:524-529.

HIGH RESOLUTION MAPPING OF CEREBRAL BLOOD FLOW IN ALZHEIMER'S DISEASE

Sidney, K. Wolfson Jr., David Gur, Howard Yonas, Walter Good, Gutti Rao, Manfred Boehnke, and Francois Boller

Departments: Neurological Surgery, Radiology, and Neurology
University of Pittsburgh
Montefiore Hospital, Presbyterian University Hospital
Veteran's Administration Hospital
Western Psychiatric Institute and Clinic
Pittsburgh, PA 15213 USA

An increased knowledge of local CNS blood flow patterns in dementia may ultimately prove highly significant in the diagnosis and in the understanding of pathophysiologic states of this related group of diseases. Since an important prevalent condition, multi-infarct dementia (MID), has cerebral circulatory implications and must be differentiated from other dementias, including Alzheimer's type (AD), it is obvious that elucidation of cerebral blood flow (CBF) changes will be important in its differentiation. Other, perhaps more subtle, circulatory changes may occur in the other dementias which will be of equal or greater importance. Reduced CBF having a distribution similar to that of the neuropathologic changes has been described in AD [1]. The advent of a method for local blood flow measurement which is noninvasive, employing a nontoxic, respirable indicator (stable xenon), which has anatomical resolving power greater than most other methods and approaching that of computed axial tomography (CT), and which is readily adapted to imaging techniques of presentation, has provided the means for a detailed study of local blood flow in the dementias, Alzheimer's in particular. Currently, at the University of Pittsburgh, we are engaged in a multidisciplinary, longitudinal study of 300 subjects including 200 with a presumptive diagnosis of AD and 100 age-matched controls. The stable xenon local CBF method, developed in our laboratories [2-5], is employed for the study of several aspects of AD and related dementias.

Among the many factors and hypotheses regarding the causes and characteristics of the various forms of "senile" and "presenile" dementia are genetic traits, genetically transmitted susceptibility to viral or other transmissible agents, transmissible agents alone, immunologic hypotheses, neurochemical aberrations, synthesis of abnormal proteins, toxic or environmental factors, abnormal blood flow and evergy metabolism, and socio-psycologic hypotheses. It is possible that the end result may be an interaction of multiples of the above factors and possibly others not yet mentioned. Since CBF can now be measured noninvasively with high resolution, its role becomes more amenable to study.

A number of investigators have attempted to study CBF in relation to different brain syndromes. This has ranged from purely functional problems such as depression to the organic syndromes of interest here -- including AD and MID. Soon after Kety and Schmidt [6] developed the N_2O method of CBF measurements, Freyhan, Woodford, and Kety [7] undertook a study of CBF in mental diseases including "psychoses and senility". They found a significant decrease in global CBF, metabolism, and O_2 consumption in these conditions. Scheinberg [8] reported that patients with cerebral arteriosclerotic disease had decreased CBF when compared with normals and that elderly patients having impaired mental status had even lower CBF and decreased metabolism. Using these methods, others have made similar findings in the ensuing years. We find reports by Melamed et al [9] that ^{133}Xe rCBF and brain size were decreased in dementia, but that the decrease in size could not be quantitatively correlated with the decrease in CBF. In a recent report, Barclay et al [10] found that repeated measurements in the same patients indicated a progressively decreasing flow in 15 AD patients--in rCBF (^{133}Xe) studies the Initial Slope Index (ISI) had a mean rate of change of -0.6/mo. ISI declined at a rate of only -0.013/mo in 30 control subjects measured once each and compared by regression analysis. The CBF rates of decline correlated with the rate of decline in functional impairment scores.

Using multiprobe, highly columnated apparatus to map the flow in the cerebral cortex, Lassen et al [11], again found that reduced CBF does not play an important role in normal aging. Both decreased global and regional CBF were noted, however, in patients with cerebral arteriosclerosis and in patients with dementia. Gustafson et al [12], using a 16-probe hemispheric approach found that AD and Pick's disease (PD) patients exhibited more or less symmetrical changes with general decrease in rCBF, while MID is globally hemispheric and/or regionally right-left asymmetric. AD patients generally showed a decrease in rCBF, but had a relatively increased flow in precentral and decreased flow in postcentral regions. PD patients, in general, exhibited the opposite: also had a general decrease in CBF but with a relative decrease in rCBF in the precentral gyrus and an increase postcentrally. Patients with affective disorder exhibited insignificant changes in rCBF.

The blood flow studies thus far described have been confined either to global flow or to region flow involving cerebral cortex. A report by Olsen et al [13] discusses the errors to be encountered in sophisticated 2-dimentsional ^{133}Xe methods involving a 254 detector gamma camera. The conclusion was that the 2-dimensional isotope technique is not reliable for quantifying focal ischemic lesions. These methods tended to overestimate ischemic regional blood flow levels. As a result of these limitations, especially the restriction of regional flow measurements to cortical regions, data is available concerning frontal, precentral and postcentral gyri, occipital, but not calcarine, regions, etc. We read very little about thalamus, limbic system, striatum, medulla, etc., because the noninvasive methods heretofore available do not provide information about these deep lying structures. On the other hand, biopsy and autopsy studies in AD indicate that the lesions of this disease are widespread and are significantly represented both neurochemically and neuroanatomically by changes in the deeper brain structures. Moreover, some of the reports do not agree as to the locations of regional decreases in flow or even to its existence.

Positron emission tomography (PET) [14-16] is not subject to the spatial limitations noted above. This method, in common with the stable xenon method and SPECT, uses tomography to "cut" through the tissue and provide information at depth. It can also be used for measurement of metabolic parameters for such important substances as glucose and O_2. This is not readily accomplished at the same time as CBF, however. PET depends upon very short-lived positron emitting radionuclides such as $^{15}O_2$ and thus must be carried out in close proximity to (very expensive) sources of these substances. The tomograph itself is equally expensive. The anatomic resolution is theoretically limited by physical constraints to perhaps, 50X less than presently achieved resolution of the Xe/CT method.

Single photon emission tomography (SPECT) was described initially by Lassen and associates [17] and others [18]. In this method increased detector sensitivity is combined with computerized tomographic technique or a gamma camera to provide blood flow and metabolism data for any depth but with limited resolution. This method is considerably more economical than PET and can thus be widely used.

Because the ultimate anatomical resolution and specificity of the Xe/CT method used in our work is that of CT itself, it is as well-suited for measurement of blood flow in deeper structures as in the cortical regions. Since deep metabolic and circulatory changes may not be symmetrical and/or mimic those of the cortex, it is important that blood flow studies include these regions. We are able to construct local cerebral blood flow maps in sections of brain at different levels which will be easily compared with equivalent CT images and even overlayed upon actual autopsy slices when available. When biopsy material is available, we can get preliminary blood flow information in the same regions using noninvasive methods.

THE Xe/CT BLOOD FLOW TECHNIQUE

Our work on the stable xenon CT method for cerebral blood flow began prior to 1977. Early work employed washout curves of inhaled xenon in baboons. The method depends upon time-dependent changes in enhancement of the CT image caused by a diffusable, radiodense gas that crosses the blood/brain barrier. By combining the radiodensity of xenon, its free diffusion characteristics, and the anatomical resolution of CT, we have the ability to construct high resolution maps of regional blood flow. This concept has been advanced and the method evolved employing rapid scanning (4 sec) and programmable automated table incrementation with Xe washin. This permits us to obtain blood flow maps of 1-6 levels through nearly the entire intracranial contents from a single 3-6 minute xenon breathing session.

Because the technique was developed in the baboon, it became necessary to study the CT anatomy of this animal and similarities were noted between these animals and humans. The CBF method was tested and reported for normal baboons and for two differnt stroke models [19]. We have reported good correlation of medium and high flow in both Xe/CT and microsphere autoradiography [20]. We now have experience with xenon inhalation and scanning in over 500 humans [3, 5, 21, 22]. Other investigators have also been experimenting with the xenon method both in animals and in man [23-26]. The main concerns with humans, as opposed to animals which are studied under anesthesia, have to do with the effects of movement and radiation dose. The former is especially important for demented subjects who, in the more advanced stages, may not have the capacity to cooperate.

In the animal work, we avoided movement by using a light anesthesia and neuromuscular blockade. The human subjects studies thus far have largely been cooperative, but we have also been able to work with comotose subjects. Early AD and MID subjects are cooperative. All understood what was being done and what was expected of them. They were able to give their own informed consent. To ease the burden of lying perfectly still for 10 minutes, we used a moldable plastic holder and an evacuable bead-filled plastic sack both form-fitted for each subject. The advanced AD subjects were more difficult. We selected subjects without involuntary movements, but could not get acceptable data in some cases. The most abnormal subjects, however, were often nearly immobile, and gave surprisingly good results. Adherence to a standardized anatomical register is not as important in this group as in the 3-year study subjects. It is possible to use a computer algorithm to correct rotational misregistration, but other types of motion are not easily overcome. The concentration of xenon used (33%) is subanesthetic and produces a number of usually not unpleasant symptoms [21]. These were explained to the subjects when obtaining consent and again just prior to the study.

The principal radiation exposure is restricted to the brain tissue selected for study. The dose with the GE 9800 scanner is about 3 rad per scan or a total of 12 rad for a 4-scan study. If multilevel studies are carried out the dose increases by about 40% to 17 rads/study for a center slice with a somewhat lower value for nonbiadjacent slices because there is less scattered radiation. These levels are within tolerable ranges especially for subjects in the elderly age group of this study and since the brain is one of the more radioresistant tissues of the body such doses are not uncommonly encountered in diagnostic CT scanning especially if both enhanced and nonenhanced views are taken. Lower cuts, when made, were obtained by adjusting the gantry angle so as to avoid the eyes.

Xenon has been reported to increase CBF [27]. But in animal experiments with concentrations even higher than those used here, we found this effect very limited during the period of measurement [20]. The effect of 33% xenon was small and not significant in the context of these studies.

STUDY PLAN

This is a report of work in progress and thus is not intended to provide conclusions, but rather to create a forum for discussion of the approach, methodology, and of the significance of problems encountered early on. A pilot study was carried out in advanced AD subjects to help determine just what levels and regions may be of greatest interest in the main study. These subjects were recruited outside the 200 participants in the longitudinal study. Multilevel Xe/CT blood flow measurements in all subjects were made as described below.

Table 1. List of Subjects Studied Thus Far

NO	CATEGORY	SEX	AGE RANGE
5	Advanced	Male	63 - 78
2	Longitudinal Study	Male	70 - 75
8	Longitudinal Study	Female	62 - 72
5	Control	Male	60 - 78
2	Control	Female	70 - 72
22	Total		60 - 78

We have performed the first of two studies in about half of the 40 subjects expected. Each surviving subject will be studied again after 3 years. Table I is a breakdown of those already seen. No correlations with the neurochemistry or neuropathology results have yet been possible. Rather than attempt any form of randomized selection we thought it more meaningful in the context of such an early probing assessment to choose 30 demented subjects to provide the best representation of the desired diagnostic categories. We included 10 from the 100 control subjects of the 3-year study to be age-matched to the 30 chosen. At the end of the study and prior to final interpretation of blood flow data, the subjects will be regrouped as above according to all information known about them at that time. Some of the diagnoses may be fairly certain because of biopsy or autopsy results and others because of the added 3 years of clinical observation. When the initial set of studies is complete for the entire group, the results will be compared to determine any immediately apparent diagnostic clues and to assess the value of this procedure in diagnosis. This is one area where benefits might accrue in advance of completion of the study. Eventually, all data will be scored in terms of diagnostic value and correlation with neurochemical, morphological, and EEG findings.

For the purposes of classifying subjects in this study, the following definitions were established:

Advanced AD: Severe motor and affective disorders; inability to care for ones needs; positive neurologic findings.

Multi-infarct dementia: Identified by the presence of arteriosclerotic disease especially of the extracranial cerebral circulation; coexisting severe hypertension; history of multiple small icti, e.g.TIA's; amaurosis fujax; mini or maxistrokes; etc.; CT evidence for this condition; and evaluation in the "ischemic score" of Hachinski.

Early AD: Apathy; loss of initiative with some decline in general performance; early cognitive deficiencies.

Age-matched Controls: Individuals in the senile (>65 years) and presenile (50-65 years) age category who are not ostensibly suffering from mental disease and who do not have severe medical problems. These are ambulatory individuals -- spouses of subjects, members of local AD interest groups or those seen in the clinic for a variety of relatively minor, not stressful conditions, e.g. dermatologic, orthopedic, endocrine, or GI problems.

Procedure for Blood Flow Determinations

Because the use of stable xenon in local cerebral blood flow mapping has been a rapidly evolving dynamic field of research and the duration of this research project is considerable (5 years), we expected that considerable improvement and refinement of technique would occur during the course of the work. In fact, the accomplishment of these improvements is one of the goals of this project. Such advances have indeed occurred as a result of experimentation and development at our institution and at other institutions. Significant improvements that have been incorporated to the extent that they remain compatible with the earlier work in terms of comparison and interpretation are described below. The specifics of measurement will be described here in terms of both past and current knowledge, technique, and available equipment. Further modification will be made when appropriate.

The first 10 subjects were studied using a GE GT/T 8800 scanner with a 320 x 320 matrix and 5 mm columnation. This unit is capable of programmed automatic interscan table incrementation. The basic slice was a nearly transverse plane connecting the upper orbit with the petrous ridges. Other levels were cut parallel to this plane. Exposure factors were established for each subject at time of study. A Hewlett-Packard CO_2 analyzer and a Gow Mack leak detector (calibrated for Xe/O_2 mixtures) were connected to the mask or mouthpiece to estimate end-tidal CO_2 and Xe respectively (Fig. 1). The subjects were mildly restrained using a plastic mold cast of Hexeplast (Hexell Medical Co., Dublin, CA 94566) and shaped for each subjects head individually. The head itself rested in a bag of plastic beads (Olympic Vac-Pac, Olympic Medical, Seattle, WA 98108) which becomes rigid when evacuated.

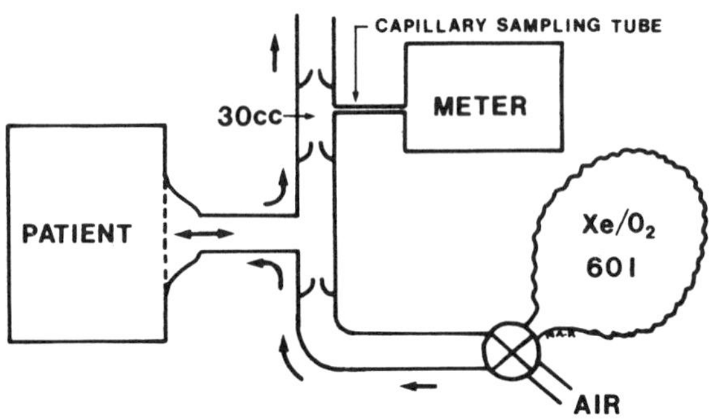

Fig. 1. Block diagram of Xe breathing apparatus. The bag may contain either Xe/O_2 or Xe/air. Expired gas os aspirated at a high valocity through the capillary and this permits the thermal conductivity meter to measure expired gas Xe concentration curves. The end-tidal Xe levels are used for the blood flow computations.

After making a scout image and an initial series of scans to select appropriate levels, two sets of nonenhanced scans were obtained during O_2 breathing. This put the subject through the sequence of table movement, acquainted him with the mask or mouthpiece and the actual study sequence and served as a baseline for the enhanced scans to follow. Xenon breathing commenced via the semiclosed system and the automatic scan sequence was repeated at 1, 1.5, 2, 3 and 5 minutes during Xe buildup or washin. A 10-20 mm table incrementation occurred between scans during an interscan delay of 6 sec. The principle upon which this method depends is that of Kety [28]:

$$C_i(t) = \lambda_i k_i \int_0^t C_a(u)\, e^{-k_i(t-u)} du \qquad (1)$$

$$\text{Blood flow} = \lambda_i k_i \qquad (2)$$

The variables are obtained from endtidal Xe and tissue Xe enhancement data. λ is calculated or extrapolated from these data. One of the more important features of this method is the ability to derive a partition coefficient (λ) for each anatomical locale of interest. The computational methods have been described and discussed elsewhere [2,3].

As predicted, the method underwent modifications during the course of the study. The most important changes included switching to the 9800 System scanner and the development of a semiautomated hardware and software system in collaboration with the General Electric Company. The 9800 System has a number of advantages, notably greatly improved signal to noise characteristics and more sensitive detectors. Scanning time was 4 sec, at 80 KV and 200 mA using a 256 x 256 matrix. The hardware package includes the Xe delivery system, Xe calibration and monitioring, acquisition of the end-tidal Xe concentration data and its transfer to the CT computer. The software permits automated computation of CBF for each pixel by deconvolution of the washin Xe curves of end-tidal and tissue concentrations. It also presents a gray scale blood flow image where flow is depicted pixel by pixel. While additional improvements in data handling are anticipated, we do not see imminent significant changes in the technique of flow measurement.

RESULTS

The nature of the Xe enhanced CT techniques for local CBF is such that data is collected during a single brief Xe inhalation session for **CT** voxel-sized units in matrices of slices over a large portion of the brain. Specific regions of interest can be defined and appropriate blood flows calculated at a later time in conjunction with other available information. Thus the initial data was transferrred from the CT disk pack to magnetic tape and was available for later processing. Initial results with some subjects are presented here but original scan data is preserved for further study depending upon the results of the biopsy and autopsy material as well as EEG and clinical data.

We planned to look at slices taken at levels parallel to the orbitopetrous plane described above. At least two significant representative levels were obtained so as to provide information about frontal and parietal cortex, basal ganglia, and region of 3rd ventricle. In particular we wished to assess flow regions corresponding to the neuropathologic and neurochemistry studies of these subjects: amygdala, centromedian nucleus thalamus, dorsomedian nucleus thalamus, superior or mid termporal lobe, hippocampus, superior and inferior parietal lobules, cingulate gyrus, head of caudate, putamen, calcarine cortex, and occipital pole. Nucleus basalis is not easily obtained because of surrounding dense bone.

Flow levels relative to the age-matched controls have yet to be determined and identified in conjunction with the other findings in these same regions. In consideration of all this data, the purely morphological as well as functional (response to CO_2 and/or stimuli), we are looking for patterns characteristic of one of the conditions considered and thus provide the desired diagnostic criteria.

Consideration of the changes themselves, particularly as <u>temporally</u> related to the anatomic, neurochemical, and electrical changes may provide important pathophysiologic information. The study is guided by evaluation of the following hypotheses:

a. In MID there is a scattered reduction in parenchymal blood flow that can be correlated anatomically with the vascular distribution.

b. The reduced blood flow of MID is correlated with the centers associated with the ischemic signs and symptoms observed.

c. The reported alteration in global and regional CBF observed in AD will be found to occur in association with regions of histopathologic changes: reduced flow being seen in the presence of tissue atrophy or degeneration while increased or unchanged flow is seen in association with regions of proliferative phenomena.

While looking at a portion of the advanced disease cases we found profound changes in many areas but have not yet been able to compare these with the other data. This is partly true because they were scanned using the 8800 and without the data handling capability described below. Figure 2 illustrates the CT and flow map of a subject with advanced AD. Especially noteworthy is the fact that reduced flow is seen where CT density is not diminished in the right frontal and temporal regions.

Originially, we planned to construct a 3-dimensional grid corresponding to the serial CT levels which were being acquired for brain volume studies. This grid was also registered to a published atlas [29] and was to be used both for the identification of structures sampled and for directing the computer in extracting flow data which corresponds as nearly as possible to the neuropathology and histochemical information. Experience with the first 10-12 study subjects and the several advanced cases has led us to another direction. The subjects are undergoing continued degenerative changes with consequent structural changes. As the brain atrophies, the relationships between the cranial landmarks and the neural structures are changing. Thus, each subject is deviating more and more from the normal. More importantly, over time each subject deviates from his own prior structure.

The atlas is now used as a guide rather than attempting to obtain exact registration. Each case and each examination must be individually assessed both with respect to CT cut selection during scanning and with

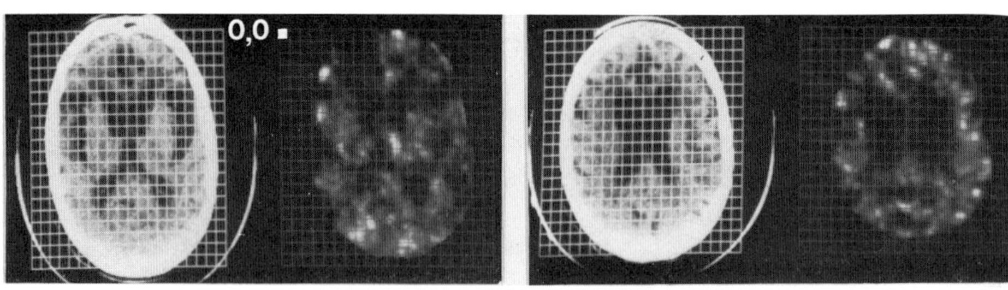

Fig. 2. CT scans and gray scale blood flow maps in a patient with advanced AD. There is profound atrophy, but reduced flow in areas of retained CT anatomy. Examples of this are seen in the comparison of ROIs (8,3), (0,4), or (15,5) CT vs flow map of the left image pair (pineal level). The most prominent reductions of flow are present in the left frontal and temporal regions.

respect to analysis of results. Regions of primary and secondary interest have been mutually established (Table 2). To minimize artifacts, scan levels are selected to provide the largest number of interesting areas without making cuts through dense bone (e.g. petrous). Although any number of cuts may be programmed, we limit the levels so as to optimize the relationship betweeen heat loading, washin curve acquisition, and amount of tissue examined. This has typically resulted in 3-5 levels for most Xe/CT work and is set to 3 for this study. While the regions of present interest are listed in the table, we wish to emphasize that flow is automatically calculated for <u>every</u> pixel in each of the 3 levels. Data is thus acquired for all possible ROIs is these slices and the selected correlations may be completely revised retrospectively at any time.

Table 2. Regions for Correlation Among CBF, Neuropathology and Neurochemistry

PRIMARY INTEREST	CT LEVEL*	SECONDARY INTEREST	CT LEVEL*
Dorsomedian nucleus thalamus	A	Caudate, (head)	A
Middle temporal lobe	A	Putamen	A
Cingulate gyrus	A	Posterior cingulate	A
Calcarine cortex	A	Occipital pole	B
Centromedian nucleus thalamus	B	Subthalamic nucleus	B
Hippocampus	B	Cerebellum	C
Amygdala	C	Substantia nigra	C

*A - Posterior margin of the anterior column of fornix at level of foramen of Munro
B - Center of pineal gland
C - Aqueduct of Sylvius

Initial analysis of the data is accomplished by individual sessions at the independent computer console. The Xe enhanced images are brought up after Xe/CT flow is calculated, and by comparison with the atlas, the 30 or so regions are identified by rectilinear coordinates on the image grid. The cursor locations are noted on hard copy, but also are marked on the image and stored in memory. The flow map corresponding to the CT image is next brought up and centered. Because there is a pixel by pixel registration between the CT scan and the corresponding flow map, the 5 x 5 mm ROI selected can be exactly represented on the flow map. It may be averaged and/or studied as a table of individual pixel values. Each pixel is 0.85 x 0.85 mm; the slice is 5 mm thick, so the voxel has a volume of 3.61 mm^3 and the typical ROI is 0.125 cm^3. This region is well within the resolution of the technique (3-4 mm full width, half max) and is small enough to permit sampling of many neurologic functional elements (nuclei and tracts). The voxel size is small enough and resolution great enough to justify a monocompartmental approach, greatly simplifying the computation. As data accumulates, the ROI value for demented subjects will be scored as to its relationship to corresponding regions of control subjects and to change in the same individual over the 3-year period of observation. These blood flow scores will then be compared with the neuropsychiatric evaluations and, of course, the scores from the neuropathologic and neurochemistry work. Several examples of the results obtained are seen in Figures 3 and 4.

Although 22 subjectes have been studied, there were changes in technique along the way and the initial examinations have not been completed in the studied group. No subject has had a second examination. The most interesting finding that seems to be coming through early on is that blood flow varies greatly in regions small enough to have distinct functional significance rather than merely following tissue density changes. Low flow has been seen in regions of high CT density and the converse. Obiously, flow is low or absent in regions of severe atrophy where brain tissue has been largely replaced by CSF. We resist the temptation to attempt to report these in detail and draw conclusions which may simply add to the somewhat confused picture already available. We are content, at this juncture, to illustrate this approach and will await completion of at least the initial exams on the full cohort before presenting a systematic result.

The final questions to be answered are: Can we recognize a definite pattern(s) of blood flow change that is (are) diagnostic for AD and/or MID? Can we make inferences from local blood flow data that fit an overall hypothesis mechanism for the pathophysiology of AD?

As mentioned above, we found that precise registration of flow maps to skeletally oriented grids or anatomic masks has a serious drawback when studying demented patients in that the atrophy encountered renders the usual relationships between neurologic structures and bony landmarks. The brain sags, shrinks, and, in general, does not fill the cranial vault. Nuclei may not only become smaller or drop out, but may also move away from (or closer to) skeletal reference points. Comparisons between "normal aging" and dementia or between "early" and "late" disease using any method that does not provide for comparing the flow scan with an anatomical or radiographic reference for the subject under study, may be misleading when looking for change in any but the very largest and general brain regions. For instance, a PET scan showing reduced blood flow or metabolism in cortical regions of those adjacent to ventricles may well reflect only the largest of the sulci or ventricles. Examples would be hippocampal gyrus or calcarine cortex whose location will necessarily shift significantly as CSF space increases and brain bulk decreases Numerous other instances of this problem exist. The work thus far highlights the advantage of Xe/CT in that the CT pinpoints the changes and the blood flow map is directly registered to the CT image allowing more precise location of the neurologic structure on the flow map.

At this stage of the work we are at the starting of an analysis that we believe will provide one of the most detailed blood flow correlations ever performed in human subjects with disease. We have worked through an early phase in which the planned approach (3-dimensional grid registered to both skeleton and to anatomical atlas) had to be modified because of the recognized effect of degeneration and atrophy. We now have a method which is practically workable, but which is much more time consuming. Because of the partially automated and standardized technique using a hardware/software package that is now available from General Electric Company, the approach can be applied by others. Then the answers to these questions may come partially from other workers as well.

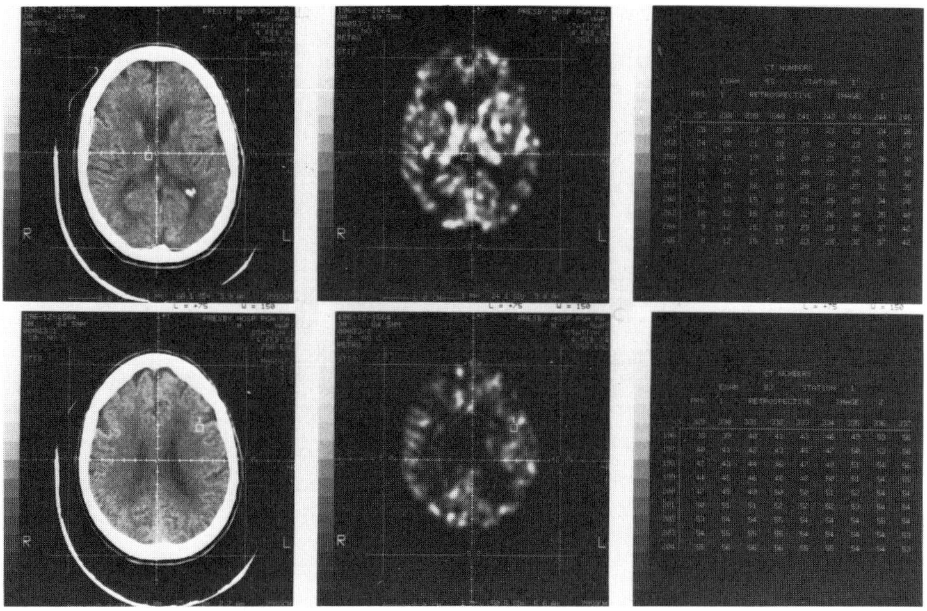

Fig. 3. Steps in anatomical analysis of flow in an AD subject. The figure contains CT images at two levels: anterior columns of fornix/foramen of Munro and the level of the body of the lateral ventricle. A 5 x 5 mm ROI has been place in the R. dorsomedian thalamic nucleus in the upper image and in the left frontal operculum in the lower image. By reference to the grid scale, these 0.125 cm^3 volumes of tissue are identified on the flow maps (center). To the right is a printout of the CBF calculated for each voxel (ml/min/100 g). This information is always computed whether requested or not. A mean and standard deviation is also calculated (as it may be for any ROI regardless of size or shape). Close inspection of the individual values reveals information about homogeneity of flow possibly indicating improper placement of the ROI or a local disturbance of flow.

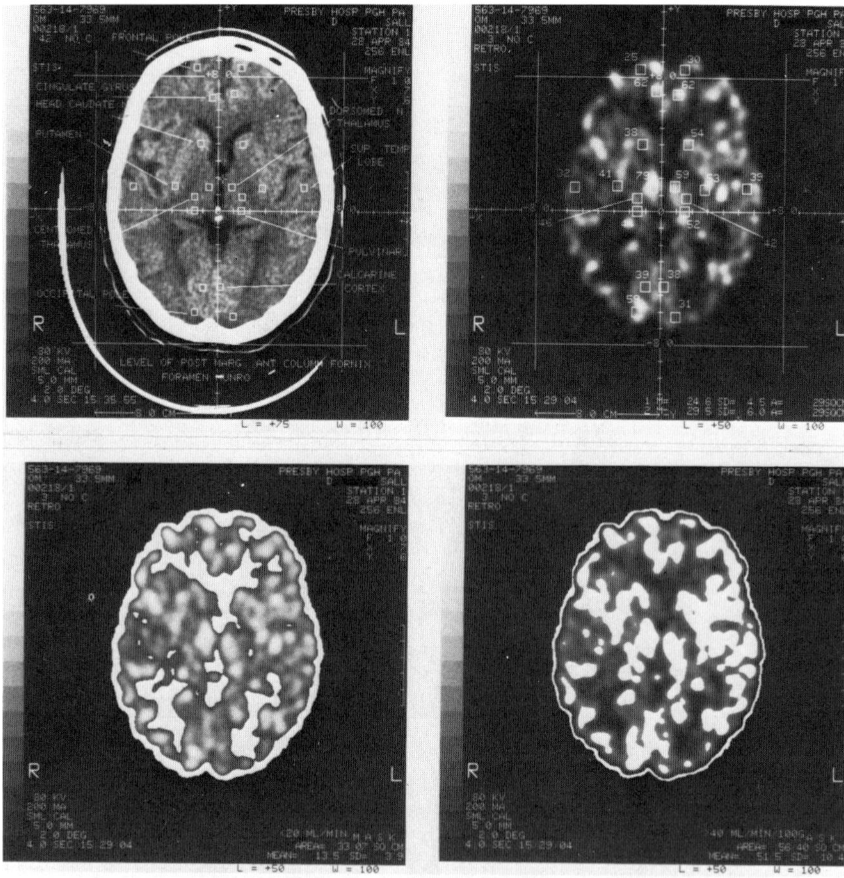

Fig. 4. Anatomic structure identification and masking in a control subject. The upper images are of a CT scan with anatomic structures identified and with corresponding ROIs registered on the accompanying flow maps. Rounded flow values are indicated right on the map next to the ROI. Although a control subject, significant differences exist between like structures on opposite sides. Another method of analysis is illustrated on the lower level. Unbalanced flow patterns are readily revealed and the degree of aberrance quantified. The left mask covers all pixels with $<$ 20 ml/min/100 g. The right masks covers all pixels with $>$ 40 ml/min/100 g. In normal subjects, there are more regions $>$ 40 than $<$ 20 and their ratio reflects the relative proportion of gray vs white matter.

ACKNOWLEDGEMENT

This work was supported in part by USPHS research grants AG03705 and HL27208 and by a Senior Investigatorship Award from the American Heart Association.

REFERENCES

1. Brun A, Gustafson L, Ingvar DH. Phatoanatomical findings in presenile dementia related to regional cerebral blood flow. Proceedings of the VII International Congress of Neuropathology, Budapest. 1975; Excerpta Medica: 101-105.
2. Gur D, Yonas H, Wolfson Jr SK, Herbert D, Kennedy WH, Drayer BP, Shabason L. Xenon and iodine enhanced cerebral CT: a closer look. Stroke. 1981; 12:573-578.
3. Gur D, Good WF, Wolfson Jr SK, Yonas H, Shabason L. In vivo mapping of local cerebral blood flow by xenon enhanced CT. Science. 1982; 215-1267-1268.
4. Wolfson Jr SK, Drayer BP, Boehnke M, Dujovny M, Cook EE. Regional cerebral blood flow by xenon enhanced computed tomography. Proceedings of the Annual Meeting of the American Association of Neurological Surgeons New Orleans. 1978; 1-3.
5. Wolfson Jr SK, Gur D, Yonas H. Cerebral blood flow determinations. In: Latchaw R, ed. Computed Tomography of the Head, Neck and Spine. Chicago, IL: Year Book Medical Publishers, Inc. 1984; 27-52.
6. Kety SS, Schmidt CF. The determination of cerebral blood flow in man by use of nitrous oxide in low concentrations. Am J Physiol. 1945; 143:53-66.
7. Freyhan FA, Woodford RB, Kety SS. Cerebral blood flow and metabolism in psychoses senility. J Nerv Ment Dis. 1951; 113:449-456.
8. Scheinberg P. Cerebral blood flow in vascular disease of the brain. Am J Med. 1950; 8:139-148.
9. Melamed E, Lavy S, Siew F, Bentin S, Cooper G. Correlation between regional cerebral blood flow and brain atrophy in dementia. J Neurol Neurosurg Psychiatry. 1978; 41:894-899.
10. Barclay L, Zemcov A, Blass JP, McDowell F. Rates of decrease of cerebral blood flow in progressive dementias. Neurology. 1984; 34:1555-1560.
11. Lassen NA, Ingvar DH. Blood flow studies in the aging normal brain and in senile dementia. Aging. 1980; 13:91-98.
12. Gustafson L, Risberg J, Silfverskiold P. Cerebral blood flow in dementia and depression. Lancet. 1981; Jan. 31, 1981:275.
13. Olsen TS, Larsen B, Skriver EB, Enevoldsen E, Lassen NA. Focal cerebral ischemia measured by the intra-arterial ^{133}Xenon method. limitation of 2-dimensional blood flow measurements. Stroke. 1981; 12:736-744.
14. Jones T, Chesler DA, Ter-Pogassian MM. The continuous inhalation of oxygen 15 for assessing regional oxygen extraction in the brain of man. Br J Radiol. 1976; 49:339-343.
15. Baron JC, Bousser MG, Comar D, Soussaline F, Castaigne P. Noninvasive tomographic study of cerebral blood flow and oxygen metabolism in vivo. potentials, limitations and clinical applications in cerebral ischemic disorders. Eur Neurol. 1981; 20(3):273-284.
16. Phelps ME, Scheldert HR, Mazziotta JC. Positron computed tomography for studies of myocardial and cerebral function.

Ann Intern Med. 1983; 98(3):339-359.

17. Stokely EM, Sveinsdottir E, Lassen NA. A single photon dynamic computer assisted tomograph (DCAT) for imaging brain function in multiple cross sections. J Comput Assist Tomogr. 1980; 4:230-240.

18. Fukuyama H, Akiguchi I, Kameyama M. A krypton-81m single photon emission tomography on the collateral circulation in carotid occlusion: the role of the circle of Willis and leptomeningeal anastomoses. J Cereb Blood Flow Metab. 1983; 3:2143-S144.

19. Yonas H, Wolfson S, Jr, Dujovny M, Boehnke M, Cook EE. Selective lenticulostriate occlusion in the primate; a highly focal cerebral ischemia model. Stroke. 1981; 12:567-572.

20. Gur D, Yonas H, Jackson DL, Wolfson Jr SK, Rockette H, Good WF, Maitz GS, Cook EE, Arena VC. Measurements of cerebral blood flow during xenon inhalation as measured by the microspheres method. Stroke. 1984; In press.

21. Yonas H, Grundy B, Gur D, Shabason L, Wolfson Jr SK, Cook EE. Side effects of xenon inhalation. J Comput Assist Tomogr. 1981; 5:591-592.

22. Yonas H, Wolfson Jr SK, Gur D, Latchaw RE, Good WF, Leanza R, Jackson DL, Jannetta PJ, Reinmuth OM. Clinical experience with the use of xenon-enhanced CT blood flow mapping in cerebrovascular disease. Stroke. 1983; 15:443-450.

23. Kelcz F, Hilal SK, Hartwell P, Joseph PM. Computed tomographic measurement of xenon brain-blood partition coefficient and implication for regional cerebral blood flow. a preliminary report. Radiology. 1978; 127:385-392.

24. Amano T, Meyer JS, Okabe T, Shaw T, Mortel KF. Stable Xenon CT cerebral blood flow measurements computed by a single compartment-double integration model in normal aging and dementia. J Comput Assist Tomogr. 1982; 6:923-932.

25. Ono H, Ono K, Mori K. Mapping of CBF distribution by dynamic Xeenhanced CT scan method. J Cereb Blood Flow Metab. 1981; 1:50-51.

26. Tachibana H, Meyer JS, Okayasa H, Shaw TG, Kandula P, Rogers RL. Xenon contrast CT-CBF scanning of the brain diffentiated normal age-related changes from multi-infarct dementia and senile dementia of Alzheimer type. J Gerentol. 1984; 39:415-423.

27. Pittenger CBEA. Clinicopathologic studies associated with xenon anesthesia. Anesthesiology. 1953; 14:10-17.

28. Kety SS. The theory and applications of the exchange of inert gas at the lungs and tissues. Pharmacol Rev. 1951; 3:1-41.

29. Roberts M, Hanaway J. Atlas of the human brain in section. Philadelphia: Lea & Febiger. 1970.

REGIONAL CEREBRAL BLOOD FLOW IN DEMENTING DISORDERS

Eldad Melamed, Mordechai Globus and Bracha Mildworf

Laboratory for Cerebrovascular Research
Department of Neurology, Hadassah University Hospital
Jerusalem, Israel

INTRODUCTION

Normal aging, Alzheimer's disease (AD), senile dementia of the Alzheimer type (SDAT) and Parkinson's disease (PD) are associated with many histological, physiological and biochemical abnormalities in the CNS but few non-invasive procedures are currently available to evaluate such changes *in vivo*. In the brain, regional cerebral blood flow (rCBF) is coupled to local tissue metabolic rates[1] and its measurement can therefore provide useful information on both cerebral hemodynamics and the metabolic-functional state[2] in these disorders. We determined the resting state rCBF in a large series of normal subjects and in patients with AD,SDAT and PD using the non-invasive and atraumatic 133 Xenon inhalation technique[3,4]. The rCBF measurements were designed to gain more insight on several important issues i.e. the natural history of the rCBF during normal aging, the extent of rCBF reductions in patients with AD and SDAT and its relation to severity of dementia and to loss of metabolically active brain tissue, the alterations in rCBF in PD patients and their relationship to severity, duration and progression of the disease, to dopatherapy and to presence of dementia and its severity.

MATERIAL AND METHODS

The rCBF was measured in 103 non-hospitalized, active, normotensive normal subjects without any evidence for neurological or intelectual deficits aged 19 to 79 years, in 46 AD and SDAT and in 110 PD patients. CT scans were evaluated for presence and severity of ventricular dilatation and cortical sulcal widening in the AD and SDAT patients. Subjects from the AD-SDAT and PD groups and controls were examined with detailed neuropsychological test battery to assess presence and extent of cognitive impairment.

The rCBF measurment was carried out in the resting state with the patient in the supine position using the non-invasive 133 Xenon inhalation method[3,4]. The radioisotope was applied through a face mask for one minute and its clearance from the brain was monitored by 16 NaI collimated scintillation detectors applied externally in a standard position over homologous regions of both cerebral hemispheres and connected on-line to a computer system. Air, drawn directly from the face mask by a vacuum pump, was continuously monitored for Xenon concentrations for later correction of the head curves for recirculation of the radioisotope[3,4]. The rCBF was computed as the Initial Slope Index (ISI) which consists predominantly of cortical gray matter flow[5].

RESULTS

In the normal subjects, there was a progressive reduction in the rCBF with advancing age (Table 1). The rates of rCBF decline were similar in both hemispheres and in the frontal, temporal, parietal and occipital regions. In the oldest (70-79) age group, CBF was reduced by a mean of 27% as compared with the youngest (19-29) subjects. The CBF decline during normal aging was not limited to the elderly subjects but already began in the younger age groups. In fact, the greatest CBF reduction (by a mean of 11%) was observed in the 30-39 years age group as compared with the youngest (19-29) subjects (Table 1).

Table 1. Effect of Normal Aging on the rCBF

Age (years)	19-29	30-39	40-49	50-59	60-69	70-79
n	44	11	12	11	17	8
CBF* (ml/100g/min)	60.8±1.2	54.2±2.4	52.2±2.0	51.0±1.6	48.1±1.7	44.1±2.1

means± S.E.M.;* mean brain CBF in this and the other tables was calculated from 16 regional flow values.

In demented patients with AD as well as in those with SDAT there were marked CBF reductions as compared with age-matched normal controls ($p<0.01$; Table 2). Decreases were more or less similar in the two groups. Also, flow reductions were almost identical in the left and right hemispheres and homogenously distributed in the various brain regions.

In our AD and SDAT patients there was no correlation between the extent of rCBF reduction and the various indices for severity of cortical atrophy and ventricular dilatation measured from their CT scans (data not shown). There was some correlation between the degree of dementia and the magnitude of rCBF decreases. In general, patients who were severely demented (Jacobs[6] minimental scores of 0-10) had greater flow reductions than those with mild cognitive impairment (Jacobs[6] score 11-21; $p<0.05$; Table 3).

The rCBF was significantly ($p<0.01$) reduced in patients with PD regardless of their age (Table 4). The rCBF decreases were similar in the two cerebral hemispheres and in the various brain regions even in PD patients with predominantly unilateral symptomatology (Table 5). There was no correlation between the magnitude of rCBF reductions and severity or duration of illness (Tables 6 and 7). Although there was a high prevalence of cognitive impairment among PD patients, there was no correlation between rCBF decline and presence and severity of dementia (Table 3).

Table 2. The rCBF in Patients with Alzhemier's Disease (AD) and Senile Dementia of the Alzheimer Type (SDAT)

Age	n	CBF (ml/100g/min)	% reduction*
50	7	44.3 $\pm$ 3.1	15.5 $\pm$ 5.6
50-59	6	39.4 $\pm$ 1.8	22.5 $\pm$ 3.3
60-69	15	37.5 $\pm$ 2.0	22.0 $\pm$ 4.1
70	18	38.0 $\pm$ 1.2	16.7 $\pm$ 2.6
Total	46	39.0 $\pm$ 1.0	18.6 $\pm$ 3.1

means $\pm$ S.E.M.;* calculated in each patient in this and in the other tables from the expected age-matched normal control values. Latter is calculated from the regression line through 103 flow values obtained in the normal subjects aged 19-79 years, see Table 1.

Table 3. Correlation Between Cognitive Impairment and rCBF Reduction in Patients with Alzheimer's Disease (AD) and Parkinson's Disease (PD).

	AD		PD	
	severe dementia	mild dementia	demented	non-demented
Jacobs score*	0 - 10	11 · 21	$<$21	$>$21
n	10	10	14	30
CBF (ml/100g/min)	37.1 $\pm$ 1.0	41.0 $\pm$ 1.5	41.4 $\pm$ 1.4	42.4 $\pm$ 1.4
% reduction**	23 $\pm$ 3	13 $\pm$ 3	14 $\pm$ 3	12 $\pm$ 3

means $\pm$ S.E.M.; * scores above 21 are normal[6]; ** from age-matched normal controls.

Table 4. The rCBF in Various Age-groups of Patients with Parkinson's Disease.

Age group	$<$50	50-59	60-69	$>$70
Mean age (years $\pm$ S.D.)	43.9 $\pm$ 5.2	54.8 $\pm$ 2.8	64.2 $\pm$ 3.0	73.6 $\pm$ 3.1
n	12	18	49	40
CBF (ml/100g/min)	46.6 $\pm$ 1.7	45.6 $\pm$ 1.7	42.1 $\pm$ 1.0	41.2 $\pm$ 1.1
% reduction*	12.4 $\pm$ 2.1	10.9 $\pm$ 1.5	12.7 $\pm$ 2.5	6.2 $\pm$ 1.8

means $\pm$ S.E.M.; * from age-matched normal controls.

Table 5. The Right and Left Mean Hemispheric CBF in Parkinsonians with Predominantly Unilateral Symptomatology.

Symptoms side	bilateral	right unilateral	left unilateral
n	81	17	21
% CBF reduction*			
Right hemisphere	9.8 ± 1.7	6.5 ± 2.0	9.0 ± 2.6
Left hemisphere	11.5 ± 1.8	11.6 ± 2.4	8.2 ± 2.3

means ± S.E.M.; * from age-matched normal controls.

Table 6. Effect of Severity of Parkinson's Disease on the rCBF.

Disease stage*	1	2	3	4
n	33	40	25	20
Mean age (years ± S.D.)	61.8 ± 11.1	64.6 ± 8.1	67.1 ± 7.7	63.4 ± 11.0
Disease duration (years ± S.D.)	2.3 ± 1.8	4.8 ± 4.0	7.3 ± 4.2	8.9 ± 4.5
% CBF reduction**	11.8 ± 2.6	9.5 ± 2.0	10.0 ± 2.1	10.6 ± 4.1

means ± S.E.M.; * according to Hoehn and Yahr[7]; ** from age-matched normal controls.

Table 7. Effect of Disease Duration on rCBF in Parkinson's Disease.

Disease duration (years)	<4	5-8	9-12	13-16
n	52	24	13	8
Mean age (years ± S.D.)	63.5 ± 8.7	63.8 ± 9.8	67.9 ± 10.3	67.1 ± 6.3
% CBF reduction*	11.8 ± 2.0	12.4 ± 2.7	6.4 ± 2.2	7.7 ± 2.5

means ± S.E.M.; * from age-matched normal controls.

The rCBF in parkinsonians was unaffected by L-dopa therapy. Severity of rCBF reduction from age-matched control values was similar in PD patients treated (n=86) or not treated (n=24) with L-dopa at time of study. In PD patients (n=26) the rCBF remained unaltered before, and 8 weeks following initiation of L-dopa therapy. In another group of PD patients on long-term L-dopa therapy (n=14), the rCBF was unchanged after drug discontinuation and when treatment was renewed. Our preliminary data suggest that in PD, the rCBF remains unchanged during disease progression. We repeated rCBF measurements, 1-2 years (1.7 ± 0.1) after first flow determination. Although this is a rather short period in the natural history of PD, severity of disease deteriorated mildly from a mean stage of 1.9 to 2.3. There was no deterioration in their mental status. However, there was no further rCBF reduction in the second measurement (Table 8).

Table 8. Effect of Disease Progression on the rCBF in Patients with Parkinson's Disease.

	n	Age (years)	Duration (years)	Stage*	Jacobs[6] score	CBF**	%reduction***
First Measurement	41	63.8±9.4	4.7±3.8	1.9±0.1	24.5±0.5	42.1±1.2	12.6±2.6
Second Measurement	41	65.5±9.4	6.5±6.4	2.3±0.1	24.2±0.5	42.5±1.4	9.8±2.4

means ± S.D. for age and disease duration, and means ± S.E.M. other parameters;* according to Hoehn and Yahr[7]; ** ml/100g/min; *** compared with age-matched normal controls.

DISCUSSION

Our study shows that the rCBF declines during normal aging. Reduction in the rCBF did not occur only in normal elderly subjects but already began, and was even more pronounced, in the younger age-groups. It seems therefore that the rCBF progressively decreases with advancing age. In demented patients with AD or SDAT, there were marked rCBF reductions that exceeded the age-dependent "normal" flow decreases (by about 20%). The extent of cerebral flow changes was similar in the AD and SDAT groups.

The causes for rCBF alterations in AD and SDAT are not yet determined. It is unlikely that they are due to changes in caliber of cerebral vessels caused by arteriosclerosis. The latter is an uncommon finding in autopsies of AD and SDAT patients[8]. In AD and SDAT, there is often cerebral atrophy manifested by cortical sulcal widening and ventricular dilatation. Since the rCBF is coupled to local cerebral metabolic rates[1,2], its reduction in demented patients could be due to loss of metabolically active brain tissue. However, we did not find a correlation between the severity of rCBF reduction and the extent of cortical atrophy measured from the CT scans. It is therefore possible that not the lost but the remaining "sick" neurons are responsible for the flow reduction because they are metabolically less active. Thus, the rCBF in AD and SDAT may secondarily decrease due to a state of reduced metabolic demand in their brains. This may be supported by our finding that there is some correlation between the severity of cognitive impairment and magnitude of rCBF decline in the demented patients. An additional theoretical mechanism may involve changes in cerebral cholinergic neurons. It is well-established that in AD and SDAT there is degeneration of cortical cholinergic heruons originating in the nucleus basalis of Meynert[9]. Cerebral microvessels are innervated by various neuronal systems and also by cholinergic neurons which participate in the control and regulation of the rCBF[10,11]. There is evidence that the cholinergic vascular neurons may cause vasodilation of cerebral arterioles[10,11]. If in AD and SDAT there is degeneration not only of the innominato-cortical cholinergic projections but also of the cholinergic neurons that innervate blood vessels, this may cause vasoconstriction and rCBF reduction. Normal aging may be associated with pathological and biochemical cnanges which are similar to those in AD and SDAT although they are of lesser magnitude and do not give rise to overt intelectual impairment[8]. Thus,similar mechanisms may be responsible for rCBF reduction during advancing age and in AD and SDAT.

Our study shows that the rCBF is also reduced in patients with PD. The causes for this phenomenon are not yet clear. Although the pathogenesis of PD is linked mainly to progressive degeneration of the nigrostriatal dopaminergic projections[12], there is accumulating evidence for involvement of the cerebral cortex in this common neurological disorder. This is supported by pneumoencephalographic, CT and postmortem findings of cortical atrophy, autopsy evidence for neuronal loss and "Alzheimer-like" changes in cortex, and a high prevalence of dementia among PD patients[13-19]. Decline of rCBF is an additional marker for participation of the cerebral cortex in the pathogenesis of PD. The cause for this flow reduction could be linked to reduced dopaminergic neurotransmission in brains of PD patients. It was recently shown that there is a degeneration not only of the nigrostriatal but also of the nigrocortical dopaminergic neurons[20]. In that case, there should have been a direct correlation between the amount of dopaminergic neuronal loss and the severity of rCBF reduction in PD patients. However, we did not find any correlation between the magnitude of rCBF decreases and the severity (stage) duration and progression of PD. Furthermore, in patients with predominantly unilateral parkinsonian symptomatology, depletions in central dopamine content are more pronounced in the contralateral hemisphere[21]. However, even in such PD patients, the extent of rCBF decreases was similar in the two cerebral hemispheres. Treatment with exogenous L-dopa corrects the deficient dopamine concentrations in the brain[21]. Therefore, if flow reduction in PD is due to dopamine deficiency, it should be reversed by L-dopa therapy. Our study indicates that the rCBF is unaltered by administration of L-dopa. Taken together, all these data suggest that the rCBF reductions in PD are not caused by diminished dopaminergic neurotransmission.

It is argued that the dementia in PD may be due to superimposed AD[14,18,19]. There is a high prevalence of "Alzheimer-like" changes including senile plaques and neurofibrillary tangles in parkinsonian brains[14,18,19]. As in AD, there is also degeneration of the innominato-cortical cholinergic projection in PD[22] and there is correlation between the severity of cognitive impairment and loss of cortical cholinergic neurons[23]. Therefore, rCBF reduction in PD and AD may share a common underlying mechanism. However, unlike in AD and SDAT, we found no correlation between the presence and severity of dementia and the magnitude of rCBF reduction in our PD patients. The techniques used may not be sufficiently sensitive to detect such correlation. Alternatively, rCBF reductions in PD may be due to a different causative factor than that in AD and SDAT. At present, it does not seem that deficiencies in central dopaminergic or cholinergic neurotransmissions are responsible and further studies should be undertaken to investigate this question. Our study indicates that rCBF measurement is an important and useful tool in the evaluation of patients with dementing neurological disorders.

ACKNOWLEDGEMENT

Supported , in part, by the Jacob and Hilda Blaustein Foundation Inc.

REFERENCES

1. N.A. Lassen, Cerebral blood flow and oxygen consumption in man, Physiol. Rev. 39:183 (1959).
2. E. Melamed and B. Larsen, Cortical activation pattern during saccadic eye movements in humans: Localization by focal cerebral blood flow increases. Ann. Neurol. 5:79 (1979).
3. W.D. Obrist, H.K. Thompson, C.H. King and H.S. Wang, Determination of regional cerebral blood flow by inhalation of 133 Xenon, Circ.Res. 20:125 (1967).
4. W.D. Obrist, H.K. Thompson, H.C. Wang and W.E. Wilkinson, Regional cerebral blood flow estimated by 133 Xenon inhalation, Stroke, 6: 245 (1975).
5. J. Risberg, Z. Ali, E.M. Wilson, and J.H. Halsey, Regional cerebral blood flow by 133 Xenon inhalation - preliminary evaluation of a initial slope index in patients with the unstable flow compartments, Stroke 6:142 (1975).
6. J.W. Jacobs, M.R. Bernhard, A. Delgado and J.J. Strain, Screening for organic mental syndromes in the medically ill, Ann. Int. Med. 86: 40 (1977).
7. M.M. Hoehn and M.D. Yahr, Parkinsonism: Onset, progression and mortality, Neurology 17:427 (1967).
8. B.E. Tomlinson, G. Blessed and M. Roth, Observation on the brains of non-demented old people, J. Neurol. Sci. 7:331 (1968).
9. P.J. Whitehouse, D.L. Price, E.G. Struble, A.W. Clark, J.T. Coyle and M.R. Delong, Alzheimer's disease and senile dementia- loss of neurons in the basal forebrain, Science 215:1237, (1982).
10. O.U. Scremin, A.A. Rovers, A.C. Raynald and A. Giardini, Cholinergic control of blood flow in the cerebral cortex of the rat, Stroke 4:232 (1973).
11. L. Edvinsson, B. Falck and C.H. Owman, Possibilities for cholinergic nerve action on smooth musculature and sympathetic axons in brain vessels mediated by muscarinic and nicotinic receptors, J. Pharmacol. Exp. Ther. 200:117 (1977).
12. J.G. Greenfield and F.D. Bosanquet, The brain stem lesions in parkinsonism, J. Neurol. Neurosurg. Psychiat. 16:213 (1953).
13. G. Selby, Cerebral atrophy in parkinsonism, J. Neurol. Sci. 6:517 (1968).
14. E.C. Alvord, The pathology of parkinsonism: II. An interpretation with special reference to other changes in aging brain, in Recent Advances in Parkinson's Disease, F.H. McDowell and C.H. Markham, eds., F.H. Davis, Philadelphia (1971), pp 131-161.
15. M. Pollack and R.W. Hornabrook, The prevalence, natural history and dementia of Parkinson's disease, Brain 89:429 (1966).
16. A.W. Loranger, H. Goodell and F.H. McDowell, Intelectual impairment in Parkinson's disease, Brain 95: 405, (1972)
17. R. Mayeux and Y. Stern, Intelectual dysfunction and dementia in Parkinson disease, in:The Dementia, R. Mayeux and W.G. Rosen, eds. Raven Press, New York (1983) pp 211-227.
18. A.M. Hakim and G. Mathieson, Dementia in Parkinson's disease: A neuropathologic study, Neurology 29:1209 (1979).

19. F. Boller, T. Mizutani, U. Roessman and P, Gambetti, Parkinson disease, dementia and Alzheimer disease: Clinicopathological correlation, Ann. Neurol. 7:329 (1980).
20. J.F. Agid and Y. Agid, Is the mesocortical dopaminergic system involved in Parkinson's disease? Neurology 30: 1326 (1980).
21. Bernheimer, W. Birkmayer, D. Hornkiewicz, P. Riederer and R. Jellinger, Brain doapmine and syndromes of Parkinson and Huntington: Clinical,morphological and neurochemical correlations, J. Neurol. Sci. 20:415 (1973).
22. P.J. Whitehouse, J.C. Hedreen, C.L. White and D.L. Price, Basal forebrain neurons in the dementia of Parkinson disease, Ann. Neurol. 13:243 (1983).
23. M. Ruberge, A. Ploska, J.F. Agid and Y. Agid, Muscarinic binding and choline acetyltransferase activity with reference to dementia, Brain Res. 232:129 (1982).

THE EARLY STAGES OF PRESENILE AND SENILE ALZHEIMER'S DISEASE: INITIAL STUDIES OF DISEASE SEVERITY AND CEREBRAL BLOOD FLOW

I. Prohovnik, G. Smith, H.A. Sackeim, R.Mayeux and Y. Stern

Departments of Psychiatry & Neurology, Columbia University

722 W. 168th Street, New York, N.Y. 10032

ABSTRACT

Previous work has documented that the common dementing diseases are associated with reductions of cerebral blood flow. Moreover, the reductions appear mostly in cortical regions, and may show sufficient regional specificity to serve as accurate diagnostic discriminators among various etiologies of dementia. We here report initial results from a study that extends these previous investigations in several directions. The present study employs a new technology for the measurement of regional Cerebral Blood Flow (rCBF). Moreover this is the first study to carefully document the severity of dementia on several dimensions, and examine rCBF abnormalities in relation to such indices of severity. Finally, all previous studies were performed on patients with severe demential of relatively long duration; we report the extension of the findings to patients at the early stages of the disease.

Studies of regional Cerebral Blood Flow (rCBF) by the ^{133}Xe inhalation method were performed on 10 patients (mean age 67) with a tentative diagnosis of Alzheimer's Disease (AD), and a control group of 13 elderly, unmedicated patients with major depressive disorder (mean age 66). The AD patients were carefully evaluated for age at onset (before and after 65), duration of the disease, severity of cognitive impairment (by the Blessed Demential Scale). They were further divided into a presenile (n=4, mean age 58) and a senile subgroup (mean age 74).

The AD group was found to have lower flows than the age-matched depressed group; the greatest flow reductions were found in the parietal lobes. Within the AD group, the younger presenile patients demonstrated dramatically lower global flows than the older senile patients. A focal parietal deficit in the presenile group was also present, compared to the senile group. There were no significant differences between the two subgroups in any measure of severity.

These findings suggest that the previously-reported rCBF abnormalities in AD may be detectibel as early as one or two years after symptom onset, and thus may contribute significantly to differential diagnosis at the early stages of the disease. Moreover, they suggest that presenile onset of the disease is associated with a far greater disruption of rCBF, and, by inference, cerebral metabolism. This would be consistent with clinical and neuropathological observations, and may provide and may provide a physiological marker of disease severity that would be more sensitive to underlying biochemical deficits than the observed impairments of cognition and behavior.

INTRODUCTION

Primary degenerative dementia of the Alzheimer type has been shown to be associated with deficits in regional Cerebral Blood Flow (rCBF), most likely reflecting reductions of cortical metabolism. The cerebral flow abnormality is mostly cortical (Frackowiak et al., 1981; Friedland et al., 1983), and consists of a global reduction (Yamaguchi et al., 1980) with focal accentuations (Gustafson and Risberg, 1979). These reported abnormalities can be of diagnostic value. Using rCBF, patients with Alzheimer's Disease can be differentiated from normals with high accuracy (Zemcov et al., 1983), and even from patients with other dementias, such as Multi-Infarct dementia or Pick's disease (Risberg and Gustafson, 1983).

Previous studies, attempting to document the diagnostic utility of rCBF, maximized the magnitude of the differences by employing patients with severe dementia of relatively long duration. However, previous investigators typically did not explicitly document severity and duration. This chapter describes initial findings of a study that attempts to address these issues. We study patients with relatively mild dementia, to test the limits of diagnostic sensitivity of rCBF. In addition, our preliminary findings indicate that the abnormalities detectible in rCBF are related to the severity of the disease. Unfortunately, there has been little systematic study of the quantification of disease severity in this context, and there is no well-established method for its measurement. In an attempt to circumvent this problem, and to examine the relationships among the several possible dimensions of severity in Alzheimer's disease, we collect data in 3 dimensions, all theoretically linked to the construct of severity. We quantify severity by 3 independent measures: estimated disease duration, cognitive impairment, and disruption of daily-living activities. All 3 are concordant with accepted definitions of the disease (c.f., DSM III and McKhahn et al., 1984), have high face validity, and are congruent with clinical experience and post-mortem neuropathological and biochemical findings. However, our initial experience indicates that the three dimensions do not demonstrate substantial overlap. The proportion of shared variance among them is typically less than 50%, and there is considerable heterogeneity in symptomatic presentation and rate of deterioration among patients. Therefore, we consider all 3 necessary at this point for a thorough documentation of severity.

Finally, we examine the dimension of Age-At-Onset (AAO) in relation to rCBF abnormalities. The postulated dichotomy between presenile and senile onset is controversial. Although it is a feature acknowledged by diagnostic criteria, its epidemiological and pathophysiological validity is still being debated. The DSM III, for example, acknowledges this distinction as a variant, but does not recognize it as pathognomonic. Some investigators (e.g., Reisberg, 1983) maintain that there is no evidence for such a distinction. Most authors, however appear to agree that patients with early AAO demonstrate a more virulent course and more rapid deterioration of the disease. There is also some evidence for greater severity of post-mortem neuropathological and biochemical deficits in patients with presenile onset (e.g., Whitehouse et al., 1983; Bird et al., 1983), as well as shorter survival (Barklay et al., 1985), compared with later onset. We have examined this variable in relation to rCBF abnormalities, and used the common cutoff age of 65 to classify our patients.

METHODS

Subjects: Ten patients were admitted with a clinical diagnosis of

Alzheimer's disease, in accordance with the procedures outlined in DSM III. Their mean age was 67.3 (SD=9.69), with a mean disease duration of about 2 years (range 6 months to 6 years). Six of these patients were studied within 1 year of estimated symptom onset. They were compared to a group of 13 elderly, unmedicated patients meeting Research Diagnostic Criteria for primary major depression. These patients were all studied prior to initiation of treatment, and their mean age was 65.88 (SD+9.90). The sex distribution was different in the 2 samples: there were 6 (60%) demented males but only 3 (23%) depressed males.

Patient Ratings: A traditional cutoff was used for the presenile/senile classification, with AAO<65 termed presenile. Cognitive capacity was quantified by our modification of the Mini-Mental State (Folstein et al., 1975); the modification is described in Mayeux et al. (1981). Disruption of behavior and capacity for activities of daily living were quantified by the Blessed Demential Rating Scale (Blessed et al., 1968). This scale has been well validated against post-mortem neuropathology, and it is appropriate for the complete range of dementia.

rCBF Measurement: We used the Novo Cerebrograph 32C, with 32 detectors over both cerebral hemispheres, mounted in a helmet-like device. Two physiological models were employed for data analysis, and 5 parameters with each model. Discussion of the various parameters and models is beyond the scope of the present report. We have chosen to report the results of the ISI parameter, derived by the M2 model, based on considerations of sensitivity and reliability (for details of the rationale and calculations, see Prohovnik et al., 1983 and Prohovnik et al, 1985). This parameter yields an estimate of flow dominated by grey-matter, and it is known to be more stable at the low-flow conditions typical of dementia than pure measures of grey-matter flow. The ISI is conservatively reported as arbitrary units; assuming a blood-brain partition coefficient for Xenon on 1.0, these units correspond to ml/100g/min.

The measurement procedure is completely noninvasive, and no blood samples are necessary for quantification. The patient is required to lie on the stretcher for 10-15 mins, breathing through a face mask or mouthpiece. All patients studied so far could tolerate this procedure with no sedation.

RESULTS

The AD group demonstrated lower cerebral blood flows than the elderly depressed group. As illustrated in Fig. 1, there was a global reduction of hemispheric mean flows of about 5%, using this parameter. The somewhat greater abnormality on the left side is contributed by a single patient, and will be discussed below. The rCBF pattern we find in the early stages of AD is characterized by an inferior parietal flow reduction, surrounded by relatively preserved flow in the occipital pole and the central sulcus. There is a weaker flow reduction in the frontal lobes. These findings were consistent across all parametrs and both models, but their magnitude was greater with the M2 model.

Striking differences of cerebral blood flow were found between the presenile and senile patients. These two samples differed significantly (p<.01) in age and age at onset, by definition, but not in the measures of severity. Duration of the disease and cognitive status indicated somewhat greater severity in the presenile group, whereas behavioral impairment was somewhat greater in the senile group (none of these differences reached significance). As illustrated in Fig. 2, the younger presenile patients demonstrated lower flows and greater regional abnormalities. Note that the greater left hemisphere lesion is determined by a single patient (case #4033). This patient was completely aphasic. As expected his rCBF demonstrated an extensive lesion in the left hemisphere, coverning most of the parietal and posterior temporal areas. This patient was untestable on the mMMS, and was scored as 0, although his true capacity is probably greatly underestimated. This also caused the disparity in mMMS scores between the

Table 1: AD Group Patient Characteristics

Case #	Age	Sex	AAO[a]	Duration[b]	mMMS[c]	BDRS[d]
Presenile:						
4032	51	M	50	1	35	8
4033	58	M	52	6	0[e]	11
4072	57	F	55	2	37	5.5
4075	64	F	61	3	45	4
Mean±SD	57.50±5.32		54.50±4.79	3.0±4.67	29.25±19.97	7.13±3.07
Senile:						
4024	67	F	66	1	23.5	8
4026	72	M	71	1	50.5	9
4028	77	M	76	1	18.5	18.5
4031	71	M	69	2	50	13.5
4034	75	M	74	1	40	4.5
4074	81	F	80	1	47	9.5
Mean±SD	73.83±4.91		72.67±5.05	1.17±0.41	38.25±13.97	10.5±4.87
TOTAL	67.3±9.69		65.4±10.48	1.9±1.59	34.65±16.22	9.15±4.39

a: AAO is estimated age at onset, in years.
b: Duration is estimated by a relative, and rounded to the nearest year.
c: modified Mini-Mental State; higher scores indicate better functioning (aged normals score 52).
d: Blessed Dementia Rating Scale; higher scores indicate poor function.
e: this patient was aphasic, and therefore untestable on the mMMS. His underlying capacity is probably better than the score indicates.

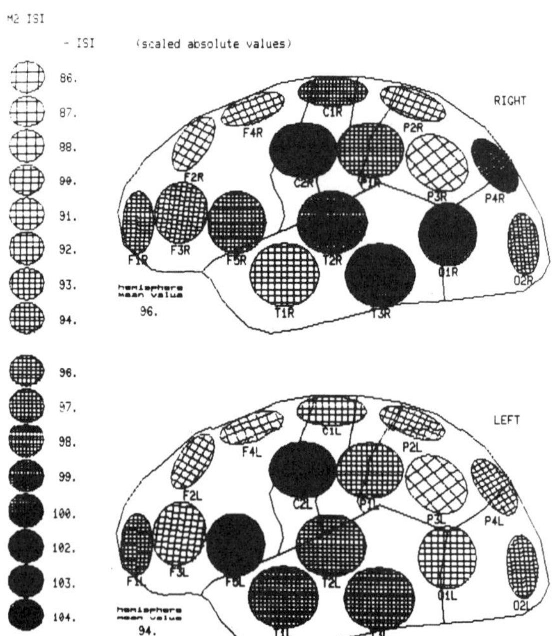

Figure 1: rCBF of the AD group, expressed as % of the depressed group (100 indicates equal values; values below 100 indicate lower flow in the AD group). The scale on the left identifies the regional flows. Hemispheric means are numerically denoted below the hemispheres.

two dementia subgroups. Again, the rCBF findings were consistent across models and parameters, but revealed greater differences with the M2 model.

Age was positively correlated with flow values within the dementia group, and negatively within the depressed group. These correlations did not reach statistical significance, but they suggest that depressed patients show the normal age-related decline of cerebral blood flow, whereas the demented patients show an opposite trend due to the greater disruption in the younger, presenile patients.

DISCUSSION

Our initial findings confirm previous work in demonstrating global and focal cerebral blood flow deficits in Alzheimer's disease. The interpretation of these flow deficits as reduced metabolic activity is supported by recent PET findings (Frackowiak et al., 1981; Friedland et al., 1983), and by evidence that the blood-brain partition coefficient for Xenon is not changed in normal aging or degenerative dementia (Amano et al., 1982). Despite the small sample sizes, we suggest that these findings indicate significant directions of development, if confirmed in larger samples.

Our findings are novel in that they were obtained in a sample with carefully-documented short disease duration, i.e., in the early stages of the disease. To the extent that there exists a difficulty in differential diagnosis of AD from major depression (e.g., Wells, 1979), this problem is most severe in the early stages of the disease. Our data suggest that even within the first one or two years (after symptom onset), there are measurable deficits in rCBF that may aid in differential diagnosis. These deficits are similar in direction and distribution to those observed later in the course of the disease (e.g., Risberg et al., 1981), but their magnitude, as expected, appears smaller. Our demented and depressed groups did not differ in blood pressure, but the demented group had significantly higher

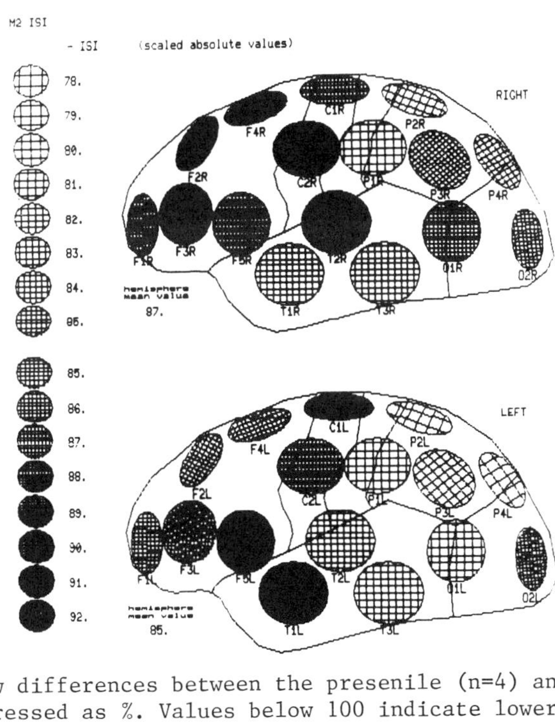

Figure 2: Flow differences between the presenile (n=4) and senile (n=6) subgroups, expressed as %. Values below 100 indicate lower flow in the presenile patients.

end-tidal PCO_2 value. Had we corrected for this $PeCO_2$ difference, the rCBF differences would have been much greater. As illustrated by case# 4033, and as previously suggested by others, the lesion visible in rCBF is not totally invariant; its extent and precise distribution are related to the nature and extent of cognitive impairment. Although the main lesion we found to typify AD was in the parietal lobes, we also report a weaker frontal flow deficit, which has not been previously observed. This finding may be the result of symptomatic presentation in our material, or other factors; its significance is yet to be determined.

Contrary to common-sense expectations, our findings indicate greater deterioration of rCBF in the patients with presenile disease onset, despite their significantly younger age. Normally, cerebral blood flow declines with age, as also suggested in our depressed control group. Indeed, Risberg and Gustafson (1983) reported lower flows in a senile group, compared to presenile. Their samples were larger than ours and somewhat older. Unfortunately, these authors did not report disease duration or quantitative severity measures. It is therefore possible that severity differences in their samples counteracted the AAO effects.

Our younger presenile patients demonstrated about 15% lower mean flow (p .05) and focal flow reductions of about 20%, which reached significance in several parietal and frontal locations. In fact, the flow differences between the two dementia subgroups were greater than between the total dementia sample and the depressed sample. This difference cannot be explained by BP or $PeCO_2$ effects: the younger presenile patients had higher $PeCO_2$ (40.30 mmHg, compared to 38.35) and both subgroups had similar, normal blood pressure values. Nor can the flow differences be easily explained by duration of the disease: both groups had relatively early Alzheimer's disease, and the difference in duration between them did not reach statistical significance (four new presenile patients, recently admitted and not included in the present analysis, show the same low flows with shorter durations). Likewise, our measures of cognitive and behavioral imairments did not reveal significant differences. Both scales employed here, the modified MMS and the Blessed Dementia Scale, are frequently used and well validated. It is still conceivable, however, that there is a dimension of severity,untapped by our three indices, which would explain the rCBF differences.

Such a difference may exist in underlying pathology, structural or biochemical. Several authors have recently suggested that presenile onset of AD is associated with greater severity of post-mortem cell loss and biochemical deficits (e.g., Whitehouse et al., 1983; Bird et al., 1983) and with shorter survival (Barclay et al., 1985). It is conceivable that rCBF directly correlates with this underlying disruption of cerebral function, more than behavioral and cognitive rating scales. Thus, rCBF may not only provide greater diagnostic precision in the early stages of the disease, but also more accurate staging and severity assessment. We are continuing our studies with this possibility in mind.

REFERENCES

Amano, T., Meyer, J.S., Takashi, O., Shaw, T. and Mortel, K.F., 1982, Stable Xenon CT cerebral blood flow measurements in normal aging and dementia, J Comp Ass Tomog, 6:923.

Barclay, L.L., Zemcov, A., Blass, J.P., and McDowell, F.H., 1985, Factors associated with duration of survival in Alzheimer's disease, Biol Psychiat, 20:86.

Bird, T.D., Stranahan, S., Sumi, S.M. and Raskind, M., 1983, Alzheimer's disease: cholineacetyltransferase activity in brain tissue from clinical and pathological subgroups, Ann Neurol, 14:284.

Blessed, G., Tomlinson, B.E. and Roth, M., 1968, The association between quantitative measures of dementia and of senile changes in the cerebral gray matter of elderly subjects, Br J Psychiat, 114:797.

Folstein, M.F., Folstein, S.E. and McHugh, P.R., 1975, Mini-mental State: a practical method for grading the cognitive state of patients for the clinician, J Psychiat Res, 12:189.

Frackowiak, R.S., Pozzilli, C., Legg, N.J., Boulay, G.H., Marshall, J., Lenzi, G.L. and Jones, T., 1981, Regional cerebral oxygen supply and utilization in dementia, Brain, 104:753.

Friedland, R.P., Budinger, T.F., Ganz, E., Yano, Y., Mathis, C.A., Koss, B., Ober, B.A., Huesma, R.H. and Derenzo, S.E., 1983, Regional cerebral metabolic alterations in dementia of the Alzheimer type. J Comp Ass Tomog, 7:590.

Gustafson, L. and Risberg, J., 1979, Regional cerebral blood flow measurements by the 133-Xe inhalation technique in differential diagnosis of dementia, Acta Neurol Scand, 60(Suppl. 72):546.

Mayeux, R., Stern, Y., Rosen, W. and Leventhal, J., 1981, Depression, intellectual impairment and Parkinson's disease, Neurology, 31:645.

McKhann, G., Drachman, D., Folstein, M.F., Katzman, R., Price, D., and Stadlan, E.M., 1984, Clinical diagnosis of Alzheimer's disease, Neurology, 34:939.

Prohovnik, I., Knudsen, E. and Risberg, J., 1983, Accuracy of models and algorithms for determination of fast-compartment flow by noninvasive 133-Xe clearance, in: "Functional Radionuclide Imaging of the Brain", P. Magistretti, ed., Raven Press, New York (1983).

Prohovnik, I., Knudsen, E. and Risberg, J., 1985, Theoretical evaluation and simulation test of the initial slope index for noninvasive rCBF, in: "Measurement of Cerebral Metabolism in Man", A. Hartmann, ed., Springer Verlag, in press.

Reisberg, B., 1983, "Alzheimer's Disease: The Standard Reference", The Free Press, New York.

Risberg, J. and Gustafson, L., 1983, 133-Xe Cerebral blood flow in dementia and in neuropsychiatry research, in: "Functional Radionuclide Imaging of the Brain", P. Magistretti, ed., Raven Press, New York.

Risberg, J., Gustafson, L. and Prohovnik, I., 1981, rCBF measurements by 133-Xe inhalation: applications in neuropsychology and psychiatry, in: "Progress in Nuclear Medicine, Volume 7", O. Juge and A Donath, eds., Karger, Basel.

Wells, C.E., 1979, Pseudodementia, Am J Psychiat, 136:895.

Whitehouse, P.J., Hedreen, J.C., White, C.L., Clark, A.W. and Price, D.L., 1983, Neuronal loss in the basal forebrain cholinergic system is more marked in Alzheimer's disease than in senile dementia of the Alzheimer type, Ann Neurol, 14:149.

Yamaguchi, F., Meyer, J.S., Yamamoto, M., Sakai, F. and Shaw, T., 1980, Noninvasive regional cerebral blood flow measurements in dementia, Arch Neurol, 37:410.

Zemcov, A., Risberg, J., Barclay L.L., and Blass, J.P., 1983, A double blind study of rCBF in the differential diagnosis of the dementias, Eur Neurol, 22(Suppl.):20.

LASER MICROPROBE MASS ANALYZER (LAMMA) - A NEW APPROACH TO THE STUDY OF THE ASSOCIATION OF ALUMINUM AND NEUROFIBRILLARY TANGLE FORMATION

Daniel P. Perl, David Muñoz-Garcia,
Paul Good and William W. Pendlebury

Department of Pathology
University of Vermont
Burlington, Vermont 05405

INTRODUCTION

Along with senile plaques, the neurofibrillary tangle (NFT) represents one of the hallmarks of the pathologic changes which characterize Alzheimer's disease and senile dementia of the Alzheimer's type. The density of NFTs in the brain at autopsy has been correlated with the presence and severity of dementia during life (Tomlinson et al, 1970). NFTs are not restricted to Alzheimer's disease, but have been found in association with several other neurologic diseases (Wisniewski et al, 1979), including repeated trauma (Corsellis et al, 1973), viral infections (Mandybur et al, 1976), lead intoxication (Niklowitz and Mandybur, 1975), or hereditary disorders (Hirano et al, 1968). The presence of abundant cortical and subcortical NFTs, unaccompanied by senile plaques, are prominent pathological findings in the brains of patients dying with either amyotrophic lateral sclerosis (ALS) (Malamud et al, 1961) or parkinsonism-dementia (PD) (Hirano et al, 1961) in the native population living on the island of Guam, where these neurodegenerative diseases have an unsually high incidence. The variety of circumstances under which NFTs are found suggests shared pathogenetic mechanisms, the unraveling of which will certainly contribute to the understanding of Alzheimer's disease.

In 1965, Klatzo and co-workers (1965) and Terry and Peña (1965) reported that the administration of aluminum salts into the cerebral spinal fluid of rabbits results in the widespread formation in the perikarya of central nervous system neurons of structures resembling NFTs under the light microscope, and these results have been confirmed by several investigators. The aluminum-induced NFTs consist of accumulations of normal-appearing straight neurofilaments (Terry and Pena, 1965; Selkoe et al, 1979), and thus differ ultra structurally from Alzheimer-type NFTs, which are made up of paired helical filaments (PHF)(Kidd, 1964; Wisniewski et al, 1976). Both Alzheimer-type and aluminum-induced NFTs share antigenic determinants with normal neurofilaments (Anderton et al, 1982; Gambetti et al, 1983; Selkoe et al, 1979), and in both cases phosphorylated neurofilament epitopes are abnormally present in the perikarya (Sternberger and Sternberger, 1984; Muñoz-Garcia et al, in preparation). However, Alzheimer type NFTs also contain additional antigenic determinants which are not present in the aluminum-induced NFT (Ihara et al,1983). Moreover, unlike aluminum-induced NFTs, the Alzheimer-type NFTs are insoluble in protein solvents (Selkoe et al, 1982).

Despite these differences, this animal model stimulated Crapper and coworkers to measure the aluminum content of tissue samples dissected from the brain of patients dying with Alzheimer's disease (Crapper et al, 1973, 1976). They found evidence of significantly increased amounts of aluminum in the Alzheimer's disease brain tissues, when compared to non-affected controls. These studies have been difficult to replicate (Trapp et al, 1978; McDermott et al, 1979; Markesbury et al, 1981) and this subject remains controversial (Wisniewski et al, 1980). These approaches employed assay techniques which are inherently tissue destructive (atomic absorption spectrometry and neutron activation analysis) and require relatively large bulk samples. In a situation of focal accumulation of an element in association with certain cellular lesions, dilution of the element of interest within the relatively large total sample being analyzed may result in an inability to detect significant differences between affected tissues and uninvolved controls. Moreover, bulk analysis methods do not control for the atrophy of the tissue, which modifies the denominator of the concentrations ratios. Finally, exogenous contamination by such a common element as aluminum always remains a possibility.

Using scanning electron microscopy in conjunction with x-ray energy-dispersive spectrometry (SEM-XES), our laboratory has developed highly sensitive techniques for the analysis of trace elemental constituents of the nervous system at the cellular level of resolution. These methods have enabled us to identify intraneuronal accumulations of aluminum in association with neurofibrillary tangle formation in the hippocampus of patients with senile dementia of the Alzheimer's type (Perl and Brody, 1980a, b; Perl and Pendlebury,1984), and cases of PD and ALS as seen in the Guamanian Chamorro (Perl et al, 1982). Adjacent, tangle-free neurons in these cases, or in age-matched controls, failed to show a similar degree of intraneuronal aluminum accumulation. Our techniques have permitted us to simultaneously evaluate several other elements within the tissues being probed. Aluminum represents the only element which was consistently altered in relationship to the presence, in a neuron, of a neurofibrillary tangle. There was a parallel tendency for increased calcium to be found within tangle-bearing neurons in most cases examined. However, a few cases have shown tangle-bearing neurons without evidence of calcium accumulation. The accumulation of aluminum and calcium in the tangled neurons of Guamanian Chamorros has been recently confirmed by an independent research group using a different technique (Garruto et al, 1984).

Despite the success we have had in employing these SEM-XES approaches to this problem, several problems inherent to the SEM-XES method have interfered with further progress with this research. First, this technique utilizes the secondary electron or surface images to locate a particular cell of interest for elemental analysis. This image can be difficult to interpret in regions of the brain which do not contain the large, regularly arranged neurons of the hippocampus. Secondly, the use of relatively thick (20 μm) tissue sections, forced by the detection limits of the X-ray spectrometry equipment, does not permit precise intracellular localization of elements. Finally, SEM-XES is not suitable for quantification, and is an extremely slow and laborious method. We now report the use of the laser microprobe mass analyzer (LAMMA), a new instrument that lacks most of the inherent limitations of SEM-XES methods discussed above, in the investigation of the association of aluminum to neurofibrillary tangle formation.

MATERIAL AND METHODS

The LAMMA 500 Instrument

The laser microprobe mass analyzer or LAMMA 500 is a recently developed analytical instrument manufactured by the Leybold-Heraeus Company of Cologne, W. Germany, which combines an optical microscope with a time-of-flight mass spectrometer. A comprehensive technical description is given by Heinen et al,

(1980), and only the essential details will be provided here. The light microscope of the instrument permits observation of the specimen to be analyzed. The specimen is typically a semithin (0.2-1 um) section cut from a plastic-embedded block of tissue. The section may be stained with toluidine blue for visualization of histologic features and is mounted on a standard 3 mm. in diameter electron microscopy copper mesh grid. The grid is placed in a high vacuum behind a high-purity quartz cover-slip which is mounted on a movable specimen holder. The instrument generates a high energy laser pulse (a Nd:YAG laser provides a 2 mJoule pulse to the specimen within the 15 nanosecond laser pulse interval) that is focused on the specimen by the objective of the optical microscope. The interaction of the laser with the tissue vaporizes/ionizes a portion of the section with a diameter in the range of 1 micron. The high energy laser is directed to the point of interest by a collinear He-Ne low energy laser beam which appears as a red spot on the tissue section. Mounted behind the specimen is the 1.8 meter long column of the time-of-flight mass spectrometer. Ions produced by the perforation of the section by the focussed high energy laser beam pulse pass down the evacuated column of the time-of-flight spectrometer where they are separated and detected according to their mass number. The principle relied upon is that the lighter mass fragments travel down the column faster than the heavier ions and thus arrive sooner at the detector. With each laser shot through the tissue, a complete mass spectrum is produced for either positive or negative ions.

Our instrument is linked to a dedicated Micro PDP 11 computer using an RT-11 operating system. Specific programs have been written to allow for the transfer and storage of mass spectra, calibration of spectra, peak identification and peak height integration, spectral averaging and plotting.

Prior to analysis of tissue sections, the instrument is calibrated by analyzing a thin section of Spurr's low viscosity medium doped with 10 mM each of Li, Na, K, Sr, and Pb, prepared as crown ether complexes. The spectral position of any two elements are fed to the computer which calibrates all subsequent spectra according to the ratios of mass number to time-of-flight.

Tissues

Analyses were carried out on the hippocampal neurons of a 67 year old Guamanian Chamorro who died of ALS after a 14 year course, and on a 44 year old Chamorro who was free of neurological disease and died acutely following perforation of a peptic ulcer. The brain of the ALS patient showed, in addition to degeneration of the pyramidal tracts and loss of anterior horn motor neurons, numerous NFTs in the hippocampus and a moderate number in the neocortex. The brain of the control patient did not show any significant pathologic changes.

LAMMA Analysis

Blocks of the pyramidal layer of the H1 sector of the hippocampus were osmicated and embedded in Spurr's low viscosity medium. Semi-thin sections (0.3 μm) were cut with a diamond knife, mounted on 3mm copper 300 mesh EM grids, stained with toluidine blue and subjected to LAMMA observation and analysis. Neurons were chosen for analysis if the cell nucleus was present in the plane of section. Each selected neuron was first evaluated by light microscopy for the presence or absence of a neurofibrillary tangle. Multiple-point LAMMA analysis was performed in the nucleus and cytoplasm of each selected neuron, as well as in the adjacent neuropil. Five laser shots were taken in each of these three areas from each selected neuron and the resultant mass spectra were collected and analyzed. The height (in millivolts) of the peaks at mass numbers 27 (corresponding to aluminum) of 40 laser shots derived from each region was averaged. The calculated means of each area were compared by the Tukey's multiple comparison test.

RESULTS

Figure 1 shows a tangle bearing neuron with multiple perforations produced by the laser beam in the course of LAMMA analysis. This shows the degree of accuracy with which each cell is identified as well as the precision of localization of each laser. Figure 2a shows a representative mass spectrum obtained from a shot through the tangle-bearing cytoplasm, showing the presence of a prominent aluminum peak. The height of this peak is markedly reduced in the spectrum shown in figure 2b, obtained from the cytoplasm of an adjacent tangle-free neuron in the same section.

Table 1 shows the means and standard error of the mean of the height in millivolts of the peaks corresponding to aluminum in each area analyzed. Analysis of variance of these data yielded an F of 35.6, with corresponding $p < 0.0001$. The means were then compared by the Tukey's test for multiple comparisons, which showed that the aluminum-related peak from the cytoplasm within NFT-bearing cells were significantly different from all others, with $p < 0.01$. Although calcium appeared to be increased in the cytoplasm of the tangle-bearing neurons, these differences did not quite reach statistical significance.

DISCUSSION

The main purpose of this paper is to introduce a new technology that has already proven its value in extraneural tissues (Verbueken et al, 1984 b) and, we believe, can be applied to the study of the pathogenesis of the neurofibrillary tangle. This is supported by the presentation of data demonstrating its capabilities for such a study. Although the data provided are preliminary in nature, they demonstrate selective accumulation of aluminum, and perhaps calcium, in the cytoplasm of neurons bearing neurofibrillary tangles of a Guamanian Chamorro. The superior spatial resolution afforded by LAMMA allows for greater precision that that obtainable by SEM-XES, with which only broad "nuclear region" and "cytoplasmic region" could be identified within probed neurons.

LAMMA spectra are not subjected to interference by the presence of other elements. Thus, it is possible to osmicate the tissue in order to demonstrate the presence or absence of neurofibrillary tangles in the neurons by

Table 1. Means ± standard errors of the height of the aluminum-related peak (mass number 27) of the number of laser shots for each area indicated in parentheses.

	Guam ALS	Guam Control
Nucleus	170 ± 26 (40)	291 ± 47 (20)
Cytoplasm with NFT	639 ± 62 (40)	-
Cytoplasm without NFT	138 ± 13 (80)	211 ± 35 (20)
Neuropil	113 ± 22 (40)	124 ± 18 (40)

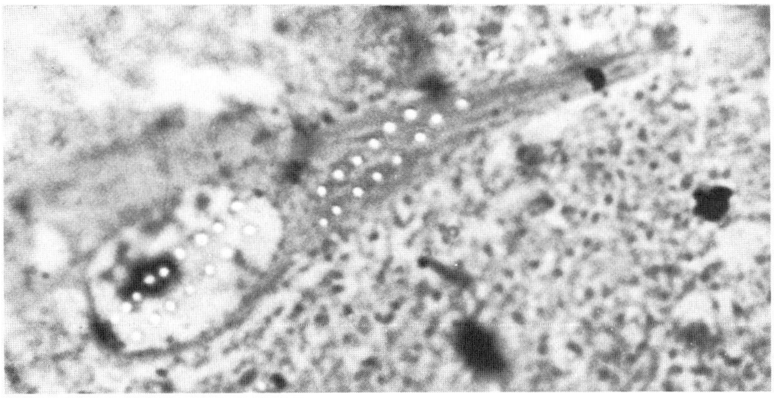

Figure 1

Photomicrograph of tangle-bearing neuron showing multiple perforations produced during LAMMA analysis. Plastic-embedded, 0.3 μm section stained with toluidine blue

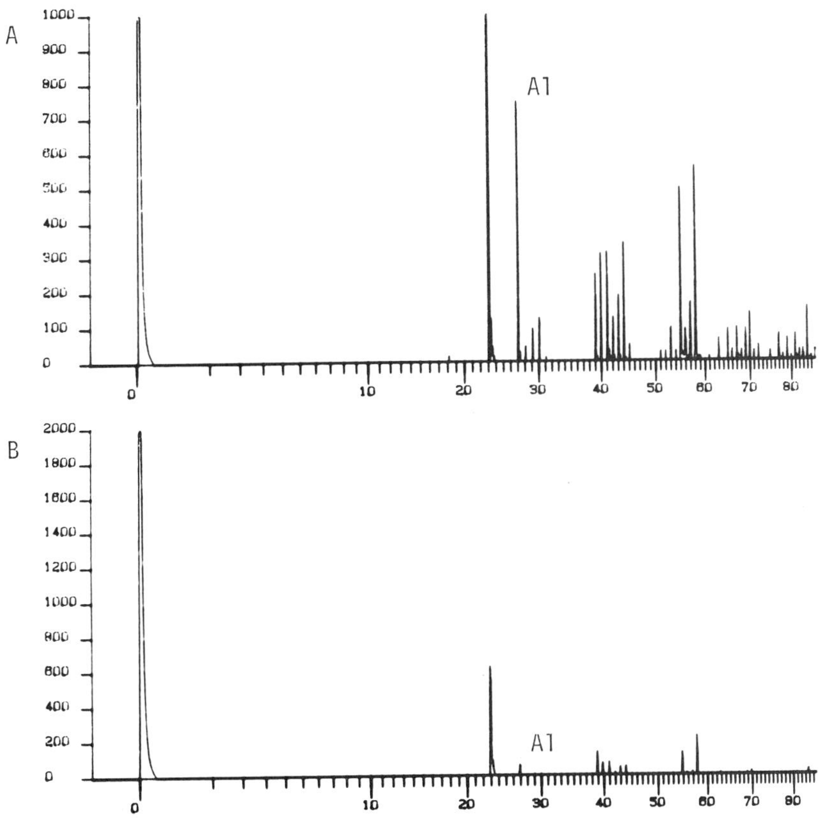

Figure 2

Partial mass spectrum from laser shots taken of the cytoplasm of a tangle-bearing neuron (A) and an adjacent tangle-free neuron (B) from a case of Guam ALS.

ultrastructural examination following LAMMA analysis. It is also important to note that no other element was noted to accumulate in the tangle-bearing neurons to the degree seen with aluminum. Although the height of the aluminum-related signal has been shown to be proportional to the concentration of the element (Verbueken et al,1984 a), quantification with LAMMA does present certain difficulties, notably the matrix effect on the heights of the peaks of the elements, as well as interference by organic fragments with the same nominal mass number as the element of interest. In spite of these problems, absolute quantification of elements in tissue sections has been recently achieved in the retina using a LAMMA instrument (Schroeder and Fain,1984). One of the aims of our present research is to achieve reliable quantification of aluminum and calcium in the neurofibrillary tangle-bearing neuron.

The significance of the selective accumulation of aluminum in tangle-bearing neurons remains unknown and its subcellular cytoplasmic localization was unexpected. The specificity of the accumulation of an element in direct association with a distinct pathology deserves consideration of the role of aluminum in the pathogenesis of neurofibrillary tangle. It is significant in this regard that epidemiological studies of ALS and Parkinsonism-dementia in Guam and the other high incidence foci show a pattern of incidence suggestive of the etiological role of the physical environment, in particular the elemental composition of the soil and water (Gajdusek and Salazar, 1982; Gajdusek, 1982). We feel that the introduction of LAMMA technology to these studies represents a major advance in this area of research.

ACKNOWLEDGEMENTS

This study was performed with the support of the John D. French Foundation, the Sandoz Corporation, and grant AG-01415 from the NIH. We thank J. Kessler for her excellent technical support and Mrs. Marceau for secretarial assistance.

REFERENCES

Anderton, B.H., Breinburg, D., Downes, M.J., Green, P.J., Tomlinson, B.E., Ulrich, J., Wood, J.N., and Kahn, J., 1982, Monoclonal antibodies show that neurofibrillary tangles and neurofilaments share antigenic determinants. Nature, 298:84.

Corsellis J.A.N., Burton, C.J., and Freeman-Browne, D., 1973, The aftermath of boxing. Psychol Med, 3:270.

Crapper, D.R., Krishnan, S.S., and Dalton, A.J., 1973, Brain aluminum distribution in Alzheimer's disease and especially neurofibrillary degeneration, Science, 180:511.

Crapper, D.R., Krishnan, S.S., and Quittkat, S., 1976, Aluminum, neurofibrillary degeneration and Alzheimer's disease, Brain, 99:67.

Gajdusek, D.C., and Salazar, A.M., 1982, Amyotrophic lateral sclerosis and Parkinsonian syndromes in high incidence among the Auyu and Jakai people of West New Guinea., Neurology, 32:107.

Gajdusek, D.C., 1982, Foci of motor neuron disease in high incidence in isolated populations of East Asia and the Western Pacific, in: "Human Motor Neuron Diseases, Advances in Neurology", L.P. Rowland ed., Vol 36, Raven Press, New York.

Gambetti, P., Shecket, G., Getti, B., Hirano, A., and Dahl, D., 1983 Neurofibrillary changes in human brain. An immunocytochemical study with a neurofilament antiserum. J Neuropathol Exp Neurol 42:69.

Garruto, R.M., Fukatsu, R., Yanagihara, R., Gajdusek, D.C., Hook, G. and Fiori, C.E., 1984, Imaging of calcium and aluminum in neurofibrillary tangle-bearing neurons in parkinsonism-dementia of Guam. Proc Natl Acad Sci USA, 81:1875.

Hirano, A., Tuazon, R., and Zimmerman, H.M., 1968, Neurofibrillary changes, granulovacuolar bodies and argentophilic globules observed in tuberous sclerosis., Acta Neuropath (Berl.), 11:257.

Hirano, A., Malamud, N., and Kurland, L.J., 1961, Parkinsonism-dementia complex, an endemic disease on the island of Guam: II. Pathological features., Brain, 84:662.

Heinen, H.J., Hillenkamp, F., Kaufmann, R., Schroder, W., and Wechsung, R, 1980, LAMMA: A new laser microprobe mass analyzer for biomedicine and biological materials analysis, in: "Recent Developments in Mass Spectrometry in Biochemistry and Medicine 6", Frigerio A, McCamish M (eds). Elsevier, Amsterdam.

Ihara, Y., Abraham, C., and Selkoe, D.J., 1983, Antibodies to paired helical filaments in Alzheimer's disease do not recognize normal brain proteins. Nature, 304:727.

Kidd, M., 1964, Alzheimer's disease - an electron microscopical study., Brain, 87:307.

Klatzo, I., Wisniewski, H., and Streicher, E., 1965, Experimental Production of neurofibrillary degeneration. I Light Microscopic observations., J Neuropath Exp Neurol, 24:187.

Malamud, N., Hirano, A., and Kurland, L.T., 1961, Pathoanatomic changes in amyotrophic lateral sclerosis on Guam: Special reference to the occurrence of neurofibrillary changes., Arch Neurol, 19:573.

Mandybur, T.I., Nagpaul, A.S., Pappas, Z., and Niklowitz, W.J., 1976 Alzheimer neurofibrillary change in subacute sclerosing panencephalitis., J Neuropath Exp Neurol, 35:300.

Markesbury, W.R., Ehmann, W.D., Hossain, T.I.M., Allauddin, M., and Goodin, D.T., 1981, Instrumental neutron activation analysis of brain aluminum in Alzheimer's disease and aging., Ann Neurol, 10:511.

McDermott, J.R., Smith, A.I., Iqbal, K., and Wisniewski, H.M., 1979, Brain aluminum in aging and Alzheimer disease, Neurology, 29:809.

Niklowitz, W.J., and Mandybur, T.I., 1975, Neurofibrillary change following childhood encephalopathy., J Neuropath Exp Neurol, 34:445.

Perl, D.P., and Brody, A.R., 1980a, Alzheimer's disease: x-ray spectrometric evidence of aluminum accumulation in neurofibrillary tangle-bearing neurons., Science, 208:297.

Perl, D.P., and Brody, A.R., 1980b, Detection of aluminum by SEM - x-ray spectrometry within neurofibrillary tangle-bearing neurons of Alzheimer's disease, Neurotoxicology, 1:133.

Perl, D.P., Gajdusek, D.C., Garruto R.M., Yanagihara, R.T., and Gibbs, C. J.,Jr., 1982, Intraneuronal aluminum accumulation in amyotrophic lateral sclerosis and parkinsonism dementia of Guam., Science, 217:1053.

Perl, D.P., and Pendlebury, W.W. 1984, Aluminum (Al) accumulation in neurofibrillary tangle (NFT) bearing neurons of senile dementia Alzheimer's type (SDAT)-detection by intraneuronal x-ray spectrometry studies of unstained tissue sections. J Neuropathol Exp Neurol 43:349.

Schroder, W.H., and Fain, G.L. 1984, Light-dependent calcium release from photoreceptors measured by laser micro-mass analysis, Nature, 309:268.

Selkoe, D.J., Ihara, Y., and Salazar, F.J. 1982, Alzheimer's disease: Insolubility of partially purified paired helical filaments in sodium dodecyl sulfate and urea, Science 215:1243.

Selkoe, D.J., Liem R.K.H., Yen S-H, and Shelanski M.K. 1979, Biochemical and immunological characterization of neurofilaments in experimental neurofibrillary degeneration induced by aluminum, Brain Res 163:235.

Sternberger, L.A., and Sternberger, N.H. 1984, Monoclonal immunocytochemistry of posttranslational change in neurofilaments. J Neuropathol Exp Neurol 43:308.

Terry, R.D., and Peña, C. 1965, Experimental production of neurofibrillary degeneration. 2. Electron microscopy, phosphatase histochemistry and electron probe analysis. J Neuropathol Exp Neurol, 24:200.

Tomlinson, B.E., Blessed, G., and Roth, M., 1970, Observations on the brains of demented old people, J Neurol Sci, 11:205.

Trapp, G.A., Miner, G.D., Zimmerman, R.L., Mastri, A.R., and Heston, L.L., 1978, Aluminum levels in brain in Alzheimer's disease, Biol. Psychiatry, 13:709.

Verbueken, A.H., Van Grieken, R.E., Paulus, G.J., and de Bruijn, W.C. 1984 a, Embedded ion exchange beads as standards for laser microprobe mass analysis of biological specimens, Anal Chem 56:1362.

Verbueken, A.H., Van de Vyver, F.L., Van Grieken, R.E., Paulus, G.J. Visser, W.J., D'Haese, P., and De Broe, M.E., 1984 b, Ultrastructural localization of aluminum in patients with dialysis-associated osteomalacia. Clin Chem, 30:763.

Wisniewski, H.M., Narang, H.K., and Terry, R.D., 1976, Neurofibrillary tangles of paired helical filaments, J Neurol Sci, 27:173.

Wisneiwski, K., Jervis, G.A., Moretz, R.C., and Wisniewski, H.M., 1979, Alzheimer neurofibrillary tangles in diseases other than senile and presenile dementia., Ann Neurol, 5:288.

Wisniewski, H.M., Iqbal,K., and McDermott, J.R., 1980, Aluminum-induced neurofibrillary changes: Is relationship to senile dementia of the Alzheimer's type. Neurotoxicol 1:121.

NORMAL PRESSURE HYDROCEPHALUS (NPH) AS A CAUSE OF PRE-SENILE AND SENILE DEMENTIA: THE COMPLEMENTARY ROLE OF RADIONUCLIDE CYSTERNOGRAPHY (RNC) AND CRANIAL COMPUTED TOMOGRAPHY (CCT) IN THE EARLY RECOGNITION OF THE TREATABLE PATIENTS

I. Garty, D. Steinmetz, J. Braun,
B. Dubnov, and E. Flatau

Departments of Nuclear Medicine, Family Medicine, Neurology and Internal Medicine B, Central Emek Hospital, Afula and Department of Diagnostic Radiology, *Rambam Medical Center Haifa, Israel

The possibility that hydrocephalus which is associated with normal pressure of the cerebro-spinal fluid (CSF) may be a treatable form of dementia has aroused renewed interest in radionuclide cysternography (RNC) for the dynamic study of CSF circulation. Improvement of imaging devices and the development of better radiopharmaceuticals have greatly increased the value of this study with the possibility of an accurate diagnosis of communicating hydrocephalus in general and NPH in particular. The diagnosis can be reinforced by CCT study. The latter study is also useful in excluding brain atrophy as a cause of dementia and thus direct the neurosurgeon towards the decision of shunt operation with the possibility of a dramatic improvement of the demented patient. We believe that the combination of these two studies is an important tool for diagnosing NPH, predicting success of shunt operations and following up the patients' post-surgical improvement and shunt patency. These conclusions are based on a study of 26 cases with dementia which form the basis of this report.

MATERIALS AND METHODS: Twenty-six patients with typical clinical picture of dementia underwent RNC by intrathecal administration of 99m-Tc-DTPA and serial scintigrams after 1, 4 and 24 hours. Ten of them (38.5%) who showed typical signs of NPH underwent subsequent CCT. Five patients were over 70 years of age at the time of diagnosis, the youngest patient was 55 years old and the oldest was aged 79 years. In five patients an indication for divertional shunt surgery was established.

RESULTS: All 10 patients with typical signs of NPH on RNC study were presented with mental deterioration, four of them were incontinent. Ataxia was found in 9 patients. Nine patients showed enlargement of ventricles by CCT with variable degress of brain atrophy. Only one patient showed severe brain atrophy on CCT with no signs of NPH. Of the 9 patients with signs of ventricular dilatation on CCT, only 5 had minimal to moderate brain atrophy, with indication for shunt surgery. All 5 operated patients showed marked mental improvement as well as improvement of gait disturbances and incontinence. Five other patients with marked brain atrophy were considered non-operable.

All the operated patients underwent periodical RNC. Only one patient showed post-surgical shunt obstruction. This patient was also complicated by post-surgical subdural hematoma. In summary, of 26 patients with signs of dementia, 9 patients (34.6%) were diagnosed as NPH by combined positive

Table 1. Causes of Dementia

1) Cerebral atrophy, mainly Alzheimer and Pick diseases
2) Vascular causes (multi infarcts, vasculitis, emboli, arteriosclerotic dementia)
3) Space occupying lesions (tumors, chronic subdural hematomas, abscesses)
4) Normal pressure hydrocephalus (NPH)
5) Chronic drug intoxication (medications, alcohol, bromides, arsenic)
6) Metabolic diseases (hypo or hyperthyroidism , pernicious anemia, electrolyte imbalance, Cushing disease, vitamin B12 Niacine and Thiamine deficiencies and others)
7) Infectious disease: neurosyphilis, tuberculosis, cryptococcosis and viral diseases
8) Specific neurological syndromes e.g. Huntington's chorea, multiple sclerosis, Wilson's disease, Parkinson disease and others
9) Pseudodementias especially depression

results of RNC and CCT studies. Five patients (19.2%) were considered operable and were treated by shunt operation with marked post-surgical improvement.

DISCUSSION: Dementia is a clinical syndrome composed of loss of intellectual function, especially failing memory and changes in personality and certain non intellectual behavioral abnormalities. Dementia is usually caused by chronic progressive degenerative disease of the brain, but there are many other related abnormalities, some of which are treatable and share the same clinical picture (1). The major causes of dementia are summarized in Table 1. Since some forms of dementia are treatable (e.g. neurosyphilis, cryptococcosis, chronic subdural hematoma, some brain tumors, chronic drug intoxication, vitamin deficiencies, certain metabolic and endocrine disorders, depression and NPH), a great effort should be made to recognize these forms and treat them as soon as possible, which could result in a dramatic improvement in some cases.

Radionuclide cysternography (RNC): Study of the distribution of various substances introduced into subarachroid spaces has been termed cysternography. This method was initially introduced by Bauer et al in 1953 and developed into widespread clinical use by Di-Chiro et al (2). This procedure was proved to be useful for detecting abnormalities in the pathway of cerebrospinal fluid (CSF) flow (3). CSF is produced primarily in the choroid plexus of cerebral ventricles. Other less important sources of CSF are the ventricular ependyma and the arachroid. It then flows through the third ventricle and aquaduct of sylvius into the fourth ventricle. Some of the CSF leaves the brain and enters the subarachroid space of the spinal canal. It goes down and then up around the spinal cord until it re-enters the cranial valut. On its return into the cranium, the CSF travels through the subarachroid space, filling the cysternal spaces. CSF also flows through the interhemispheric fissure on its route to the vertex, where absorption takes place in the paccionian's granulations (Fig. 1). Alteration of either of the events of movement or absorption of the radiopharmaceutical should be a sign of altered CSF production, distribution or absorption (4).

Techniques of RNC: The radiopharmaceutical is injected into the lumbar intrathecal subarachroid space. The injected material mixes with the CSF and ascends within the spinal canal to the brain. The most commonly used radiopharmaceutical is technetium-99m (99m-Tc) bound to the inorganic chelating agent diethylenetriaminepentaacetic acid (DTPA). This large non diffusable molecule remains in the CSF as long as the examination takes place. Other materials in use are Indium-111 and Yb-169 bound to the same chelating agent (3).

Serial scintigraphic images in the sequence of 1, 4 and 24 hours after injection are obtained. Imaging time is short and can be completed in 1 to 3 minutes. Typically posterior and lateral views are obtained at each of the intervals noted above (Fig. 2).

The normal RNC study: In the early part of the examination (i.e. up to 4 hours after injection) the activity is found mainly in the basal cysterns and thus is limited to the lower part of the brain. Late in the examination (24 hours after injection) most of the activity is found in the upper part of the image, with diffusion into brain tissue. If the study is normal, activity should be demonstrated in the lateral ventricles at any stage of the study (4).

Communicating hydrocephalus: Hydrocephalus is a pathological increase of the CSF volume associated with enlargement of the ventricles. The term 'communicating hydrocephalus' (CH) denotes free communication between the subarachroid space and the ventricles. CH can be diagnosed cysternographically by the appearance of the tracer in the ventricles. Usually ventricular enlargement is also demonstrated (Fig. 2). Ventricular reflux is associated with failure of the tracer to completely ascend around the cerebral convexities with delayed retention of the radiopharmaceutical in the ventricles up to 24 hours (Fig. 2).

Normal pressure hydrocephalus (NPH) and cerebral atrophy: The association of characteristic neurological symptoms, CSF pressure of less than 180mmH2O and ventricular enlargement has been termed normal pressure hydrocephalus. The syndrome was initially described by Adams et al in 1965 (5). NPH should be considered in cases showing the clinical triad of fluctuating dementia, spastic gait and urinary incontinence progressing to coma in acute conditions (6). NPH may be secondary to previous head trauma or following a history of subarachroid hemorrhage or meningitis, or may be idiopathic. Since normal pressure hydrocephalus is a treatable form of dementia, the accurate early diagnosis of this condition is mandatory. Many tests have been in the diagnostic evaluation of patients with suspected NPH. These include pneunonencephalography, contrast angiography, radionuclide cysternography, computed tomography, the CSF infusion test, continuous CSF pressure recording, electroencephalography, and measurements of regional cerebral blood flow. In general the results of these tests cannot predict with a high degree of certainty the outcome of ventricular shunting (7). The results of our study emphasize the value of combined CCT and RNC as a valuable tool for diagnosing NPH and selecting the patients with the best indication for a successful ventricular shunt operation. By cysternography, the syndrome of NPH has the general appearance of communicating hydrocephalus described above: enlarged visualized ventricles with a block to the flow of the CSF around the cerebral convexities in most cases. The ventricles are still visualized after 24 hours and more (Fig. 2). It has been postulated that the cases which respond most favorably to neurosurgical intervention have the most persistent activity in the ventricles (8). However, if severe cerebral atrophy is associated, there is no indication for shunt operation, since no improvement is expected by this procedure.

Cerebral atrophy (hydrocephalus ex vaccuo): This pathology results from loss of brain substance by a degenerative process (9). Clinically, cerebral atrophy usually presents a picture of dementia, often identical to NPH. A finding of brain atrophy with or without compensatory ventricular enlargement does not call for any surgical action. Radionuclide cysternography is considered the best non-invasive diagnostic procedure to distinguish NPH from cerebral atrophy. The most common RNC pattern in these cases is delayed tracer ascent with or without convexity block and without ventricular reflux.

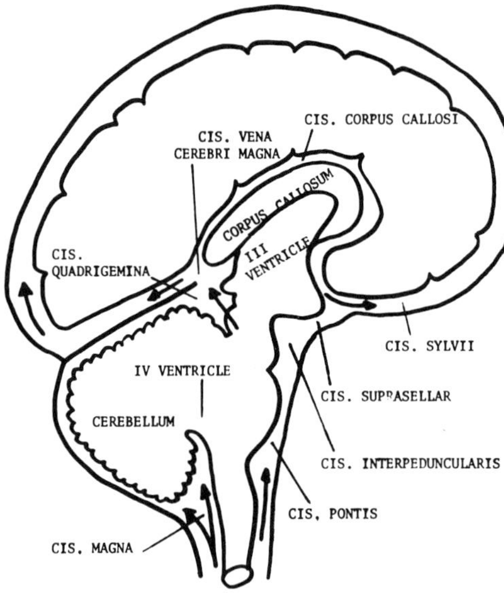

Fig. 1. Circulation of cerebrospinal fluid (see text)

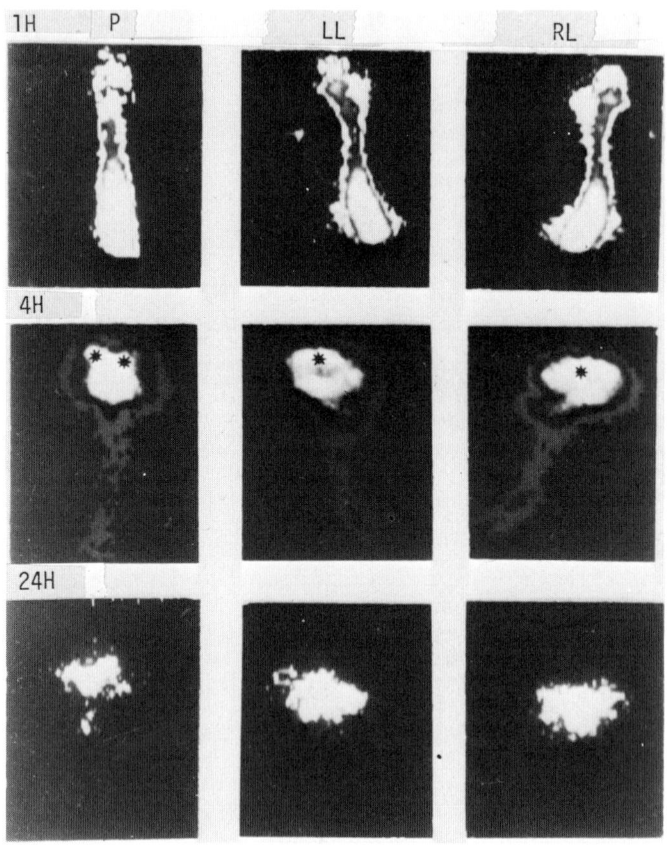

Fig. 2. Communicating hydrocephalus. Marked activity within the enlarged ventricles is demonstrated (see markers). Ventricular activity persists after 24 hours (bottom images). No activity over the convexities is evident in this stage. P-posterior view, LL-left lateral, RL-right lateral

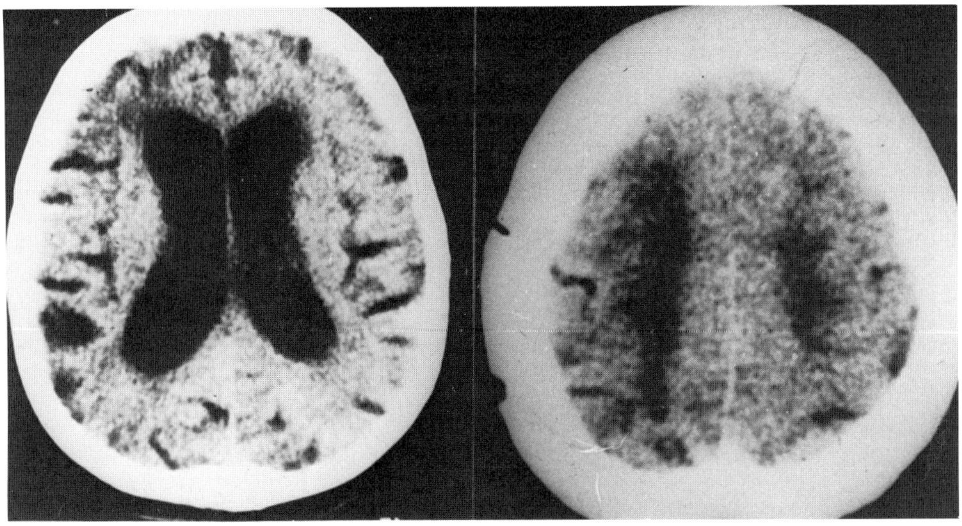

Fig.3. CCT of a patient with normal pressure hydrocephalus. Left - the lateral ventricles are markedly widened. Right - at the level of the cerebral convexity the brain sulci are relatively narrowed and decreased in number

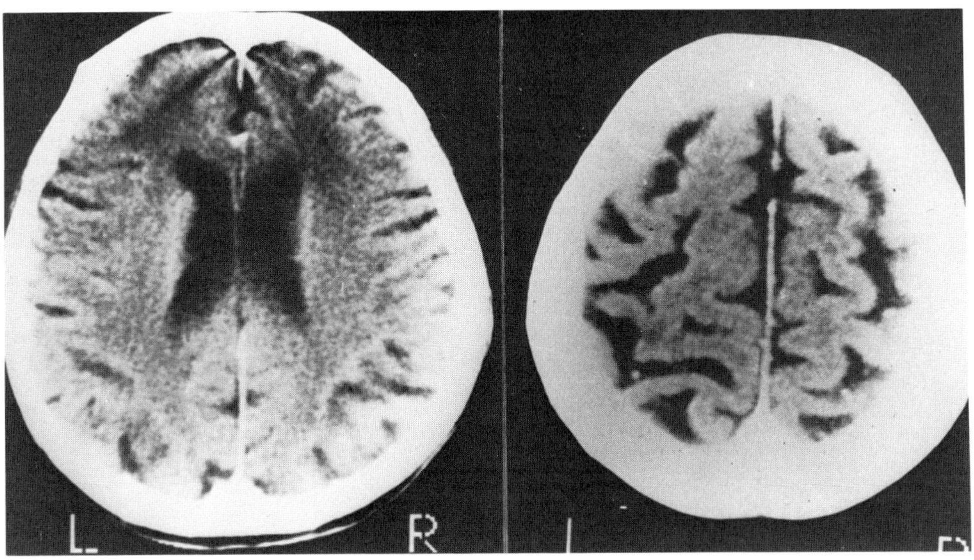

Fig.4. CCT of a patient with marked cerebral atrophy. Left - the lateral ventricles are mildly widened. Note moderate widening of the sulci. Right - at the level of the cerebral convexity there is marked widening of the brain sulci.

<u>The role of CCT in the differential diagnosis of dementia</u> : CCT is considered an accurate diagnostic method in defining CSF space, because of the relatively great density difference between CSF and brain parenchima. This is the best screening test for patients with dementia. Table 1 summarizes the principle causes of dementia. The CT is sensitive in detecting most of them. It provides information concerning the size, shape and position of the CSF space. The most characteristic CCT findings is lateral ventricular dilation, dilatation of fourth ventricles and absence of sulcal enlargement (Fig. 3). A low degree of ventricular dilatation and high

degree of sulcal prominence is a classic appearance of cerebral atrophy (Fig. 4).

The complementary role of CCT and RNC in the diagnosis of NPH: CCT provides much information about the size of the ventricles. Thus ventricular dilation can be determined by this method. However, CCT does not provide a physiological dynamic information about CSF flow, offered by the cysternogram. It is in estimating the CSF clearance capacity that cysternography is more useful. Patients with the classical clinical triad of dementia, with CCT findings of dilated ventricles and ventricular reflux and stasis on cysternography are expected to respond to CSF diversion shunt (Figs. 2,3). On the other hand, if atrophy is clearly apparent by CCT (Fig. 4), these patients are not likely to respond to shunting and will not require cysternography. However, in cases of significant ventricular dilatation without atrophy (Fig. 3) cysternography should be performed. In these cases the demonstration of ventricular reflux by RNC supplies the proof that the hydrocephalus is communicating (Fig. 2). In that way CCT and RNC are complementary for the evaluation of patients with dementia (10).

Shunt patency studies by RNC: Diversionary CSF shunt is widely employed in the treatment of hydrocephalus. Once the shunt has been place, it must be monitored periodically, since a number of complications may occur. The most frequent complication is shunt obstruction. Several methods determining shunt patency have been advised, but only the RNC has been proven to be highly accurate in the diagnosis of shunt obstruction and in localization of the probable site of obstruction. The diagnosis of patent shunt after intrathecal injection of radiopharmaceutical is made by the rapid appearance of activity within the ventricles. If the shunt is blocked the radiopharmaceutical will stream around the cerebral convexities, instead of entering the ventricles (11).

In summary: Dementia is a clinical syndrome composed of loss of intellectual function, and changes in personality. Since normal-pressure-hydrocephalus is one of the single treatable forms of dementia, the accurate diagnosis based on clinical manifestations and complementary findings from CCT and RNC is mandatory.

REFERENCES

1. R. D. Adams and M. Victor, The dementias and Korsakoff's psychosis, in: Principles of neurology, McGraw-Hill Book Company, New York, 2nd ed. p 285 (1981).
2. G. Dichiro, P. M. Reames, and W. B. Matthews, RISA-ventriculography and RISA-cysternography, Neurology 14: 185 (1964).
3. E. V. Staab, and A. Shirkhoda, Cerebro-spinal fluid scanning, Clin Nucl Med 6: 103 (1981).
4. F. H. De Land, and H. N. Wagner, Jr, Cysternography, in: Atlas of nuclear medicine, vol 1, W. B. Saunders Company, Philadelphia, London, Toronto, p 177 (1969).
5. R. D. Adams, C. M. Fisher, S. Hakim, R. G. Ojemann, W. H. Sweet, Symptomatic occult hydrocephalus with "normal" cerebro-spinal-fluid pressure: a treatable syndrome, N Engl J Med 273: 117 (1965).
6. D. F. Benson, M. LeMay, D. H. Patten, and A. B. Rubens. Diagnosis of normal-pressure hydrocephalus, N Engl J Med 283: 609 (1970).
7. D. C. McCullough, J. C. Harbert, G. Di Chiro, and A. K. Ommaya, Prognostic criteria for CSF shunting from isotope cysternography in communicating hydrocephalus, Neurology 20: 594 (1970).
8. D. L. Gilday, C. D. Maynard, K. A. McKusick, C. L. Partain, B. A. Siegel and E. V. Staab. Central nervous system, in: Kirchner P. T. (Ed). Nuclear Medicine Review Syllabus, Society of Nuclear Medicine, p 195 (1980).

9. Leading article: Cerebral atrophy or hydrocephalus? Br Med J 280: 348, (1980).
10. M. H. Gado, R. E. Coleman, K. S. Lee, M. A. Mikhael, P. O. Anderson, and C. R. Archer, Correlation between computerized transaxial tomography and radionuclide cysternography in dementia, Neurology 26: 555 (1976).
11. R. W. Hayden, T. G. Rudd, and D. B. Shurtleft, Radionuclide evaluation of suspected cerebrospinal fluid shunt malfunction: clinical correlation, J Nucl Med 20: 621 (1979).

MEASLES VIRUS INFECTION OF HUMAN NEURAL CELL LINES AS A MODEL FOR PERSISTENT VIRAL INFECTION OF THE CENTRAL NERVOUS SYSTEM *

Y.L. Danon[1], B. Rager-Zisman[3], B. Garty[1] and N. Gadoth[2]

[1]Div.of Pediatric Immunology,Dept. of Pediatrics A and [2]Neurology, Rogoff-Wellcome Medical Research Institute Beilinson Medical Center, Tel-Aviv University Medical School, Petah-Tikva, and [3]Dept. of Microbiology and Immunology ,Ben-Gurion University of the Negev,Israel

Introduction

Measles virus is a ubiquitous human pathogen member of the genus morbillivirus. Acute measles caused by the virus is commonly regarded as a childhood self limited and relatively innocuous disease. However, serious parainfectious complications of measles may occur. In about 1 in 1000 cases, acute encephalomyelitis with perivascular inflammatory and demyelinating damage, may lead to death in 10-20% of patients.[1] At least one third of the affected are left with major neurological residua, such as recurrent seizures, mental retardation, hyperkinesis and perceptual disorders.[2] In spite of the wide use of live attenuated measles virus vaccine, this exanthem is still a major public health problem.

The mechanism by which parainfectious encephalitis (PE) evolves has not yet been clearly established. However, the similarity between the neuropathology of PE and experimental allergic encephalomyelitis (EAE) implies an immune mediated disorder as a causative mechanism for PE.[3] An association between morbillivirus infection, multiple sclerosis (MS) and subacute sclerosing panencephalitis (SSPE) has been suggested and supported by a variety of epidemiological and serological data.[4] Neurotropism is common to measles, distemper and other viruses and they frequently cause inflammatory demyelination. Recently Hasse et al. [5] have obtained direct evidence for such an association. Using a measles genome cDNA probe they could detect complementary intracellular measles nucleotide sequences by <u>in-situ</u> hybridization, in sections from brains of 4 out of 10 patients with MS and in high percentage of patients with SSPE.

*Supported in part by the Shauder Foundation for Medical Research, Tel-Aviv University, Sackler School of Medicine.

The nature of viral persistence in the CNS has become crucial to the understanding of a variety of chronic demyelinating CNS disorders. In the present paper we describe a model of chronic persistent measles virus infection of human neural cells in vitro. We hope that our model may help in the study of measles virus replication and its effect on host neural cells.

Materials and Methods

Virus: The wild type Edmonston strain of measles virus[6] and previously described cold sensitive mutants of measles virus[7], were grown in Vero cells and had a titer of 10^6 plaque forming units (PFU)/ml.

Antisera: Antimeasles hyperimmune serum was prepared by immunization of rabbits with purified Edmonston measles virus grown on Vero cells. Monoclonal antibodies against measles virus hemagglutinin (HA) and nucleocapsid (NP) were prepared as previously described.[8,9] Monoclonal antibodies against measles fusion (F) and matrix (M) polypeptides were donated by Dr. E. Norrby (Karolinska University,Stockholm).[10] Anti-α-interferon serum (ENZO Co. New-York, USA) was used for interferon assay.

Cell lines: The following human neuroblastoma cell lines were used as target cells: LA-N-1,LA-N-2,LA-N-5,CHP-100,CHP-134,IMR-32,SK-N-SH, SK-N-MC. Human glioma cell lines:U-273-MG and U-254-MG[11] were also used. Cells were grown in a monolayer to a confluency in a Leibovitz L-15 medium or RPMI medium (Maagar Biologic Industries,Beth Haemek,Israel) containing 200 mmol/ml of L-Glutamine (Gibco Laboratories Grand Island, NY USA) and 15% fetal calf serum (Bio-lab Laboratories,Jerusalem,Israel).

Infection and infective titration: Cells grown in 24 well plastic dishes (Linbro Scientific Corp. Hamden, Conn USA) were inoculated with viruses at a multiplicity of infection (MOI) starting with 0.1. To titrate infectivity, we used the semiquantitative plaque assay[12] or infectious center assay.[13]

Immunochemical analysis of measles polypeptides: Persistently infected cell lines after cloning were tested by indirect immuno-fluorescence assay to visualize viral antigen expression as described before.[7] Radioimmunoprecipitation[14] served to demonstrate measles specific proteins by the heteroantisera and monoclonal antibodies described above.

Results and Discussion

All ten different human neuroblastoma and glioma cell lines: LA-N-1, LA-N-2, LA-N-5, CHP-100, CHP-134, SK-N-SH, SK-N-MC, IMR-32 and gliomas U-273-MG and U-251-MG, were infected with a wild type Edmonston measles virus at MOI of 1. After 60 min. of absorption at 33°C, cultures were incubated at 37°C.

Under normal conditions, human neuroblastoma cells grow in tissue culture to a confluency comprising a heterogenous population of cells. The majority are round small cells, while generally less than 2% of the cells are well differentiated and contain developed neurites (Fig.1). By 4-5 days after infection, cultures manifest cytopathic effects characterized by cell fusion, multinucleated giant cells, dendrite extension and cytolysis. Morphologic cell differentiation was noted as soon as 120 hours after measles virus absorption (Fig. 2).

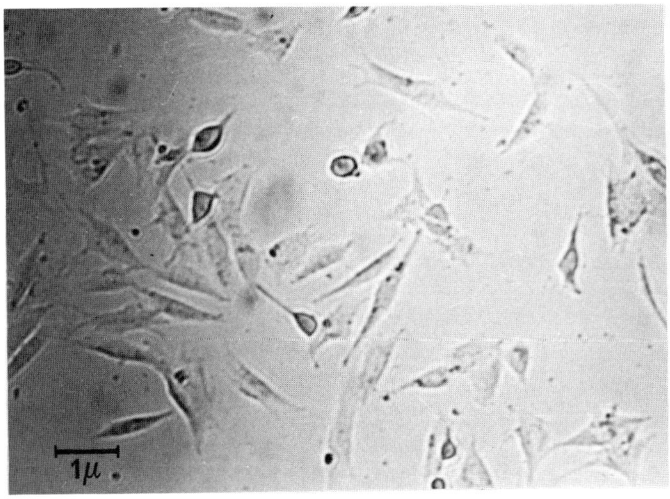

Fig. 1: Control culture of LA-N-1 human neuroblastoma cells, grown in a monolayer, in a Leibovitz, L-15 medium, containing 15% fetal calf serum and 200 mmol/ml of L-Glutamine. The cells grow in clusters and appear round, elongated and contain few processes.

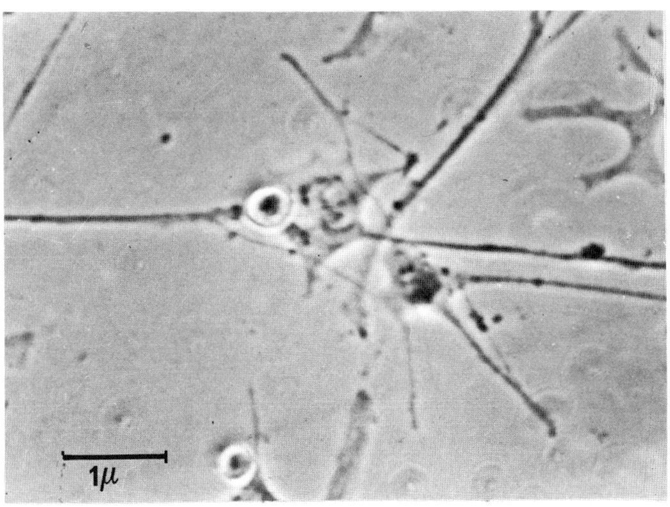

Fig. 2 : LA-N-1 human neuroblastoma cells, 3 months after infection with wild type Edmonston measles virus, and several subcultures. The cells are flattened, contain inclusion bodies and long processes .

An acute cytolytic crisis caused rapid destruction of the following human neuroblastoma and glioma cell lines: LA-N-2, CHP-100, CHP-134, SK-N-MC, IMR-32, U-273-MG and U-251-MG. In the other cell lines: LA-N-1, LA-N-5 and SK-N-SH, following the acute crisis a small number of cells survived and grew into colonies within two to three weeks.Those colonies contained well differentiated cells with significantly reduced growth rate.

During subculturing, some cycles of crisis and cytolysis were observed after trypsinization and before the cultures stabilized as a persistently infected cells. These that survived the lytic cycle and are persistently infected cell lines, now grow for more than 14 months in culture.

Use of the measles cold sensitive mutant resulted in development of chronic persistent measles infection in glioma cell line (U-273-MG) and additional two neuroblastoma cell lines CHP-134;IMR-32. The infection with the cold sensitive mutant resulted in the development of a persistently infected cell line without the lytic crisis and cytopathic effect seen with the acute Edmonston measles virus infection.

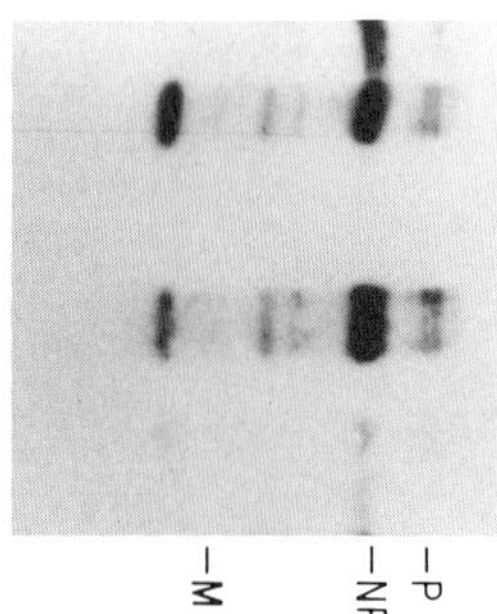

Fig.3: Immunoprecipitation and SDS-PAGE of [^{35}S] methionine labeled cells. The cells were infected with the Edmonston wild virus and labeled with [35S] methionine for 12 hrs. The lysates were subjected to immunoprecipitation with monoclonal antibodies to measles proteins. P: measles phosphoprotein; NP: nucleocapsid protein; M: matrix protein. Note positive results with LA-N-1, LA-N-5, and SK-N-SH lines. CHP-100 and U-273-MG are negative, while measles isolate and the IP-3-Ca cell line serve as positive controls. IP-3-Ca is a SSPE virus carrier cell line in which viral matrix protein is the only measles structural protein not routinely detected.[15]

Indirect immunofluorescence with polyclonal antimeasles antibodies indicated that 60-90% of the different cell lines produced detectable measles virus antigens. Immunoprecipitation using monoclonal antibodies to measles virus proteins is shown in fig. 3.

The persistently infected cell lines maintained at 37°C produced negligible amounts of interferon. These results might be related to the persistence of measles virus infection in the cell lines.

Measles virus is known to persist in the central nervous system in the form of the so-called "slow virus" disease,SSPE. In addition morbillaviruses were isolated from brains of patients with MS. There is a considerable amount of evidence to support the view that measles viruses can persist in the CNS of man and experimental animals.[4,5,16] The exact mechanisms of persistent infection, virus replication and host interaction in the CNS are not clear. From the study of measles virus persistently infected culture cells, the mechanisms of persistence of viral infection in vitro might be studied in relevance to the persistent infection in vivo including the ability to explore the possibility of developing virus mutants,[7] host restrictions on viral replication,[15,17] immunologic restriction or defective interfering particles.

In the study of Semliki forest virus (SFV) in murine model in vivo and in neuroblastoma cells in vitro, a differential tropism to CNS of various mutants was described.[18] Similar to our results, neuroblastoma cells infected with SFV mutants survived while wild virus caused cytolysis.

The advantage of our system is the possibility to explore mechanisms of persistence of measles virus infection in human neural cell lines that have been well characterized electrophysiologically, and their neurotransmitter receptors, enzymes, hormonal receptors,and karyotype have all been precisely worked out.[19,20,21] The present model enables the study of the effects of virus infection on specialized neural cell functions in vitro, and may help to clarify pathophysiologic mechanisms involved in slow virus infection of the CNS. This model might be used in the research of Alzheimer's disease (AD) as there are views suggesting that increased chromosome aneuploidy in AD might be a consequence of infection by a virus or virus-like agent.[22]

References

1. K.P. Johnson, J.S. Wolinsky and A.H. Ginsberg, Immune mediated syndromes of the nervous system related to virus infections. In: Handbook of Clinical Neurology, P.J. Vinken and G.W. Bruyn, ed, Vol. 34, Elsevier-North Holland, Amsterdam (1978).
2. J.H. Menkes, In: Textbook of child neurology. 2nd Edition. Lea and Feibiger, Philadelphia (1980).
3. H.E. Gendelman, J.S. Wolinsky, R.T. Johnson, N.J. Pressman, G.H. Pezeshkpour and G.F. Boisset, Measles encephalomyelitis: Lack of evidence of viral invasion of the central nervous system and quantitative study of the nature of demyelination. Ann. Neurol., 15: 354 (1984).
4. F.E. Payne, J.V. Baublis and H.H. Itabashi, Isolation of measles virus from cell cultures of brain from a patient with subacute sclerosing panecephalitis. New Engl. J. Med.,281: 585 (1969).
5. A.T. Haase, P. Ventura, C.J. Gibbs,Jr. and W.W. Tourtellotte, Measles virus nucleotide sequences: Detection by hybridization in-situ. Science, 212: 672 (1981).
6. V. ter Meulen and W.W. Hall, Slow virus infections of the nervous system: Virological, immunological and pathogenic considerations. J. Gen. Virol, 41:1 (1978).
7. B. Rager-Zisman, J.E. Egan, Y. Kress and B.R. Bloom, Isolation of cold sensitive mutants of measles virus from persistently infected murine neuroblastoma cells. J. Virol., In Press (1985).
8. M.J. Birrer, S. Udem, S. Nathenson and B.R. Bloom, Antigenic variants of measles virus. Nature, 293: 67 (1981).

9. M.J. Birrer, B.R. Bloom and S. Udem, Characterization of measles polypeptides by monoclonal antibodies. Virology, 108:381 (1981).
10. E. Norrby, S.N. Chen, T.Togashi, H.Shesberadaran and K.P. Johnson, Five measles virus antigens demonstrated by use of mouse hybridoma antibodies in productively infected tissue culture cells. Arch. Virol, 71:1 (1982).
11. R.C. Seeger, Y.L. Danon, P.M. Zeltzer, Y.E. Maidman and S.A. Rayner, Expression of fetal antigens by human neuroblastoma cells. Prog. Cancer Res. Therapy, 12:199 (1980).
12. B. Rager-Zisman and T.C. Merigan, A useful quantitative semimicromethod for viral pluques assay. Proc.Soc.Exp.Biol.Med., 142: 1174 (1973).
13. M. Nowakowski, J.D. Feldman, S. Kano and B.R. Bloom, The production of vesicular stomatitis virus by antigen or mitogen stimulated lymphocytes and continuous lymphoblastoid lines. J. Exp. Med., 137:1042 (1973).
14. M. Sakaguchi, Y. Yoshikawa and K. Jamshouchi, Growth of measles and subacute sclerosing panencephalitis viruses in human neural cell lines. Microbiol. Immunol., 28:461 (1984).
15. W.W. Hall, R.A. Lamp and P.W. Choppin, Measles and subacute sclerosing panencephalitis virus proteins: Lack of antibodies to the M protein in patients with subacute sclerosing panencephalitis. Proc. Natl. Acad. Sci. USA, 76: 2047 (1979).
16. R.T. Johnson, The possible viral etiology of multiple sclerosis. Adv. Neurol, 13: 1 (1975).
17. W. Hall,R. Lamp and P.W. Choppin, Measles virus proteins in the brain tissue of patients with subacute sclerosing panencephalitis:Absence of the M protein. New Engl. J. Med., 12: 690 (1981).
18. G. J. Atkins and B.J. Sheahan, Semliki forest virus neurovirulence mutants have altered cytopathogenicity for central nervous system cells. Infect. Immunity, 36: 333 (1982).
19. J.L. Biedler,R.A. Ross,S. Shanske,B. Spengler and A.E. Evans, Human neuroblastoma cytogenetics. Proc.Cancer Res.Therapy,12:81 (1980)
20. R.A. Ross,J.L. Biedler,B.A. Sprengler and D. Reis, Neurotransmitter enzymes in human neuroblastoma cell lines. Cell. Med. Neurobiol.,1: 301 (1981).
21. G.J. West, J. Uki, H.R. Herschman and R.C. Seeger, Adrenergic cholinergic and inactive human neuroblastoma cell lines with the action potential Na^+ ionophore. Cancer Res, 37: 1372 (1977).
22. L.J. Whalley, The dementia of Down's syndrome and its relevance to aetiological studies of Alzheimer's disease. In: F. Marott Sinex, C.M. Merril (Eds). Alzheimer's disease, Down syndrome, and aging. New York, Acad. Sci, New-York (1982).

BRAIN IRON AND DOPAMINE D_2 RECEPTORS IN THE RAT

Dorit Ben-Shachar and
Moussa B. H. Youdim

Rappaport Family Institute
and Department of Pharmacology
Faculty of Medicine
Technion
Haifa, Israel

INTRODUCTION

Iron deficiency (ID), the most prevalent nutritional disorder in the world (1,2), is characterized by haematological changes and stunted growth (3). In man, ID causes behavioural alterations which include pica eating, low I.Q. and reduction in attention, learning capacity and cognition, sleep disturbances and EEG changes (4-9). In rats made iron deficient the behavioural changes include significant reduction in maze learning ability, in responsiveness to environmental stimuli and learned task performance (10,11).

The biochemical changes in the rat brain following ID suggest an abnormality of the dopaminergic system. Our previous studies have shown that nutritional iron deficiency in the rat caused a significant reduction of brain non-haem iron (30%) accompanied by a 40-60% reduction in dopamine D_2 receptor (maximum number of binding sites-Bmax) in the rat caudate nucleus membrane homogenates. This correlates with reduced behavioural response to directly acting dopamine agonist, apomorphine (12,13). The effect of ID is specific for the dopamine D_2 receptors since ID has no effect on dopamine D_1 receptor (14) and other neurotransmitter receptors (α and β adrenergic, cholinergic, muscarinic, serotonergic and benzodiazepines) (13). Almost all the behavioural and biochemical effects caused by ID can be reversed in adult rats by an adequate iron supplementation. However, if ID is induced early in life it has a long term consequence which persists after peripheral iron status (serum iron, haemoglobin and other iron proteins) has been restored to normal (15). Thus new born rats (10 days) made ID never fully recover their brain non-haem iron levels, dopamine receptor sites and apomorphine induced behaviour (15,16). Dallman et al. (16) and Weinberg et al. (11) had shown that a period of early ID followed by a 3 month of iron supplementation in new born rats produced a persistent reduction of whole brain non-haem iron in adulthood. These rats were less responsive than the controls in mildly aversive novel situations, they ambulated less in exploratory tasks and had reduced learning capacity. Since iron plays an important role in many physiological processes including enzymatic activities, membrane structures, protein and lipid synthesis (3), a period of early ID in young rats may have a permanent effect on the natural postnatal development of neurons that govern the above behaviours.

The above evidence strongly suggested that iron may have a role in dopamine D_2 receptor biochemistry or function. This is reinforced by the observation that ID-like chronic neuroleptics (haloperidol, chlorpromazine and fluphenazine) treatment causes a) high significant increase in serum prolactin as well as prolactin receptor number in the liver (17,18), b) reduced behavioural responses to presynaptic (amphetamine) and postsynaptic (apomorphine) dopaminergic acting drugs (14), and c) an inhibition of amphetamine induced hypothermia, a function associated with mesolimbic dopamine system (19). Further indirect evidence for iron having a role in dopaminergic neurotransmission is its uneven distribution in the brain, showing a pattern similar to that of dopamine and neuropeptides (20,21). Furthermore Csernansky et al. (22) have shown that direct injection of $FeCl_3$ into the brain results in dopamine D_2 receptor supersensitivity as measured by behavioural response to apomorphine as well as ^{3}H-spiperone binding. In order to further understand iron dopamine D_2 receptor relationship, the effect of iron chelators and iron salts on ^{3}H-spiperone binding <u>in vitro</u> was investigated.

IN VITRO EFFECTS OF IRON SALTS AND CHELATORS ON DOPAMINE D_2 RECEPTORS

Iron-chelators, 1,10-phenanthroline, 2,4,6-tripyridyl-s-triazine (TPZ), 2,2'-bipyridyl and desferrioxamine when preincubated with caudate nucleus membrane preparations prior to the addition of the ligand, ^{3}H-spiperone, inhibited the binding of the latter (Fig. 1). The inhibitory potency of the chelators are in the range of their chelating capacity. In contrast other bivalent iron chelators such as EDTA and nitrilotriacetic acid had no effect on ^{3}H-spiperone binding to dopamine D_2 receptors. From the preliminary studies that have been carried out it is apparent that the action of iron-chelator, 1,10-phenanthroline, on dopamine D_2 receptor is rather specific. This chelator was without effect on ^{3}H-dihydroalprenolol binding to β-adrenoreceptor sites in the caudate nucleus.

The inhibition of ^{3}H-spiperone binding by 1,10-phenanthroline is non-competitive and reversible. This would suggest that although iron may be important for dopamine D_2 receptors it may not be part of the specific binding site. Iron may be involved in a more complex fashion in the regulation of dopamine D_2 receptor. This is supported by the fact that <u>in vitro</u> iron salts (Fe^{++} or Fe^{+++}) do not modify ^{3}H-spiperone binding to caudate nucleus preparations from control and iron deficient animals. Furthermore, the inhibitory actions of 1,10-phenanthroline cannot be prevented in the presence of excess iron salts. In contrast, we have reported that iron-chelator complex is even more potent in its inhibition of ^{3}H-spiperone binding than 1, 10-phenanthroline alone. It is well known that metal-chelator complexes can induce lipid peroxidiation which would result in irreversible membrane damage (23). This phenomenon may explain why iron-chelator complex action on dopamine D_2 receptor binding sites was intensified. Similar effect was also observed with Cu-phenanthroline complex.

MPTP AND DOPAMINE D_2 RECEPTOR

The Parkinson disease inducing neurotoxic compound, N-methyl-4-phenyl 1,2,5-6-tetrahydropyridine (MPTP) is thought to be metabolized by monoamine oxidase B to N-methyl-4-phenyl-1,2,pyrimidium ion (MPP^+) (24-27). Because of their chemical structural resemblance to certain iron chelating agents and the highly localized iron in striatum their effect on ^{3}H-spiperone binding was examined. While MPTP was a potent inhibitor of ^{3}H-spiperone binding to the caudate nucleus membrane preparations, MPP^+ was without action (Fig. 2). The presence of iron salts in the assay did not alter their specificity and unlike the action of 1,10-phenanthroline the MPTP effect was irreversible.

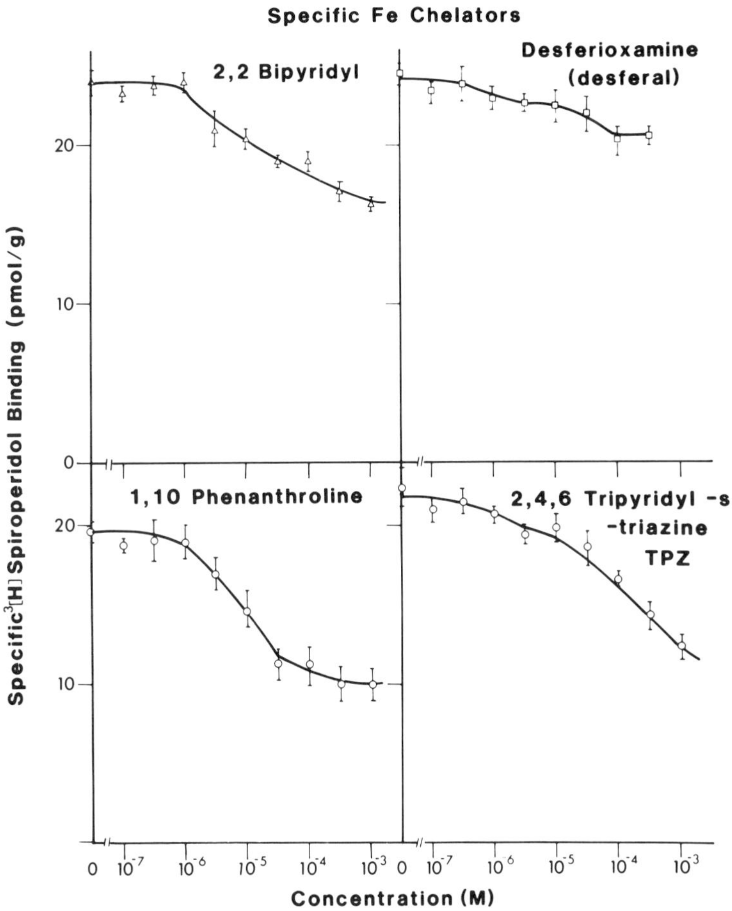

Fig. 1. Inhibition of ^{3}H-spiroperidol binding to caudate nucleus membrane homogenates by various iron chelators. Caudate nucleus membrane homogenates were incubated for 15 min in 37°C with various concentrations (10^{-7}-10^{-3}M) of iron chelators prior to addition of 1nM ^{3}H-spiroperidol. Specif ^{3}H-spiroperidol binding was determined in the presence or absence of 10μM haloperidol. Values are means ±SEM of 5 experiments.

DISCUSSION

The reversible non-competitive inhibition of ^{3}H-spiperone binding by 1,10-phenanthroline would suggest that if iron is important for the ligand binding to dopamine D_2 receptor, it may not necessarily be a part of the binding site. If it is a part of the dopamine D_2 receptor it must be involved in a more complex fashion, since simple addition of iron salts in vitro ($FeCl_2$ or $FeCl_3$) to caudate nucleus membrane homogenates from iron deficient rats did not restore the binding of ^{3}H-spiperone to normal. The fact that ^{3}H-spiperone binding is specifically reduced by iron chelators and not by other bivalent ion chelators may support the latter notion. There are other possible ways by which iron may effect the dopamine D_2 receptor function.

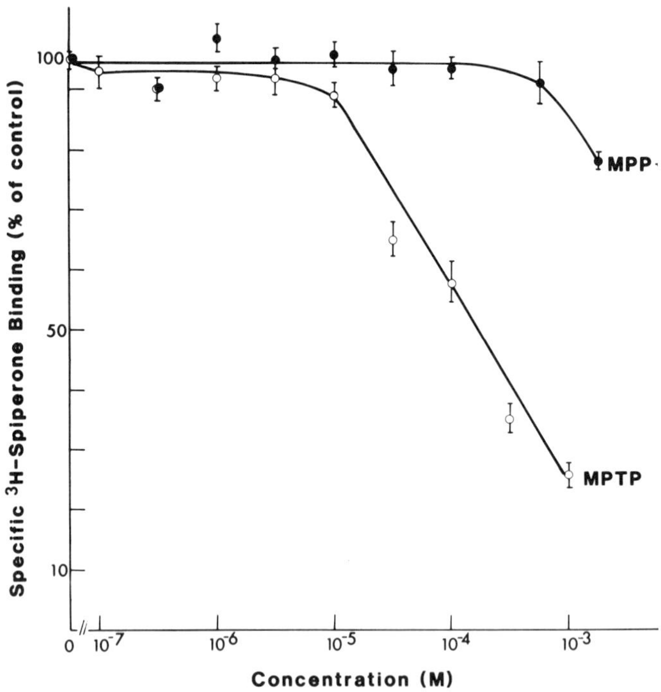

Fig. 2. Inhibition of ^{3}H-spiroperidol binding to caudate nucleus membrane homogenates by MPTP or MPP^+. Caudate nucleus membrane homogenates were incubated for 15 min in 37°C with various concentrations (10^{-7}-10^{-3}M) of MPTP or MPP^+ prior to addition of 1nM ^{3}H-spiroperidol. Specific ^{3}H-spiroperidol binding was determined in the presence or absence of 10μM haloperidol. Values are expressed as percentage of control and are means ±SEM of 3 experiments.

Iron is known to be an important constituent of the membrane components. It may thus confer a special conformation to the DA D_2 receptor which when removed as is the case in iron deficiency would result in altered receptor function. However, membrane fluidity of the caudate nucleus membrane preparation was not changed as a result of iron deficiency. The third suggestion is that iron may be important for the enzyme responsible for the synthesis of the dopamine D_2 receptor, and may actually be incorporated into it. The latter suggestion is in part supported by the <u>in vivo</u> effects of ID and the recovery process which are time and age dependent.

It is apparent that the effect of early iron deficiency on the biochemical and behavioural changes in rats are irreversible even after long term treatment with iron supplementation (15). Thus, the long term consequence of early iron deficiency leading to minimal brain damage in children with this common nutritional disorder should be examined more seriously. Recent studies (28) have shown that certain children with iron deficiency anaemia do not respond to iron therapy even after 4 years of treatment. The similarity in the uneven distribution of brain iron, dopaminergic neurons and neuropeptides on the one hand and the fact that iron can modify dopaminergic

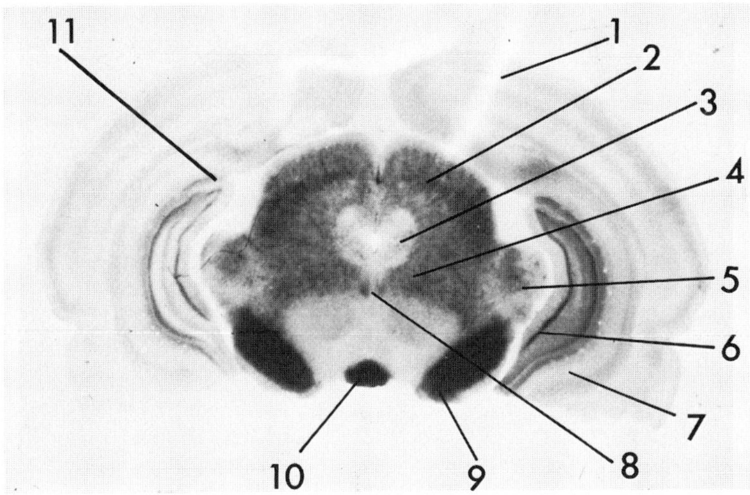

Fig. 3. Distribution of iron in the rat brain at the level of substantia nigra. The dark-stained areas represent iron-deposits as identified by Perls' DAB histochemical method (20).
1. Cortex; 2. superior colliculus; 3. central gray; 4. reticular formation; 5. medial geniculate nucleus; 6. Ammon's horn; 7. hippocampus; 8. oculmotor nucleus; 9. substantia nigra; 10. interpenduncular nucleus; 11. dentate gyrus.

neurotransmission on the other suggests a much more important physiological role for iron than hitherto considered.

Although decreased brain iron-metabolism can affect dopaminergic neurotransmission, both biochemically and behaviourally, the role of this metal should also be considered in Parkinson's disease and Alzheimer's disease. Such a proposal is not far fetched since extraordinary high concentration of iron deposits are present in the substantia nigra, caudate nucleus, globus pallidus and hippocampus-dentate gyrus (Fig. 3) (29), the regions specifically affected in these age related disorders. It is well known that in the brain iron has a very slow rate of turnover (29). Haeme and nonhaeme iron together with the ferritin comprise only a small fraction of the total iron present in brain tissue. The greater fraction of brain iron occurs in as yet unidentified or functional form. Neurotoxins have been suspected in the pathogenesis of Parkinson's and Alzheimer's disease. One such neurotoxin N-methyl-4-phenyl-1,2,5,6-tetrahydropyridine (MPTP) is known to cause Parkinsonism in human subjects and animals (24,26,27,30,31) and inactivates dopamine D_2 receptor in vitro (Fig. 2). This compound is a substrate for monoamine oxidase type B and is oxidized to N-methyl-4-phenyl 1,2-dipyrimidium ion (MPP^+) with the generation of H_2O_2 (31). Transition metals e.g. iron, are involved in the formation and reactivity of oxygen radicals. Such radicals are known to be formed from H_2O_2 and can caused deleterious effects on many systems (23,32,33). Homolytic fission of the O-O and in H_2O_2 produces hydroxyl radicals, $^{\cdot}OH$. A simple mixture of H_2O_2 and iron (II) salts also forms the $^{\cdot}OH$ radicals (Fenton reaction). Therefore, a whole series of radical reactions can be provoked by iron which catalyses the decomposition of H_2O_2 leading to increased lipid peroxidation reactions (32,33).

In view of the damaging effects of oxygen radicals and the presence of high iron concentrations in substantia nigra and hippocampus-dentate gyrus and Ammon's horn cones, the study of brain iron and metabolism in the above diseases should be investigated. Thus Hallervorden-Spatz disease is associated with excessive accumulation of iron pigments resulting in demelinization and neuronal loss in the iron rich globus pallidum (34-37). In general such patients suffer from dementia (37) as well as severe dystonia and hypokinetic rigid motor disturbances. Whether similar changes in transition or other metal metabolism occurs in Alzheimer's disease remains unanswered.

REFERENCES

1. L. Garby, Iron deficiency: definition and prevalence, in: "Clinics in Haematology," S. T. Collender, ed., W. B. Saunders, London (1973).
2. Nutrition Canada, Nutrition Canada National Survey, Canadian Department of National Health and Welfare, Publ. No. H-58-36 (1973).
3. A. Jacobs and M. Worwood, eds., in: "Iron in Biochemistry and Medicine," Academic Press, London (1974).
4. R. L. Leibel, D. B. Greenfield and E. Pollitt, Iron deficiency: behaviour and brain biochemistry, in: "Iron Deficiency Brain Biochemistry and Behaviour," E. Pollitt and R. L. Leibel, eds. Raven Press, New York (1982).
5. P. R. Dallman, E. Beutler and C. A. Finch, Effect of iron deficiency exclusive of anaemia, Br. J. Haematol., 40:179 (1978).
6. E. Pollitt and R. L. Leibel, Iron deficiency and behaviour, J. Pediatr., 88:372 (1976).
7. F. A. Oski and A. M. Honig, The effect of therapy on the developmental scores of iron deficient infants, J. Pediatr., 92:21 (1977).
8. T. E. Webb and F. A. Oski, Iron deficiency anemia and scholastic achievement, behavioural stability and perceptual sensitivity of adolescents, J. Pediatr., 82:827 (1973a).
9. D. M. Tucker, H. H. Sandstead, J. G. Penland, S. L. Dawson and D. B. Milne, Iron status and brain function: serum ferritin levels associated with asymmetries of cortical electrophysiology and cognitive performance, Am. J. Clin. Nutr., 39:105 (1984).
10. J. Weinberg, S. Levine and P. R. Dallman, Long term consequences of early iron deficiency in the rat, Pharmacol. Biochem. and Behaviour, 11:631 (1979).
11. J. Weinberg, P. R. Dallman and S. Levine, Iron deficiency during early development in the rat. Behavioural and physiological consequences, Pharmacol. Biochem. and Behaviour, 12:493 (1980).
12. R. Ashkenazi, D. Ben-Shachar and M. B. H. Youdim, Nutritonal iron and dopamine binding sites in the rat brain, Pharmacol. Biochem. and Behaviour 17 (Suppl. 1) 43 (1982).
13. M. B. H. Youdim, D. Ben-Shachar, R. Ashkenazi and S. Yehuda, Brain iron and dopamine receptor function, in: "CNS Receptors - From Molecular Pharmacol to Behaviour," P. Mandel and F. V. De Feudis, eds., Raven Press, New York (1983).
14. M. B. H. Youdim and A. R. Green, Biogenic monoamine metabolism and functional activity in iron deficient rats: behavioural correlates, in: "Iron Metabolism," Ciba Symposium No. 51, Elsevier, Amsterdam (1977).
15. M. B. H. Youdim and D. Ben-Shachar, Brain iron and dopamine receptors function, Fed. Proc., 43:4973 (1984).
16. P. R. Dallman, M. A. Siimes and E. C. Manies, Brain iron persistent deficiency following short-term iron deprivation in the young rat, Br. J. Haematol., 31:209 (1975).
17. T. Amit, R. J. Barkey, D. Ben-Shachar and M. B. H. Youdim, Characterization of hepatic prolactin receptors induced by chronic iron deficiency and neuroleptics, Eur. J. Pharmacol., (1985) submitted.

18. R. J. Barkey, D. Ben-Shachar, T. Amit and M. B.H. Youdim, Increased hepatic and reduced prostatic prolactin binding in iron deficiency and neuroleptic treatment: correlation with changes in serum prolactin and testosterone, Eur. J. Pharmacol., 109:193 (1985).
19. M. B. H. Youdim, S. Yehuda and A. Ben-Uriah, Iron-deficiency induced circadian rhythm reversal of dopaminergic-mediated behaviours and thermoregulation in rats, Eur. J. Pharmacol., 74:295 (1981).
20. J. M. Hill and R. C. Switzer, The regional distribution and cellular localization of iron in the rat brain, Neurosci. 11:595 (1984).
21. M. Quick and L. L. Iversen, Regional study of ^{3}H-spiroperidol binding and DA-sensitive adnylate cyclase in the rat brain, Eur. J. Pharmacol., 56:323 (1979).
22. J. C. Csernansky, C. A. Holman, K. A. Bonnet, K. Grabowsky, R. King and L. E. Hollister, Dopaminergic supersensitivity at distant sites following induced epileptic foci, Life Sci., 32:385 (1983).
23. J. M. C. Gutteridge and B. Halliwell, The role of superoxide and hydroxyl radicals in the degradation of DNA and deoxyribose induced by copper phenanthroline complex, Biochem. Pharmacol., 31:2801 (1982).
24. S. P. Markey, J. N. Johannessen, C. C. Chiueh, R. S. Burns and M. A. Herkenham, Intraneuronal generation of a pyridinium metabolite may cause drug induced Parkinsonism, Nature, 311:464 (1984).
25. O. Hornykiewicz, Dopamine in the basal ganglia: its role and therapeutic implications, Brit. Med. Bull., 29:172 (1973).
26. R. E. Heikkila, L. Manzino, F. S. Cabbat and R. C. Duvoisin, Protection against the dopaminergic neurotoxicity of 1-methyl 1-4-phenyl-1,2,5,6-tetrahydropyridine by monoamine oxidase inhibitors, Nature, 311:467 (1984).
27. M. B. H. Youdim, Oxidation of N-methyl-4-phenyl 1,2,5,6-tetrahydropyridine (MPTP) by rat brain coupled to tetrazolium nitro blue. Eur. J. Pharmacol. (1985) in press.
28. R. J. Cantwell, The long term neurological sequelae of anemia in infancy, Pediatr. Res., 8:342 (1974).
29. M. B. H. Youdim, Brain iron metabolism: biochemical and behavioural aspects in relation to dopaminergic neurotransmission, in: "Handbook of Neurochemistry,"Vol. 10, New Series, A. Lajath, ed. Plenum Press, New York (1985).
30. See Kopin et al. this volume.
31. See Youdim et al. this volume.
32. B. Halliwell and J. M. Gutteridge, Oxygen toxicity, oxygen radicals, transition metals and disease, Biochem. J., 219:1 (1984).
33. T. F. Slater, Free radical mechanisms in tissue injury, Biochem. J., 222:1 (1985).
34. J. Hallervorden and H. Spatz, Eigenartige Erkrankung im extrapyramidalen system mit besonderer beliligung des globus pallidus den substantia nigra, Z. Neurol. Psychiat., 79:254 (1922).
35. J. Szanto and F. Gallyas,A study of iron metabolism in neuropsychiatric patients. Hallervorden-Spatz disease, Arch. Neurol., 14:438 (1966).
36. J. M. Wigboldus and G. W. Bruyn, Hallervorden-Spatz disease, in:"Handbook of Clinical Neurology", P. J. Vinken and G. W. Bruyn, eds., North Holland, Amsterdam (1969).
37. C. Kessler, K. Schwechheimer, R. Reuther and J. A. Born, Hallervorden-Spatz syndrome restricted to the pallidal nuclei, J. Neurol., 231:112 (1984).

DOWN'S SYNDROME AND ALZHEIMER'S DISEASE: ARE COMMON GENES FROM HUMAN CHROMOSOME 21 INVOLVED IN BOTH DISORDERS?

Y.Groner, N.Dafni, L.Sherman, D.Levanon, Y.Bernstein, E.Danciger, O.Elroy-Stein and A.Neer

Department of Virology, The Weizmann Institute of Science
Rehovot, Israel 76100

INTRODUCTION

Why do most victims of Down's syndrome (D.S.) develop Alzheimer's dementia (A.D.) in middle age? The intriguing links between D.S, an inborn chromosomal disorder, and A.D, a condition that develops late in life in individuals with no obvious genetic abnormality were recognized many years ago. Nevertheless, the actual metabolic faults underlying both these conditions are still unknown (1-3).

Down's syndrome, by far the most common genetic abnormality, results from the presence of an extra chromosome 21, a condition technically known as trisomy 21 (4). It is characterized by severe mental retardation, as well as a wide variety of physiological defects including reduced viability, abnormalities of morphogenesis, increased incidence of leukemia, high susceptibility to infections and some signs of premature aging (5-7). In addition, clinical and pathological studies of adult patients with D.S. reveal that many of these individuals develop a progressive dementia and a variety of neurological abnormalities closely resembling the clinical picture of A.D. Thus an association has been suggested between the two conditions (8-14), i.e., genes on chromosome 21 might play a role in the development of Alzheimer's disease (15-17).

The causative factor for the trisomy is generally considered to be ovarian nondisjunction, at meiosis; the more recent studies have indicated that a nondisjunction of paternal origin occurring at the first or second meiotic division probably accounts for approximately 20% of D.S. (18). In most cases, patients with Down's syndrome have a karyotype with 47 chromosomes (46 plus one additional 21). However, cases of D.S. have been identified in which only a portion of chromosome 21 is present in triplicate, usually translocated to another chromosome. This finding has permitted the localization of the region "responsible" for the syndrome on segment 21q22 - the distal portion of the long-arm of chromosome 21 (19-27).

Although the relationship of trisomy 21 to Down's syndrome has been known for 25 years (4), there is no effective treatment and very little is known about the way in which the additional chromosomal segment (21q22) causes the disease or whether it is connected to Alzheimer's dementia (1,2,7). Similarly, the biochemical basis of presenile dementia itself is unknown, although epidemiological studies show that A.D. can be familial and apparently hereditary (28), another indication of a genetic cause. In D.S. it is assumed that the extra 21q22 segment codes for normal products and that the abnormalities found in the syndrome are produced by a gene dosage effect. That is, overproduction of certain proteins encoded by 21q22 distorts the delicate balance of biochemical pathways which are important for the proper development and function of the organs affected in the syndrome (2,7). The validity of this assumption is emphasized by recent findings that certain oncogenes are, in fact, normal cellular genes that contribute to the malignant transformation of cells by the irregularity of their expression, involving either overproduction of their gene products or mistiming of expression during cell cycle and development (29).

Seven genes have been assigned, so far, to human chromosome 21; ribosomal RNA (rRNA) (30,31); interferon receptor (IRFC)(32); Cu/Zn-superoxide dismutase (SOD-1)(32);glycineamide phosphoribonucleotide synthetase (GARS) (33,34); aminoimidazol ribonucleotide synthetase (AIRS)(34); liver-type phosphofructokinase (PFKL)(35), and more recently, the gene coding for cystathionine β-synthase (CBS)(36). Of these, IFRC, SOD-1, PFKL and GARS have been localized to 21q22, the chromosomal region involved in D.S.(37-43). The four genes residing at the 21q22 segment show various levels of increased activity in trisomy 21 cells; erythrocytes, white blood cells and cultured fibroblasts of D.S. patients exhibited an increase of about 50% in SOD-1 activity due to higher levels of SOD-1 protein (44-54). Similar observations have been made for GARS (55,56) and PFKL (35,57). As for IFRC, trisomy 21 cells were three to seven times more sensitive to the effects of exogenous interferon than normal cells (58). Although, at present, there is no satisfactory explanation for this amplification of a 1.5-fold gene dosage effect into a 3-7 fold protective effect, it should be kept in mind that the functional consequences may not necessarily be directly proportional to the gene dosage.

While various other genes residing in 21q22 are undoubtedly involved in the etiology of the Down's phenotype, two of the genes from this region (SOD-1 and PFK-L) may be implicated in the reported neuropathological changes and/or electrophysiological abnormalities of trisomy 21 nerve cells (59). Cu/Zn-superoxide dismutase (SOD-1) catalyses the dismutation of free O_2^- radicals to yield hydrogen peroxide and oxygen: $O_2^- + O_2^- + 2H^+ \rightarrow O_2 + H_2O_2$. Gene dosage response of SOD-1 in trisomy 21 has been shown in blood cells and cultured fibroblasts (44-54). It has been suggested that the increase of SOD-1 activity in trisomy 21 could lead to an increased production of H_2O_2. The accumulation of peroxides in the cell might exert effects by oxidizing sulphydryl groups and by peroxidation of polyunsaturated fatty acids (60,61). In Down's syndrome, erythrocytes, catalase levels are normal (62), but gluthathionine peroxidase (GSHPx) activity is significantly increased (63-65). This is believed to be an adaptive response to the elevated levels of hydrogen peroxides produced by the augmented SOD-1 activity, rather than a gene dosage effect, since the gene coding for GSHPx is located on human chromosome No. 3 (66). However, as was reported by Brooksbank and Balazs (67) this adaptive mechanism does not function in the brain of D.S. fetuses and GSHPx activity is not elevated along with that of SOD-1. Brain cells may be in general more susceptible than other cells to alterations in the steady-state levels of superoxides (O_2^-) and hydrogen peroxides (H_2O_2). The increased activity of SOD-1 in D.S. brains, where it is not compensated for by an increase in GSHPx, will therefore result in elevated levels of H_2O_2 and other active oxygen species ($^1O_2$ and HO·), which can react directly with polyunsaturated fatty acids to form hydroperoxides (68). Also, the arachidonic acid cascade, leading to the biosynthesis of prostaglandins, and involving cooxidation of unsaturated fatty acids, is modulated by the intracellular oxidative environment (69). Therefore, the higher SOD-1 activity may explain the reported increase in lipoperoxidation by cerebral homogenates of D.S. fetuses (67) and the decrease in unsaturated fatty acids content in D.S. brains (70). Alterations in lipid peroxidation may be the basis of the reported abnormalities in membrane functions, i.e. a decrease in Na^+/K^+ ATPase and serotonin uptake in D.S. platelets (71), as well as abnormal electric membrane properties of D.S. neurons in cell culture (72).

Phosphofructokinase (PFK), the key regulatory enzyme of glycolysis, catalyzes the phosphorylation of fructose-6-phosphate to fructose 1,6 diphosphate. The human enzyme is a tetrameric protein with a M.W. of approximately 340,000. Vora et al., (73-76) have established the existence of a trigenic isozyme system for human PFK. Three structural loci, PFK-M (muscle), PFK-P (platelet), and PFK-L (liver) on chromosomes 1, 10 and 21, respectively encode the distinct PFK subunits. The gene coding the L subunit was assigned to chromosome 21 and has subsequently been mapped to the 21q22 region (42). A tissue may express, one, two or all three genes, and the various subunits randomly form tetramers whose catalytic activity is influenced by their composition. Accordingly, the isozymes proportion in different organs reflects the relative activity of glycolysis versus gluconeogenesis; the M-type subunit predominates in organs like skeletal muscle, heart and brain whose energy metabolism depends mainly on glycolysis, whereas, the L-type predominates in organs with active gluconeogenesis, i.e. liver and kidney (for rev. see 77,78). In the brain of developing embryos all three subunits are expressed at almost the same level. At mid gestation, the relative amount of the L-subunit declines, so that near-term brain contains mainly M and P subunits and only minor amounts of the L-subunit (79). In erythrocytes of Down's syndrome patients PFK activity is elevated due to gene dosage effect. Analysis of the subunit composition revealed that in contrast to normal red blood cells which contain approximately 10% L_4-type isozyme, PFK from trisomy 21 cells showed a striking increase in L-type isozyme and an absence of M_4 (80). If similar alterations in PFK isozyme composition occur in D.S. brain the rate of glycolysis may be decreased and the rate of gluconeogenesis increased. An opposite isozyme shift was reported in cancerous cells, where there is an extra demand for glycolysis; the relative expression of the P-subunit increased, followed in some cases by an increase in the M-subunit (77). Since brain metabolism is heavily dependent upon glucose utilization, alteration in the glycolysis/gluconeogenesis ratio may be associated with the neuropathological changes observed in D.S. and constitute the basic underlying cause of the mental retardation. In the context of a common "responsible" gene for the D.S. and the A.D. phenotypes, it is intriguing that a 90% reduction in the activity of PFK was observed in brains of individuals who died from A.D. (81). More recently, abnormalities of PFK in cultured fibroblasts from patients with A.D., as well as in trisomy 21 fibroblasts, were also reported (16).

With recent advances in the techniques and applications of recombinant DNA research it has become feasible to approach the molecular biology of the chromosomal region responsible for D.S. in an attempt to isolate and identify the gene or genes involved in the pathology associated with the syndrome. A gene involved in D.S. should fulfill the following criteria (a) reside at the 21q22 segment, (b) be over-expressed in all or certain tissues of D.S. fetuses, and (c) show a connection between its overproduction or mistiming of expression and clinical symptoms of D.S.

As a part of our long-term research effort to elucidate, at the molecular level, how an excess of the 21q22 chromosomal region results in abnormality of morphogenesis and mental function, we have studied the gene coding for SOD-1. A cDNA clone was constructed and the active SOD-1 gene residing at the 21q22 region was isolated (82,83). The molecular structure of the gene was analyzed and polymorphic markers (RFLPs) within the gene were identified. More than 100 Kb of chromosomal DNA from the vicinity of the gene were isolated and characterized (84,85). To determine the dosage effect, the expression of the SOD-1 gene was examined in trisomy 21 cells and in the organs of aborted D.S. fetuses. Normal cells containing extra copies of the SOD-1 gene and thus expressing higher levels of SOD-1 protein were constructed by gene transfer experiments. The effects exerted on cellular metabolism by the elevated levels of SOD-1 in these cells were studied, and correlated with the clinical symptoms of D.S. (86).

RESULTS

Construction of a cDNA Clone for Human Cu/Zn Superoxide Dismutase (SOD-1)

Poly(A)-containing RNA enriched for human Cu/Zn superoxide dismutase (SOD-1) mRNA was isolated, used to synthesize double-stranded cDNA, which was inserted into the endonuclease PstI site of the plasmid pBR322. The chimeric molecules were used to transform *Escherichia coli*. Two clones containing SOD-1 cDNA inserts were identified by their ability to hybridize with SOD-1 mRNA. Each of these clones carried a 650 base-pair insert, as was determined by restriction enzyme digestion and electron microscopic heteroduplex analysis. One clone, designated pS61-10, was sequenced (Fig.1). It contained 459 nucleotides representing the entire coding region and 95 nucleotides of the 3' untranslated region. The AAUAAA hexanucleotide found approximately 20 nucleotides upstream from the 3' poly(A)-tract in eukaryotic cellular mRNAs is absent, being replaced by AUUAAA. The predicted amino acids represented by the pS61-10 insert agree with the published amino acid sequence of human SOD-1 with few exceptions. Once the plasmid containing the SOD-1 cDNA insert was identified, it was used as a probe on genomic DNA blots and on RNA blots to obtain information about the SOD-1 gene and the SOD-1 mRNA. The results showed that the probe reacted with several genes in human cells and with two species of poly(A)-containing RNAs.

```
    1   2   3   4   5   6   7   8   9   10  11  12  13  14  15  16  17  18  19  20  21  22  23  24  25  26
    ALA THR LYS ALA VAL CYS VAL LEU LYS GLY ASP GLY PRO VAL GLN GLY ILE ILE ASN PHE GLU GLN LYS GLU SER ASN
G32 ATG,GCG,ACG,AAG,GCC,GTG,TGC,GTG,CTG,AAG,GGC,GAC,GGC,[illegible]A,GTG,CAG,GGC,ATC,ATC,AAT,TTC,GAG,CAG,AAG,GAA,AGT,AAT,
          40        50             60              70           80              90         100        110

27  28  29  30  31  32  33  34  35  36  37  38  39  40  41  42  43  44  45  46  47  48  49  50  51  52  53
GLY PRO VAL LYS VAL TRP GLY SER ILE LYS GLY LEU THR GLU GLY LEU HIS GLY PHE HIS VAL HIS GLU PHE GLY ASP ASN
GGA,CCA,GTG,AAG,GTG,TGG,GGA,AGC,ATT,AAA,GGA,CTG,ACT,[illegible]AA,GGC,CTG,CAT,GGA,TTC,CAT,GTT,CAT,GAG,TTT,GGA,GAT,AAT,
      120        130        140                150           160        170              180        190

54  55  56  57  58  59  60  61  62  63  64  65  66  67  68  69  70  71  72  73  74  75  76  77  78  79  80
THR ALA GLY CYS THR SER ALA GLY PRO [illegible]S PHE ASN P[illegible] [illegible]U SER ARG LYS HIS GLY GLY PRO LYS ASP GLU GLU ARG HIS
ACG,GCA,GGC,TGT,ACC,AGT,GCA,GGT,CCT,CAC,TTT,AA[illegible],CCT,[illegible]A,TCC,AGA,AAA,CAC,GGT,GGG,CCA,AAG,GAT,GAA,GAG,AGG,CAT,
    200            210        220        230            240        250        260              270

81  82  83  84  85  86  87  88  89  90  91  92  93  94  95  96  97  98  99  100 101 102 103 104 105 106 107
VAL GLY ASP LEU GLY ASN VAL THR ALA ASP LYS ASP GLY VAL ALA ASP VAL SER ILE GLU ASP SER VAL ILE SER LEU SER
GTT,GGA,GAC,TTG,GGC,AAT,GTG,ACT,GCT,GAC,AAA,GAT,GGT,GTG,GCC,GAT,GTG,TCT,ATT,GAA,GAT,TCT,GTG,ATC,TCA,CTC,TCA,
    280        290             300        310        320               330        340              350

108 109 110 111 112 113 114 115 116 117 118 119 120 121 122 123 124 125 126 127 128 129 130 131 132 133 134
GLY ASP HIS CYS ILE ILE GLY ARG THR LEU VAL VAL HIS GLU LYS ALA ASP ASP LEU GLY LYS GLY GLY ASN GLU GLU SER
GGA,GAC,CAT,TGC,ATC,ATT,GGC,CGC,ACA,CTG,GTG,GTC,CAT,GAA,AAA,GCA,GAT,GAC,TTG,GGC,AAA,GGT,GGA,AAT,GAA,GAA,AGT,
  360       370           380              390       400          410          420         430

135 136 137 138 139 140 141 142 143 144 145 146 147 148 149 150 151 152 153
THR LYS THR GLY ASN ALA GLY SER ARG LEU ALA CYS GLY VAL ILE GLY ILE A[illegible]A GL[illegible] STOP
ACA,AAG,ACA,GGA,AAC,GCT,GGA,AGT,CGT,TTG,GCT,TGT,GGT,GTA,ATT,GGG,ATC,GCC,C[illegible], TAAACATTCCCTTGGATGTAGTCTGAGG
440        450        460        470            480          490          500        510        520

CCCCTTAACTCATCTGTTATCCTGCTAGCTGTAGAAATGTATC[illegible]GATAAACATTAAACACTGTAATCTTAA[illegible]AAAAAAC17
     530        540        550        560        570        580        590        600
```

Fig. 1. DNA sequence of SOD-1 cDNA clone (83).

The Cu/Zn-SOD mRNAs

Two SOD-1 mRNAs of 0.7 and 0.9 kilobases (Kb) were found in a variety of human cells (Fig. 2). These two species were also present in monkey cells, whereas mouse cells contained only a 0.7 Kb RNA. In the mouse/human hybrid line WAV4dF9-4a that contains chromosome 21 as the only human chromosome, the two human SOD-1 RNAs were detected indicating that both are encoded by this chromosome. These RNAs were found in poly(A)-containing polysomal RNA and were translated *in vitro* to immunoprecipitable SOD-1 polypeptides, indicating that they are functional mRNAs. The SOD-1 mRNA

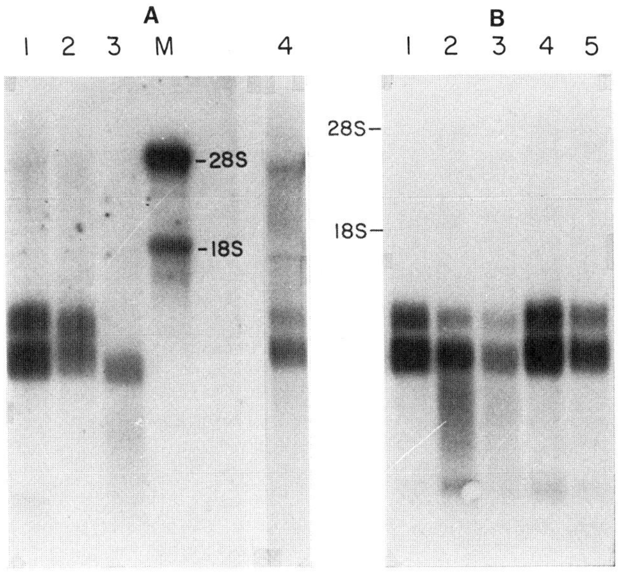

Fig. 2. Detection of SOD-1 mRNAs.
(A) RNA extracted from the following sources: lane 1 - SV80 human cells; lane 2 - COS monkey cells; lane 3 - A9 mouse cells; lane 4 - poly(A)-containing nuclear RNA.
(B) RNA extracted from various human cell lines: lane 1 - GM-137; lane 2 - HL60; lane 3 - U937; lane 4 - SV80; lane 5 - FS-11. Analyses were carried out as described previously (84).

content was quantitated by the dot-blot hybridization procedure. The single-stranded DNA insert of pS61-10 subcloned in bacteriophage M13 was used as a reference. Quantitative analysis by this technique showed that both normal fibroblasts (FS-11) and transformed cells (SV-80) contain between 0.002 and 0.006% SOD-1 mRNA. Because the proportion of mRNA varied between different poly(A)-containing RNA preparations, it was essential to use an internal standard for comparison. RNA samples were hybridized to both SOD-1 cDNA (pS61-10) and to HLA-B cDNA. The highest amount of SOD-1 mRNA was found in cells from a Down's syndrome patient (K193), which contained 1.6-3 times more SOD-1 RNA than normal fibroblasts (FS-11) or SV-80 transformed cells. This increase is probably related to the presence of three copies of chromosome 21 in K193 cells; accordingly, GM-137 cells, which are monosomic for chromosome 21, contained the least amount of SOD-1 mRNA (70% of FS-11), indicating a gene dosage response of SOD-1 transcription.

Isolation of the SOD-1 gene (see below) revealed that the two SOD-1 mRNAs are transcribed from the same gene. The major 0.7 Kb species is approximately four times more abundant than the minor 0.9 Kb mRNA. These two mRNAs differ in the length of their 3'-untranslated region and both have 5' multiple ends. The longer transcript contains 222 additional nucleotides beyond the 3'-polyadenylated terminus of the short mRNA. S_1 nuclease mapping and sequence analysis showed that these extra 222 nucleotides are specified by sequences contiguous to those shared by the two SOD-1 mRNAs. The 5'-termini of the two SOD-1 mRNAs were identified and mapped by both primer extension and S_1 mapping. The majority of SOD-1 molecules (90-95%) have a 5'-start site located 23 base pairs (b.p) downstream of the hexanucleotide -TATAAA- (see Fig. 3). The rest of the SOD-1 mRNA molecules have 5'-termini 30, 50 and 65 b.p. upstream from the major start region.

Several lines of evidence support the conclusion that the two SOD-1 mRNAs are transcribed from a unique gene. First, hybridization experiments with defined restriction fragments of SOD-1 cDNA clone showed that both mRNAs contain sequences of the entire coding region plus the 95 nucleotides representing the 3'-untranslated region of the small SOD-1 mRNA. Second, primer extension and S_1 mapping experiments with genomic DNA probes from the 5' and 3'-ends of the SOD-1 gene indicated that the DNA sequences encoding the large transcripts are contiguous to those shared by the two mRNA species. Thirdly, only one region of human DNA with nucleotide sequences identical to the SOD-1 cDNA was detected (see below).

Anatomy of the Chromosomal Locus Encoding the Cu/Zn SOD

The SOD-1 gene locus, including more than 100 Kb of chromosomal DNA from the 21q22 region were isolated and characterized (see Fig. 4). Human genomic libraries in lambda Ch4A were screened with the cloned SOD-1 cDNA and several overlapping recombinant phages containing the whole SOD-1 gene were isolated. Heteroduplex analysis and DNA sequencing (Fig. 3) reveals five rather small exons and four introns that interrupt the coding region. This gene is present as a single copy per haploid genome and the DNA regions present in the isolated phages λA-2 and λB-1 are the only ones with nucleotide sequences idential to the SOD-1 cDNA. We therefore concluded that this region represents the unique SOD-1 functional gene. The gene is approximately 11 Kb in length and is interrupted by four introns. In proportion to the sizes of the two SOD-1 mRNAs (0.7 and 0.9 Kb) this is a large gene because it is over 12 times the length of the longer mRNA species. In addition to this gene we have isolated four SOD-1 related processed pseudogenes. Experiments with a genomic library of human chromosome 21 have indicated that the processed genes do not reside on this chromosome. Genomic blots of human DNAs isolated from cells trisomic for chromosome 21 shows the normal pattern of bands after digestion with EcoRI, PstI or BglII and hybridization to the SOD-1 cDNA probe. This is as expected, since it is assumed that the additional chromosome 21 is not defective and codes for the normal cellular proteins and that the abnormalities observed in Down's syndrome are due to an excess of some of these gene products. All the protein coding regions and part of the introns of the SOD-1 gene were sequenced as well as 300 b.p. of the 5'-flanking region and 220 b.p. of the 3'-flanking region (Fig. 3). In the donor sequence of the first intron a T to C transition occurred and hence it deviates from the 5'GT....AG 3' consensus. The unusual 5'-G-C donor site is not an artifact of the cloning procedure because it was detected in both λA2- and λB-1 which represent the two alleles of the SOD-1 gene (see below). Since this is the only functional SOD-1 gene present in the genome there is no reason to assume that the G-C- donor site is not functional *in vivo*. In fact, we have inserted an 11 Kb fragment, derived from λB-1, which contains the SOD-1 gene, into a plasmid vector carrying the bacterial phosphotransferase (neo) gene that can inactivate the aminoglycoside antibiotic G418 (87,88), and used it to transfect mouse L-cells. Many of the transformants resistant to the antibiotic G418 synthesized immunoprecipitable human SOD-1 polypeptides at relatively high efficiency indicating that indeed the G-C variant is functional. As indicated above, the λA-2 and λB-1 recombinants were isolated from the library of human fetal liver DNA and both contained the entire SOD-1 gene (Fig. 4). When hybridized to each other they formed a stable DNA duplex across their overlapping region. The restriction maps of that region are identical except for one BglII site (marked by the asterisk in Fig. 4) which is missing in λB-1. When the two phage DNAs were cut by BglII, blotted and probed with the SOD-1 cDNA clone, the λA-2 generated three fragments: a 4.1 Kb, a 3.6 Kb and a 1.5 Kb. The 3.6 Kb and 1.5 Kb BglII fragments were missing from the digest of λB-1, instead it contained one 5.1 Kb fragment. To test whether λA-2 and λB-1 are alleles of the same locus, 7 different human DNA samples from unrelated individuals were digested with BglII and analyzed by Southern blot hybridization. Two out of the 7 samples contained the 1.5 Kb fragment which is diagnostic for the λA-2 form of the gene. We, therefore, concluded that the

```
-270 -240 -210
GTACCCTGTT TACATCATTT TGCCATTTTC GCGTACTGCA ACCGGCGGGC CACGCCGTGA AAAGAAGGTT GTTTTCTCCA CAGTTTCGGG GTTCTGGACG TTTCCCGGCT
-180 -150 -120 -90
GCGGGGCGGG GGGAGTCTCC GGCGCACGCG GCCCCTTGGC CCGCCCCAGT CATTCCCGGC CACTCGCGAC CCGAGGCTGC CGCAGGGGGC GGGCTGAGCG CGTGCGAGGC
mRNA start site
-60 -30
CATTGGTTTG GGGCCAGAGT GGGCGAGGCG CGGAGGTCTG GCCTATAAAG TAGTCGCGGA GACGGGGTGC TGGTTTGCGT CGTAGTCTCC TGCAGGTCTG GGGTTTCCGT
50 80 Ala Thr Lys Ala Val Cys Val Leu Lys Gly Asp Gly Pro Val Gln Gly Ile
TGCAGTCCTC GGAACCAGGA CCTCGGCGTG GCCTAGCGAG TT ATG GCG ACG AAG GCC GTG TGC GTG CTG AAG GGC GAC GGC CCA GTG CAG GGC ATC
Ile Asn Phe Glu Gln Lys 150 240
ATC AAT TTC GAG CAG AAG GCAAGGGCTG GGACCGGGAG GCTTGTGTTG CGAGGCCGCT CCCGACCCGC TCGTCCCCCC GCGACCCTTT GCATGGACGG GTCGCCCGCC
250 300
AGGG·····························CCTAGAGCAGT TAAGCAGCTT GCTGGAGGTT CACTGGCTAG AAAGTGGTCA GCCTGGGATT TCGGACACAG ATTTTTCCAC
350 400 Glu Ser Asn
TCCCAAGTCT GGCTGCTTTT TACTTCACTG TGAGGGGTAA AGGTAAATCA GCTGTTTTCT TTGTTCAGAA ACTCTCTCCA ACTTTGCACT TTTCTTAAAG GAA AGT AAT
Gly Pro Val Lys Val Trp Gly Ser Ile Lys Gly Leu Thr Glu Gly Leu His Gly Phe His Val His Glu Phe Gly Asp Asn Thr Ala
GGA CCA GTG AAG GTG TGG GGA AGC ATT AAA GGA CTG ACT GAA GGC CTG CAT GGA TTC CAT GTT CAT GAG TTT GGA GAT AAT ACA GCA G GTGG
600 Gly Cys Thr Ser Ala Gly Pro His Phe Asn Pro Leu
GT·······························CATAATTTAG CTTTTTTTTC TTCTTCTTAT AAATAG GC TGT ACC AGT GCA GGT CCT CAC TTT AAT CCT CTA
Ser Arg Lys His Gly Gly Pro Lys Asp Glu Glu Arg 710 770
TCC AGA AAA CAC GGT GGG CCA AAG GAT GAA GAG AG GTAACAAGAT GCTTAACTCT TGTAATCAAT GGCGATACGT TTCTGGAGTT CATATGGTAT ACTACTTGTA
800 880
AATATGTGCC TAAGATAATT CCGTGTTTCC CCCACCTTTG CTTTTGAACT TGCTGACTCA TGTGAAACCC TGCTCCCAAA TGCTGGAATG CTTTTACTTC CTGGGCTTAA
900 950 990
AGGAATTGAC AAATGGGCAC TTAAAACGAT TTGGTTTTGT AGCATTTGAT TGAATATAGA ACTAATACAA GTGCCAAAGG GGAACTAATA CAGGAAATGT TCATGAACAG
1000 1045 His Val Gly Asp Leu Gly
TACTGTCAAC CACTAGCAAA ATCAATCATC ATT··································TGATGCTTTT CATATAG G CAT GTT GGA GAC TTG GGC
Asn Val Thr Ala Asp Lys Asp Gly Val Ala Asp Val Ser Ile Glu Asp Ser Val Ile Ser Leu Ser Gly Asp His Cys Ile Ile Gly Arg
AAT GTG ACT GCT GAC AAA GAT GGT GTG GCC GAT GTG TCT ATT GAA GAT TCT GTG ATC TCA CTC TCA GGA GAC CAT TGC ATC ATT GGC CGC
Thr Leu Val 1170 1250
ACA CTG GTG GTAAGTTTTC ATAAAGGATA TGCATAAAAC TTCTTCTAAC AGTACAGTCA TGTATCTTTC ACTTTGATTG TTAGTCGCGA ATTCTAAGAT CCAGATAAAC
1270 1320
TGT··············································GTTTCTGCTT TTAAACTACT AAATATTAGT ATATCTCTCT ACTAGGATTA ATGTTATTTT
1350 1400 Val His Gly
TCTAATATTA TGAGGTTCTT AAACATCTTT TGGGTATTGT TGGGAGGAGG TAGTGATTAC TTGACAGCCC AAAGTTATCT TCTTAAAATT TTTTACAG GTC CAT GAA
Lys Ala Asp Asp Leu Gly Lys Gly Gly Asn Glu Glu Ser Thr Lys Thr Gly Asn Ala Gly Ser Arg Leu Ala Cys Gly Val Ile Gly Ile
AAA GCA GAT GAC TTG GGC AAA GGT GGA AAT GAA GAA AGT ACA AAG ACA GGA AAC GCT GGA AGT CGT TTG GCT TGT GGT GTA ATT GGG ATC
Ala Gln STOP 1550 I 1600
GCC CAA TAAACATTCC CTTGGATGTA GTCTGAGGCC CCTTAACTCA TCTGTTATCC TGCTAGCTGT AGAAATGTAT CCTGATAAAC ATTAAACACT GTAATCTTAA
Poly A 1650 II 1700 III
AAGTGTAATT GTGTGACTTT TTCAGAGTTG CTTTAAAGTA CCTGTAGTGA GAAACTGATT TATGATCACT TGGAAGATTT GTATAGTTTT ATAAAACTCA GTTAAAATGT
1750 1800 IV Poly A
CTGTTTCAAT GACCTGTATT TTGCCAGACT TAAATCACAG ATGGGTATTA AACTTGTCAG AATTTCTTTG TCATTCAAGC CTGTGAATAA AAACCCTGTA TGGCACTTAT
1850 1900 1950
TATGAGGCTA TTAAAGAAT CCAAATTCAA ACTAAATTAG CTCTGATACT TATTTATATA AACAGCTTCA GTGGAACAGA TTTAGTAATA CTAACAGTGA TAGCATTTTA
V 2000 2050
TTTTGAAAGT GTTTTGAGAC CATCAAAATG CATACTTTAAAACAGCAGGTC TTTTAGCTAA AACTAACACA ACTCTGCTTA GACAAATAGG CTGTCCTTTG AAGCTT
```

Fig. 3. Nucleotide and amino acid sequences of the SOD-1 gene (85).

The sequence of all coding regions and adjacent nucleotides are shown with 110 bases per line. The "TATA", "CAT" and polyadenylation sequences are boxed. The splice junctions are underlined. The exons were identified by comparison with the cDNA sequences. The sites of initiation of transcription and poly(A)-tail are indicated. The arrows mark the two 9 nucleotides direct repeats at the 3' non coding region.

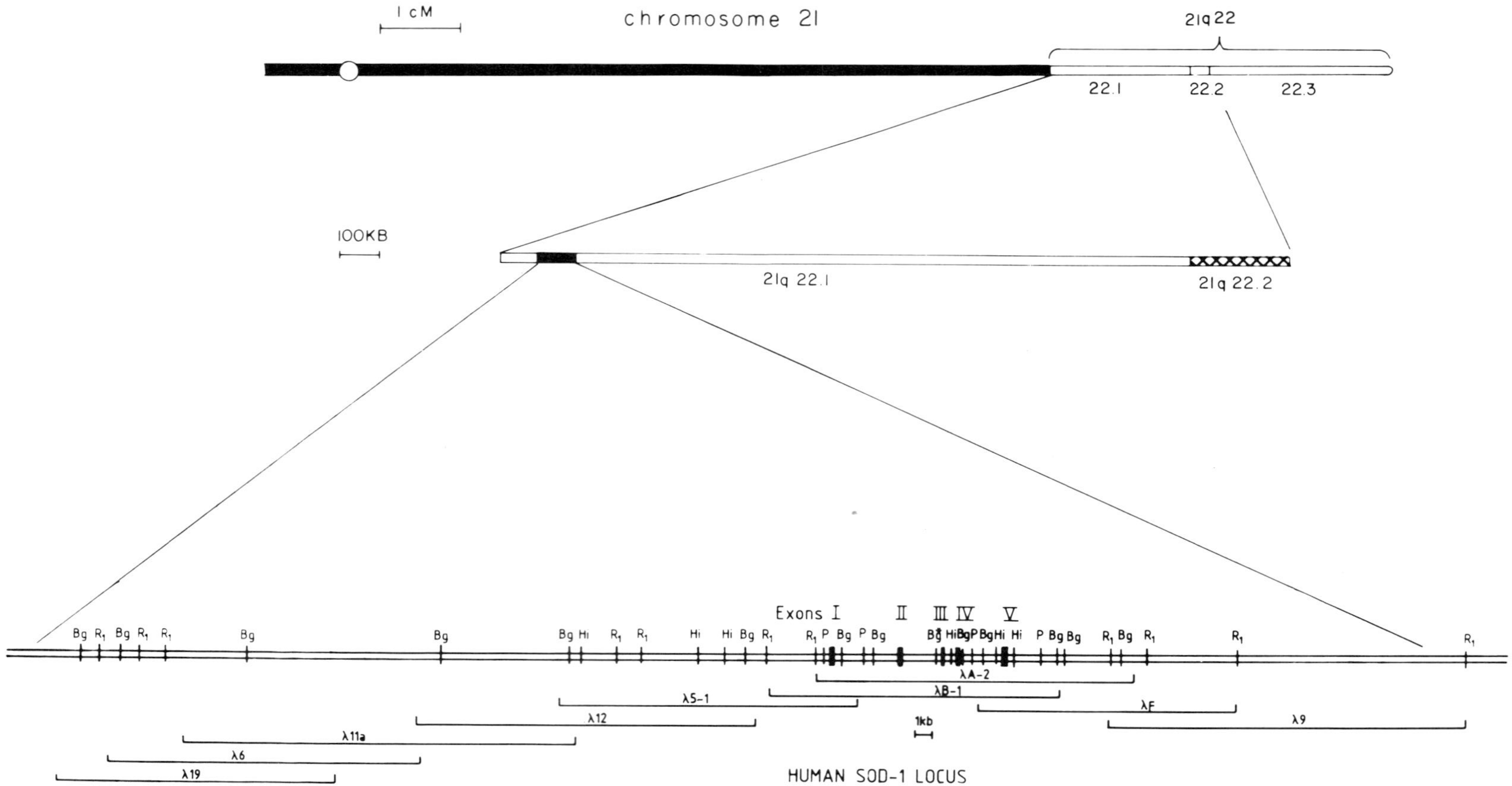

Fig. 4. A simplified representation of human chromosome 21 depicting the regine 21q22 responsible for Down's syndrome and the SOD-1 gene.

λA-2 and λB-1 contain the two alleles of the SOD-1 gene and that the additional BglII site was created by an alteration in the nucleotide sequence which causes restriction fragment length polymorphism (RFLPs)(89,90). The Mendelian inheritance of the BglII RFLP, as well as additional polymorphic markers present in the SOD-1 locus, were determined by analyzing the segregation patterns in informative families (Antonarakis et al., unpublished results). This information was used to construct a linkage map on chromosome 21 which in the future may be applied for analyses of a possible genetic predisposition in A.D. Variations in DNA sequences that occur in only one of the homologous chromosomes and thus result in alteration of the length of restriction fragments (RFLPs) have been detected at various human gene loci. The Mendelian inheritance of the RFLPs make them important genetic markers for studies of inherited diseases.

Biological Assay for Genes that may be Involved in Down's syndrome

Trisomy 21 cells display a variety of phenotypic changes. Documented examples include: hyper responsiveness of D.S. fibroblasts to β-adrenergic stimulation (91), decrease in Na^{+}/K^{+} ATPase activity and serotonin uptake (71), increased adhesiveness of D.S. fetal fibroblasts in culture (92), decrease in unsaturated fatty acids content in D.S. brain (70), alteration in mobility and redistribution of cell membrane macromolecules similar to those observed in aging cells (93), and abnormal electric membrane properties of D.S. neurons in cell culture (72). It was also reported that fibroblast cultures from D.S. patients grow slower and have a shorter lifespan than normal fibroblasts (94,96). All these defects may result from an excess of gene products coded by the extra copy of chromosome 21 and may thus reflect the *in vivo* abnormalities associated with the syndrome. We set out to develop these phenomena into a biological assay for genes that may be involved in D.S. Since an elevated activity of Cu/Zn SOD can be considered as a symptom of D.S. we first examined the effects produced by overexpression of the SOD-1 gene. The experimental approach was to introduce the human SOD-1 cDNA clone which contains the entire coding region (Fig. 1) into human disomy cells as part of a plasmid vector pMSV2-SOD-Neo carrying the bacterial phosphotransferase gene (neo) which confers resistance to neomycin (87,88)(Fig. 5-A). A similar vector containing the cellular SOD-1 gene isolated from the phage λB-1 was also constructed (Fig. 5-B). Both human and mouse cells were used as hosts for the vector SOD-1 constructs. Cells were transfected by the calcuium phosphate precipitation method and selected initially for G418 resistance. Only those cells that express the bacterial phosphotransferase gene (neo) survived. A number of cell lines that overexpress the vector-derived human SOD-1 were isolated from the G418 resistance transformants. Those cell lines are now being examined for phenotypic changes that may result from the elevated expression of SOD-1. The question we ask is, would normal cells which were programmed to express high levels of SOD-1 also acquire some altered properties? If so, would the process be reversed by inhibiting the expression of the vector derived SOD-1 and hence lowering the amounts of SOD-1 produced in those high SOD-1 cell lines? Inhibition of thymidine kinase gene expression in mouse L-cells by microinjection of antisense RNA was recently reported (97) and translational inhibition by complementary RNA transcript was shown to regulate the expression of ompF in *E. coli* (98). To test this possibility we have constructed a recombinant vector carrying the SOD-1 cDNA in an inverted orientation. This anti-SOD vector when transfected into cells should generate an "antisense" RNA. This "antisense" RNA should bind to the native SOD-1 messenger, prevent it from being translated and thus lower the production of SOD-1 within those cells.

To understand how trisomy 21 produces Down's syndrome the gene or genes involved in the pathology associated with the syndrome should be identified. "Chromosome walking" from the SOD-1 locus will hopefully lead to the isolation and identification of the SOD-1 neighboring genes.

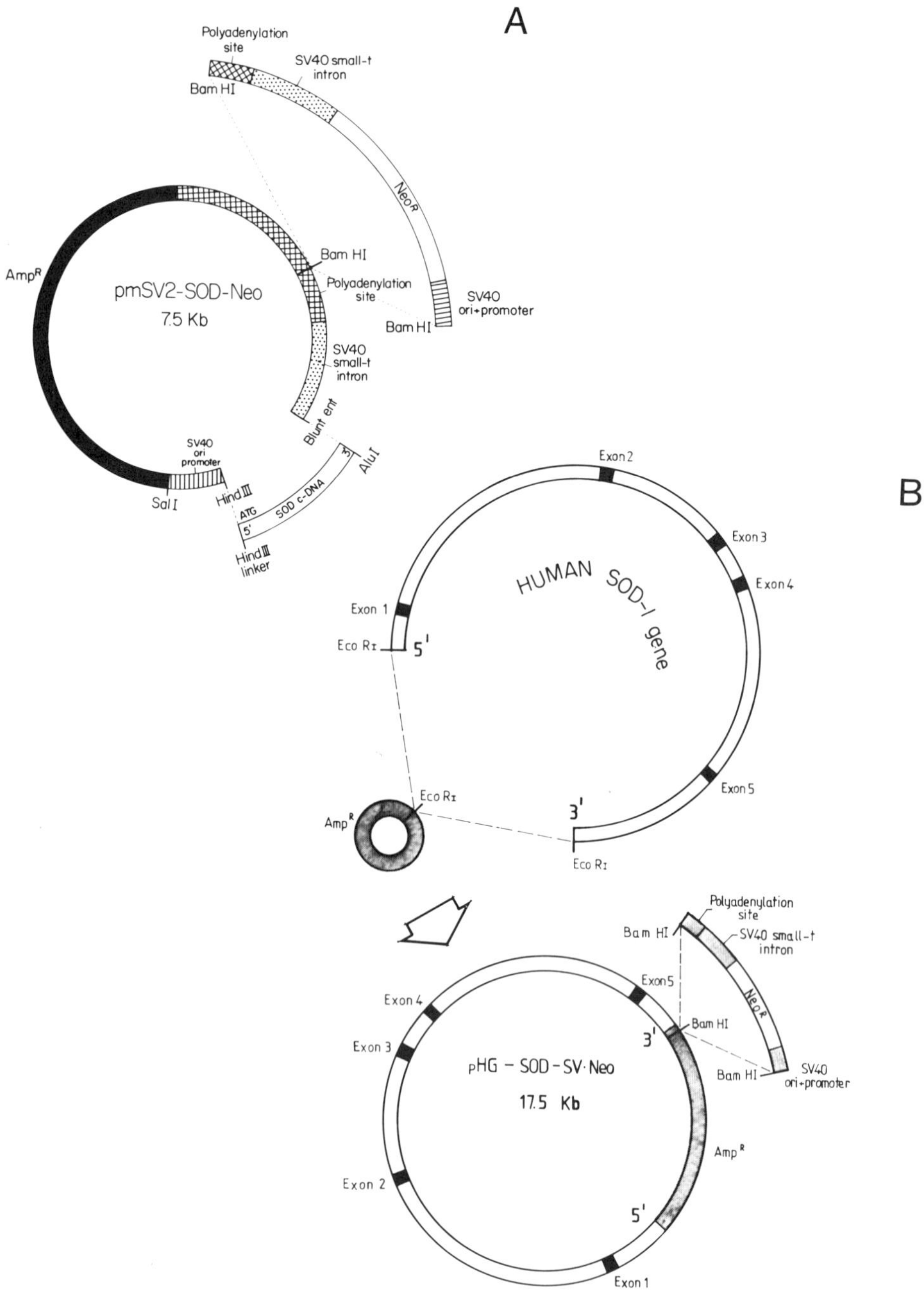

Fig. 5. Structure of SOD-1 DNA transducing vectors.

A - pBR322 DNA is represented by the solid black element. The open arcs represent either the neo gene or the SOD-1 cDNA. The hatched segment contain the SV40 origin of DNA replication and early promoter.
B - pBR322 DNA is represented by grey segments. The solid black regions are the exons of the SOD-1 gene. The open arc represents the neo gene. The SOD-1 expression in this vector is regulated by the native regulatory elements of the gene.

Besides the SOD-1, three other genes have been localized to the 21q22 and a few more will probably be assigned to this region in the future. We intend to isolate and characterize as many genes as possible from the 21q22 segment, to examine their expression in various tissues of D.S. abortuses and to study their effect when overexpressed in normal cells. This approach should provide the means to identify those genes on 21q22 that are involved in Down's syndrome and possibly Alzheimer's dementia.

This work was supported by a Basic Research Grant No. 1-906 from the March of Dimes Birth Defects Foundation, by Biotechnology General Corp., Israel, by the Weizmann Institute Leo and Julia Forchheimer Center of Molecular Genetics and by the Minerva Foundation, Munich/Germany.

REFERENCES

1. R. Katzman, ed., in: "Biological Aspects of Alzheimers Disease" Banbury Report No. 15, Cold Spring Harbor Laboratory, New York (1983).
2. F.M. Sinex and C.R. Merrill, eds., in: "Alzheimer's Disease, Down's Syndrome and Aging" New York Academy of Sciences, New York (1982).
3. R.J. Wartman, in: "Alzheimer's Disease" Scientific American 252:48-56 (1985).
4. J.M. Lejeune, M. Gautier, and R. Turpin, Etudes des chromosomes somatiques de neuf enfants mongoliens, Compt.Rend.Acad.Sci. 248: 1721-1722 (1959).
5. G.M. Martin, Genetic syndromes in man with potential relevance to the pathology of aging, Birth Defects Orig. Article Series XIV (1) 5-39 (1978).
6. G.R., Burgio, M. Fraccaro, L. Tiepolo, and U. Wolf, eds., Trisomy 21 Springer-Berlin, (1981).
7. F.F. de la Cruz, and P.S. Gerald, eds., Trisomy 21 (Down Syndrome) Research Perspective. University Park Press, Baltimore (1981).
8. G.A. Jervis, Early senile dementia in mongoloid idiocy, Am. J. Psychiatry. 105:102-106 (1948).
9. P.C. Burger, and F.S. Vogel, The development of the pathologic changes of Alzheimer's disease and senile dementia in patients with Down's syndrome, Am. J. Pathol. 73:457-476 (1973).
10. W.G. Ellis, J.R. McCullogh, and C.L. Corley, Presenile dementia in Down's syndrome: Ultrastructural identity with Alzheimer's disease, Neurology 24:101-106 (1974).
11. W.M. Hooper, and F.S. Vogel, The limbic system in Alzheimer's disease: Neuropathological investigation, Am. J. Pathol. 85:1-13 (1976).
12. A.H. Ropper, and R.S. Williams, Relationship between plaques, tangles, and dementia in Down syndrome, Neurology 30:639-644 (1980).
13. G. Solitare, and J. Lamarche, Alzheimer's disease and senile dementia as seen in mongoloids: Neuropathological observations, Am. J. Ment. Dis. 70:840-848 (1966).
14. D.R., Crapper, A.J. Dalton, M. Skopitz, P. Eng, J.H. Scott, and V. Hachimski, Alzheimer degeneration in Down's syndrome. Electrophysiological alterations and histopathologic findings, Arch. Neurol. 32:618-623 (1975).
15. C.J. Epstein, Down's syndrome and Alzheimer's disease: Implications and approaches, in: "Biological Aspects of Alzheimer's Disease", R. Katzman, ed., Cold Spring Harbor Laboratory, N.Y. 169-182 (1983).
16. S. Sorbi, and J.P. Blass, Fibroblast phosphofructokinase, in: "Alzheimer's disease and Down's Syndrome" ibid p. 297-305,(1983).
17. G.G. Glenner, and C.W. Wong. Alzheimer's disease and Down's syndrome sharing a unique cerebrovascular amyloid fiber protein, Biochem. Biophys Res. Comm. 122:1131-1135 (1984).
18. J.F. Mattei, M.G. Mattei, S. Aymes, and F. Giraud, Origin of the extra chromosome in trisomy 21, Hum. Genet. 46:107-110 (1979).
19. E. Niebuhr, Down's syndrome. The possibility of a pathogenic segment on chromosome 21, Hum. Genet. 21:99-100 (1974).

20. J.D. Williams, R.L. Summit, P.R. Martens, and R.A. Kimbrell, Familial Down's syndrome is due to t(10,21) translocation: evidence that the Down's syndrome phenotype is related to trisomy of a specific segment of chromosome 21, Am. J. Hum. Genet. 27:478-481 (1975).
21. J. Cervenka, R.J. Gorlin, and G.R. Djavadi, Down's syndrome due to partial trisomy 21q. Clin. Genet. 11:119-121 (1977).
22. R.A. Pfeiffer, E.K. Kessel, and K.H. Soer, Partial trisomies of chromosome 21 in man. New observations due to translocations 19:21 and 4:21, Clin. Genet. 11:207-213 (1977).
23. M. Poissonier, B. St. Paul, B. Dutrillaux, M. Chassegne, M. Gruyer, and G. Bligniers,-Strouk, Trisomy 21 partiello (21q21 to 21q22.2), Ann. Genet. 19:69-73 (1976).
24. P.M. Sinet, J. Coutourier, B. Dutrillaux, M. Poissonier, O. Raoul, M.O. Rethore, D. Allard, J. Lejeune, and H. Jerome, Trisomic 21 et superoxide dismutase, tentative de localisation sur la sous bande 21q21.1, Exp. Cell Res. 97:47-55 (1976).
25. A. Hagemeijer, and E.M.E. Smith, Partial trisomy 21. Further evidence that trisomy of band 21q22 is essential for Down's phenotype, Hum. Genet. 38:15-23 (1977).
26. T. Philip, J. Fraisse, P.-M. Sinet, B. Lauras, J.M. Roberts, and F. Freycon, Confirmation of the assignment of the human SOD gene to chromosome 21q22, Cytogenet. Cell Genet. 22:521-523 (1978).
27. R.L. Summitt,Chromosome 21 specific segments that cause the phenotype of Down syndrome, in: Trisomy 21 (Down Syndrome) Research Perspectives, F.F. de la Cruz and P.S. Gerald, eds. University Park Press, (1981).
28. L.L. Heston, Dementia of the Alzheimer type: A perspective from family studies, in: "Biological Aspects of Alzeheimer's Disease",R. Katzman, ed., Cold Spring Harbor Laboratory p 183-191, N.Y. (1983).
29. H.E. Varmus, The Molecular Genetics of Cellular Oncogenes, Ann. Rev. Genet. 18:553-612 (1984).
30. H.J. Evans, R.A. Buckland, and M.L. Pardue, Location of the genes coding for 18S and 28S ribosomal RNA in the human genome, Chromosome 48:405-426 (1974).
31. R.D. Schmickel, and M. Knoller, Characterization and localization of the human genes for ribosomal ribonucleic acid, Pediat. Res. 11: 929-935 (1977).
32. Y.H. Tan, J. Tischfield, and F.H. Ruddle, The linkage of genes for the human interferon-induced antiviral protein and inophenol oxidase-B traits to human chromosome G-21, J. Exp. Med. 137:317-330 (1973).
33. E.E. Moore, C. Jones, F.-T. Kao, and D.C. Oates, Synteny between glycinamide ribonucleotide synthetase and superoxide dismutase (soluble), Am. J. Hum. Genet. 29:389-396 (1977).
34. D. Patterson, S. Graw, and C. Jones, Demonstration, by somatic cell genetics, of coordinate regulation of genes for two enzymes of purine synthesis assigned to human chromosome 21, Proc.Natl.Acad. Sci. USA 78:405-409 (1981).
35. S. Vora, and U. Franke, Assignment of the human gene for liver-type-6-phosphofructokinase isozyme (PFK_L) to chromosome 21 by using somatic cell hybrids and monoclonal anti-L antibody, Proc.Natl.Acad.Sci. USA 78:3738-3742 (1981).
36. F. Skoby, N. Krassikoff, and U. Franke, Assignment of the gene for cystathionine β-synthase to human chromosome 21 in somatic cell hybrids, Hum. Genet. 65:291-294 (1984).
37. P. Garber, P.-M. Sinet, H. Jerome, and J. Lejeune, Copper/zinc SOD activity in trisomy 21 by translocation, Lancet ii:914-918 (1979).
38. J.M. Emberger, R. Lloret, and D. Rossi, Trisomic 21 partielle a 45 chromosomes par translocation de deux 21 sur le 14: 45,XX,-14,-21+t (14q21q21q), Ann. Genet. 23:179-180 (1980).
39. N. Crosti, A. Rigo, R. Stevanato, J. Bajer, G. Neri, R. Bova, and A.Serra, Lack of position effect on the activity of SOD/ Cu/Zn gene in subjects with 21/D and 21/G Robertsonian translocation, Hum.Genet. 57:203-204 (1981).

40. A. Jeziorowska, L. Jakubowski, A. Armatys, and B. Kaluzewski, Copper/zinc superoxide dismutase (SOD-1) activity in regular trisomy 21, trisomy 21 by translocation and mosaic trisomy 21, Clin. Gen. 22: 160-164 (1982).
41. L.B. Epstein, and C.J. Epstein, Localization of the gene AVG for the antiviral expression of immune and classical interferon to the distal part of the long arm of chromosome 21, J. Infect. Dis. (Suppl.) 133:A56-A62 (1976).
42. D.R. Cox, H. Kawashima, S. Vora, and C.J. Epstein, Regional mapping of SOD-1 PRGS and PFK-L on human chromosome 21: implications for the role of these genes in the pathogenesis of Down Syndrome, Am. J. Hum. Genet. 35:118A (1983).
43. B. Chadefaux, D. Allard, M.O. Rethore, O. Raoul, M. Poissonier, S. Gilgenkrantz, C. Cheruy, and H. Jerome, Assignment of human phosphoribosylglycinamide synthetase locus to region 21q22.1, Hum. Genet. 66:190-192 (1984).
44. S. Sichitiu, P.-M. Sinet, J. Lejeune, and J. Frezal, Surdosage de la forme dimerique de l'indophenoloxydase dans las trisomic 21, secondaire au surdosage genique, Hum. Genet. 23:65-72 (1974).
45. P.-M. Sinet, D. Allard, J. Lejeune, and H. Jerome, Augmentation d' activite de la superoxyde dismutase erythrocytaire dans la trisomic pour le chromosome 21, C.R. Acad. Sci (Paris) 278:3267-3270 (1974).
46. A.W. Erikson, R.F. Frants, and P.H. Jongbloet, Quantitative immunological studies on cytoplasmic superoxide dismutase: High concentration in red cells of Down syndrome, Abstr. Amer. J. Hum. Genet. 27: 33A (1975).
47. P. Benson, Gene dosage effect in trisomy 21, Lancet ii:584 (1975).
48. R.R. Frants, A.W. Eriksson, P.H. Jongbloet, and H.J. Hamers, Superoxide dismutase in Down syndrome, Lancet ii:42-43 (1975).
49. N. Crosti, A. Serra, A. Rigo, and P. Viglino, Dosage effect of SOD-A gene in trisomy 21 cells, Hum. Genet. 31:197-203 (1976).
50. A.D. Tamarkina, G.A. Annenkov, I.K. Filippoy, and T. Lamchingin, Dosage effect of cytoplasmic SOD-1 gene in the erythrocytes of patients with Down's syndrome, Genetika 13:929-932 (1977).
51. W.W. Feaster, L.W. Kwok, and C.J. Epstein, Dosage effects for superoxide dismutase-1 in nucleated cells aneuploid for chromosome 21, Am. J. Hum. Genet. 29:563-570 (1977).
52. Y. Yamamoto, N. Ogasawara, A. Gotoh, H. Komiya, H. Nakai, and Y. Kuroki, A case of 21q-syndrome with normal SOD-1 activity, Hum. Genet. 48: 321-327 (1979).
53. J.M. Berg, H.A. Gardner, R.J.M. Gardner, E.G. Goh, V.D. Markovic, N.E. Simpson, and R.G. Worton, Dic(21;21) in a Down's syndrome child with an unusual chromosome 9 variant in the mother, J. med. Genet. 17: 144-155 (1980).
54. N.J. Leschot, R.M. Slater, H. Joenje, M.J. Becker-Bloemkolk, and J.J. de Nef, SOD-A and chromosome 21. Conflicting findings in a familial translocation (9p24;21q214), Hum. Genet. 57:220-223 (1981).
55. C.H. Scoggin, J. Bleskan, J.N. Davidson, and D. Patterson, Gene expression of glycinamide ribonucleotide synthetase in Down syndrome, Clin. Res. 28:31A (1980).
56. J.A. Bartley, and C.J. Epstein, Gene dosage effect for glycinamide ribonucleotide synthetase in human fibroblasts trisomic for chromosome 21, Biochem. Biophys. Res. Commun. 93:1286-1289 (1980).
57. R.B. Layzer, and C.J. Epstein, Phosphofructokinase and chromosome 21, Am. J. Hum. Genet. 24:533-543 (1972).
58. L.B. Epstein, S.H.S. Lee, and C.J. Epstein, Enhanced sensitivity of trisomy 21 monocytes to the maturation-inhibiting effects of interferon, Cell Immunol. 50:191-194 (1980).
59. B.S. Scott, L.E. Becker, and T.L. Petit, Neurobiology of Down's syndrome Prog. Neurobiol. 21:199-237 (1983).

60. P.M. Sinet, J. Lejeune, and H. Jerome, Trisomy 21 (Down's syndrome) glutathione peroxidase hexose monophosphate shunt and I.Q, Life Sci. 24:29-34 (1979).
61. P.M. Sinet, Metabolism of oxygen derivatives in Down's syndrome in Alzheimer disease and aging, F.M. Sinex, and C.R. Merill, eds, Ann. New York Acad. Sci. 396:83-94 (1982).
62. S.N. Pantelakis, A.G. Karaklis, D. Alexion, E. Vardas, and T. Valaes, Red cell enzymes in trisomy 21, Am. J. Hum. Genet. 22:184-193 (1972).
63. H. Frischer, L.K. Chu, T. Ahmad, P. Justice, and G.F. Smith, Superoxide dismutase and glutathione peroxidase abnormalities in erythrocytes and lymphoid cells in Down's syndrome, Progr. clin. biol. Res., 55:269-283 (1981).
64. J. Kedziora, R. Lukaszewicz, M. Koter, G. Bartosz, B. Pawlowska, and D. Aitkin, Red blood cell glutathione peroxidase in simple trisomy 21 and translocation 21/22, Experientia, 38:543-544 (1982).
65. P.M. Sinet, A.M. Michelson, A. Bazin, J. Lejeune, and H. Jerome, Increase in glutathione peroxidase activity in erythrocytes from trisomy 21 subjects, Biochem. biophys. Res.Commun, 67:910-915 (1975).
66. L.M.M. Wijnen, M. Monteba-Van Heusel, P.L. Pearson, and P.M. Khan, Assignment of a gene for glutathione peroxidase (GPX1) to human chromosome 3, Cytogenet. Cell Genet, 22:232-235 (1978).
67. B.L. Brooksbank, and R. Balazs, Superoxide dismutase, gluthathione peroxidase and lipoperoxidation in Down's syndrome fetal brain, Devel. Brain Res., 16:37-44 (1984).
68. J.A. Bedweg, and M.L. Karnovsky, Active oxygen species and the functions of phagocytic leukocytes, Ann. Rev. Biochem., 49:695-726 (1980).
69. L.J. Marnett, Hydroperoxide-dependent oxidations during prostaglandin biosynthesis, in: Free Radicals in Biology, W.A. Pryor, ed., V1 p.64-90, Academic Press, N.Y. (1984).
70. S.N. Shah, Fatty acid composition of lipids of human brain myelin and synaptosomes: Changes in phenylketonuria and Down syndrome, Int. J. Biochem., 10:477-482 (1979).
71. E.E. McCoy, and L. Enns, Sodium transport quabain binding and (Na^+/K^+) ATPase activity in Down's syndrome platelets, Pediat. Res., 12:685-689 (1978).
72. B.S. Scott, T.L. Petit, L.E. Becker, and B.A.V. Edwards, Abnormal electric membrane properties of Down's syndrome DRG neurons in cell culture, Devel. Brain. Res. 2:257-270 (1982).
73. S. Vora, L. Corash, W.K. Engel, S. Durham, C. Seaman, and S. Piomelli, The molecular mechanism of the inherited phosphofructokinase deficiency associated with hemolysis and myopathy, Blood 55:629-635 (1980).
74. S. Vora, C. Seaman, S. Durham, and S. Piomelli, Isozymes of human phosphofructokinase: Identification and subunit structural characterization of a new system, Proc.Natl.Acad.Sci. USA 77:62-66 (1980).
75. S. Vora, Isozymes of human phosphofructokinase in blood cells and cultured cell lines: Molecular and genetic evidence for a trigenic system, Blood 57:724-731 (1981).
76. S. Vora, Isozymes of phosphofructokinase, in: "Isozymes: Current Topics in Biological Medical Research", M.C. Rattazzi, J.G. Scandalios, G.S. Whitt, eds., New York, Alan R. Liss, Vol. 6, pp. 119-167 (1982).
77. S. Vora, Isozymes of human phosphofructokinase: Biochemical and genetic aspects, Isozymes:Curr. Top. Biol. Med. Res., 11:3-24 (1983).
78. G.A. Dunaway, A review of animal phosphofructokinase isozymes with an emphasis on their physiological role, Molec. Cell. Biochem., 52: 75-91 (1983).
79. M. Davidson, M. Collins, J. Byrne, and S. Vora, Alterations and phosphofructokinase isozymes during early human development, Biochem. J. 214:703-710 (1983).
80. S. Vora, and U. Francke, Assignment of the human gene for liver-type 6-phosphofructokinase isozyme (PFKL) to chromosome 21 by using somatic

cell hybrids and monoclonal anti-L antibody, Proc.Natl.Acad.Sci. USA 78:3738-3742 (1981).

81. D.M. Bowen, P. White, J.A. Spillane, M.J. Goodhart, G. Curzon, P. Iwangoff, W. Meyer-Ruge, and A.M. Davison, Accelerated aging or selective neuronal loss as an important course of dementia, Lancet ii:11-15, (1979).

82. J. Lieman-Hurwitz, N. Dafni, V. Lavie, and Y. Groner, Human cytoplasmic superoxide dismutase cDNA clone: A probe for studying the molecular biology of Down's syndrome, Proc.Natl.Acad.Sci. USA 79:2808-2811 (1982).

83. L. Sherman, N. Dafni, J. Lieman-Hurwitz, and Y. Groner. Nucleotide sequence and expression of human chromosome 21-encoded superoxide dismutase mRNA, Proc.Natl.Acad.Sci. USA 80:5465-5469 (1983).

84. L. Sherman, D. Levanon, J. Lieman-Hurwitz, N. Dafni, and Y. Groner, Human Cu/Zn superoxide dismutase gene: Molecular characterization of its two mRNA species, Nucleic Acid Res., 12:9349-9365 (1984).

85. D. Levanon, J. Lieman-Hurwitz, N. Dafni, M. Wigderson, L. Sherman, Y. Bernstein, Z. Laver-Rudich, E. Danciger, O. Stein, and Y. Groner, Architecture and anatomy of the chromosomal locus in human chromosome 21 encoding the Cu/Zn superoxide dismutase, EMBO J, 4:77-84 (1985).

86. Y. Groner, J. Lieman-Hurwitz, N. Dafni, L. Sherman, D. Levanon, Y. Bernstein, E. Danciger, and O. Elroy-Stein, Molecular structure and expression of the gene locus on chromosome 21 encoding the Cu/Zn superoxide dismutase and its relevance to Down's syndrome, Ann. New York Acad. Sci. In press.

87. R.C. Mulligan, and P. Berg, Expression of a bacterial gene in mammalian cells, Science 209:1422-1427 (1980).

88. P.J. Southern, and P. Berg. Transformation of mammalian cells to antibiotic resistance with a bacterial gene under control of the SV40 early region promoter, J. Molec. App. Genet. 1:327-341 (1982).

89. Y.W. Kan, and A.M. Dozy, Polymorphism of DNA sequence adjacent to the human β-globin structural gene: Relationship to sickle cell mutation, Proc.Natl.Acad.Sci. USA 75:5631-5635 (1978).

90. D. Botstein, R.L. White, M. Skolnick, and R.W. Davis, Construction of a genetic linkage map in man using restriction fragment length polymorphisms, Amer. J. Hum. Genet. 32:314-331 (1980).

91. J.D. McSwigan, D.R. Hanson, A. Lubiniecki, L.L. Heston, and J.R. Sheppard, Down syndrome fibroblasts are hyper-responsive to β-adrenergic stimulation, Proc.Natl.Acad.Sci. USA 78:7670-7673 (1981).

92. T.C. Wright, R.W. Orkin, M. Destrempes, and D.M. Kurnit, Increased adhesiveness of Down syndrome fetal fibroblasts *in vitro*. Proc.Natl.Acad.Sci. USA 81:2426-2430 (1984).

93. F. Naeim, and R.L. Walford, Disturbances of redistribution of surface membrane receptors on peripheral mononuclear cells of patients with D.S. and of aged individuals, J. Gerontology 35:650-655 (1980).

94. E.L. Schneider, and C.J. Epstein, Replication rate and lifespan of cultured fibroblasts in Down's syndrome, Proc.Soc.Exp.Biol. Med., 141:1092-1094 (1972).

95. D.J. Segal, and E.E. McCoy, Studies on Down's syndrome in tissue culture, J. Cell. Physiol. 83:85-90 (1974).

96. J. Boue, C. Deluchat, H. Nicolas, and A. Boue, Prenatal losses of trisomy 21, in: Trisomy 21, G.R. Burgio, H. Fraccaro, L. Tiepolo, and U. Wolf, eds, pp. 183-193, Springer-Verlag, New York (1981).

97. J.G. Izant, and H. Weintraub, Inhibition of thymidine kinase gene expression by antisense RNA: A molecular approach to genetic analysis, Cell 36:1007-1015 (1984).

98. T. Mizuno, M.Y. Chou, and M. Inouye, A unique mechanism regulating gene expression: Translational inhibition by a complementary RNA transcript (mic RNA), Proc.Natl.Acad.Sci. USA 81:1966-1970 (1984).

THE NATURAL HISTORY OF ALZHEIMER'S FAMILIES: AN UNDERUTILIZED METHOD FOR EXPLORING BASIC AND THERAPEUTIC STRATEGIES IN AGE-RELATED NEUROPSYCHIATRIC DISORDERS

Gail Ann Thoen

University of Minnesota Hospitals
Department of Psychiatry
Minneapolis, Minnesota 55455 U.S.A.

"We're so relieved that mother has Alzheimer's disease.
At least now we know what it is..."

INTRODUCTION

Biological researchers studying basic and therapeutic strategies in Alzheimer's disease (AD) and other age-related neuropsychiatric disorders have noted the critical need for interdisciplinary studies describing the untreated natural history of families of dementia patients (Heston, 1984; Clayton, 1984; Knopman, 1984).

Only a small portion of research about DAT deals with the impact of this progressive, irreversible, dementing disease on the proband's family. Of the research which has been done, much of it focuses on various aspects of home care as compared to institutional care, particularly with respect to caregivers (Martinson, 1984). The practical application of this research has been published in three popular books which have become "Bibles" for those interested in the caregiver role: Mace and Rabins (1981) THE 36-HOUR DAY, Reisberg's (1983) A GUIDE TO ALZHEIMER'S DISEASE FOR FAMILIES, SPOUSES, AND FRIENDS, and Heston and White's (1983) DEMENTIA: A PRACTICAL GUIDE TO ALZHEIMER'S DISEASE AND RELATED ILLNESSES.

No study known to this author has utilized the traditional participant observation method to describe disturbance in mood in Alzheimer's probands and their relatives spanning three generations of family members. A primary aim of this study is to fill that gap. Hypotheses will be generated to be tested in follow-up studies. Far from regarding the project as a definitive study on the impact of DAT on family members, we hope it will serve as an exploratory pilot study.

The author wishes to thank Drs. Leonard L. Heston, William Schofield, and Barry D. Garfinkel who provided suggestions on an earlier draft of the manuscript and Dr. Paula J. Clayton and Janice W. Feinberg, M.S.W., for their encouragement and support. This study was supported in part by the Department of Psychiatry, University of Minnesota Hospitals.

SUBJECTS

Three generations of family members (proband, adult children, grandchildren, and spouses) in two unrelated Alzheimer's families were interviewed and observed by a psychologist (G.A.T) for minimum of two and a half hours for each subject. See Figures 1 and 2 for age and sex composition and additional data. An adult child in each family, who also served as the key informant, was interviewed and observed for a minimum of eleven hours. Medical records for each proband were reviewed by the author and a psychiatrist to verify that the work up used to assign a probable diagnosis of Alzheimer's disease (DAT) conformed to current clinical diagnostic criteria. Work ups included computed tomography (CT), EEG, comprehensive blood chemistry analyses, and neuropsychological testing. It should be noted that the diagnosis in most cases of dementia depends on postmortem examination or brain biopsy, and that the diagnoses are presumptive.

Contact with the families was made through the key informant. The families were not known to the author; in both cases, the informant was referred by a colleague. The two cases were chosen from a larger pool of possible families with the intent of matching probands as closely as possible for severity (moderate), date of diagnosis (May, 1984), age (>70), race (white), sex (female), education (<college graduate), and socio-economic status (middle class). Additional inclusionary criteria determined by the research design required that: (a) one proband have a relative with senile dementia (parent or sibling) while the other did not and (b) one adult child reside <100 miles away from the proband and the other reside >500 miles away from the proband. Volunteers were normal in the sense that each was an independent, community-dwelling individual who did not have a current medical condition that would interfere with full participation in the study. Data was collected between December, 1984 and February, 1985.

METHODS

The study combined traditional participant observation in the subject's natural environment (home and community) with a one-hour psychological interview conducted by the author, a written questionnaire, and self-administered Minnesota Multiphasic Personality Inventory (MMPI). The MMPI's (Hathaway and McKinley, 1943) were scored by a computer service; results of the written data and the field work were discussed with a psychiatrist (L.L.H.), a psychologist (W.S.) and a social worker (J.W.F.). Two home visits to each family were designed to observe (a) the proband interact with family members during mealtime and (b) family members interact during mealtime when the proband was not present. A minimum of bi-weekly telephone contact with the key informants was maintained throughout the study. Excepting for one grandchild in the familial DAT case who was not available to participate in the study, and two grandchildren in the non-familial case, who participated in the written part of the study but were not available for interview, all subjects were investigated according to the procedures described above.

THE FAMILIES: AN OVERVIEW OF THREE GENERATIONS OF TWO ALZHEIMER'S FAMILIES

The Lancaster Family - The Lancaster family has its roots divided between a large midwestern city, a rural midwestern town and the Pacific

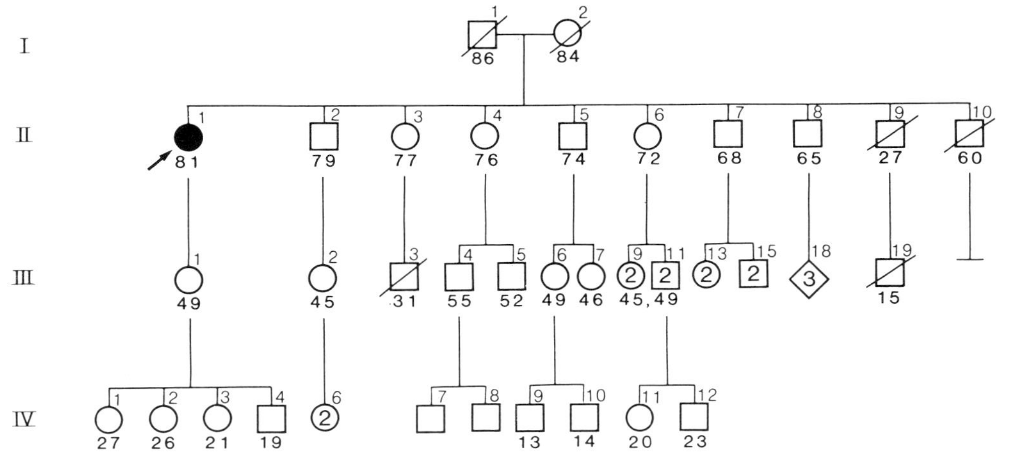

I: (1) "heart attack" (2) probable Alzheimer's disease, 8-year illness

II: (1) Alzheimer's disease, May, 1984 diagnosis; severe rheumatoid arthritis:

Disalcid, Tolectin, Plaquinal, Prednisone, and Cortisone injections of some of her joints

(2) prostate cancer (5) prostate cancer (9) suicide (10) "heart attack"

III: (3) accident (19) accident

Figure 1. Lancaster Family

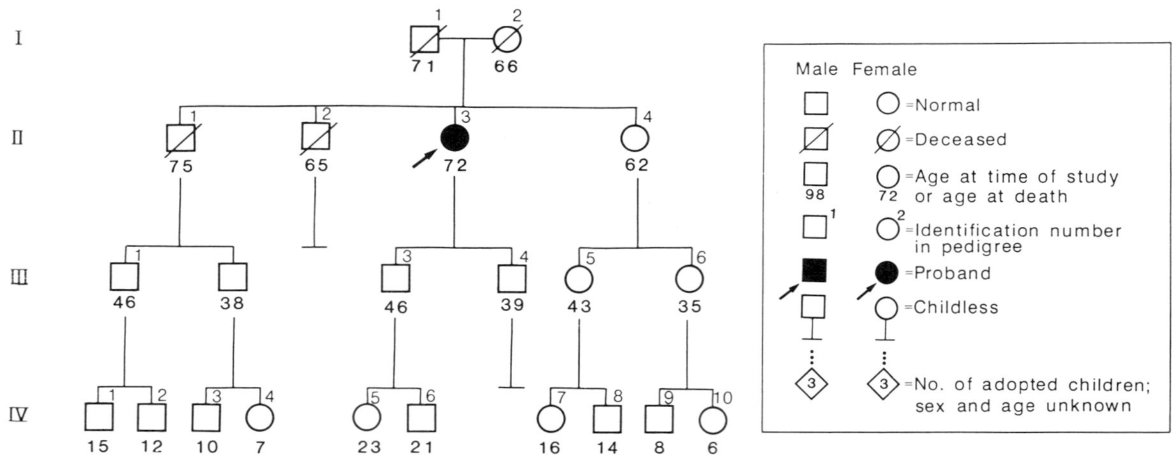

I: (1) "hardening of the arteries"

(2) cancer, type unknown

II: (1) "heart attack" (2) "heart attack"

(3) Alzheimer's disease, May, 1984 diagnosis; Xanax

Figure 2. Oswald Family

Northwest. The age and sex composition of the family and additional data is presented in Figure 1. The proband and her husband, both white and nominally protestant, grew up, married, and established their own home in the same farming community. At the time of marriage, the proband was a 21 year old unskilled worker; her husband, a 25 year old farmer. Her only pregnancy produced a normal child at age 30. The proband worked throughout her 49 year marriage, primarily as a psychiatric aid in a state hospital for the deaf. Her late husband worked as a farmer and small businessman. By all reports the marriage was extremely happy.

Daughter reports that her the proband was of average intelligence before the onset of Alzheimer's disease. She was one of ten children who had to quit school after the eighth grade to work on the family farm. The proband has been widowed for eight years and has been living alone for the past year in a one-bedroom apartment in a senior citizen's building in the community where she lived most of her life. Daughter reports that the proband is aware of the decline in her memory abilities but that "...she has no idea that she has Alzheimer's, so please don't mention it in front of her." The proband has felt depression which she attributes to memory loss, arthritis, and aging. She is able to continue living alone because of the extensive support system organized by her daughter, which includes weekly visits and phone calls; respite care by a LPN, who gives the proband a weekly bath; and several other family members, friends, and neighbors who stop by to visit and to be sure that she has taken her medicine (see Figure 1).

The Lancasters appear as the "quintessential American family"--middle class, upwardly mobile, healthy, educated, close-knit, and fun-loving. The family exudes a strong moral fiber coupled with a zest for life.

The proband's daughter, the key informant in this case study, is a full-time homemaker and high school graduate. She has been married for 29 years and lives in a middle class suburban home near a large midwestern city located 60 miles from her mother. She resides with her husband, a small businessman, and their adolescent son, who attends college. Two unmarried daughters (one a nurse; the other a college student) have established their own homes nearby and visit frequently. The eldest daughter is married and lives 350 miles away with her husband of one year.

<u>The Oswald Family</u> - The Oswald family has its roots divided between two urban midwestern cities. The age and sex composition of the family and additional data is presented in Figure 2. The proband and her husband, both white and Jewish, reside in a upper middle class condominium home.

The proband's first husband, a small businessman, also white and Jewish, died in 1956 of a "heart attack." Her current husband of nearly 20 years, although in excellent health, retired last year from his work as a photographer to care for the proband. He has not sought respite help. The proband has a high school education. Before her remarriage, she worked at unskilled jobs in order to support her two minor children. Her sons report that she was of average intelligence before the onset of Alzheimer's disease, and while she is aware of her failing memory, "...she has absolutely no idea that she has Alzheimer's...we never mention it in front of her." Until her illness interfered, the proband led an active life as a full-time homemaker and enjoyed travelling extensively with her husband.

Her oldest son, a high school graduate and small businessman, his wife and their two unmarried adult children (both college students) live near the proband. They visit her less than once a month. Telephone calls are infrequent and brief. Her younger son, the key informant in the case study, is a college graduate and salesman. He is unmarried and lives 600 miles away in a large city. He visits his family about four times a year and telephones about twice a month.

The family unanimously condemns itself for not being close-knit, rather secretive, and--for as long as they can remember--"...somehow always missing out on the best things that life has to offer..."

INTERVIEW RESULTS

Severity of Alzheimer's Disease in the Proband and its Impact on the Families

As illustrated in Figure 3, the diversity of global ratings regarding the severity of Alzheimer's disease in the proband is remarkably variable within and between families. Each family member was asked on the questionnaire and during one or more interview sessions to rate the proband's illness as "mild," "moderate," or "severe." These stages roughly correspond to Reisberg's (1982) seven-point Global Deterioration Scale wherein a rating of "mild" in this study would be assigned to stage 1, 2, or 3; a rating of "moderate" would be assigned to stage 4 or 5; and a rating of "severe" would be assigned to stage 6 or 7. (Reisberg reports that many patients are not brought or do not come for treatment until stage 5, at which time they can still dress themselves, but most have their clothes laid out for them because they are no longer able to select, appropriate and matching attire.) The physician's rating was taken from extensive medical records forwarded to the author by the neurologists who made the initial diagnoses in May, 1984.

In the Lancaster family, Daughter (No. 1) rates the severity of her mother's illness as far less severe than other raters. Her daughter, grandchild No. 5, rates her grandmother's illness as far more severe than other raters. Mace and Rabins' (1981) classic work, THE 36-HOUR DAY, gives us a starting point from which to examined this discrepancy. They report that Alzheimer's makes a victim of the family as well as the patient because of the enormous physical and emotional toll disease takes on caregivers. They also stress that families need respite care to relieve the feeling that they "just can't go another day" caring for the patient. Although Daughter (No. 1) is her mother's only child and primary caregiver, she has organized an effective support system including hiring an LPN to help care for the proband on a weekly basis, particularly to bathe her. She and her husband have also worked out a system of packaging the proband's medication for her arthritis in plastic pouches and taping her daily dosage to a calendar which the proband checks every day (see Figure 1). Other family members, friends, and neighbors, as well as her spouse and children (Nos. 2-6), aid her in the physical and emotional burden of caring for her mother. It is possible that because the primary caregiver is not overburdened, and because the proband is currently comfortable and stable in her own apartment, Daughter does not perceive her mother's illness to be as advanced as do other raters. Indeed, on my first home visit she remarked, "We're so relieved to know that mother has Alzheimer's. At least now we know what it is."

The entire Lancaster family agreed that one of the most stressful periods in the history of the illness and its impact on the family was the year prior to May, 1984--before the diagnosis of DAT was made. Daughter

Table 1. Psychological Assessment of Three Generations of Family Members

No.	Family Member	Age	Sex	Physician Report	MMPI	Questionnaire	Self Report	Family Report	Psychological Interview	Participant Observation
				Source of Data						
	Lancaster Family:									
1	Proband	81	F	X			0	X	X	X
2	Adult Child†	49	F			0	0	0	0	0
3	Spouse	54	M				0		0	0
4	Grandchild	27	F				0		0	0
5	Grandchild	26	F					0		
6	Grandchild	21	F				0	0	0	0
7	Grandchild	19	M				0	0	0	0
	Oswald Family:									
8	Proband	72	F	X			0	X	X	X
9	Spouse	75	M	X	X	X	X	0	X	X
10	Adult child	46	M		X	0	0	X	X	X
11	Spouse	38	F	X	X	X	X	X	X	X
12	Grandchild	23	F		X	0		X		
13	Grandchild	21	M		X	0		0		
14	Adult child†	39	M		0	0	0	0	0	0

X Significant psychological disturbance
0 Emotional distress
† Informant in case study

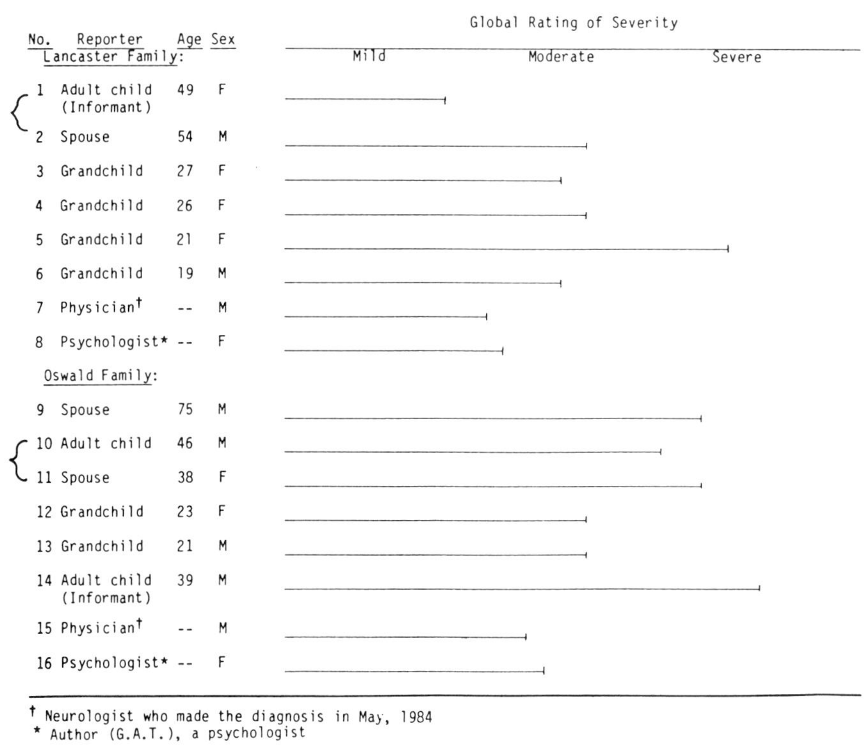

† Neurologist who made the diagnosis in May, 1984
* Author (G.A.T.), a psychologist

Figure 3. Severity of Alzheimer's Disease in Proband As Reported By Three Generations of Family Members, Physician, and Psychologist

vividly recalled that prior to the diagnosis, a critical incident occurred which "forced" family members to acknowledge to themselves that "...something was terribly wrong with grandma..." The critical event revolved around the wedding of the proband's eldest grandaughter (No. 3), a time daughter pointed out when the proband clearly illustrated that she could no longer dress herself appropriately or join in festivities in a socially acceptable manner. "Her failing memory became obvious to everyone...Before the wedding, we just all made excuses for her behavior." Daughter also recalled her anger at the family physician from whom she had sought help prior to this critical incident; she felt that he had abruptly dismissed her concerns about the proband's failing memory as "just a normal part of old age."

Grandaughter No. 5 gave me a clue as to why she perceived her grandmother's illness as quite severe during one home visit when I participated in a Sunday family brunch. The informant and her husband (Nos. 1-2) were hosts for this event at which all the grandchildren (Nos. 4-6) except No. 3 (who lives out of town) were present to help with the study and to review a rough draft of the Lancaster family pedigree. As the family discussion proceeded around the breakfast table, grandaughter No. 5 remarked, "I guess I know now that we have it good! I was talking to my friend the other day and found out that her grandmother has got Alzheimer's, too. But she is really a basketcase...they have her living at home with them." The grandchild continued to clarify that she thought that her grandma was pretty "bad off" until her friend educated her about the progressive nature of the disease.

This incident is reminicent of Mace and Rabins' (1981) suggestion that providing families with information about the disease and its ramifications is one of the greatest needs of Alzheimer's families so that they can plan for the patient's future needs. Knowing what to expect may help relieve anxiety.

The Oswald family's rating of the severity of the proband's illness presents a markedly different picture from the Lancaster family. The most severe ratings of the patient's illness were made by her spouse (No. 9), who is also her sole caregiver; her youngest son (No. 14), who lives 600 miles away and sees his family about four times a year; and her daughter-in-law (No. 11), who lives nearby with the patient's eldest son and their two adult children (Nos. 12-13). The daughter-in-law describes her husband and her brother-in-law as "...completely turning their backs on their responsibility to their mother and leaving it all their stepfather." She concurred with both sons' report that they were never close to their mother while they were growing up and have "no real relationship" with her as adults. The daughter-in-law also noted that the proband was never close to her grandchildren, even though they have always lived in nearby neighborhoods. She also concurred with the sons that while their stepfather was a very decent and sensitive man, he could never replace their "real" father.

Much like the Lancaster family described earlier, a critical incident also occurred in the Oswald family history which "forced" the proband's husband to acknowledge to himself that something was terribly wrong with his wife and to seek a medical opinion. Whereas the Lancaster family took the proband to a neurologist, Mr. Oswald took the proband to a psychiatrist. Mr. Oswald recalled vividly the psychiatrist calling him into his office while his wife waited outside: "He told me outright that there was nothing he could do for my wife...that she probably had dementia...and that he would like to refer her for a complete medical examination." Unlike the Lancaster family, who reported being relieved at the diagnosis, the proband's husband and two sons stressed their feelings of loss and anger.

In contrast to the Lancaster family, the Oswalds were extremely knowledgable about the progressive nature of Alzheimer's and the enormous demands that caring for the proband was placing on her spouse. In spite of this awareness, both sons and the daughter-in-law steadfastly maintained that they "...would stay out of it unless he asks for our two cents." Indeed, on the airplane flight home from a visit to the proband, the younger son asked the author if she thought that he was justified in considering his mother "gone" and best to leave the details to his step-dad.

In thinking about the foregoing data, I could not help but be struck by Freud's "Mourning and Melancholia" (1957) in which he hypothesized that grieving might become melancholia if the lost object was too ambivalently cathected and hostility to the object was unconscious. The proband's sons, although thinking of themselves as faithful and dutiful--if not loving sons--made statements to indicate that they had "stored up" decades of resentment against their mother for real and imagined transgressions. This resentment and, perhaps guilt, contributed to their selective assessment of the proband's condition (and no doubt affected their own emotional state, which is discussed in the following section).

Like his stepsons, Mr. Oswald (No. 9) had ambivalent feelings about his wife, whom he married when he was in his fifties. "I swear that she had Alzheimer's right after we were married," he confided in me. "She was so emotional and unpredicable then, and its just gotten worse in recent years." Embarrassed perhaps by his outburst, Mr. Oswald stressed that he felt duty and honor-bound to take care of his wife in their own home until he could no longer care for her. He was conflicted, however, because the proband's physician had told him that very week that his own blood pressure was very high and that "it wouldn't help his wife if he were to have a heart attack taking care of her." The physician also indicated his concern about Mr. Oswald's own emotional state, as well as his physical well being. Mr. Oswald described himself as "depressed and angry" about the situation.

Goldman and Luchins (1984) point out in their article on depression in spouses of Alzheimer's patients that "because of the progressive loss of intellectual function, and, often, of personality in demented individuals, the impact on the family has been characterized as similar to bereavement." Perhaps the burden of reversing roles and having to care for his ailing wife had become excessive for Mr. Oswald.

Psychological Assessment of Three Generations of Family Members in Two Alzheimer's Families

As illustrated in Table 1, the intensity of psychological distress is high in both families in this study. Table 1 is for descriptive purposes only; no causal relationships are implied. Family members were assessed by the measures in Table 1 as to whether or not they were experiencing "significant psychological disturbance" (SPD), "emotional distress" (ED), both or neither. SPD is operationally defined as an emotional state meeting American Psychiatric Association (1980) DSM-III criteria for a psychiatric diagnosis. ED is operationally defined as an emotional state not meeting American Psychiatric Association DSM-III criteria for a psychiatric diagnosis, but nonetheless distressing.

"Family Report" refers to comments made by a family member about another member's emotional state. An example from the Lancaster family illustrates this type of interchange: the informant and her spouse were describing the two-hour round trip by automobile which the informant makes at least weekly to visit and care the proband. Her spouse volunteered that this trip was becoming increasing stressful for his wife; she was always worried about what condition she would find her mother in when she got there. He added, "At least the phone calls at all hours of the night have stopped; they were really upsetting for _______________. It was often difficult for her to get back to sleep."

As indicated in Table 1, every family member in both families experienced SPD or ED. I regard the reported distress as minimal. The implications for mental health professionals who care for Alzheimer's patients are clear: Routine inquiries should be made emotional state, particularly mood, in caregivers and other family members. Goldman and Luchins (1984) suggest that treatment of such distress not only relieves the suffering of affected family members; it also enhances the care they can provide for the dementia patient.

DISCUSSION

A salient feature of these two case histories is the incidence and nature of the variance within and between families regarding the impact of having a close genetic relative with DAT. It is also notable that, in agreement with Mace and Rabins (1981), findings suggest that "Alzheimer's makes a victim of the family as well as the patient because of the enormous emotional and physical toll this disease takes on the caregiver." The evidence suggests that all family members experienced some degree of psychological distress with marked exacerbations in some family members.

The findings may, of course, be interpreted differently and organized into any number of theoretical frameworks. Taken alone they are certainly not definitive. Future studies might address these questions: How does the impact of DAT on family members compare to the impact of other chronic diseases (for example, rheumatoid arthritis, Huntington's chorea, or cancer)? How does the level of emotional distress in family members interface with the impact of DAT on the family? Are there common critical events which confront DAT families? If so, what role do they play? How does the presence or absence of familial versus non-familial DAT impact on the family? And finally, what methods are best suited to study the impact of DAT on the family? These and other worthy questions remain to be investigated.

REFERENCES

Clayton, P.J., November 9, 1984, personal communication, Minneapolis, University of Minnesota Hospitals.

Diagnostic and Statistical Manual of Mental Disorders (Third Edition), 1980, American Psychiatric Association, Washington, D.C.

Goldman, L.S. and Luchins, D.J., 1984, Depression in the spouses of demented patients, Am J Psychiatry 141:11.

Hathaway, S.E. and McKinley, J.C., 1943, Minnesota Multiphasic Personality Inventory Manual, The Psychological Corporation, New York.

Heston, L.L., November 9, 1984, personal communication , Minneapolis, University of Minnesota Hospitals.

Heston, L.L. and White, J.A., 1983, Dementia: A Practical Guide to Alzheimer's and related diseases, Freeman, San Francisco.
Knopman, D., November 9, 1984, personal communication, Minneapolis, University of Minnesota Hospitals.
Mace, N.L. and Rabins, P.V., 1981, The 36-hour Day, The Johns Hopkins University Press, Baltimore.
Martinson, I., 1984, Unpublished manuscript, San Francisco, University of California.
Reisberg, B., 1983, A Guide to Alzheimer's Disease, The Free Press, New York.
Reisberg, B., Ferris, S.H., DeLeon, M.J. and Crook, T., 1982, The global deterioration scale for assessment of primary degenerative dementia, Am J Psychiatry 139:9.

BIOLOGICAL MARKERS FOR ALZHEIMER'S DISEASE

John Blass, Andrea Baker, Arthur Balin, Laurie Barclay
Gary Gibson, Christine Peterson, and Neil Sims

Cornell Medical College and Rockefeller University
Burke Rehabilitation Center, 785 Mamaroneck Ave
White Plains, NY 10605

INTRODUCTION

The classical biological marker for Alzheimer disease is that originally described by Alois Alzheimer: the histological appearance of the cortex, nowadays defined precisely in terms of numbers of the characteristic plaques and tangles in appropriate regions of brain (McKahn et al., 1984). The other widely accepted marker at the present time is deficiency of cholinergic markers in affected cortex, notably choline acetyltransferase (CAT) activity (Bowen et al., 1982). Neither, however, is entirely specific for Alzheimer disease. We and others have seen brains at autopsy which contained the requisite numbers of plaques and tangles but which came from people who were clinically clearly not demented at the time they died (Ulrich, 1985). A number of groups have demonstrated profound cholinergic deficiencies and even damage to the nucleus basalis complex in patients who had dementing syndromes other than Alzheimer disease (Arendt et al., 1983). The first observation may reflect "preclinical disease," and the second the importance of cholinergic systems in a variety of dementias. It is important to note, however, that neither of these accepted biological markers of Alzheimer disease would turn out to be "specific" if they were to be tested in conventional prospective studies. Their importance is their meaning in the appropriate clinical context and their relevance to the pathophysiology of the disorder (Perry et al., 1978). Biological "markers" in other areas of medicine have analogously complex relations to the disorders with which they are associated. Diabetes is not the only condition in which blood sugar is elevated; Tay-Sachs disease is not the only clinical condition associated with a genetic deficiency of hexosaminidase A (Johnson, 1981). Indeed, hexosaminidase A deficiency has even been reported in a few clinically normal people (Navon et al., 1976). Both of these abnormalities are, however, clearly important and diagnostically useful in the appropriate clinical context, because they relate directly to the pathophysiology of the specific disorder with which they are associated.

The search for other biological markers for Alzheimer disease is thus a search for pathophysiologically significant changes which can be meaningfully interpreted in the context of the clinical syndrome. Other articles in this volume discuss biological changes in the nervous system and cerebrospinal fluid of patients with Alzheimer disease, and these topics will not be covered systematically here. This discussion focusses on potential biological markers or more precisely on possible leads to the discovery of potential biological markers in non-neural tissues.

OBSERVATIONS

Plasma/Serum

Two groups have reported increases in cholinesterase activity in Alzheimer serum relative to controls (Smith et al., 1982b; Perry et al., 1982). The enzyme involved is presumably a pseudocholinesterase, and the relationship of these changes to changes in the cholinergic compartment of the brain remain to be elucidated. It would be particularly interesting to examine the relationship, if any, between the elevation of the plasma activity and the loss of the intermediate form of cholinesterase from Alzheimer brain reported by Atack et al. (1983).

In searching for possible clues to mechanisms in Alzheimer disease, we have examined the levels of amino acids in serum. The only statistically significant change was a slight elevation in serume alanine (Table 1). There was a tendency for ratios of glutamine/glutamate to be slightly elevated, but this did not reach statistical significance.

Table 1: Amino Acids in Alzheimer and Control Sera

	Number	Alanine	Glutamine/Glutamate
Controls	26	341 ± 19	7.8 ± 0.8
Alzheimer	20	408 ± 17*	9.5 ± 0.6

(Values are mean ± SEM; *, P<0.05.)

The controls include patients with other types of dementia including multi-infarct dementia. These values were gathered prospectively, but the subjects were not under dietary control. The obvious follow-up is to measure blood ammonia and pyruvate and lactate. Prospective studies now underway at our institution suggest that pyruvate dose tend to be elevated in the blood of patients with Alzheimer disease, and ammonia more variably so. Gottfries et al (1974) have reported elevations of lactate in the CSF of some Alzheimer patients, and Adolfson et al (1980) reported accelerated clearance of infused glucose from the blood of Alzheimer patients. These findings are, of course, not specific, but they do agree with other evidence discussed below that an abnormality in carbohydrate catabolism may occur in a subgroup of Alzheimer patients.

Red Blood Cells

There are at least nine reports of abnormalities in RBC from patients with Alzheimer disease. They cluster into two groups, one indicating some sort of membrane abnormality and the other suggesting an abnormality of choline metabolism. The first report, [which proposed the "possibility that this disorder may have more widespread membrane involvement than was originally thought]," was by Markesbery et al (1980). They described alterations in the electron spin resonance signal from a particular probe (MAL-6) in RBC ghosts from patients with Alzheimer disease. Subsequent studies have reported an increase in Na-Li countertransport (Diamond et al., 1983) and an impairment of ouabain binding (McHarg et al., 1983). Both Chipperfield et al. (1981) and Perry et al (1982) reported decreases in RBC cholinesterase activities (although these were not found by Markesbery et al., 1980). Three groups have reported increases in RBC choline content in at least a subgroup of patients with Alzheimer disease (Friedman et al., 1981; Hanin et al., 1984; Blass et al., in press).

These may relate to a decrease in choline efflux (Butterfield et al., 1984) rather than to an increase in choline influx (Sherman et al., unpublished). There are a variety of speculative mechanims by which one could relate the alterations in membranes and in choline metabolism, and no evidence to choose among them at present.

Although we suspect the alterations in choline levels are at best a soft marker for more important changes, it was interesting to see if the Alzheimer patients with high choline values differed significantly from those with normal RBC cholines. In the Burke series, elevations of RBC choline above 2.8 were associated with less severe cognitive impairment and fewer neurological abnormalities but with a signficantly greater prevalence of family history of dementia: 65% vs 32%, $P<0.01$ (Barclay et al., 1985). Whether or how the RBC abnormalities might relate to a genetic predisposition to Alzheimer disease is completely unknown.

Platelets

A recent brief report by Zubenko et al (1984) indicated the existence of a membrane abnormality in Alzheimer disease platelets as well - specifically, in the repolarization of a fluorescent hexatriene membrane probe. Two other reports of platelet abnormalities concern subtle changes in enzyme activities (Smith et al., 1982a; Blass and Zemcov, 1984).

Lymphocytes

At least four reports indicate aberrations in chromosomal stability in Alzheimer disease lymphocytes (Nordenson et al., 1980; Moorehead and Heyman, 1983; Robbins et al., 1983; Fishman et al., 1984). Whether or not these changes in lymphocytes might relate in some way to the alterations in chromatin structure recently reported in Alzheimer brain (Crapper-McLachlan et al., 1984) is entirely conjectural. There are other reports of functional abnormalities of lymphocyte functions in Alzheimer patients (Miller et al., 1981; Kraus, 1983), but these have not been independently confirmed.

Granulocytes

Jarvik et al. (12) reported that leukocytes from Alzheimer patients move less in response to heat than do control cells. In subsequent studies they suggested that this effect was due to a factor in Alzheimer serum (Matsuyama et al., 1983). These studies have also not yet been independently confirmed.

Fibroblasts

Cultured cells including skin fibroblasts provide a useful tool for studying diseases with a genetic component. They are a standard tool for molecular biological studies at the level of DNA, and permanent cultures of lymphocytes and cultures of fibroblasts are being accumulated from patients with familial forms of Alzheimer disease at the Mutant Genetic Cell Repository specifically to be available for such studies. In those cases where the gene product is expressed in the cells in culture, they can also be used to study the cellular pathophysiology of the disorder. Identification of such cellular abnormalities can be critical for two reasons. A number of genetic disorders are known - certain thalassemias being the classic examples - in which a variety of changes at the DNA level lead to changes in a single protein. In such disorders, knowledge of the gene product is very helpful in working out the molecular genetic abnormalities. Furthermore, identification of the aberrant gene product(s) may have relatively direct implications for unravelling the cellular pathophysiology and therefore potentially for designing rational interventions. Mapping of the human genome has not yet reached the point where one can often hope to identify the gene product from identification of a linkage marker or even of the gene itself. A number of recent studies indicate that Alzheimer disease has an important genetic component in a significant proportion of patients (Larsson et al., 1965; Breitner and Folstein, 1984; Barclay et al., this volume). If the gene is expressed in cultured fibroblasts, they will provide a particularly useful tool for studying this age-related disease, since the cultured skin fibroblast is a classical tool for investigating the cell biology of human aging (Cristofalo, 1975; Schneider and Mitsui, 1976).

Several brief reports over the last decade have indicated the existence of subtle abnormalities in Alzheimer disease fibroblasts, but none has as yet proven readily reproducible. Andia-Waltenbaugh and Puck (1977) proposed the existence of a microtubular defect, but Harper et al (1979) using different methods failed to confirm it. We reported a deficiency in the activity of the enzyme phosphofructokinase (PFK) in Alzheimer disease fibroblasts (Sorbi and Blass, 1983) but subsequent studies indicated that this change was at best a soft marker for some other more fundamental abnormality in the patient cells (Kseziak-Reding and Blass, in preparation). Moshowitz et al. (1983) reported a decreased response to interferon in some Alzheimer cells, but this finding has not been extended or independently confirmed.

Recent studies do, however, continue to indicate the existence of subtle but potentially significant abnormalities in Alzheimer fibroblasts. Two are of particular interest because they might prove to be related to changes which might be of importance in the brain (Table 2).

Table 2: Alterations in Alzheimer Disease Fibroblasts.

	^{45}Ca Uptake	$^{14}CO_2$ Production
Controls (6)	0.17 $\pm$ 0.01	21 $\pm$ 1
Alzheimer (6)	0.11 $\pm$ 0.01*	29 $\pm$ 3*

(Values are mean $\pm$ SEM of the number of lines indicated in parentheses; *, $p<0.05$.)

The decrease in uptake of radioactive calcium was specifically in the portion taken up into the cells, not in superficial binding (Peterson et al., in press). Since a number of workers have proposed that alterations in cellular calcium homeostasis may play a critical role in the development of Alzheimer disease (Khachaturian, 1984; Gibson and Peterson, 1982; Sheu et al., in press), emphasizing the potential pathophysiological importance of such a change. The increase in oxidation of [U-^{14}C]glucose to $^{14}CO_2$ in the fibroblasts parallels a change reported by Sims et al. (1983) in Alzheimer brain biopsies, suggesting that changes in carbohydrate catabolism in the brain in this disease not only reflect the pathophysiology but may be an inherent cellular characteristic of this disorder (Blass and Zemcov, 1984).

One possible mechanistic link between these two abnormalities could be some form of inherent mitochondrial abnormality. Mitochondria carry out oxidative metabolism and also play a key role in the maintenance of intracellular calcium homeostasis. In brain, mitochondrial calcium pumping seems closely linked to the utilization of pyruvate (Baudry et al., 1983). These considerations and others led us to study the pyruvate dehydrogenase complex (PDHC) as a mitochondrial marker in Alzheimer disease fibroblasts. Previous studies indicated that PDHC was of reduced activity but normal structure in both affected and unaffected areas of

Alzheimer cortex (Sheu et al., in press) and in two studies, of normal activity in Alzheimer fibroblasts (Sorbi et al., 1983). More recent studies have indicated that this mitochondrial marker may, indeed, be reduced in Alzheimer fibroblasts studied under conditions chosen to bring out mitochondrial abnormalities (Table 3).

Table 3: Pyruvate Dehydrogenase Complex Activity in Fibroblasts

Alzheimer	2.6 ± 0.9 (7)
Control	5.3 ± 0.3 (17)

(Values are mean nmol/min/mg protein ± SEM; P<0.001.)

Again, what makes this result of some interest is the parallel to the changes found in the brain. Of course, all these results need to be extended and independently confirmed before much can be made of them.

One of the questions which has concerned students of Alzheimer disease ever since his original report is whether or not this disease can usefully be considered a form of accelerated aging (Alzheimer, 1911). This question can be phrased more precisely as whether or not Alzheimer disease is a form of generalized accelerated cellular aging. The cells which die prematurely in the nervous system could be said to have "aged" prematurely, but the same could be said of the neurones which die prematurely in any degenerative disease of the nervous system, including diseases of early adult life. This question can be approached usefully with cultured skin fibroblasts, since their replicative capacity is perhaps the most widely accepted marker of human biological age (Schneider et al., 1976). Recent studies at both Burke and the Rockefeller Institute indicated that the time until phase out, ability of cells to incorporate tritiated thymidine (Cristofalo index), and growth curves were the same in Alzheimer cells and controls matched for chronological age and for passage number (Table 4).

Table 4: Properties of Fibroblasts

	Control	Alzheimer
Number	4	4
Chronological age	66 ± 7	66 ± 6
Female:Male	3:1	3:1
Cristafolo index	30 ± 5	27 ± 8
Passages to phase out	14.5 ± 1.8	17 ± 2.0

While these studies were done with relatively few cell lines, they suggest strongly that whatever else Alzheimer disease may be, it is not a form of <u>generalized</u> accelerated cell aging. This conclusion is in agreement with the common clinical observation that in the earlier stages of their course, patients with Alzheimer disease often look if anything young for their age and in robust general health. These patients do look prematurely old in the latter stages of their illness, when they are deathly ill. The results in Table 4 also indicate that age-,sex-, and passage-matched control cells are appropriate controls for Alzheimer fibroblasts. Differences observed between control and patient cultures can be attributed to the disease rather than to the Alzheimer cells being "physiologically older."

IMPLICATIONS

The search for biological markers in Alzheimer disease has several goals. These include at least defining diagnostically useful measurements, providing information about the pathophysiology of the disorder, and guiding further research.

The study of non-neural tissues has not yet achieved signal advances toward the first goal. None of the changes described so far and no combination of them appear specific enough for Alzheimer disease to seem diagnostically useful.

The multiple abnormalities described in non-neural tissues do, however, have implications for the pathophysiology of Alzheimer disease. So many have now been described that it is fair to say that at the cellular level, Alzheimer disease has systemic manifestations. This is one of several lines of evidence that have led to the suggestion that Alzheimer disease may meaningfully be considered a systemic disease (Nordenson et al., 1980; Markesbery et al., 1980; Blass and Zemcov, 1984). Another is the evidence that the major risk factor for Alzheimer disease is genetic, in several populations (Larsson et al., 1963; Breitner and Folstein, 1984; Heyman et al., 1984; Barclay et al., this volume). The aberrant gene(s) must exist in every cell at some stage of its development, even in the precursor cells of mature erythrocytes and platelets. The issue then becomes not whether nonneural cells are "abnormal" at the molecular level, but the extent to which the gene(s) of interest express. The third type of evidence is entirely clinical. It is the profound weight loss which frequently accompanies the later stages of Alzheimer disease, even in patients in favored economic and social circumstances who are fed a more than adequate diet by devoted and often well-paid caretakers. The combination of adequate or excessive caloric intake with weight loss in the absence of malabsorption suggests inefficient utilization of calories or, at the cellular level, mitochondrial uncoupling.

The implication of these studies for further research is that readily available non-neural cells including cultured cells provide a valid tool for studying the fundamental cellular abnormalities in Alzheimer disease. Indeed, they have the advantage that alterations which persist in anatomically normal structures and particularly in culture can not be attributed to secondary effects of the disease or of toxins, drugs, or "malnutrition" (Blass et al., 1977). Two caveats should, however, promptly be raised. The first is that changes in peripheral tissues are obviously of interest only if they can be related to changes in the tissue responsible for the clinical illness, namely the brain. The changes in fibroblasts discussed above are of interest in large part because they parallel documented or proposed changes in Alzheimer brain. The second caveat is that study of extraneural tissues has had chequered success in the clinical neurosciences. It has proven of great use in the study of mental retardation and of a variety of other neurologically defined syndromes, which have proven on close examination to be related to a series of inborn errors of metabolism (Rowland, 1984). It has as yet provided little useful information in the study of such nosologicaly confused conditions as the schizophrenias (Blass et al., 1977).

The critical question obviously is what the pathophysiologically important changes in Alzheimer cells are. Studies of both red cells and platelets have led to the suggestion that there is a generalized abnormality in membrane transport processes in Alzheimer cells (Markesberry et al., 1980; Zubenko et al., 1984). Other studies including our own have led us to propose an intrinsic abnormality in mitochondria, perhaps relating to calcium accumulation (Sheu et al., in press). These abnormalities may well prove to be secondary to some more fundamental cellular change, but even so they may prove to be pathophysiologically significant. Membrane transport is a particularly critical function of neurones, and the brain shows a second-to-second dependence on efficient carbohydrate oxidation unequalled by any other tissue. Mild uncoupling of mitochondria or some other subtle variant of "histotoxic hypoxia" might well lead to premature death of particular populations of neurones. These considerations have led to a proposal that Alzheimer disease may have characteristics of a systemic metabolic encephalopathy (Blass and Zemcov, 1984; Table 5).

Table 5: Formulation of Alzheimer Disease

Hypothesis 1: Alzheimer disease is a late onset system degeneration, characteristically invo lving cholinergic neurones of the nucleus basalis complex but usually involving other populations of neurones as well.

Hypothesis 2: At least at a molecular level, Alzheimer disease is a systemic disease which can usefully be studied not only by examining brain but also by studying non-neural tissues.

Hypothesis 3: Biologically, Alzheimer disease shares a number of characteristics with metabolic encephalopathies.

Hypothesis 4: Abnormalities in cereberal metabolic rate in Alzheimer disease reflect not only altered neuronal activity but also intrinsic abnormalities in the nerve cells.

CONCLUSION

The "biological markers" which have been described so far in non-neural tissues from Alzheimer patients are not specific for Alzheimer disease and have little if any diagnostic use. They may, however, provide valuable clues to the fundamental cellular pathophysiology of Alzheimer disease. Non-neural tissues may also provide valuable and easily excessible tools for elucidating these processes.

ACKNOWLEDGEMENT

These studies were supported by the Will Rogers Institute, the Altshul Laboratory for Dementia Research, Alzheimer's Disease and Related Disorders Association-Westchester Division, and the National Institute of Aging (NA 03583).

REFERENCES

Adolfson, R., Bucht, G., Liithner, F. and Windblad, B., 1980, Hypoglycemia in Alzheimer's disease, Acat. Med. Scand., 208:387.

Alzheimer, A., 1911, On a unique disease of old age (German), Z. Ges. Neurol. Psychiat., 4:356.

Andia-Waltenbaugh, A.M. and Puck, T.T., 1977, Alzheimer's disease: Further evidence of a microtubule defect, J. Cell Biol., 75:279a.

Ardendt, T., Bigl, V., Arendt, A. Tennstedt, A., 1983, Loss of neurones in the nucleus basalis of Meynert in Alzheimer's disease, paralysis agitans, and Korsakoff's disease, Acta Nauropath (Berl.), 61:101.

Atack, J.R., Perry, E.K., Bonham, J.R., Perry, R.H., Tomlinson, B.E. Blessed, G. and Fairbairn, A., 1983, Molecular forms of acetylcholinesterase in senile dementia of the Alzheimer type: Selective loss of the intermediate (10S) form, Neuroscience Lett., 40:199.

Barclay, L.L., Kheyfets, S., and Zemcov, A., 1985, Red cell/plasma choline as a marker of severity and genetic predisposition in Alzheimer disease, In preparation.

Baudry, M., Gall, C., Kessler, M., Alapour, H. and Lynch, G., 1983, Denervation-induced decrease in mitochondrial calcium transport in rat hippocampus, J. Neurosci., 3:252.

Blass, J.P. and Zemcov, A., 1984, Alzheimer disease - A metabolic systems degeneration? Neurochem. Path., 2:103.

Blass, J.P., Milne, J.A. and Rodnigh, R., 1977, Newer concepts of psychiatric diagnosis and biochemical research on mental illness, Lancet, 1:738.

Blass, J.P., Hanin, I., Barclay, L.L., Kopp, U. and Reding, M.J., 1985, Red blood cell abnormalities in Alzheimer disease, J. Amer. Geriat. Soc., 33:401-405.

Bowen, D.M., Benton, J.S., Spillane, J.A., Smith, C.T.T. and Allen, S.J., 1982, Choline acetyltransferase activity and histopathology of frontal neocortex from biopsies of demented patients, J. Neurol. Sci., 57:191.

Breitner, J.C.S. and Folstein, M.F., 1984, Familial Alzheimer dementia: A prevalent disorder with specific clinical features, Psychol. Med. 14:63.

Butterfield, D.A., Nicholas, M. and Markesbery, W.R., 1984, Decreased rate of choline efflux across erythrocyte membranes in Alzheimer disease, Neurology, 34:S121.

Chipperfield, B., Newman, P.M. and Moyes, I.C.A., 1981, Decreased erythrocyte cholinesterase activity in dementia, Lancet 2:199.

Crapper-McLachlan, D.R., Lewis, P.N., Lukin, W.J., Sima, A., Bergeron, C. and DeBoni, U., 1984, Chromatin structure in dementia, Ann. Neurol., 15:329.

Cristafolo, V.J., 1975, Thymidine labelling index as a criterion of aging in vitro, Gerontologia, 22:9.

Diamond, J.M., Matusyama, S.S., Meier, K. and Jarvik, L.F., 1983, Elevation of erythrocyte countertransport in Alzheimer's dementia, N. Eng. J. Med., 309:161.

Fischman, H.L., Reisberg, B., Albu , P., Ferris, S.H. and Rainer, J.D., 1984, Sister chromatid exchanges and cell cycle kinetics in Alzheimer disease, Biol. Psych. 19:319.

Friedman, E., Sherman, K.A., Ferris, S.H., Reisberg, B., Bartus, R.T. and Schneck, M.K., 1981, Clinical response to choline plus piracetam in senile dementia: relation to red cell choline levels, New Eng. J. Med., 304:1490.

Gibson, G.E. and Peterson, C., 1982, Biochemical and Behavioral Paralels in Aging and Hypoxia, in: "The Aging Brain: Cellular and Molecular Mechanisms of Aging in the Nervous System, E. Giacobini et al., eds, Raven Press, N.Y.)

Hanin, I., Reynolds, C., Kupfer, D.J., Kopp, U., Taska, L.S., Hoch, C.C., Spiker, D.G., Sewitch, D.F., Martin, D., Marin, R.S., Nelson, J.P., Zimmer, B. and Morycz, R., 1984, Elevated red blood cell/plasma choline ratio in dementia of the Alzheimer type: Clinical and polysomnographic correlates, Psychiatry Res., 13:167.

Harper, C.G., Buck, D., Gonatas, N.K., Guilbert, B. and Avrameas, S., 1979, Skin fibroblast microtubule network in Alzheimer's disease, Ann. Neurol., 6:548.

Heyman, A., Wilkinson, W.E., Stafford, J.A., Helms, M.J., Sigmon, A.H. and Weinberg, T., 1984, Alzheimer's disease: A study of epidemiological aspects, Ann. Neurol., 15:335.

Jarvik, L.J., Matsuyama, S.S., Kessler, J.O., Fu, T.K., Tsai, S.Y. and Clark, E.O., 1982, Philothermal response of polymorphonuclear leukocytes in dementia of the Alzheimer type, Neurobiol. Aging, 3:93.

Johnson, W.G., 1981, The clinical spectrum of hexosaminidase deficiencies, Neurology, 31:145.
Khachaturian, Z.S., Towards theories of brain aging, in: "Handbook of Studies on Psychiatry and Old Age", D.W. Kay and G.D. Burrows, eds., Elsevier, New York.
Kraus, L.J., 1983, Decreased natural killer cell activity in Alzheimer disease, Neurosci. Abstr., 9:115.
Larsson, T., Sjogren, T. and Jacobson, G., 1963, Senile dementia - A clinical, sociomedical, and genetic study, Acta Psychiat. Scand., 167:1.
Markesbery, W.R., Leung, P.K. and Butterfield, D.A., 1980, Spin label and biochemical studies of erythrocyte membranes in Alzheimer disease, J. Neurol. Sci., 45:323.
Matsuyama, S.S. and Fu, T.K., 1983, Inhibition of normal polymorphonuclear leukocyte response by serum from dementia of the Alzheimer type patients, Age, 6:72.
McHarg, A., Naylor, G.J. and Ballinger, B.R., 1983, Erythrocyte ouabain binding in dementia, Gerontology, 29:140.
McKhann, G., Drachman, D., Folstein, M., Katzman, R.D., Price, D. and Stadlan, E.M., 1984, Clinical diagnosis of Alzheimer's disease: Report of the NINCDS-ADRDA work group under the auspices of the Department of Health and Human Services Task Force on Alzheimer's disease, Neurology, 34:939.
Miller, A.E., Neighbour, P.A., Katzman, R., Aronson, M. and Lipkowitz, R., 1981, Immunologic studies in senile dementia of the Alzheimer type: Evidence of enhanced suppressor cell activity, Ann. Neurol., 10:506.
Moorhead, P., and Heyman, A., 1983, Chromosome studies of patients with Alzheimer disease, Amer. J. Hum. Genet., 14:545.
Moshowitz, S.L., Dawson, G.J. and Elizan, T.S., 1983, Antiviral response of fibroblasts from familial Alzheimer's disease and Down's syndrome to human interpheron alpha, J. Neural Transmission, 57:121.
Navon, R., Geiger, B., Ben-Yosef, Y. and Rattazzi, M.C., 1976, Low levels of β-hexosaminidase A in health individuals with apparent deficiency of this enzyme, Am. J. Hum. Gen., 28:339.
Nordenson, I., Adolfson, R., Beckman, G., Bucht, G. and Winblad, B., 1980, Chromosomal abnormality in dementia of Alzheimer type, Lancet, 1:481.
Perry, E.K., Tomlinson, B.E., Blessed, G., Bergman, K., Gibson, P.H. and Perry, R.H., 1978, Correlation of cholinergic abnormalities with senile plaques and mental test scores in senile dementia, Brit. Med. J., 2:1457.
Perry, R.H., Wilson, I.D., Bober, M.J., Atack, J., Blessed, G., Tomlinson, B.E. and Perry, E.K., 1982, Plasma and erythrocyte acetylcholinesterase in senile dementia of Alzheimer type, Lancet 1:174.
Peterson, C., Gibson, G.E. and Blass, J.P., 1985, Altered calcium uptake in cultured skin fibroblasts from patients with Alzheimer disease, New. Eng. J. Med. 312:1063.
Robbins, J.H., Otsuka, F., Tarone, R.E., Polinsky, R.J., Brumback, R.A., Moshell, A.N., Nee, L.E., Ganges, M.B. and Cayeux, S.J., 1983, Radiosensitivity in Alzheimer disease and Parkinson disease, Lancet, 1:468.
Rowland, L.P., 1983, Molecular genetics, pseudogenetics, and clinical neurology, Neurology, 33:1179.
Schneider, E.L. and Mitsui, Y., 1976, The relationship between in vitro cellular aging and in vivo human age, Proc. Natl. Acad. Sci. USA, 73-3584.

Sheu, K.F.R., Kim, Y.Y., Blass, J.P. and Weksler, M.E., 1985, An immunochemical study of the pyruvate dehydrogenase deficit in Alzheimer's disease brain, Ann. Neurol. 17:444.

Sims, N., Bowen, D.M., Neary, D. and Davison, A.N., 1983, Metabolic processes in Alzheimer's disease: Adenine nucleotide content and production of $^{14}CO_2$ from [U-14C]glucose *in vitro* in human neocortex, J. Neurochem., 41:1329.

Smith, R.C., Ho, B.T. and Kralik, P., 1982a, Platelet monoamine oxidase in Alzheimer disease, J. Gerontol., 37:572.

Smith, R.C., Ho, B.T., Hsu, L., Vroulis, G., Claghorn, J. and Schoolar, J., 1982b, Cholinesterase enzymes in the blood of patients with Alzheimer disease, Life Sci. 30:543.

Sorbi, S. and Blass, J.P., 1983, Fibroblast phosphofructokinase in Alzheimer disease and Down's syndrome, Banbury Report, 15:297.

Ulrich, J., 1985, Alzheimer changes in nondemented patients younger than sixty-five: Possible early stages of Alzheimer's disease and senile dementia of Alzheimer type, Ann. Neurol., 17:273.

Zubenko, G.S., Cohen, B.M., Growdon, J., and Corkin, S., 1984, Cell membrane abnormality in Alzheimer disease, Lancet, 2:235.

ACETYLCHOLINE METABOLISM IN BRAIN: IS IT REFLECTED BY CSF CHANGES?

Giacobini, E., Becker, R., Elble, R., Mattio, T. and McIlhany, M.

Depts. of Pharmacology, Psychiatry, Medicine and Surgery
Southern Illinois University School of Medicine
Springfield, IL 62708 USA

THE ORIGIN OF ACETYLCHOLINESTERASE IN CEREBRAL SPINAL FLUID (CSF)

The soluble acetylcholinesterase (AChE) which is localized in the cell bodies of cholinergic as well as non-cholinergic neurons (Giacobini, 1959) is transported to the periphery as a mobile fraction by axoplasmic flow at a relatively rapid rate (Lubinska and Niemerko, 1971; Fig. 1). Acetylcholinesterase is also present in peripheral nerve endings of cholinergic neurons (Giacobini, 1959) where it represents 20% of the total neuronal activity as compared to 69% for the cell body and 11% for the axon (Giacobini et al., 1979). Acetylcholinesterase decreases in response

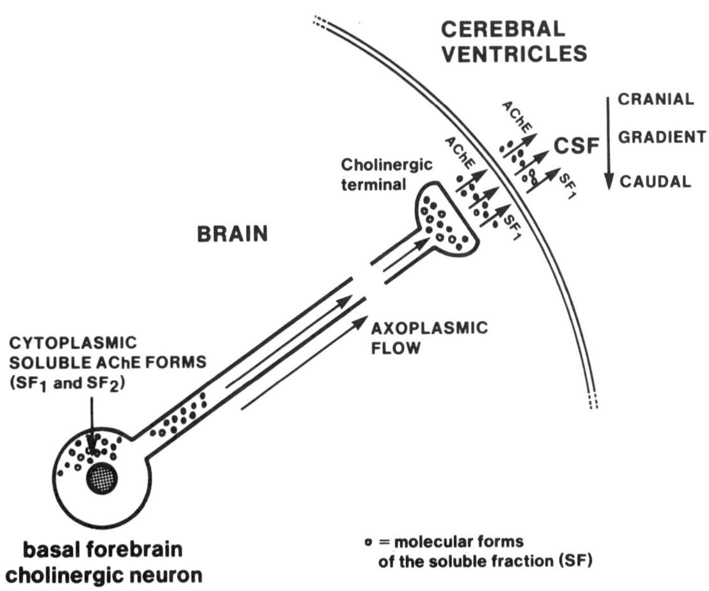

FIGURE 1. Secretory Hypothesis of AChE in Dog CSF (Bareggi and Giacobini, 1978; Scarsella et al, 1979)

Table I
Acetylcholinesterase Activity in CSF and Plasma of the Dog

	Total ChE Activity (µmole ACh hydrol/ml/hr)	AChE Activity (µmole ACh hydrol/ml/hr)	Protein (mg/ml)	AChE specific Activity (µmole ACh hydrol/hr/mg protein
Plasma	42.3 ± 1.4 (3)	9.3 ± 0.2 (3)	53.8 ± 2 (3)	0.17 ± 0.009 (3)
CSF				
Ventricular	2.3	1.2 ± 0.2 (4)*	0.55 ± 0.1 (4)*	2.18 ± 0.2 (4)*
Cisternal		4.4 + 0.3 (6)*	0.68 ± 0.2 (6)*	6.5 ± 2.5 (6)*

All values are mean ± S.E.M. Numbers in parenthesis indicate number of samples. All statistical values in the table are relative to the corresponding plasma value. * $p < 0.1$

to denervation and its levels are regulated by trans-synaptic effects (Giacobini et al., 1979). Its activity has also been demonstrated in extracellular fluids such as plasma and CSF of several species (Augustinsson, 1963) including man (Plattner and Hintner, 1930). Plasma AChE activity in dog is significantly higher than in either ventricular or cisternal CSF (Table I). However, since protein levels in plasma are about 100-fold higher than in CSF, the specific activity of AChE is lower in plasma than in CSF (Bareggi and Giacobini, 1978 and Table I). Acetylcholinesterase activity in plasma represents only 22% of total cholinesterase activity while in ventricular CSF it is about 50%. Scarsella et al. (1979) compared the activity of AChE and butyrylcholinesterase (BuChE) in the cisternal CSF, plasma and brain of beagle dogs and described the characteristics of the molecular forms of both enzymes. Based on their distribution and similarities it was concluded that the single soluble form of AChE present in the CSF corresponds to the slower of the two forms found in the soluble fraction from brain tissue (Fig. 2) and, therefore, it could be expected to be present in the CSF as a result of leakage or secretion from the nervous tissue (Fig. 1). Massoulié and Bon (1982) reported that in normal human subjects only one molecular form of AChE, the globular tetramer G_4 is present. In SDAT (senile dementia of Alzheimer type), Atack et al. (1983) reported a selective loss of the intermediate (10S) form in brain. A combined origin from blood plasma and brain tissue appears to be probable for the BuChE of the CSF. Additional evidence for the neuronal origin of AChE in CSF is the significant increase in AChE specific activity seen by Bareggi and Giacobini (1978) in the CSF following the administration of chlorpromazine (10 mg/kg i.v.), a drug which increases acetylcholine (ACh) turnover and ACh output. Taking these results together, we proposed (Bareggi and Giacobini, 1978) that in the dog, AChE activity present in CSF is mostly of cerebral origin and may reflect changes in neuronal AChE activity. Further evidence for this hypothesis are the findings of Chubb and Smith (1975)in the perfusate from the ox adrenal gland, of Chubb et al. (1974, 1976) in the rabbit CSF and of Gisiger and Vigny (1977) in perfusate from stimulated sympathetic ganglia. As for the origin of the single form of AChE found in blood plasma (Fig. 2) it appears most likely that its source is the CSF while a combined origin from both blood plasma and brain tissue (soluble fraction) appears to be probable for the BuChE of the CSF. Our results have also

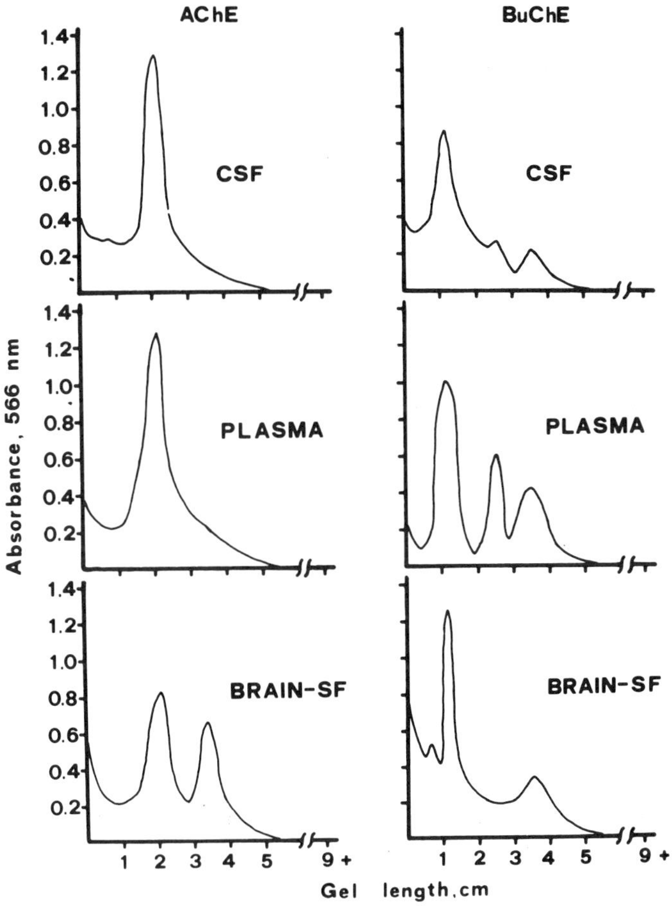

FIGURE 2: Pattern of AChE and BuChE Molecular Forms in Dog CSF, Plasma and Brain (mod. Scarsella et al., 1979)

demonstrated a craniocaudal (i.e. ventricular vs. cisternal) gradient of AChE activity. The gradient reflects the different locations of the sites of AChE input from the brain into CSF (Fig. 1), mostly the lateral and the fourth ventricles and the sites of their secretion from CSF to blood, mostly the subarachnoidal spaces. We suggest that there is a continuous, rather low rate of exit of AChE into the CSF resulting in an accumulation of the soluble enzyme form along the ventricular system (Fig. 1). The demonstration of such a gradient for AChE in canine CSF is in agreement with our hypothesis of a cerebral origin of AChE. In this case, CSF on its way from the lateral ventricles to subarachnoidal spaces would receive a continuous input of AChE from brain tissue.

EFFECT OF ACETYLCHOLINESTERASE INHIBITION ON ACETYLCHOLINESTERASE ACTIVITY IN CSF

In order to further substantiate the validity of our hypothesis, we monitored the levels of AChE activity in dog CSF and plasma following i.v. (intravenous) or i.c.v. (intracerebral ventricular) administration of various doses (20 µg to 1,000 µg) of the cholinesterase inhibitor, physostigmine. Adult male beagle dogs (8-10 kg b.w.) carried an implanted reservoir (Rickam) which communicated with the lateral ventricle through a silastic catheter (Codman). Both single and double reservoirs were used, so that CSF could be sampled or drug injected in the awake, non-anesthetized dog from the same or from the contralateral ventricle. The time of infusion (i.v. or i.c.v.) was 90 seconds. Symptoms of cholinergic hyperactivity and behavior were recorded. Each experiment lasted 24 hrs, during which AChE activity was monitored both in plasma and CSF at fixed intervals.

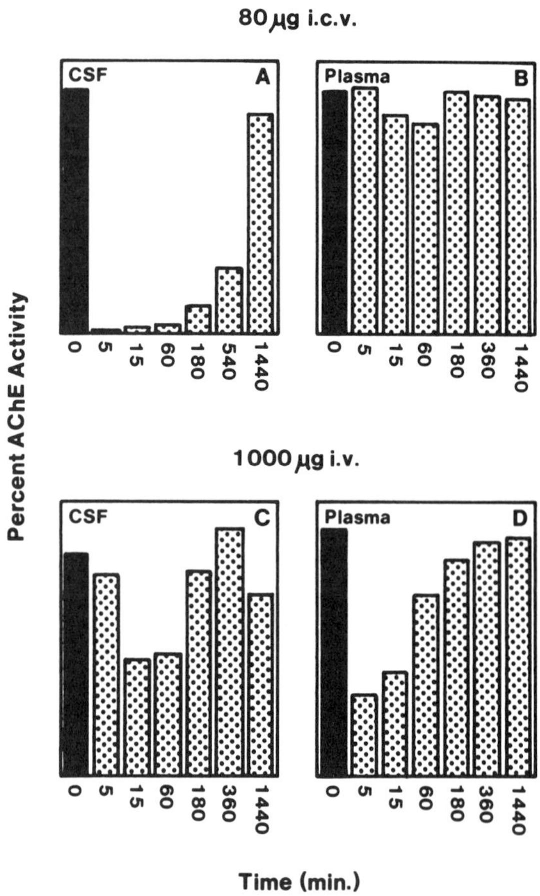

FIGURE 3: Effect of physostigmine on AChE activity of plasma and CSF in the dog. A and B, 80 µg i.c.v.; C and D, 1000 µg i.v. Time 0 (=control) equals 100% of AChE activity.

The effects of two routes of administration (i.c.v. and i.v.) of physostigmine (Phy) on AChE activity in CSF and plasma of dogs are shown in Fig. 3. Acetylcholinesterase activity after 80 µg i.c.v. was reduced more than 90% at 5 min in the CSF (Fig. 3A). At 9 hrs, AChE activity was still 70% inhibited. The CSF showed a steady return of activity with values reaching control level by 24 hrs. Acetylcholinesterase activity in plasma was decreased slightly at 15 and 60 min (Fig. 3B). Two dogs showed symptoms of cholinergic, central and peripheral hyperactivity such as: hypersalivation, laryngospasm, bronchospasm, tremor and hind-leg rigidity. These symptoms appeared at 5 min after injection and lasted 20 min. Two other dogs showed only moderate hypersalivation at this dosage.

Intravenous administration of Phy (1000 µg) produced a different profile of AChE inhibition in CSF and plasma (Fig. 3C,D). Maximal inhibition was seen at 15 min and was 50% of control. By 180 min AChE activity had returned to control values. In plasma, maximal inhibition (65%) was seen at 5 min. Activity in plasma steadily recovered to normal levels at approximately 180-360 min. All four dogs tested showed symptoms of central cholinergic hyperactivity of a less severe degree than with i.c.v. (80 μg) administration. Hypersalivation, laryngospasm, bronchospasm, generalized tremor and rigidity, coughing and sneezing were observed.

The administration of an equivalent dose (100 μg/kg i.v.) in the rat produces a maximal inhibition of brain AChE activity of 64% at 5 min. This is followed by a rapid recovery which will bring the activity back to 90% at 60 min. Plasma BuChE is 50% inhibited at 5 min but is still 40% inhibited at one hour. A six-fold higher dosage of Phy (650 μg/kg i.m.) administered to the rat produces a maximal 75% inhibition of AChE activity and a significant 130-150% increase in ACh levels in brain (Hallak and Giacobini, 1985).

In comparing routes of administration, i.v. was much less effective in reducing AChE activity in CSF than i.c.v. Also the time of AChE inhibition was much longer with the i.c.v. route. Intracerebral administration appears to be the route of choice of Phy, if maximal central AChE inhibition is the goal for the treatment. Also, peripheral symptoms of cholinergic hyperactivity seems to be less severe with i.c.v. than i.v. administration, while the opposite is true for central symptoms.

CHOLINERGIC MARKERS IN THE CSF OF NORMAL ELDERLY AND SDAT PATIENTS

Our longitudinal studies on animals (Giacobini, 1982; Giacobini et al., 1984) have shown that the cholinergic terminal is selectively vulnerable to the process of aging and that presynaptic mechanisms are more affected than postsynaptic ones (Giacobini, 1982). In particular, two membrane-related mechanisms are affected by age. First, an early failure in the uptake mechanism (V_{max}) for choline (Ch) occurs which is followed by a decreased synthesis of ACh. Second, the senescent cholinergic synapse releases, under experimental conditions, significantly less ACh than the adult one (Giacobini et al., 1984). These biochemical data correlate well with the EM morphometric data which demonstrate that two important features for neurotransmitter storage and release, total vesicular volume and appositional membrane, are decreased (Giacobini et al., 1984). These results, obtained in the normal aging animal support the hypothesis that cholinergic transmission is an age-dependent phenomenon which declines in conjunction with increasing age (Giacobini, 1983).

The marked reduction in synaptosomal high affinity Ch transport recently found in SDAT patients by Rylett et al. (1983) could be indicative of degenerative process in cholinergic nerve terminal boutons resulting from an overall decrease in the number of carrier sites per nerve terminal as demonstrated in our experiments in aging animals (Giacobini, 1982, 1983).

Acetylcholinesterase activity in CSF is shown as a function of age in 23 normal control subjects (age range from 3 to 83) in Fig. 4. The figure shows a tendency for the average AChE activity to increase with age. Over the 80 year span, the average AChE activity increases in CSF by a factor of 1.5. This result confirms the finding of Tune et al. (1985).

As shown in Fig. 5C, the mean AChE activity in CSF does not differ between normal age matched controls and early and/or low dementia group patients (Group I, n=9). A slight but clear decrease is seen if the more severe groups of dementia (Groups II, n=5 and III, n=1) are compared with controls. However, the number of patients examined (6) is still too small for allowing any statistical conclusion. With regard to cholineacetyltransferase (ChAc) activity (Fig. 5A), an increase in enzyme activity is seen between normal age matched controls and SDAT patients (Groups I, n=5;

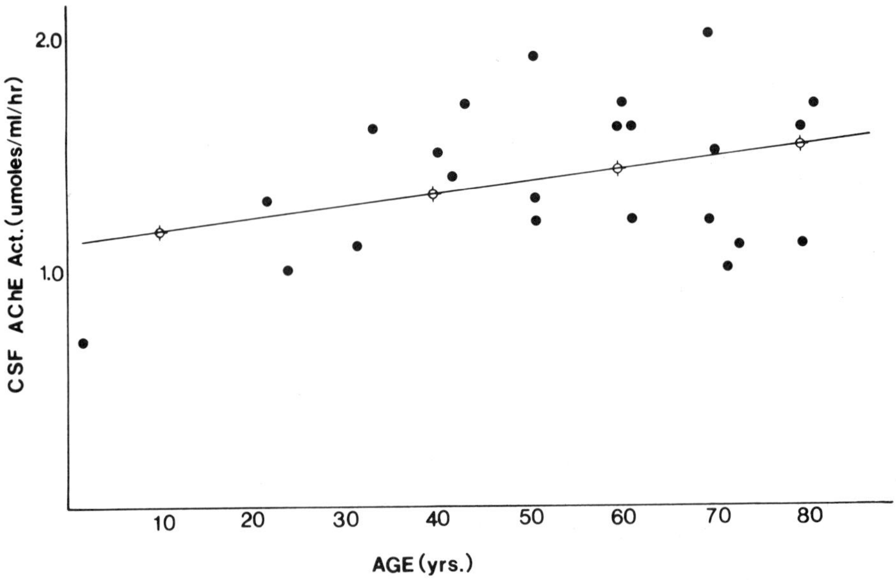

FIGURE 4: AChE Activity in CSF as a Function of Age in Normal Subjects.

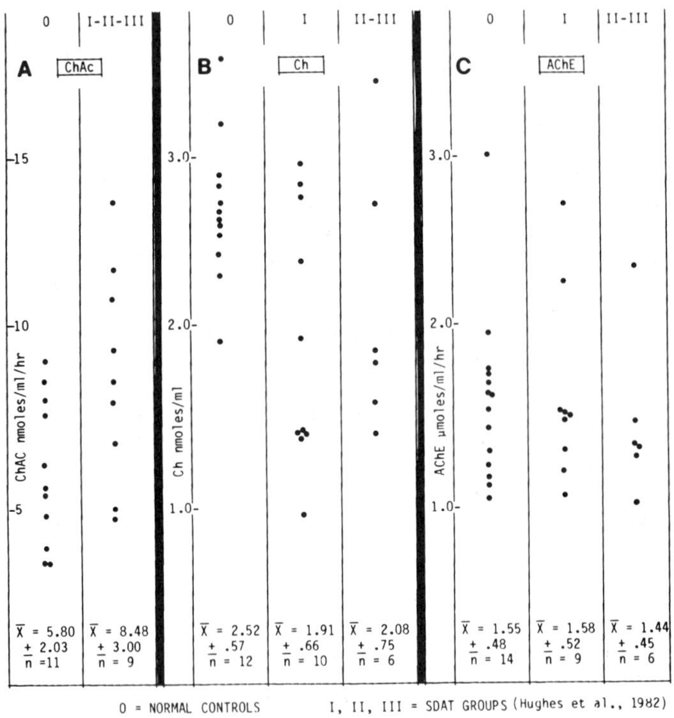

FIGURE 5: AChE and ChAc Activity as well as Ch Levels in CSF of Healthy Age-Matched Controls and SDAT Patients.

II, n=3 and III, n=1 together). Choline (Fig. 5B) by contrast shows a decrease ($p < .01$) when normal controls are compared with Groups I (n=10); II (5=1) and III (n=1) diagnostic categories. These preliminary results from our laboratory indicate that changes in all three CSF parameters studied may occur in SDAT patients. However, it is necessary to extend our study to a larger number of patients to draw any definitive conclusions. The data found in the literature for AChE activity are mainly based on relatively small groups of controls and patients and often no relationship has been established with the grade of severity of the diagnoses and/or with the progression of the disease. Our preliminary results show that when CSF was re-examined in the same patient following a period of one month, the levels of AChE activity were found to be highly reproducible (less than 6% difference). On the other hand, when a larger interval (3-6 months) between CSF analysis was used, indicative changes in one direction, increase for Ch and decrease for ChAc and AChE were seen.

The changes seen in Ch and ChAc after a 3-6 month follow-up may be indicative of the progression of the disease. Measurable ACh levels found by us in the CSF were in the range of 100 to 800 pmole/ml. By using new approaches, we are presently attempting to conclusively determine whether the ACh we have measured in the CSF of both normals and SDAT patients is of CNS origin.

ACKNOWLEDGEMENTS

Supported in part by funds for pilot project from S.I.U. School of Medicine; E.F. Pearson Foundation and S.I.U. Alzheimer Research Fund. The authors gratefully acknowledge the technical skills of Virginia Hoban and Diana Smith for typing the manuscript.

REFERENCES

Atack, J.R., Perry, E.K., Bonham, J.R., Perry, R.H., Tomlinson, B.E., Blessed, G. and Fairbairn, A., 1983, Molecular forms of acetylcholinesterase in senile dementia of Alzheimer type: selective loss of the intermediate (10S) form, Neurosci. Letters, 40:199-204.

Augustinsson, K.B., 1963, Classification and comparative enzymology of the cholinesterases and methods for their determination, Handb. Exp. Pharmakol., 15:89-128.

Bareggi, S.R. and Giacobini, E., 1978, Acetylcholinesterase activity in ventricular and cisternal CSF of dogs, J. Neurosci. Res., 3:335-339.

Chubb, I.W. and Smith, A.D., 1975, Isoenzymes of soluble and membrane-bound acetylcholinesterase in bovine splachnic nerve and adrenal medulla, Proc. R. Soc. Lond. (Biol.), 191:245-261.

Chubb, I.W., Goodman, S. and Smith, A.D., 1974, Increased concentration of an isoenzyme of acetylcholinesterase in rabbit cerebrospinal fluid after peripheral stimulation, J. Physiol. (Lond.), 242:118-120P.

Chubb, I.W., Goodman, S. and Smith, A.D., 1976, Is acetylcholinesterase secreted from central neurons into the cerebrospinal fluid? Neuroscience, 1:57-62.

Giacobini, E., 1959, The distribution and localization of cholinesterases in nerve cells, Acta Physiol. Scand., 45(Suppl 156):1-45.

Giacobini, E., 1982, In: "Aging of the Brain: Molecular and Cellular Mechanisms of Aging", Raven Press, New York, pp. 271-284.

Giacobini, E., 1983, In: "Aging of the Brain", Raven Press, New York, pp. 197-210.

Giacobini, E., Pilar, G., Suszkiw, J. and Uchimura, H., 1979, Normal distribution and denervation changes of neurotransmitter related enzymes in cholinergic neurones, J. Physiol., 286:233-253.

Giacobini, E., Mussini, I. and Mattio, T., 1984, Aging of cholinergic synapses in the avian iris, In: "Developmental Neuroscience: Physiological and Pharmacological Control of Nervous System Development", F. Caciagli, E. Giacobini and R. Paoletti, ed., Elsevier, pp. 89-93.

Gisiger, V. and Vigny, M., 1977, A specific form of acetylcholinesterase is secreted by rat sympathetic ganglia, FEBS Lett., 84:253-256.

Hallak, M.E. and Giacobini, E., 1985, Effects of physostigmine on cholinesterase activity, choline and acetylcholine levels in rat brain, Abst. Intl. Meeting Soc. Neurochem.

Hughes, C.P., Berg, L., Danziger, W.L., Coben, LA. and Martin, R.L., 1982, A new clinical scale for the staging of dementia, Br. J. Psychiatry, 140:566-572, 1982.

Lubinska, L. and Niemerko, S., 1971, Velocity and intensity of bidirectional migration of acetylcholinesterase in transected nerves, Brain Res., 27:329-342.

Massoulié, J. and Bon, S., 1982, The molecular forms of cholinesterase and acetylcholinesterase in vertebrates, Ann. Rev. Neurosci., 5:57-106.

Plattner, F. and Hintner, H., 1930, Die spaltung von acetylcholin durch organextrakte and koperflussigkeiten, Pflug Arch. Ges. Physiol., 225:19-25.

Rylett, R.J., Ball, M.J., Colhoun, E.H., 1983, Evidence for high affinity choline transport in synaptosomes prepared from hippocampus and neocortex of patients with Alzheimer's disease, Brain Res., 289:169-175.

Scarsella, G., Toschi, G., Bareggi, S.R. and Giacobini, E., 1979, Molecular forms of cholinestereases in cerebrospinal fluid, blood plasma, and brain tissue of the beagle dog, J. Neurosci. Res., 4:19-24.

Tune, L., Gucker, S., Folstein, M., Oshida, L. and Coyle, J.R., 1985, Cerebrospinal fluid acetylcholinesterase activity in senile dementia of the Alzheimer type, Ann. Neurol., 17(1):46-48.

ACETYLCHOLINESTERASE ACTIVITY AND SOMATOSTATIN-LIKE IMMUNOREACTIVITY IN LUMBAR CEREBROSPINAL FLUID OF DEMENTED PATIENTS

Gomez S.[1], Davous P.[2], Faivre-Bauman A.[3], Valade D.[2], Jeannin C[2]., Rondot P.[2] and Puymirat J.[2,3]

1 Laboratoire de Biochimie du Pr COHEN, Bd Raspail, Paris France
2 Service de Neurologie du Pr RONDOT, Hôpital Ste-Anne, Paris France
3 Laboratoire de Neuroendocrinologie Cellulaire, Collèoge de France, Paris, France

INTRODUCTION

Recent studies on post-mortem and brain biopsies have provided good evidence for a central cholinergic deficit in presenile and senile dementia of the Alzheimer type (AD/SDAT).(Bowen et al. 1976; Davies 1979).More recent results suggest that the deficit in the central nervous system is not limited to cholinergic neurons. Indeed Somatostatin-like immunoreactivity (SLI) and presynaptic markers of Nor-adrenergic and serotoninergic systems have also been reported to be reduced in post-mortem cerebral cortex from cases of AD/SDAT (Bowen et al.1983; Yates et al. 1983; Araï et al.1984). In contrast, no consistent involvement of Dopaminergic, Gabaergic, Substance P, Vasointestinal peptide (VIP), Thyrotropin-Releasing-Hormone (TRH) and Cholecystokinin (CCK) systems have been found in AD/SDAT(See rev. by Rossor and Emson 1982)

Somatostatin-like immunoreactive material and Acetylcholinesterase (AchE) activities are present in human cerebrospinal fluid (CSF) (Patel et al. 1977; Oram 1981). A reduction of SLI levels in the CSF of AD/SDAT patients, with contradictory results concerning AchE activities have been reported (Davies 1979,Oram et al. 1981;Francis et al.1984, Soininen et al.,1984; Wood et al.1984;;Gomez et al.1985).

In this study, we have measured SLI and AchE in the CSF of documented demented patients.Furthermore, in few cases, we have compared the CSF-SLI and AchE activity levels with the SLI concentration and Choline-acetyl transferase (ChAT) activities in the frontal cortex obtained by biopsy.

PATIENTS

Patients.CSF was obtained by lumbar puncture from 83 subjects, 18 controls and 65 demented patients.

The control group was composed of 10 women (mean age 78.2±4.5 years old) and 8 men (mean age 57.1±5.9).All control patients were non-medicated, presented no sign of cerebral involvement and were hospitalized for neuropathy or functionnal disorders.

The demented patients were divided in three groups:

Group 1: Patients (10 women, 8 men, mean age 61.9±1.2, range 53-70 years), with probable Alzheimer's disease (AD) were studied. Diagnosis was established from Hachinsky score, DMS III criteria, normal metabolite and spinal fluid studies, C.T scan showing diffuse cerebral atrophy. In two cases , the diagnosis was established by cerebral biopsy. All the patients had complete neuropsychological evaluation including mental status questionnaire(M.S.Q), simple reaction time, verbal memory and evolutionnal tests, and when possible, psychometric evaluation by Wechsler memory H.Q and Raven matrices P.M 38 or P.M 47. Global disability was evaluated on a scale scored from 0 to 24 maximum.10 patients received neuroleptics, 8 were free of treatment.

Group 2: 37 patients(women only, mean age 85, range 71 to 91 years), with senile dementia of the Alzheimer type (SDAT) were studied. In this group, the diagnosis was based on clinical grounds: early appearance of memory disorders, presence of aphasia and apraxia, progressive course (more than 7 years) of followed up, lack of focal neurological sign, lack of hypertension or coronary heart disease. Hachinsky score was 4 or less. All patients were free of treatment.

Group3: 5 patients (4 females ,1 male,mean age:71.8±8.4 years old) with the diagnosis of Multi Infarctus Dementia (MID).The diagnosis was based on clinical grounds,C.T. scan.All have an Hachinski score of $\geqslant 6$

Lumbar puncture.

All lumbar punctures were performed between 9 and 10 a.m in patients in the sitting position after an overnight fast and 8 hours of bed rest. The punctures were made between the 3rd and the 4th, or between the 4th and the 5th vertebras.10 ml CSF were collected in 1 ml HCL 1N,for SLI determination;the next ml was collected in a dry tube for AChE assay.All the samples were stored at -20°C until assay.An aliquot was used for determination of total protein, cell count and immunoglobulin.Specimen blood stained containing more than 50 red cells/mm^3 were discarded.

Tissue samples:Samples of right frontal cerebral cortex with underlying white matter were removed from 7 patients after craniotomy and divided for histological and biochemical analysis. Two female patients, 57 and 58 years old had an history of rapid progressive dementia without significant atrophy on C.T scan. Typical changes of histopathological examination confirmed the clinical diagnosis of Alzheimer's disease. One male patient , 34 years old had a history of subacute dementia during 8 months followed by myoclonia, ataxia,and incontinence. EEG was grossly abnormal but did not show any periodic activity. C.T scan was normal. Pathological examination revealed spongiosis typical of Creutzfeldt-Jakob disease. The fourth patient , 32 years old,had a typical depression since 3 months when appeared limb apraxia and memory disturbances. His condition quickly deteriorated with epileptic fits and incontinence. AIDS was suspected on immunological data. Pathological examination confirmed a multifocal progressive leucoencephalopathy and cerebral toxoplasmosis.The fifth patient,69 years old,had an history of familial dementia with sub-cortical lesions at histological level. The two last patients were men operated for a metastatic tumor located in the right frontal cerebral cortex and served as control.

Tissues were divided into aliquots and immediately frozen in liquid nitrogen. For SLI determination, brain tissues were homogenized in H Cl 0.1N. The extracts were centrifugated for 1 hour at 100,000g in a SW 50 Rotor (Beckman L 50) and the supernatant was tested for SLI. For ChAT assay, brain tissue was homogenized in Phosphate buffer 10mM pH 7.4 containing Triton X100 0.2%. The extracts were centrifugated for 10 min. at 15,000g and an aliquot of the supernatant was used for the assay.

Permission for diagnosis biopsies was obtained in all cases after informed consent of the families.

METHODS

Somatostatin radioimmunoassay. RIA of immunoreactive Somatostatin was performed as described previously using an antisomatostatin antiserum (36-38), ^{125}I-Tyr-0-S-14 and synthetic standard S-14 (Gomez et al 1985)The sensitivity was around 3pg and the sensibility 15pg.

Cholinergic markers assay. Acetylcholinesterase activity was measured by the colorimetric assay of Ellman et al (1961).The specificity of the reaction was studied using BW 284 C51 10^{-5}M as a specific inhibitor of Acetylcholinesterase and Ethopropazine (10^{-5}M) as a specific inhibitor of Butyrylcholinesterase, (Gomez et al. 1985). Choline-acetylTransferase activity was determined according to the technique of Fonnum (1975).

Protein were determined by the method of Lowry et al (1951). Results are expressed as mean ± SEM. Student's t test was used for statistical analysis.

RESULTS

Total Cholinesterase activity (ChE) present in human CSF was essentially Acetyl Cholinesterase (AChE) since the reaction was inhibited by B.W.284C51 (around 80-90%) and no more than 20% by Ethopropazine (Table I). Thus, no correcting factors have been usualy applied for AChE assay. Human CSF, AChE activity was independent of patient sex (Table I) and age at least between 50 and 90 years old. In patients with AD/SDAT disease,CSF-ChE activity was 68% of that observed in controls (TableII). This decrease was not due to the presence of an endogenous inhibitor of AChE in the CSF of demented patients since its addition to control CSF failed to reduce its activity. Futhermore, in AD/SDAT, AChE activity decreases rapidly between 60 and 70 years and more slowly thereafter (Fig.I). Although, AChE activities are higher in Alzheimer's dementia(17.5±1.7) than in Senile Dementia of the Alzheimer Type(14.9±0.8),there is a significant decrease of each group compared to controls ($P<.05$,$P<.001$). At last, AChE was not correlated with the duration and the score of the disease.

The concentration of SLI in CSF from AD/SDAT patients was significantly reduced by 25% compared with controls($p<0.01$)(TableII). There was no correlation between CSF-SLI level and sex, patient groups(A.D.22.5±5.1, SDAT:25.6±1.3),duration of the disease and the score of the dementia. Futhermore, we found no correlation between CSF-SLI levels and CSF-AChE activity.A similar ratio AChE/SLI was observed in controls and AD/SDAT patients:0.68 and 0.62 respectively.

TABLE 1 Acetyl Cholinesterase activity in the CSF of control patients results are in nM/min/ml

	MALE n=8	FEMALE n=10
mean age	57±8	78±4
Total ChE	21.4±1.2	22.5±3
AChE	17.7±1	19.5±2
BuChE	3.7±6	3.7±6

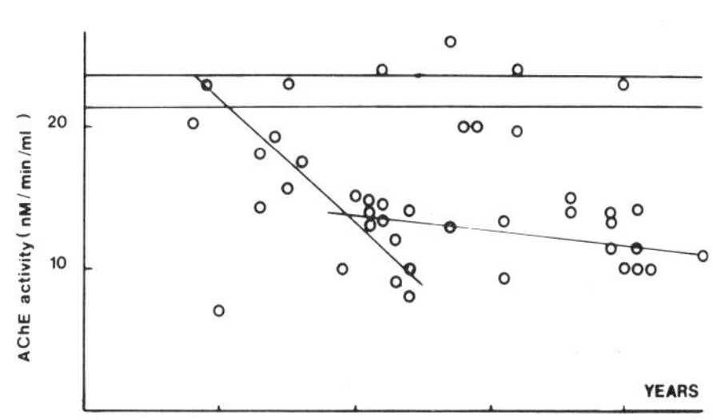

Figure 2 AChE activity in the CSF of patients with SDAT as function of age

TABLE II:AChE and SLI LIKE IMMUNOREACTIVITY IN THE CSF OF DEMENTED PATIENTS

	CONTROLS n=18	AD/SDAT n=55	MID n=5	H.D. n=2	OTHERS 1 n=1	2 n=1	3 n=1
ChE nM/mn/ml	22.2±2.2	15.1±0.7 **	16±1.7 **	18.2±7.8	N.D.	18.7	N.D.
SLI pg/ml	32.3±2.6	24.3±1.6*	24±5.6	27±4	54	40	13
ChE /SLI	0.68	0.62	.71	.67		0.47	

MID=MultiInfarctusDementia;H.D.=HuntingtonChorea;1=Creutzfeldt-Jakob
2=Sub-Cortical Dementia;3=Dementia type Gerstmann Straussler.
Significatively different from controls:*($p<0.01$) ;**($p<0.001$)

A significant decrease of AChE but not of SLI was found in the CSF of 5 cases of Multi Infarctus Dementia (Table II).In contrast,in 2 cases of Huntington Chorea,we found no change of AChE and SLI.At last, in 2 cases of non Alzheimer's dementia ,the CSF-SLI remain unchanged.

In few cases,the CSF-SLI levels and CSF-AChE were compared with the SLI concentration and ChAT activity in the frontal cortex obtained by biopsy.ChAT activity was reduced in 2 cases of Alzheimer's disease and remained unchange in 2 cases of non Alzheimer's diseases (one case of Creutzfeldt-Jakob and one case of Sub- Cortical dementia (TableIII).In three patients,the level of AChE in the CSF does not agree well with the level of ChAT in the frontal cortex compared to controls .In cortical tissue ,SLI was reduced in 2 cases of Alzheimer's disease and in one case of Sub Cortical Dementia.No change was observed in one case of Creutzfeldt-Jakob. However,in two cases,the value of SLI in the CSF agree with the cortical SLI levels compared to controls.Moreover,in one case the SLI is more affected in the CSF than in the frontal cortex (TableIII)

TABLE III:CHOLINERGIC AND SOMATOSTATINERGIC ACTIVITIES IN THE CEREBRAL CORTEX AND THE CSF OF DEMENTED PATIENTS

N°	HISTOLOGICAL DIAGNOSIS	CEREBRAL TISSUE ChAT pM/h/mg	SRIF pg/mg	CSF AChE nM/mn/ml	SRIF pg/ml
1	TUMOR	407	35	N.D.	N.D.
2	TUMOR	252	N.D.	N.D.	N.D.
3	ENCEPHALITIS	N.D.	27	N.D.	N.D.
4	ALZHEIMER	35	18	N.D.	4
5	ALZHEIMER	170	5	20.5	N.D.
6	CREUTZFELDT-J.	354	29	9.7	54
7	SUBCORT.DEM.	570	19	25.2	40

N.D not determined

DISCUSSION

This study shows that more than 80% of Cholinesterase activity present in the CSF samples from controls and AD/SDAT is true Acetylcholinesterase.The decrease of CSF-AChE activity reported here agrees with the results obtained by Soininen et al.(1984)while it differs from those of Wood et al.(1982)and Davies(1979).These differences may be explained by differences in the age of either the control or the demented group.Indeed,in the study of Wood(1982) the mean age of controls was 48 years old and it is therefore possible that AChE activity varied depending of the age.On the other hand,our study shows that the decrease of AChE activity in AD/SDAT patients is more prononced in older than in younger demented patients.This may explain the absence of reduction of AChE observed by Davies(1979)in patients with Pre Senile Dementia.

The decrease of SLI in the CSF of patients with AD/SDAT agrees with others studies(Soininen et al.1984;Wood et al.1982;Francis et al.1984).However the decrease reported here is smaller than those reported previously.These discrepancy may be partly due to differences in diagnosis of AD/SDAT disease as suggest the recent work of Francis et al.(1984).

The simultaneous decrease of AChE and SRIF in the CSF is relatively specific for AD/SDAT disease. Indeed,we found a decrease of AChE activities but not of SLI in M.I.D.and no change of these two activities in 2 cases of Huntington Chorea and in 2 non Alzheimer's disease.However,these results contrast with the decrease of CSF-SLI in MID and Huntington's Chorea reported by others groups (Cramer et al,1981,Wood et al.1982)

The reduction of ChAT activity in the frontal cortex obtained by biopsy only in patients with Alzheimer's disease suggests that the degenerescence of cholinergic neurons is not a general feature of dementia.The comparison of the value of SLI and AChE in the CSF with the level of SLI and ChAT in the frontal cortex of the same patients may suggest that CSF-SLI and CSF-AChE are not a parfait index of frontal cortex activity.

In conclusion, our study shows that CSF-SLI and CSF-AChE are reduced in AD/SDAT disease and remained unchange in two cases of Huntington's Chorea and in 2 cases of non Alzheimer's disease.These results taken together with those obtained in cortical biopsy seem to indicate that the cholinergic and somatostatinergic deficits are probably not a general feature of dementia.Further study are necessary to confirm this hypothesis and to clarify the relationship between these activities in the CSF and the clinical state.

ACKNOWLEDGEMENTS:The authors wish to thank the hospital nurses from the department of Neurology for technical assistance. We also wish to thank Pr J.P. Caron and Dr C. Goujon (Creteil Hospital) who have provided us cortical biopsies and the department of Pr Potel (Champcueil) for CSFsamples .This work was supported by Ministere de la Recherche et de l'Industrie.

REFERENCES

Arai H.,Kosaka K.and Iisuka R.,1984,Changes in biogenic amines and their metabolites in post mortem brain from patients with Alzheimer type dementia.J. Neurochem.,43,388

Bowen,D.M.,SmithC.B.,WhiteP.,andDavison A.N.1976,Neurotransmitter-related enzymes and indices of hypoxia in senile dementia and other abiotrophies.Brain,99,459.

Bowen,D.M.Allen S.J.,Benton J.S.,Goodhardt M.J.,Haan E.A.,Palmer A.M.,Sims N.R.,Smith C.C.T.,Spillane J.A.,Esiri M.E.,Neary D.,

Snowdon J.S., Wilcok G.K. and Davison A.N., 1983. Biochemical assessment of serotoninergic and cholinergic dysfunction and cerebral atrophy in Alzheimer's disease. J. Neurochem. 41, 2.

Cramer, H., Kobler, G., Oepen, G., Schomburg, G. and Schroter, E. 1981. Huntington's Chorea-Measurement of somatostatin, substance P, and cyclic nucleotides in the cerebrospinal fluid. J. Neurol. 225, 183.

Davies, p. 1979. Neurotransmitter-related enzymes in senile dementia of of Alzheimer type. Brain Res., 171, 319.

Ellman, G.L., Courtney, D.K., Anders V. and Featherstone R.M. 1961. A new and rapid colorimetric determination of acetylcholinesterase activity. Biochem. Pharmacol. 7, 88.

Fonnum, F. 1975. A rapid radiochemical method for the determination of choline acetyl transferase activity. J. Neurochem. 24, 407.

Francis, P.T., Bowen, D.M., Neary, D., Palo, J., Wikstrom, J. and Olney, J. 1894. Somatostatin-like immunoreactivity in lumbar cerebrospinal fluid from neurohistologically examined demented patients. Neurobiol. of Aging, 5, 183.

Gomez, S., Davous, P., Rondot, P., Faivre-Bauman, A., Valade, D. and Puymirat, J. 1985. Somatostatin like immunoreactivity and acetylcholinesterase activities in cerebrospinal fluid of patients with Alzheimer disease and senile dementia of the Alzheimer type. PsychoNeuroendoc. In press.

Oram, J.J., Edwardson, J. and Millard, P.H. 1981. Investigation of cerebrospinal fluid neuropeptides in idiopathic senile dementia. Gerontology, 27, 216.

Patel, Y.C., Krishna, Rao, Ph D. and Reichlin, S. 1977. Somatostatin in human cerebrospinal fluid. The New England J. of Med. 296, 10, 529.

Rossor, M.N. and Emson, P.C. 1982. Neuropeptides in degenerative diseases of the central nervous system. T.I.N.S. November, 399.

Soininen, H., Joskkonen, J.T., Riekkinainew, K.J., Hallonew, T.O., Riekkinen, P.J. 1984. Reduced cholinesterase activity and somatostatin like immunoreactivity in the cerebrospinal fluid of patients with dementia of the Alzheimer type. J. of Neurol. Sci. 63, 167.

Wood, C.M., Etienne, P., Lal, S., Gauthier, S., Cajal, S. and Nair, NPV. 1982. Reduced lumbar somatostatin levels in Alzheimer's disease. Life Sci. 31, 2073.

Yates, C.M., Simpson, J., Gordon, A., Maloney, A.F.J., Alton, Y., Ritchie, M. and Urouhard, A. 1983. Catecholamines and cholinergic enzymes in pre-senile and senile Alzheimer Type Dementia and Down Syndrome. Brain Res. 280, 119.

MONOAMINE NEUROTRANSMITTER METABOLITES AND HYDROXYLASE COFACTOR IN ALZHEIMER-TYPE DEMENTIA AND NORMALS

Peter LeWitt, Robert Levine, Walter Lovenberg, Nunzio Pomara, Michael Stanley, David Gurevich, Patricia Schlick and Richard Roberts

Neurology Department, Lafayette Clinic
951 E. Lafayette, Detroit, MI 48207

INTRODUCTION

Tetrahydrobiopterin (BH_4) is the cofactor involved in the initial and rate-limiting step of tyrosine hydroxylation. As such, it has the potential for regulating the synthesis of L-DOPA and ultimately, production of dopamine and norepinephrine. BH_4 is also the hydroxylase cofactor for serotonin synthesis, though its role in the regulation of this step has not been as thoroughly established as for the catecholamines[1]. The distribution of BH_4 in the rodent brain is not uniform, and concentrations are greatest in regions of monoaminergic neuronal terminals, such as the neostriatum[2]. The cofactor can be generated within the nervous system by a metabolic pathway starting with guanosine triphosphate[3] and involving at least one stable intermediate in primates, dihydroneopterin triphosphate.

Like metabolites of neurotransmitters, BH_4 can be measured in the CSF, and concentrations correlate well with homovanillic acid (HVA), the major metabolite of dopamine in man[4]. In Parkinson disease, in which marked depletion of nigrostriatal dopaminergic neurons evolves, there are substantial reductions also in CSF[5] and brain (striatal)[6] cofactor concentrations. Whether the decreased BH_4 content in Parkinsonism reflects decreased synthesis per each catecholaminergic neuron or only a diminished pool of neurons capable of pterin synthesis is not known at present. However, correlation between monoamine metabolites and CNS-derived biopterin cofactor may yield insight into the regulation of neurotransmitter synthesis and metabolism. Previous studies[7-9] with several neurological illnesses have implied such relationships, and this study has been conducted to evaluate for evidence of abnormalities in Alzheimer-type dementia.

MATERIALS AND METHODS

Ten healthy controls (mean age: 62, range: 44-83) underwent neurological screening and participated in a program of elective lumbar puncture for research studies. Patients did not have behavioral or clinical features of dementia, or other neurological findings compatible with CNS disease. Several were spouses of dementia patients. Lumbar punctures were performed in decubitus position after overnight bed rest and fasting, and if any CNS-active medications were in use, these had been discontinued at least two weeks earlier. Cerebrospinal fluid (CSF) was collected on ice in a standardized manner, and frozen at -70°C. Aliquots from a pooled specimen of the 3rd-17th ml were used for HVA, 5-hydroxyindoleacetic acid (5-HIAA) and 3-methoxy-4-hydroxyphenylethylene glycol (MHPG) determinations by high-pressure liquid chromatography and gas chromatography-mass fragmentometry. Cerebrospinal fluid samples from the 18th-19th ml were used for determination of biopterin and neopterin; the pterins were fully oxidized with acidified iodine to assess total biopterin (TB) and total neopterin (TN)[10]. Pterins were assayed by high-pressure liquid chromatography, using authentic standards obtained from Dr. B. Schircks, Wetteswil, Switzerland.

Fifteen patients with mild to moderate dementia were referred for further work-up and participation in these studies. In all instances, they were felt to have primary dementia consistent with "probable"[11] Alzheimer disease (AD) based on a consistent history, lack of other significant contributing factors to dementia, and neurological examinations without additional significant neurological deficits such as Parkinsonism. All patients had CAT scans of the head and routine CSF studies in support of their diagnosis. Any CNS-active medications taken had been discontinued at least two weeks earlier. Patients ranged in age from 44-83 years (mean: 62), and were otherwise in good health. None had a family history of dementing illness or Down's syndrome.

Assays were conducted on the entire group of samples in "blind" fashion, and numerical data was analyzed by conventional statistical tests for determination of significance.

RESULTS

The mean $\pm$ S.E.M. values for total biopterin (TB) in dementia, 18.1 ± 1.3 pmol/ml CSF, was substantially less than the mean value for healthy controls, 27.7 ± 1.4 ($p < 0.01$). These results are shown in Figure 1, plotted against age. Although earlier studies of BH_4 have shown a decline in CSF TB concentration in normals as a function of age[1], the four decade span of measurements in this study with both dementia and normals does not reveal any age-related trends. In contrast to the TB, CSF values of total neopterin (TN) in the dementia (42.6 ± 4.0 pmol/ml CSF) and control groups (39.8 ± 2.6) did not differ significantly.

CSF was also analyzed for the major metabolites of the three brain monoamines, dopamine, serotonin, and norepinephrine. The major metabolites of the first two, HVA and 5-HIAA, respectively, were significantly diminished in the dementia group (both comparisons significant at the $p < 0.01$ level), with reductions from controls to 65 and 72%, respectively. In contrast, the major metabolite of norepinephrine, MHPG, was reduced only to 91% of control in the dementia group, a decrease which did not reach statistical significance. The correlation coefficients between TB and MHPG reached significance at the $p < 0.05$ level, while for both 5-HIAA and HVA, the correlation between TB was highly significant at the $p < 0.01$ level.

DISCUSSION

BH_4 joins an expanding list of neurotransmitter-related substances found to be diminished in the brain in AD. The reduction in CSF TB content was of similar magnitude to that in Parkinson disease[5]. In both normals and in AD, TB was highly correlated to the major CSF metabolites of catecholamines and serotonin. Neopterin, an oxidized, dephosphorylated precursor of biopterin[3], was not diminished in parallel with TB, as would be expected if the TB reduction was due mainly to a dropout of monoaminergic neurons containing a biopterin-generating system. Hence, the CSF findings suggest impairment limited to the final step(s) of BH_4 synthesis in AD. Because of the role BH_4 plays as hydroxylase cofactor in the rate-limiting

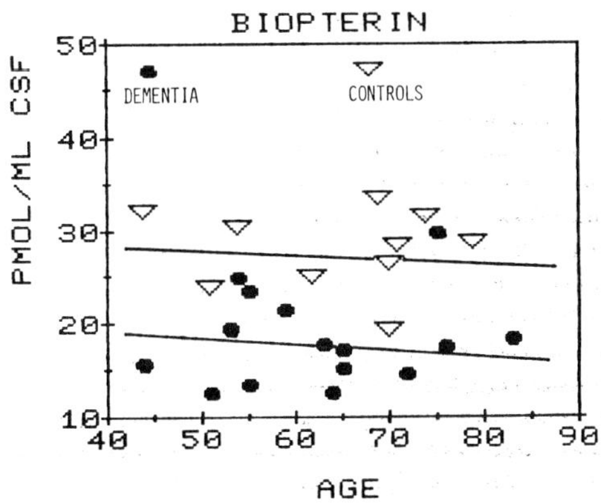

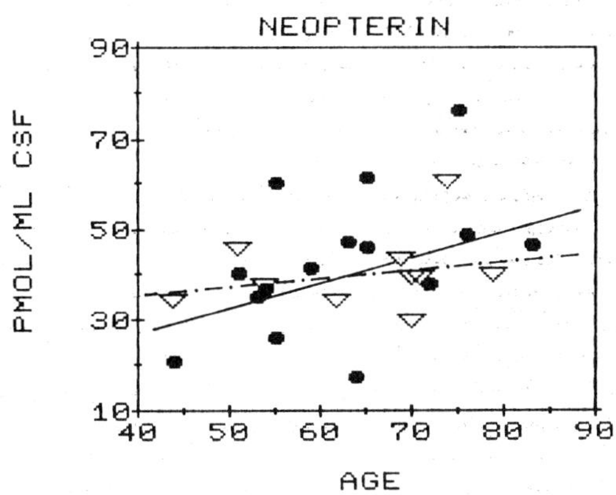

Fig. 1. Biopterin and neopterin levels in CSF from subjects with dementia (Alzheimer disease-type) and normal controls versus age (in years). The regression lines for each data group illustrate the differences found with biopterin but not with neopterin.

steps of monoamine synthesis[1], there could be a causal relationship between biopterin content and the changes seen in the CSF monoamine metabolites. Whether the diminished TB concentration is a reflection of "physiological" down-regulation of neurotransmitter synthesis or else a primary defect cannot be inferred from the data. Substantial decreases in brain monoaminergic systems, notably that of norepinephrine, have been found in several studies of AD brain[12-15], and it is possible that diminished BH_4 synthesis could be a contributing factor. It has also been hypothesized that the high concentrations of the reduced cofactor found in catecholaminergic nerve terminals[2,16] might have an additional function in a protective role against toxic by-products in neurotransmitter biosynthesis[5].

In addition to CSF studies[7,17], other evidence has pointed to abnormal BH_4 metabolism in AD. Temporal lobe specimens from AD patients had diminished enzymatic capacity to generate BH_4, as compared to control samples[18]. In these specimens, the content of TB was also decreased, despite increases over controls in TN content; dihydropteridine reductase activity (the enzyme regenerating BH_4 after its participation in hydroxylation steps) did not differ from controls. These observations are in keeping with our results suggesting a defect in the latter stage(s) of biopterin synthesis. That impaired biopterin generation might be a systemic metabolic disorder is suggested by the finding of serum biopterin[19] (but not neopterin[20]) concentrations in AD subjects to be approximately half of those in controls. Several forms of "atypical" phenylketonuria have been described with congenital omission of enzymes needed in biopterin synthesis or metabolism[21]. Whether disturbances of biopterin metabolism might also be contributing factors to the pathogenesis of AD or other neurogenerative disorders merits further study.

REFERENCES

1. R. A. Levine, D. M. Kuhn, A. C. Williams, and W. Lovenberg, Influence of aging on biogenic amine synthesis: Role of the hydroxylase cofactor, in: "Age and the Pharmacology of Psychoactive Drugs," A. Raskin, D. S. Robinson, and J. Levin, eds., Elsevier/North Holland, New York (1981).
2. R. A. Levine, D. M. Kuhn, and W. Lovenberg, The regional distribution of hydroxylase cofactor in rat brain, J. Neurochem. 32:1575-1578 (1979).
3. D. S. Duch, S. W. Bowers, J. H. Woolf, and C. A. Nichol, Biopterin cofactor biosynthesis: GTP cyclohydrolase, neopterin and biopterin in tissues and body fluids of mammalian species, Life Sciences 35:1895-1901 (1984).
4. A. C. Williams, R. A. Levine, T. N. Chase, W. Lovenberg, and D. B. Calne, Hydroxylase cofactor activity in cerebral spinal fluid of normal subjects and patients with Parkinson's disease, Science 204:624-626 (1979).
5. P. A. LeWitt, L. P. Miller, R. P. Newman, R. S. Burns, et al., Tyrosine hydroxylase cofactor (tetrahydrobiopterin) in Parkinsonism, Adv. Neurol. 40:459-462 (1984).
6. T. Nagatsu, T. Yamaguchi, T. Kato, T. Sugimoto, et al., Biopterin in human brain and urine from controls and parkinsonian patients: Application of a new radioimmunoassay, Clin. Chem. Acta 101:305-311 (1981).
7. A. C. Williams, R. A. Levine, T. N. Chase, W. Lovenberg, and D. B. Calne, CSF hydroxylase cofactor levels in some neurological diseases. J. Neurol. Neurosurg. Psychiatry 43:735-738 (1980).
8. H. C. Curtius, H. Müldner, and A. Niederwieser, Tetrahydrobiopterin: Efficacy in endogenous depression and parkinson's disease, J. Neural Transm. 55:301-308 (1982).
9. P. A. LeWitt, L. P. Miller, R. P. Newman, W. Lovenberg, R. Eldridge, and T. N. Chase, Pteridine cofactor in dystonia: Pathogenic and

therapeutic considerations, Neurology 33 (Suppl. 2):161 (1983).
10. T. Fukushima, and J. C. Nixon, Analysis of reduced forms of biopterin in biological tissues and fluids, Anal. Biochem. 102:176-188 (1980).
11. G. McKhann, D. Drachman, M. Folstein, R. Katzman, D. Price, and E. M. Stadlin, Clinical diagnosis of Alzheimer's disease: Report of the NINCDS-ADRDA work group under the auspices of Department of Health and Human Services Task Force on Alzheimer's Disease, Neurology 34:939-944 (1984).
12. R. Adolfsson, C. G. Gottfries, B. E. Roos, and B. Winblad, Changes in brain catecholamines in patients with dementia of Alzheimer type. Brit. J. Psychiatry 135:216-223 (1979).
13. R. M. Marchbanks, Biochemistry of Alzheimer's Dementia, J. Neurochem. 39:9-15 (1982).
14. A. J. Cross, T. J. Crow, J. A. Johnson, et al. Monoamine metabolism in senile dementia of Alzheimer type. J. Neurol. Sci. 60:383-392 (1983).
15. H. Arai, K. Kosaka, and R. Iizuka, Changes of biogenic amines and their metabolites in postmortem brains from patients with Alzheimer-type dementia. J. Neurochem. 43:388-393 (1984).
16. R. A. Levine, L. P. Miller, and W. Lovenberg, Tetrahydrobiopterin in striatum: Localization in dopamine nerve terminals and role in catecholamine synthesis. Science 214:919-921 (1981).
17. C. Morar, S. B. Whitburn, J. A. Blair, R. J. Leeming, and G. K. Wilcock, Tetrahydrobiopterin metabolism in senile dementia of Alzheimer type, J. Neurol. Neurosurg. Psychiatry 46:582 (1983).
18. P. A. Barford, J. A. Blair, C. Eggar, C. Hamon, C. Morar, and S. B. Whitburn, Tetrahydrobiopterin metabolism in the temporal lobe of patients dying with senile dementia of Alzheimer type, J. Neurol. Neurosurg. Psychiatry 47:736-738 (1984).
19. A. A. Aziz, R. J. Leeming, and J. A. Blair, Tetrahydrobiopterin metabolism in senile dementia of Alzheimer type, J. Neurol. Neurosurg. Psychiatry 46:410-413 (1983).
20. J. H. Young, B. Kelly, and B. E. Clayton, Reduced levels of biopterin and dihydroneopterin reductase in Alzheimer type of dementia. J. Clin. Exp. Gerontol. (1982).
21. S. Kaufman, G. Kapatos, W. B. Rizzo, J. D. Schulman, L. Tamarkin, and G. R. Van Loon, Tetrahydrobiopterin therapy for hyperphenylalanemia caused by defective synthesis of tetrahydrobiopterin. Ann. Neurol. 14:308-315 (1983).

ANTIBODIES TO CHOLINERGIC CELL BODIES IN ALZHEIMER'S DISEASE

J. Chapman*, A.D. Korczyn†, M. Hareuveni†† and D.M. Michaelson*

Departments of Biochemistry* and Microbiology††, Faculty of Life Sciences, Tel Aviv University and Department of Neurology†, Ichilov Medical Center, Tel Aviv University Sackler School of Medicine, Tel Aviv, Israel

ABSTRACT

In the present investigation we examined the possibility that patients with senile dementia of the Alzheimer type (SDAT) produce antibodies which interact with cholinergic neurons. The anticholinergic antibody contents of sera obtained from 10 SDAT patients and 5 elderly controls were assayed by means of a solid phase immunoassay (ELISA). Using purely cholinergic cell bodies isolated from the electric lobe of *Torpedo* brain as antigen, binding of SDAT sera was 156±32% of controls. Statistical analysis of the results by means of Student's t-test and Wilcoxon two-sample test found them to be significantly different ($p<0.01$). By contrast binding of SDAT sera to purely cholinergic nerve terminals isolated from the *Torpedo* electric organ did not differ statistically from those of controls. The significance of the SDAT antibodies directed against these antigens in the pathogenesis of SDAT and their potential use in diagnostic procedures is discussed.

INTRODUCTION

Senile dementia of the Alzheimer type (SDAT) is the major dementing disorder of old age. Despite the immense number of clinical cases the etiology and pathogenesis of the disease are still obscure. Furthermore, the definite diagnosis of the disease can only be made based on histopathological evidence obtained at autopsy or by biopsy (McKhann et al. 1984).

Recent studies indicate a decreased cholinergic activity in the CNS in SDAT (Rossor 1982). This is manifested both by a decrease in presynaptic cholinergic parameters (e.g. choline uptake (Rylett et al. 1983) and acetylcholine synthesis and release (Sims et al. 1983)) and by selective degeneration of certain cholinergic neurons (Coyle et al. 1983). The mechanisms underlying these changes are not known.

Several lines of evidence suggest that immunological mechanisms may be involved in the pathogenesis of SDAT. These include the presence of amyloid fibrils in the senile plaques (Eikelenboom & Stam 1982) and elevated serum immunoglobulin and increased blood-cerebrospinal fluid barrier permeability (Alafuzoff et al. 1983). Significantly higher binding of antineuronal antibodies in senile dementia have been described (Nandy 1978). Whether immunoglobulin abnormalities associated with SDAT play a part in inducing the cholinergic dysfunction is not known.

In the present communication we examined the possibility that antibodies in SDAT sera bind specifically to cholinergic neurons. This was performed by means of an enzyme linked immunoadsorbant assay (ELISA) utilizing as antigens the purely cholinergic nerve terminals and cell bodies isolated respectively from the *Torpedo* electric organ and electric lobe. Our findings suggest that sera of SDAT patients contain antibodies directed specifically against the cholinergic perikarya.

MATERIALS AND METHODS

1. Purification of cholinergic cell bodies and nerve terminals.
Nerve terminals (synaptosomes) were purified from the homogenates of fresh *Torpedo* electric organ by differential and density gradient centrifugation as previously described (Michaelson & Sokolovsky 1978). The cell bodies of the cholinergic neurons which innervate the electric organ were isolated from freshly excised *Torpedo* electric lobes as described by Dowdall et al. (1978). Both preparations (∿2 mg protein/ml) were kept at -70°C until used.

2. Preparation of antisera. Antisera to *Torpedo* synaptosomes and cholinergic perikarya (PK) were prepared by immunizing rabbits with 0.2 mg and 0.5 mg protein respectively twice at a 14-day interval as in Walker et al. (1982). Human sera were obtained from ten patients who fulfilled the criteria of SDAT (mean age 76±8) and from five elderly controls without signs of dementia or immunological disease (mean age 74±5).

3. Detection of anticholinergic antibodies. Plastic ELISA wells (NUNC Immunoplates Type II) were coated for 24 h at 4°C with 200 µl of synaptosomes (15 µg/ml) or cholinergic cell bodies (20 µg/ml) diluted in 50 mM sodium bicarbonate pH 9.6, after which they were washed (x 3) with phosphate buffered saline pH 7.5 (PBS) which contained Brij (0.1%). (This procedure resulted in the adsorbance of about 5-10% acetylcholinesterase activity (Ellman et al. 1961) associated with the antigen, which is an estimate of the amount of protein bound to the plate). Plates were then incubated for 60 min at room temperature with PBS + 1% BSA after which they were washed (x 3) with PBS + Brij. Sera to be tested were diluted in PBS containing

Brij and trasylol (250 unit/ml) after which they were placed (200 μl) in the wells and allowed to stand overnight at 4°C. The wells were then emptied and washed (x 15) with PBS + Brij. Alkaline phosphatase conjugates (1:1000 dilutions in PBS + Brij + trasylol) were added (200 μl) and incubated for 2 hrs at 37°C. Goat antirabbit IgG (Tago) and goat anti-human IgG+IgM (Sigma) were used for rabbit and human sera, respectively. Plates were then washed (x 15) with PBS + Brij after which 200 μl of substrate (paranitrophenyl phosphate 0.6 mg/ml in diethylamine-HCl pH 9.8) were added and the absorbance (410 nm) was measured by means of a Dynateck microplate reader. In experiments in which the specificity of the human antibodies was examined, some plates were coated similarly except that a *Torpedo* liver membrane fraction (Walker et al. 1982) was utilized as antigen. Protein was determined according to Bradford (1976).

RESULTS

The aim of this investigation was to search for specific abtibodies directed against cholinergic neurons, using a sensitive method which is specific for either cholinergic nerve terminals (synaptosomes) or cell bodies (PK). To this purpose, serum antibody binding to these antigens was assayed by a method of ELISA. The validity of this approach was examined by testing the binding of rabbit anticholinergic PK and antisynaptosome sera to the above antigens. As shown in Figure 1, rabbit antisynaptosome serum had half

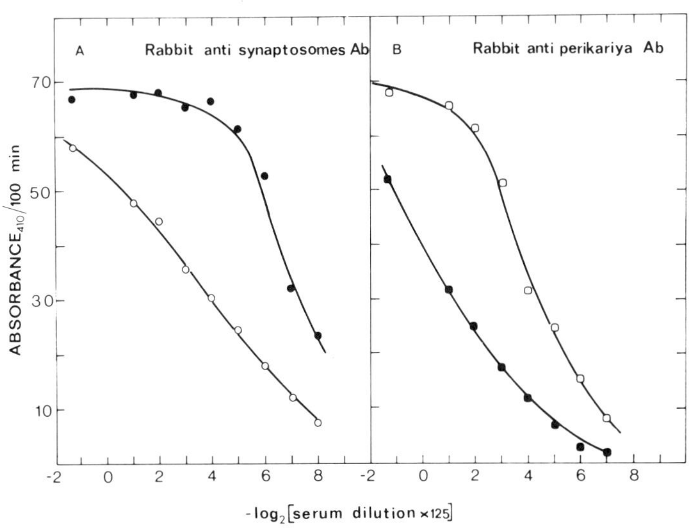

Figure 1: The cross reactivity between rabbit antibodies produced against cholinergic nerve terminals (synaptosomes) and cell bodies (PK).

A. The level of antisynaptosomal antibodies produced by rabbits immunized with *Torpedo* synaptosomes (●) and with cholinergic PK (o).

B. The level of anticholinergic PK antibodies produced by rabbits immunized with cholinergic PK (□) and with cholinergic synaptosomes (■).

Results presented were obtained by means of ELISA as described in Materials and Methods.

maximal binding to the synaptosomes at serum dilution 1:16,000 and to cholinergic PK at 1:1,000. Rabbit anti-PK serum was shown to have half maximal binding to PK at 1:2,000 and to synaptosomes of 1:250. Thus by this method anticholinergic synaptosome antibodies bind more to synaptosomes than to cholinergic cell bodies by a factor of 16, and anticholinergic cell body antibodies bind 8 times better to PK than to synaptosomes.

Having established the validity of the method we then examined the binding of serum from SDAT patients and from controls to the two cholinergic antigens. Figure 2 represents the binding to cholinergic PK of antibodies from individual sera diluted 1:80. All SDAT patients (n=10) yielded

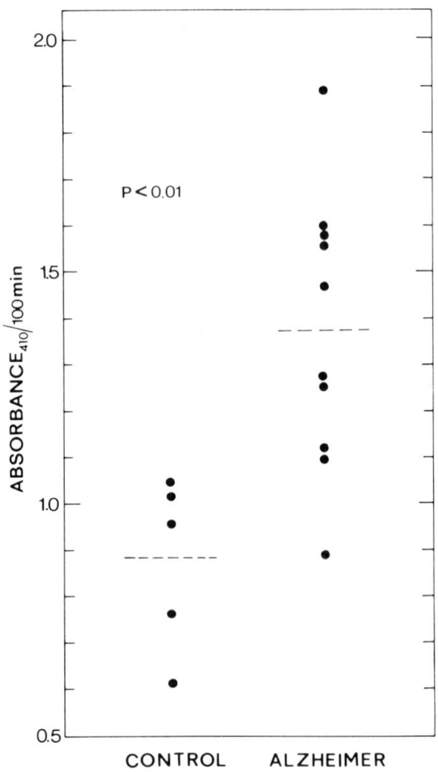

Figure 2: The level of antibodies directed against cholinergic cell body antigens in patients with SDAT. Antibody concentrations were estimated by means of an ELISA assay which utilized purely cholinergic PK isolated from the electric lobe of *Torpedo* as antigen, and human antibodies at a serum dilution of 1:80. Results presented are of ten patients and five controls.

values above the average of the controls (n=5). The average of the SDAT patients was 156±32% (mean±SD) of controls. This difference was found to be statistically significant ($p<0.01$; Wilcoxon 2 sample test and Student's t-test). It is of interest to note that the only patient under the age of 65, a case of presenile dementia, had the highest value. Binding to cholinergic PK at different serum dilutions is shown in Figure 3. The difference

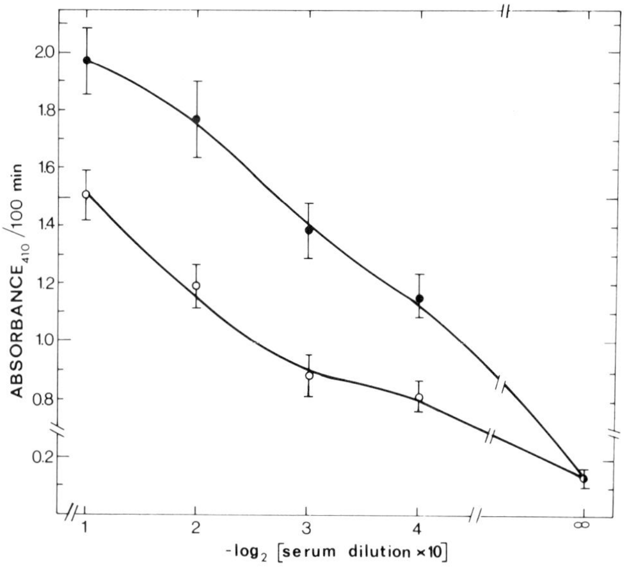

Figure 3: Titration of the level of anticholinergic cell body antibodies in patients with SDAT. Antibody concentrations were estimated at the indicated serum dilutions by ELISA as described in the legend to Fig. 2. Results presented are the mean ± SEM of ten patients (●) and five controls (o) at each serum dilution.

between control and SDAT antibody levels decreased by about 50% at serum dilution 1:160 although it was still statistically significant ($p<0.01$).

The specificity of antibodies to the cholinergic cell body in SDAT sera was investigated by determining the binding of these antibodies to other parts of the cholinergic neuron (nerve terminals) and to non-cholinergic *Torpedo* antigens (liver membranes). Table 1 illustrates the binding (mean±SD) of SDAT and control sera to these antigens. Controls are seen to bind similarly to all antigens while SDAT sera bind maximally to cholinergic PK and to a lesser extent to synaptosomes and liver membranes.

Table 1: Antibodies against *Torpedo* antigens in SDAT

Antigen / Antibody	Cholinergic cell bodies	Cholinergic nerve terminals	Liver membranes
Control (n=5)	100 ± 19	94 ± 16	83 ± 19
SDAT (n=10)	156 ± 32	127 ± 30	115 ± 30
Statistical significance	p < 0.01	n.s.	n.s.

The level of antibodies (serum dilution 1:80) produced by SDAT patients and controls against cholinergic cell body and nerve terminals and against *Torpedo* liver membranes were determined by ELISA as described in Materials and Methods. Results presented (mean ± SD) are relative to the level of control anticholinergic cell body antibodies.

It should be noted that SDAT sera bind to the cholinergic synaptosomes and the liver membranes more than controls, however this difference is smaller than that obtained with the PK and it is not statistically significant ($p>0.05$).

To investigate the specificity of antibody binding to each antigen, data obtained with different antigens were compared in pairs by subtracting for each individual the binding to one antigen from that to the other. Results at serum dilution 1:80 are depicted in Figure 4. SDAT sera contained

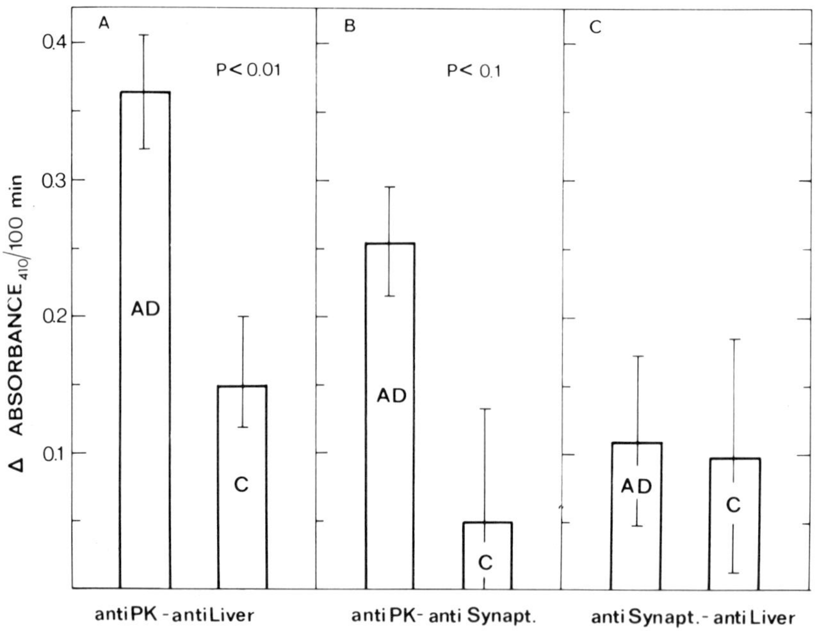

Figure 4: Antigen specificity of the antibodies produced by patients with SDAT.

A. Comparison of the level of anticholinergic PK and antiliver antibodies. The concentration of antibodies (at serum dilution of 1:80) were measured by ELISA (see legent to Fig. 1) utilizing cholinergic PK and *Torpedo* liver membranes as antigens. Results presented are the difference between the anti-PK and antiliver antibodies of each of 10 SDAT patients (mean±SEM) and five controls (mean±SEM).

B. Comparison of the level of anticholinergic PK and anticholinergic nerve terminal antibodies. Results presented were obtained as described above, except that cholinergic PK and synaptosomes were utilized as antigens.

C. Comparison of the level of anticholinergic nerve terminal and antiliver antibodies. Results presented were obtained as described above except that cholinergic synaptosomes and *Torpedo* liver membranes were utilized as antigen.

significant amounts of specific antibodies to cholinergic PK as compared to liver membranes ($p<0.01$). Most of these antibodies do not recognize the nerve terminals. No difference in binding of SDAT and control sera to synaptosomes and liver membranes was found.

DISCUSSION

Our results show that sera from patients with SDAT contain specific antibodies directed against cholinergic PK. This finding is consistent with previous reports of antineuronal antibodies in the disease (Nandy 1978) and suggests that some of these antibodies may act against cholinergic neurons.

The relevance of anti *Torpedo* PK antibodies to SDAT is not known. Cross reactivity between mammalian and *Torpedo* antigens is well established (Kushner 1984), thus the anticholinergic PK SDAT antibodies presently reported may also recognize human cholinergic neurons. In this context, our finding of anticholinergic cell body antibodies and not of anticholinergic synaptosomal antibodies is in accordance with the suggestion that cholinergic dysfunction in SDAT originates in selective degeneration of cholinergic cell bodies in the basal forebrain (Coyle et al. 1983).

It is still not known whether the antibodies described play a primary role in the pathogenesis of SDAT, since it is also possible that they develop secondarily to degeneration of cholinergic neurons and exposure of previously hidden neuronal antigens. We are currently attempting to resolve this question by immunizing laboratory animals with cholinergic cell bodies and examining the resulting effects on cholinergic function and behavior. Finally, whatever the pathogenetic role of PK specific antibodies in SDAT, we suggest their presence may serve a simple and low cost diagnostic test. The pursuit of these theoretical and practical goals will undoubtedly be furthered by purification of the antibodies and the relevant antigenic proteins. Work along these lines is currently in progress in our laboratory.

ACKNOWLEDGEMENTS

We thank Professor I. Keydar for her assistance and for valuable discussions. This work was supported in part by grants from the Dysautonomia Foundation and from the Fund for Basic Research administered by the Israel Academy of Sciences and Humanities.

REFERENCES

Alafuzoff, I., Adolfsson, R., Bucht, G. and Winblad, B., 1983, Albumin and immunoglobulin in plasma and cerebrospinal fluid, and blood-cerebrospinal fluid barrier function in patients with dementia of Alzheimer type and multi-infarct dementia. *J. Neurol Sci.*, 60:465.

Bradford, M., 1976, A rapid and sensitive method for quantitation of microgram quantities of protein utilizing the principle of protein-dye binding. *Anal. Biochem.*, 72:248.

Coyle, J.T., Price, D.L. and DeLong, M.R., 1983, Alzheimer's disease: A disorder of cortical cholinergic innervation. *Science*, 219:1184.

Dowdall, M.G., Fox, G., Wachtler, K.M., Whittaker, V.P. and Zimmermann, H., 1976, Recent studies on the comparative biochemistry of the cholinergic neuron. *Cold Spring Harbor Sym. Quant. Biol.* XL:65.

Eikelenboom, P. and Stam, F.C., 1982, Immunoglobulins and complement factors in senile plaques. *Acta Neuropathol.* (Berl) 57:239.

Ellman, G.L., Courtney, K.D., Andres, V.Jr. and Featherstone, R.M., 1961, A new and rapid colorimeter determination of acetylcholinesterase activity. Biochem Pharmacol., 7:88.

Kushner, P.D., 1984, A library of monoclonal antibodies to Torpedo cholinergic synaptosomes. J. Neurochem., 43:775.

McKhann, G., Drachman, D., Folstein, M., Katzman, R., Price, D. and Stadlan, E.M., 1984, Clinical diagnosis of Alzheimer's disease. Neurology, 34:939.

Michaelson, D.M. and Sokolovsky, M., 1978, Induced acetylcholine release from active purely cholinergic Torpedo synaptosomes. J. Neurochem., 30:217.

Nandy, K., 1978, Brain reactive antibodies in aging and senile dementia. in: "Alzheimer's Disease: Senile Dementia and Related Disorders". Aging, Vol. 7, R. Katzman, R.D. Terry and K.L. Bick, eds., Raven Press, New York.

Rossor, M.N., 1982, Neurotransmitter and CNS disease: Dementia. Lancet, ii:1200.

Rylett, R.J., Ball, M.J. and Colhoun, E.H., 1983, Evidence for high affinity choline transport in synaptosomes prepared from hippocampus and neocortex of patients with Alzheimer's Disease. Brain Res., 289:169.

Sims, N.R., Bower, D.M., Allen, S.J., Smith, C.C.T., Neary, D., Thomas, D.J. and Davison, A.N., 1983, Presynaptic cholinergic dysfunction in patients with dementia. J. Neurochem., 40:503.

Walker, J.H., Jones, R.T., Obrocki, J., Richardson, G.P. and Stadler, H., 1982, Presynaptic plasma membranes and synaptic vesicles of cholinergic nerve endings demonstrated by means of specific antisera. Cell Tissue Res., 223:101.

NICOTINIC AND MUSCARINIC BINDING SITES ON LYMPHOCYTES FROM ALZHEIMER PATIENTS

A. Adem, A. Nordberg, G. Bucht[1] and B. Winblad[1]

Department of Pharmacology, University of Uppsala, Box 591
S-751 24 Uppsala and [1]Department of Geriatric Medicine
University of Umeå, S-90187 Umeå, Sweden

INTRODUCTION

There is growing evidence that Alzheimer's disease(AD/SDAT) is a generalized disease not only confined to the brain. One way to further strengthen this assumption might be to study peripheral blood cells such as lymphocytes which have nicotinic and muscarinic like binding sites. The presence of muscarinic binding sites on intact lymphocytes(Gordon et al, 1978; Zalcman et al, 1981; Strom et al, 1981; Adem et al, 1984) as well as in lymphocyte membrane fractions has been described (Adem et al,1984). Nicotinic binding sites on lymphocytes were inferred from functional studies(Richman et al, 1979). Evidence for the presence of nicotinic binding sites on intact living lymphocytes as well as lymphocyte membrane preparation was, recently, obtained in our laboratory. In this study we present a comparison of nicotinic and muscarinic binding sites of lymphocytes as well as plasma cholinesterase activity in Alzheimer patients and age matched controls.

METHODS

The AD/SDAT patients were all institutionalized at the Psychogeriatric clinic Umedalens Sjukhus, Umea and had been under medical follow up for a long time. They all fulfilled the DSM-III criteria for AD/SDAT. All the patients were tested with Mini-Mental-Test, MMT (Folstein et al.). The mean time for hospitalization was 5.1 + 1.0 years. All controls had volunteered for an extensive general health survey and had no signs of somatic or psychiatric disease. None of the controls were smokers but one of the Alzheimer patients was a smoker (50 grams tobacco/week). Four patients were on neuroleptic drugs while the controls were drug free.

Blood samples(30-40 ml) were collected from fasting donors by venipuncture in EDTA tubes. The blood samples were kept at 4^0C overnight. Lymphocytes were isolated using Ficoll- Paque(Pharmacia Fine Chemicals) according to the method of Böyum(1968). Briefly the blood was centrifuged at 2000 rpm for 12 minutes(18 - 20 ^{0}C) after which the plasma was removed and an equal volume of Tris:Hank's balanced solution, HBS (Tris : HBS, 1:1) was added. The plasma was stored at -20 ^{0}C until determination of plasma cholinestrase activity was performed. The lymphocytes were harvested after centrifugation over a density gradient of Ficoll-Paque. The cells were then washed twice using Tris:HBS. The lymphocytes were finally suspended in Tris:HBS and protein concentration was measured.

Membrane fractions were prepared in the following way: after the second wash the lymphocytes were burst using 20 ml water (hypo- osmotic shock). An equal volume of 0.64 M sucrose solution was added. The cells were then homogenized in a glass homogenizer with a motor driven teflon pestle(10 strokes at 1500 rpm). The resulting homogenate was centrifuged at 1500 rpm for 10 minutes at 4 ^{0}C. The supernatant was taken and centrifuged at 17000 rpm for 1 hour at 4 ^{0}C. The resulting pellet ("P2") was suspended in 0.32 M cold sucrose solution, to give a final protein concentration of 1-2 mg/ml, and used for binding assays directly or kept at -20 ^{0}C until binding assays were performed. The protein concentration was measured according to Lowry et al(1951) using bovine albumin as standard.

Binding assay

In binding assays intact lymphocytes suspended in Tris:Hank (protein concentration 1-2mg/ml) were incubated with ^{3}H-quinuclidinyl benzilate (^{3}H-QNB, 5.3 nM, Sp. act. 38 Ci/mmol, NEN, UK) in 50mM Na-K phosphate buffer, pH=7.4, to a final volume of 1020ul. The incubation was performed at 25 ^{0}C for 60 min. In parallel experiments atropine was included in the incubation media (final concentration 10^{-4} M) to measure unspecific binding. After incubation the samples were chilled on ice and centrifuged in a Beckman Microfuge^R for 5 minutes. The amount of radioactivity bound was measured according to Nordberg and Winblad(1981). All measurements were performed in triplicates. Specific binding of ^{3}H-QNB was defined as the amount of ^{3}H-QNB bound in the absence of competing ligand minus the amount bound in the presence of atropine(10^{-4} M).

^{3}H-Nicotine(^{3}H-Nic, 7nM, SA 73 Ci/mmol) was incubated with intact lymphocytes in 50 mM Tris-HCl buffer(pH=8) for 10 minutes at 4 ^{0}C. The samples were centrifuged and the pellets were washed with 0.2 ml each of Tris-HCl buffer after removal of the supernatant. The specific binding was calculated by subtracting the value for nonspecific binding in the presence of 10^{-4} M unlabelled nicotine.

In similar binding experiments lymphocyte membrane fractions, (protein concentration 1-2mg/ml) were incubated with ^{3}H-QNB or ^{3}H-Nic as described above for intact cells.

Saturation studies with increasing concentrations of ^{3}H-QNB(1-20nM) were performed using intact lymphocytes and lymphocyte membrane fractions. Likewise studies with increasing concentrations of ^{3}H-Nicotine(1-20nM) were performed using membrane fractions.

Plasma Cholinesterase Activity

Plasma cholinesterase activity was determined according to the method of Augustinsson et al(1978). The procedure is based on the liberation of thiocholine from the substrate acetylthiocholine or butyrylthiocholine by the action of plasma cholinesterase. The thiocholine subsequently reacts with 4,4'-dithiodipyridine to give 4-thiopyridone which has an absorption maximum at 324mm.

RESULTS AND DISCUSSION

Saturation studies with increasing concentration of ^{3}H-QNB (1-20nM) and ^{3}H-Nic(1-20nM) were performed. Fig.1, 2 and 3 show the saturation curves of the binding of increasing concentration of ^{3}H-QNB to intact lymphocytes and membrane fractions and of ^{3}H-Nic to membrane fractions, respectively.

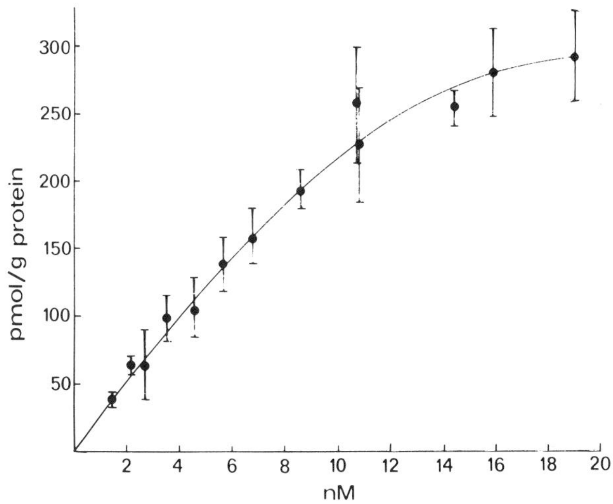

Fig.1. Specific binding of ^{3}H-QNB binding to intact lymphocytes. Intact lymphocytes (protein concentration 1-2 mg/ml) were incubated at 25 ^{0}C for 60 min. with increasing concentration of ^{3}H-QNB (1-20 nM, K_d = 26nM, B_{max} = 760pmol/g protein). Each point represents a mean $\pm$ S.E.M of duplicate results. Atropine 10^{-4} M was used to measure non-specific binding.

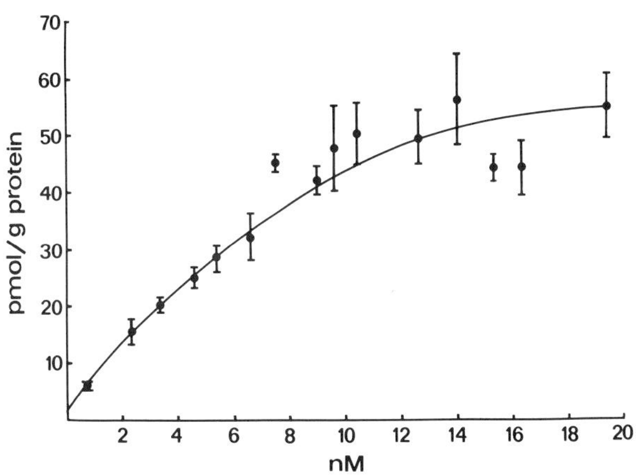

Fig.2. Saturation curve for ^{3}H-QNB binding to lymphocyte membrane fractions. Lymphocyte membrane fractions were incubated at 25^{0}C for 60 min. with increasing concentrations of ^{3}H-QNB (1-20 nM, K_d = 15nM, B_{max} = 109pmol/g protein). Each point represents mean $\pm$S.E.M value of four separate experiments each performed in duplicate. Atropine 10^{-4} M was used to measure non-specific binding.

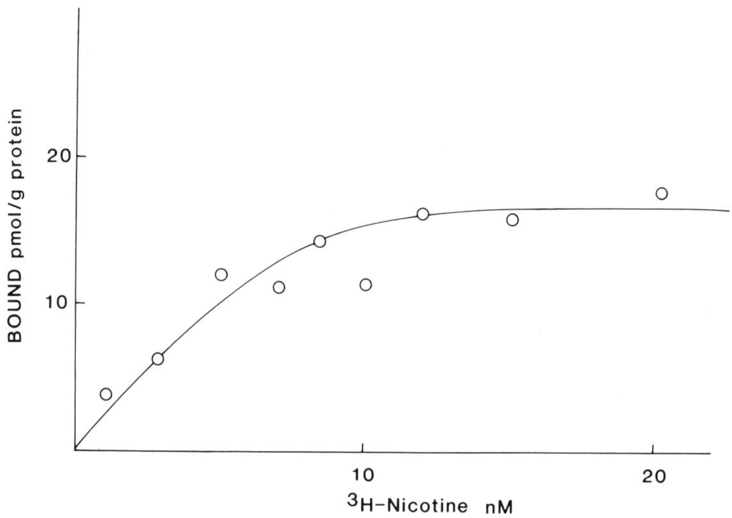

Fig.3. Saturation curve for ^{3}H-Nic binding to lymphocyte membrane fractions. Lymphocyte membrane fractions were incubated with increasing concentration of ^{3}H-Nic(1-20nM, K_d = 6.4nM, B_{max} = 23pmol/g protein) at 4°C for 10 minutes. Nicotine 10^{-4} M was used to measure unspecific binding.

The inhibition of ^{3}H-QNB binding to intact lymphocytes and membrane fractions and of ^{3}H-Nic to membrane fractions with increasing concentration of unlabelled cholinergic ligands was studied. From table 1 and 2 it can be seen that the IC_{50} values for nicotine, for example, differ thousand fold in the case of nicotinic and muscarinic receptors, thus showing the presence of specific nicotinic and muscarinic receptors on lymphocytes.

TABLE 1. IC_{50} values (molar concentration) of ^{3}H-QNB displacement by different cholinergic drugs.

Displacing Ligand	Intact Lymphocytes	Lymphocyte Membrane
Muscarinic Antagonists		
Atropine	3.0×10^{-5} (n=5)	3.1×10^{-7} (n=6)
Scopolamine	3.2×10^{-5} (n=3)	6.5×10^{-7} (n=3)
Muscarinic Agonists		
Oxotremorine	1.0×10^{-5} (n=2)	10.5×10^{-7}(n=5)
Pilocarpine		4.8×10^{-7} (n=2)
Nicotinic Agonist		
Nicotine		9.5×10^{-5} (n=2)

TABLE 2. IC_{50} values (molar concentration) of ^{3}H-Nicotine displacement by different cholinergic drugs.

Displacing Ligand	Lymphocyte Membrane fractions
Nicotine	2.4×10^{-8} (n=3)
Tubocurarine	2.3×10^{-6} (n=3)
Atropine	3.4×10^{-5} (n=3)

Table 3 shows a comparison of the nicotinic and muscarinic receptor binding in Alzheimer patients and age matched controls. As seen from table 3 a significant loss in both nicotinic (-41%, $p<0.01$) and muscarinic (-26%, $p<0.05$) receptor binding was obtained in Alzheimer patients in comparison to controls when intact lymphocytes were used. There was still a significant decrease in nicotinic receptor binding when data from the Alzheimer patient who smoked was excluded. Neuroleptic drugs did not seem to have any significant effect since data from patients on neuroleptic drugs were evenly distributed in the Alzheimer group. In the case of lymphocyte membrane fractions a slight decrease in muscarinic and nicotinic receptor binding was obtained in Alzheimer patients compared to controls. However the number of experiments performed with membrane fractions were few, due to insufficient amount of blood obtained from some of the patients and controls.

TABLE 3. Nicotinic (^{3}H-Nicotine) and muscarinic(^{3}H-QNB) receptors on lymphocytes from Alzheimer patients and age matched controls.

	AGE (years)	Nicotinic Receptors Intact Cells	Nicotinic Receptors Membranes	Muscarinic Receptors Intact Cells	Muscarinic Receptors Membranes
		pmol/g protein		pmol/g protein	
Control	76 ± 5	656 ± 53	20 ± 8	168 ± 15	37 ± 10
(7M, 6F)		(n=12)	(n=6)	(n=12)	(n=7)
AD/SDAT	78 ± 6	386 ± 50**	6.8 ± 4	124 ± 11*	28 ± 13
(3M, 7F)		(n=10)	(n=4)	(n=10)	(n=4)

Mv ± SE
n= number of individuals.
M= males; F= females.
* $p<0.05$ ** $p<0.01$

Table 4. Plasma cholinesterase activity: Hydrolysis of Butyrylthiocholine(BTC) and Acetylthiocholine(ATC) by plasma cholinesterase(see methods). The change in absorbance/minute (Δ_A) for BTC, ATC and BTC/ATC in plasma from controls and Alzheimer patients.

	BTC	ATC	BTC/ATC
	Change in absorbance per minute		
Controls (n=8)	0.851 ± 0.210	0.529 ± 0.132	1.61
AD/SDAT (n=8)	0.903 ± 0.08	0.567 ± 0.05	1.61

Mv ± SE   n= number of individuals

In parallel experiments we also investigated lymphocytes from 5 institutionalized patients with Multiinfarct dementia(MID, mean age 79 ± 3, MMT 8-21). As compared to the controls the MID patients had lower lymphocytic nicotinic (423 ± 123) and muscarinic (124 ± 16) receptor binding. Furthermore lymphocytes from ten patients with Parkinson's disease (mean age 76 ± 2) were investigated. Their MMT score varied between 15-30. Interestingly these patients showed a significant lower binding in the case of nicotinic (335 ± 50, -49%, $p<0.001$) but not muscarinic(139 ± 18) receptors. One patient, 37 years old, who has lipopolycystic osteodysplasia with dementia had surprisingly low muscarinic and nicotinic receptor binding.

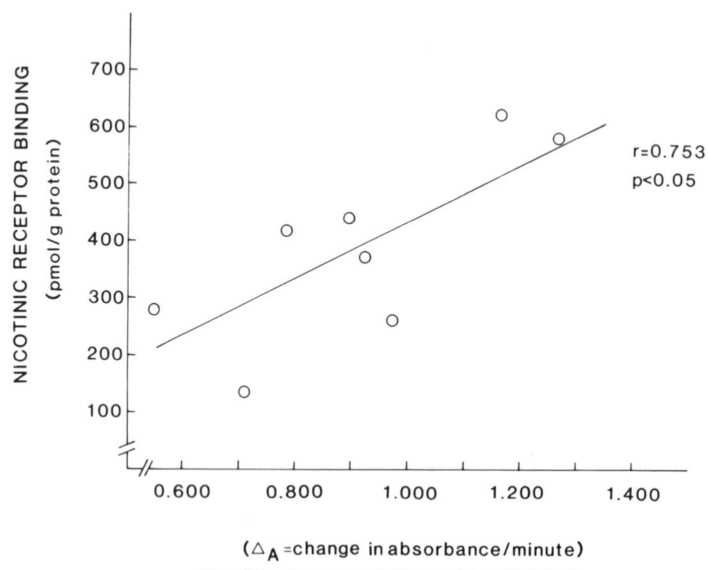

Fig. 4. Correlation between plasma cholinesterase activity and nicotinic receptor binding in lymphocytes obtained from Alzheimer patients.

The possibility of plasma cholinesterase as a peripheral marker in Alzheimer's dementia was tested. As seen in table 4 we found no difference between mean plasma cholinesterase activity in controls and Alzheimer patients. Smith et al(1981) found higher plasma cholinesterase activity in Alzheimer patients but this finding was not reproducible by others(Marquis et al, unpublished data). Cholinesterase activity in the CSF has been reported to be decreased (Soininen et al.1981,1984) or unchanged (Davies, 1979; Wood, 1982). In the brain a loss of acetylcholinesterase (Pope et al,1965; Davies, 1979, Perry, 1980; Attack et al, 1983) and increase of butyrylcholinesterase (Perry, 1980) were reported. It is interesting to note that a significant correlation between plasma cholinesterase activity and nicotinic receptor binding can be found in the Alzheimer group whereas no correlation can be found in the control group(Fig.4).

CONCLUSION

The data from our studies indicate a decrease in number of lymphocytic cholinergic receptors, muscarinic and nicotinic, in Alzheimer's disease. This new approach using lymphocytes offers the advantage that patients can be followed prospectively and biochemichal changes may be correlated to the severity of the different symptoms of the disease.

ACKNOWLEDGEMENT

This study was supported by grants from the Swedish Medical Research Council, the Swedish Tobacco Company and Loo and Hans Ostermans Foundation.

REFERENCES

Adem, A., Nordberg, A., and Slanina, P., 1984, Human lymphocyte muscarinic receptors: a comparison of the binding of ^{3}H-QNB to intact lymphocytes and lysed lymphocyte membrane fractions, Submitted.

Atack, J.R., Perry,E.K., Tomlinson, B.E., Bonham, J.R. Perry, R.H., Candy, J., Blessed, G., and Fairbain, A., 1983, Molecular forms of AChE in Senile dementia of Alzheimer: selective loss of the intermediate (10S) form, Neuroscience Letts., 40:199-204.

Augustinsson, K-B., Eriksson, H., Faijersson Y., 1978, A new approach to determining cholinesterase activities in samples of whole blood, Clinica Chimica Acta, 239-252.

Boyum, A. 1968,"Isolation of mononuclear cells and granulocytes from human blood." Scand, J. Clin. Lab. Invest. 21 Suppl. 97 (paper IV): 77-89.

Davies, P., 1979, Neurotransmitter-related enzymes in senile dementia of Alzheimer's type, Brain Res., 171: 319-327.

Gordon, M.A., Cohen, J.J., and Wilson, I.B., 1978, Muscarinic cholinergic receptors in murine lymphocytes: demonstration by direct binding, Prdoc. Natl. Sci. USA 75; 2902-2904.

Lowry, O.H., Rosenbrough, N.J., Farr, A.L , and Randall, R.J., 1951, Biol. Chem. 193: 265.

Nordberg, A., and Winblad, B, 1981, Cholinergic receptors in human hippocampus-regional distribution and variance with age, Life Sci. 29: 1937-1944.

Perry, E.K., (1980) The cholinergic system in old age and Alzheimer's disease, Age and Ageing, 9: 1-8.

Pope, A., Hess, H., and Levinm E., 1965, Neurochemical pathology of the cerebral cortex in presenile dementias, Trans. Aer. Neurol. Assoc., 89: 15-16.

Richman,D.P., and Arnason,B.G.W , 1979, Nicotinic acetylcholine receptor: Evidence for a functionally distinct receptor on human lymphocytes, Proc. Natl. Acad Sci. USA 76: 4632-4635.

Smith, R.C., Ho, B.,T., Hsu, L., Vroulis, G., Claghorn, J., Schoolar, J., 1982, Cholinesterase enzymes in the blood of patients with Alzheimer's disease, Life Sci., 30: 543-546.

Soininen, H.S., Jolkkonen, J.T., Reinikainen, K.J., Halonen, T.O., and Riekkinen, P.J., 1984, Reduced cholinesterase activity and somatostatin-like immunoreactivity in cerebrospinal fluid of patients with dementia of the Alzheimer type, J. Neurol. Sciences 63:167-172.

Soininen, H., T. Halonen and Riekkinen, P.J., 1981b, Acetylcholinesterase activities in cerebrospinal fluid of patients with senile dementia of Alzheimer type, Acta Neurol. Scand. 64: 217-224.

Strom, T.B., Lane, M.A., and George, R., 1981, The parallel, time dependent, bimodal change in lymphocyte cholinergic binding activity and cholinergic influence upon lymphocyte-mediated cytotoxicity after lymphocyte activation, J.Immunol. 127: 705-710.

Wood, P.L, Etienne, P., Lal, S., Gauthier, S., Cajal, S., and Nair, N.P.V., 1982, Reduced lumbar CSF somatostatin levels in Alzheimer's disease, Life Sci., 31: 2073-2079.

Zalcman, S.J., Neckers, L.M., Kaayalp, O., and R.J Wyatt,1981, Muscarinic cholinergic binding sites on intact human lymphocytes, Life Sci. 29: 69-73 .

CHOLINERGIC MUSCARINIC BINDING BY LYMPHOCYTES: CHANGES WITH AGE ANTAGONIST TREATMENT AND SENILE DEMENTIA

J.M. Rabey[1], L. Shenkman* and G.M. Gilad

The Center for Neuroscience and Behavioral Research
The Weizmann Institute of Science, Rehovot, Israel
and [1]Department of Neurology, Ichilov Medical Center
Tel Aviv University, Tel Aviv, Israel

INTRODUCTION

Lymphocytes respond to cholinergic agonists with increased cyclic-GMP levels, enhanced RNA and protein synthesis, and altered immune function (1-3). These induced alterations are diminished or blocked by the specific muscarinic antagonist, atropine, implying the presence of muscarinic cholinergic receptor sites on lymphocytes. Indeed, recently muscarinic receptors were demonstrated and characterized in murine lymphocytes (4-6) and in peripheral circulating human blood lymphocytes (7). These findings imply that lymphocytes may prove useful as peripheral markers for the muscarinic cholinergic system. However, it remains to be established if changes in lymphocyte muscarinic receptors can be evoked by treatment with muscarinic agonists and antagonists, similar to changes in muscarinic receptors of the brain (8-10). Further, as hypofunction of central cholinergic systems has been implicated in the deterioration of faculties during aging (11-13) and in the etiology of senile dementia (14-21), a peripheral marker for central muscarinic cholinergic function would be very useful (20-21). It is, therefore, of interest to know whether any changes occur in muscarinic binding by peripheral lymphocytes during normal aging and in senile dementia. We report here that the number of muscarinic cholinergic receptor sites on lymphocytes is increased after treatment with antimuscarinic drugs. Furthermore, there is a tendency for a continuous increase in the number of receptors with age. And, in contrast, lymphocytes derived from people with senile dementia exhibit a marked reduction in the number of muscarinic receptor binding sites.

METHODS

Animal experiments. Male Sprague-Dawley (SPD) and Lewis rats were housed 4-5 to a cage, supplied freely with food and water and maintained at 24°C with 12h light dark cycle (light 07:00-19:00h). Rats were considered adults at 4-5 months of age and old at 24 months. Atropine

* Present address: L. Shenkman, Department of Internal Medicine, C, Meir Hospital, Kfar Saba, Israel.

sulfate (20 mg/kg) in 0.9% (w/v) NaCl (saline) was injected subcutaneously (0.5 ml per rat) once a day for 14d. Rats injected with saline served as controls.

Human patients. Studies were carried out on human volunteers of both sexes. Patients treated with muscarinic agonists (prostigmine or pyridostigmine) for 4-8 months or antagonists (trihexyphenidyl or biperiden) for 4-12 months, were compared with age matched healthy volunteers. Patients with senile dementia were diagnosed on the basis of their mental status as suffering from marked confusion, disorientation, inability to concentrate and memory loss. Patients with any metabolic or cardiovascular disorders and those suffering from multi-infarct dementia (as ascertained by computerized-tomographic scans) were excluded. Age matched healthy volunteers served as controls.

Blood collections. Rats: trunk blood was collected after decapitation using heparin as anticoagulant. Humans: blood was collected by venipuncture with heparin as anticoagulant.

Isolation of lymphocytes. Both rat and human lymphocytes were isolated in the same manner on a Ficoll-Hypaque gradient (22). Following centrifugation for 45 min at 1000xg the lymphocyte layer was separated and then washed twice in RPMI 1640 nutrient medium (GIBCO). Washed lymphocytes were resuspended in RPMI, counted with a haemocytometer and their viability determined by trypan blue exclusion.

Brain dissections. Rat brains were rapidly excised after decapitation, the hippocampus dissected (23) and then frozen on dry ice and stored at $-50^{o}C$ until assayed.

$[^3H]$-quinuclidinyl benzilate(QNB) binding assay. Assays in brain homogenates: tissue samples were homogenized in 10 vol of 0.32M sucrose in a glass homogenizer fitted with a Teflon pestle, centrifuged at 1000xg for 10 min and the supernatant decanted for assay of QNB binding according to Yamamura and Snyder (24). A 20 μl aliquote was incubated with 230 μl solution of 50 mM sodium-potassium phosphate buffer, pH 7.4 containing various concentrations of QNB (spec. act. 33 Ci/mol, New England Nuclear). After incubation at room temperature for 45 min the reaction was stopped by the addition of 3 ml of ice-cold saline and the contents passed through a glass filter (Whatman GF/C) positioned over a vacuum. The filters were washed with 6 ml saline and then taken for radioactivity measurements. To determine nonspecific binding, samples were incubated for 10 min with 10 μM atropine sulfate prior to incubation with QNB.

Binding by lymphocytes: one million lymphocytes were incubated in 0.5 ml of RPMI medium containing different concentrations of QNB (5-200 nM). Incubation was at room temperature for 45 min. Specific binding was determined by pre-incubation of parallel tubes with 100 μM atropine for 15 min before adding QNB. The reaction was stopped by adding 3 ml of ice-cold saline followed by a rapid filtration on pre-wetted Whatman GF/B filters. After washing with 6 ml of saline, the radioactivity on the filters was measured by liquid scintillation spectrometry. Figure 1 illustrates a characteristic saturation curve of QNB binding by human lymphocytes. Specific binding expressed as the difference in QNB bound to lymphocytes in the presence of atropine, constitutes 50-70% of the total binding measured in the absence of atropine. One hundred fmoles bound correspond to a difference of about 2000 cpm. When Scatchard analysis was performed, binding at the lower concentrations (up to 10 mM) could not be fitted, and thus Bmax (425.4 fmol/$1x10^6$ cells) and Kd (62.2 nM) values were calculated from the linear regression line of the higher QNB concentrations (25-150 nM) (Fig. 1).

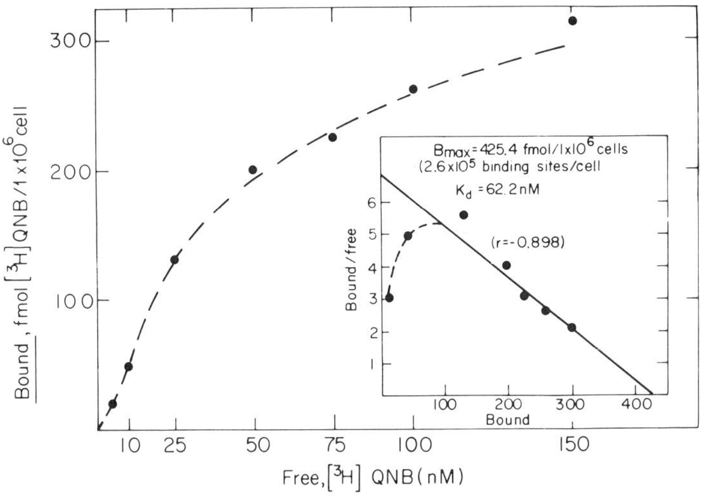

Fig. 1. Specific QNB binding to human lymphocytes from a 34 years old male as a function of concentration. Each point represents the mean value of duplicate measurements. Inset: a Scatchard plot of the results and the derived Kd and Bmax values and the number of binding sites per cell.

Maximal displacement of QNB binding was higher (70%) with atropine than with oxotremorine (50%), a muscarinic agonist. Also, atropine had a lower Ki value (35μM) than oxotremorine (52μM).

It has been suggested that retention of QNB by viable lymphocytes may be due to a process of uptake, internalization or nonspecific trapping (25). We have found this unlikely as washing the lyphocytes after the incubation with ice-cold fresh media (a 5 min process) resulted in 80-85% loss of radioactivity.

Protein determination. The protein content of brain homogenates or lymphocyte samples was determined by the method of Lowry et al. (26).

RESULTS

Increased QNB binding in rat and human lymphocytes and in rat brain after antagonist treatment. Treatment of rats with the antimuscarinic agent, atropine, and of humans with the antimuscarinic drugs trihexyphenidyl or biperiden, resulted in an increased QNB binding capacity by lymphocytes.

After atropine treatment the increase in QNB binding capacity by rat lymphocytes, which was due to both increased Bmax and decreased Kd values (Fig. 2), was paralleled by an increased binding in the hippocampus (Table I). It is important to notice the difference between QNB concentrations needed to detect and saturate binding in lymphocytes (Fig. 2) and in brain (Table I). In the brain maximal QNB binding capacity is about 100 fold higher than in lymphocytes.

In human lymphocytes, the increased binding capacity after cholinergic antagonist treatment was due to higher Bmax values, while Kd values did not change significantly (Fig. 3).

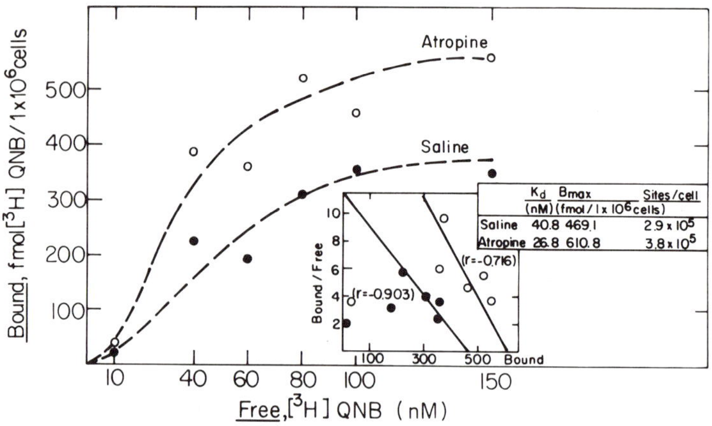

Fig. 2. Specific QNB binding to lymphocytes from SPD rats treated with saline (solid circle) or atropine (open circle) as a function of QNB concentration. Each point represents the mean value of two separate experiments, ran in triplicates, on lymphocytes pooled from 6 rats. Inset: a Scatchard plot of the results and the derived Kd and Bmax values and the number of binding sites per cell.

Table I. Specific QNB Binding to Hippocampal Homogenates After Atropine Treatment of SPD Rats

Treatment	Bmax (pmol/mg protein)	Kd (nM)
Saline	2.16 $\pm$ 0.10	0.60 $\pm$ 0.04
Atropine	2.62 $\pm$ 0.15*	0.58 $\pm$ 0.04

Results are the mean ($\pm$ SEM) values of 5-7 rats. * = $p<0.05$.

Lymphocytes from two patients treated with prostigmine and pyridostygmine, had no change in QNB binding capacity (Fig. 3).

Changes in Lymphocytes With Age and Senile Dementia. Binding capacity of QNB increases with age through adult life of rats (Fig. 4) and humans (Fig. 5).

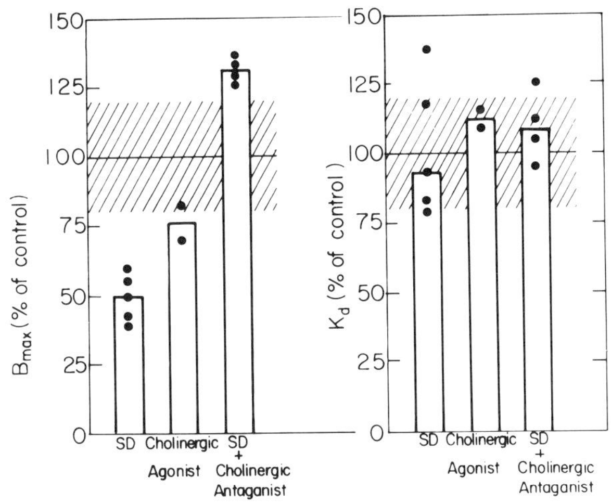

Fig. 3. Differences in Bmax (left) and Kd (right) values after Scatchard analyses of QNB binding to lymphocytes from patients with senile dementia (SD), patients treated with prostigmine and pyridostigmine (cholinergic agonists), and SD patients treated with trihexyphenidyl and biperiden (cholinergic antagonists). Results are expressed as percent of controls (shaded area). Bars represent the median value in each group.

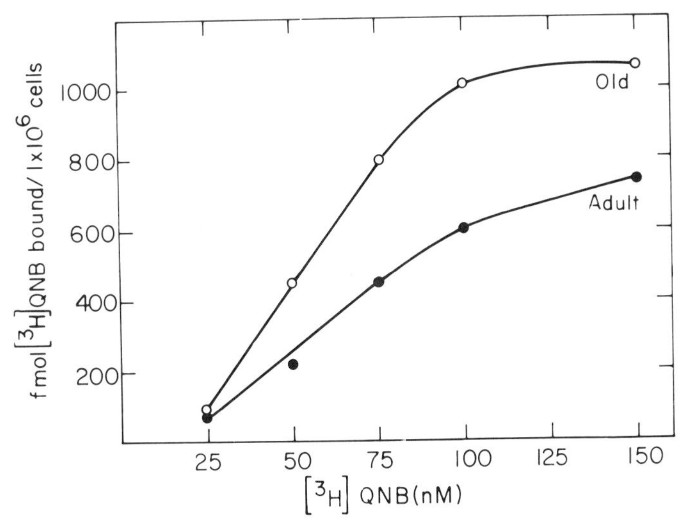

Fig. 4. Specific QNB binding to lymphocytes from adult (7 months) and old (24 months) male Lewis rats. Each point represents the mean value of two separate experiments, ran in triplicates, on lymphocytes pooled from 6 rats.

In humans (Fig. 5) the age dependent increase in binding capacity was highly correlated with increased Bmax values, indicating an age-dependent increase in the number of binding sites per lymphocyte. The values of Kd, slightly decreased after 50 years of age. Thus, a moderate age dependent decrease in Kd values, indicating increased affinity of the ligand to its receptor, also contributed to the observed increase in QNB binding capacity.

Lymphocytes from groups of patients with senile dementia had significantly lower Bmax values as compared with age matched controls while Kd values did not differ significantly (Figs. 3 and 5).

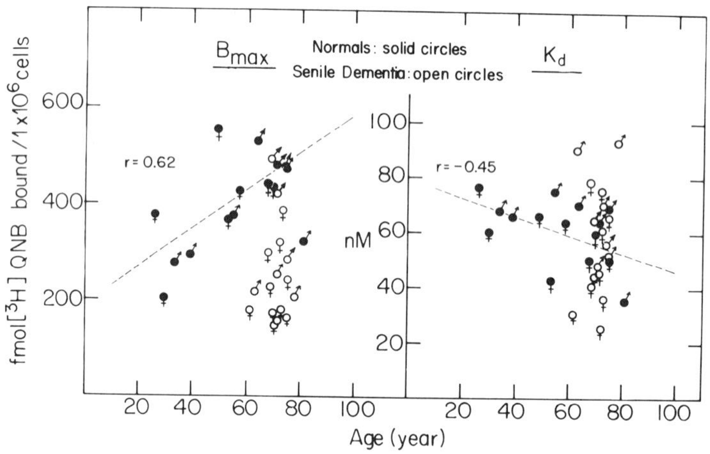

Fig. 5. Scatter diagrams of Bmax (left) and Kd (right) values determined by Scatchard analyses of QNB binding to lymphcytes from females (♀) and males (♂) of various ages (solid circles), and from patients with senile dementia (open circles). Bmax values demonstrated a high positive correlation with age (r=0.62) while senile dementia patients had lower Bmax values. Kd values demonstrated only a moderate negative correlation with age (r=-0.45) and were unchanged in senile dementia.

DISCUSSION

The present study demonstrates that a) peripheral circulating blood lymphocytes possess cholinergic muscarinic binding sites which are responsive to pharmacological treatment with antimuscarinic drugs; b) there is an age dependent increase in muscarinic binding capacity by adult lymphocytes, and c) in senile dementia there is a marked reduction in muscarinic binding capacity by lymphocytes.

The study supports the findings of others regarding the presence of muscarinic receptors on human (7), mouse (4) and rat (5) lymphocytes. The results demonstrate that the kinetics of QNB binding in human and rat lymphocytes are apparently similar, but both are quite different than that in the brain. This discrepancy holds true even when compared to measurements done in brain slices (27), indicating a much lower affinity (about 100 fold) for the ligand to muscarinic receptors on lymphocytes as compared to the brain. Yet, in spite of these kinetic differences, the response to chronic treatment with antimuscarinic drugs in lymphocytes is similar to the increased muscarinic binding observed in the rodent brain after similar treatment (8-10), suggesting functional homology.

The age-dependent increase in muscarinic binding capacity by lymphocytes is intriguing. Such an up-regulation was not observed in the brain, rather, no alteration or a reduction in receptor numbers was observed (19,20,28). The reduction in binding sites associated with senile dementia is of great interest for the following reasons: a) it indicates that the malfunction of the cholinergic system which is most often associated with senile dementia is not confined to the brain but is expressed in the periphery as well, and b) it implies that the immune system is also affected, primarily or secondarily (29-31). therefore, changes in the immune system should be considered in the diagnosis and treatment of senile dementia, as implied before (29). The changes observed in this study could, in principle, originate from different populations of B and T lymphocytes (30,31). In fact, a recent report suggests that QNB binding is greater in B than in T murine lymphocytes (6). This will have to be determined in humans as well.

The study suggests that cholinergic muscarinic binding to circulating blood lymphocytes may serve a useful peripheral marker for evaluating changes of the brain cholinergic system induced by drug treatment, as well as changes associated with aging and senile dementia.

ACKNOWLEDGEMENTS

This work was supported in part by a grant from the Israel Center for Psychobiology, Charles E. Smith Family Foundation. G.M. Gilad is an incumbent of the Paul and Gabriella Rosenbaum Career Development Chair, in perpetuity, established by Paul and Gabriella Rosenbaum Foundation, Chicago, Il.

REFERENCES

1. T.B. Strom, A.T. Sytkowski, C.B. Carpenter and J.P. Merrill, Cholinergic augmentation of lymphocyte-mediated cytotoxicity. A study of the cholinergic receptor of cytotoxic T lymphocytes, Proc. Natl. Acad. Sci. U.S.A. 71:1330 (1974).
2. G. Illiano, G.P.E. Tell, M.I. Segel and P. Cuatrecasas, Guanosine 3':5'-cyclic monophosphate and the action of insulin and acetylcholine, Proc. Natl. Acad. Sci. U.S.A. 70:2443 (1973).
3. G.R. Schreiner and E.R. Unanue, The modulation of spontaneous and anti-Ig-stimulated motility of lymphocytes by cyclic nucleotides and adrenergic and cholinergic agents, J. Immunol. 114:802 (1975).
4. M.A. Gordon, J.J. Cohen and I.B. Wilson, Muscarinic cholinergic receptors in murine lymphocytes: demonstration by direct binding, Proc. Natl. Acad. Sci. U.S.A. 75:2902 (1978).
5. W. Maslinski, K. Krzustyniak, E. Grabczewska and J. Ryzewski, Muscarinic acetylcholine receptors of rat lymphocytes, Biochim. Biophys. Acta 758:93 (1983).
6. S.F. Atweh, J.J. Grayhack and D.P. Richman, A cholinergic receptor on murine lymphocytes with novel binding characteristics, Life Sci. 35:2459 (1984).
7. S.J. Zalcman, L.M. Neckers, O. Kaayalp and R.J. Wyatt, Muscarinic cholinergic binding sites on intact human lymphcytes, Life Sci. 29:69 (1981).

8. J. Ben-Barak and Y. Dudai, Scopolamine induces an increase in muscarinic receptor level in rat hippocampus, Brain Res. 193:309 (1980).

9. A. Westlind, M. Grynfarb, B. Hedlund, T. Bartfai and M. Fuxe, Muscarinic supersensitivity induced by septal lesion or chronic atropine treatment, Brain Res. 225:131 (1981).

10. M. McKinney and J.T. Coyle, Regulation of neocrotical muscarinic receptors: effects of drug treatment and lesions, J. Neurosci. 2:97-105 (1982).

11. D.A. Drachman, Memory and cognitive function in man: does the cholinergic system have a specific role?, Neurology 27:783 (1977).

12. R.T. Bartus, R.L. Dean, B. Beer and A.S. Lippa, The cholinergic hypothesis of geriatric memory dysfunction: a critical review, Science 217:408 (1982).

13. K.L. Davies, R.C. Mohs and J.R. Finklenberg, Enhancement of memory by physostigmine, N. Engl. J. Med. 301:946 (1979).

14. P. Davis, Neurotransmitter related enzymes in senile dementia of the Alzheimer type, Brain Res. 171:319 (1979).

15. G.E. Gibson, C. Peterson and D.J. Jenden, Brain acetylcholine synthesis declines with senescence, Science 213:674 (1981).

16. P.J. Whitehouse, D.L. Price, R.G. Struble, A.W. Clark, J.T. Coyle and M.R. DeLong, Alzheimer's disease and senile dementia: loss of neurons in the basal forebrain, Science 215:1237 (1982).

17. E.K. Perry, B.E. Tomlinson, G. Blessed, K. Bergmann, P.H. Gibson and R.H. Perry, Correlation of cholinergic abnormalities with senile plaques and mental test scores in senile dementia, Br. Med. J. 2:1457 (1978).

18. J.A. Richter, E.K. Perry and B.E. Tomlinson, Acetylcholine and choline levels in post-mortem human brain tissue: preliminary observations in Alzheimer's diseases, Life Sci. 26:1683 (1980).

19. S. Corkin, Acetylcholine, aging and Alzheimer's disesase. Implications for treatment, Trend. Neurosci. 5:287 (1981).

20. M.M. Schneck, B. Reisberg and S.H. Ferris, An overview of current concepts of Alzheimer's diseases, Am. J. Psychiatry. 139:165 (1982).

21. R.C. Smith, B.T. Ho, L. Hsu, G. Vroulis, J. Claghorn and J. Schoolar, Cholinesterase enzymes in the blood of patients with Alzheimer's disease, Life Sci. 30:543 (1982).

22. A. Boyum, Isolation of mononuclear cells and granulocytes from blood, Scand. J. Clin. Invest. 21:77 (1968).

23. G.M. Gilad and V.H. Gilad, Strain-dependent differences between the septo-hippocampal cholinergic system and hippocampal size, Brain Res. 222:423 (1981).

24. H.I. Yamamura and S.H. Snyder, Muscarinic cholinergic binding in rat brain, Proc. Natl. Acad. Sci. U.S.A. 71:1725 (1974).

25. J.M. Maloteaux, A. Gossuin, C. Waterkeyn and P.M. Laduron, Lack of muscarinic and dopaminergic receptors but trapping of ^{3}H ligands on human lymphocytes: a possible artefact in binding studies on intact cells, Abstracts of the 13th Collegium Internationale Neuro-Psychopharmacologicum Congress, Vol. II: p. 462 (1982).

26. O.H. Lowry, N.J. Rosebrough, A.L. Farr and R.J. Randall, Protein measurement with the Folin phenol reagent, J. Biol. Chem. 193:265 (1951).

27. M.R. Hanley and L.L. Iversen, Muscarinic cholinergic receptors in rat corpus striatum and regulation of guanosine, cyclic 3'5'-monophosphate, Mol. Pharmacol. 14:246 (1978).

28. T.E. Reisine, H.I. Yamamura, E.D. Bird, E. Spokes and S.J. Enna, Pre-and postsynaptic neurochemical alterations in Alzheimer's disease, Brain Res. 159:477 (1978).

29. A.E. Miller, A.P. Neighbour, R. Katzman, M. Aronson and R. Lipkowitz, Immunological studies in senile dementia of the Alzheimer type: evidence for enhanced suppressor cell activity, <u>Ann. Neurol.</u> 10:506 (1981).
30. W. Augener, G. Cohnen, A. Reuter and G. Brittinger, Decrease of T lymphocytes during aging, <u>Lancet</u> i:1164 (1974).
31. A. Ben-Zvi, U. Galili, A. Russell and M. Schlesinger, Age associated changes in subpopulations of human lymphocytes, <u>Clin. Immunol. Immunopathol.</u> 7:139 (1977).

DEXAMETHASONE SUPPRESSION TEST IN SENILE DEMENTIA OF THE ALZHEIMER TYPE

P.Davous (1), M.Roudier (2), Y.Lamour (3), H.Susini de Luca (1), and C.Abramowitz (2)

1. Sainte Anne Hospital, 75014 Paris, France
2. Ch.Richet Hospital, 95400 Villiers le Bel, France
3. INSERM U 161, 75014 Paris, France

INTRODUCTION

The dexamethasone suppression test (DST) has been widely studied in depressive patients. According to Carroll (1), the average sensitivity of this test is 45% among depressed patients irrespective of the etiology of the depression. Little is known about DST results in dementia of the Alzheimer type (SDAT) and in non demented elderly patients and there are conflicting results in the literature (2-6). The purpose of the present investigation was to determine the frequency of abnormal DST responses in a population of elderly inpatients affected with SDAT compared to a group of control mentally healthy patients of similar age range.

SUBJECTS AND METHODS

The study group consisted of 35 elderly inpatients 71 to 95 year-old, free of neuroleptic or antidepressant drugs for at least 3 months. All the patients were hospitalized in the same department since at least 2 months. They were all able to walk and feed without assistance. Two groups were studied: 27 patients with SDAT and 8 controls. The diagnosis of SDAT was established according to DSM III criteria (7). All the patients were investigated by complete detailed neurological examination, standard laboratory tests, EEG and CT scan. Patients with focal neurological signs or symptoms, previous stroke history or evidence of arteriosclerosis were excluded to rule out multi-infarct dementia. Age range of SDAT patients was 71-95 (mean 84). There were 2 men and 25 women. Control elderly patients were free of hepatic or renal disease and infection. Two of them had congestive heart failure and received diuretics without spironolactone. All the control subjects were mentally healthy and free of previous history of depression. Their age range was 75-92 (mean: 85). There was 1 man and 7 women.

Patients were evaluated for dementia by the Mini Mental State (MMS). Scores on the MMS range from 30 (no impairment) to 0 (most impairment). Pathological deterioration is suspected when patients score under 20 (8). In the present study, SDAT patients had scores of 0 to 19 (mean ± SD= 7.5 ± 5.3). Control patients had scores of 22 to 27 (mean ± SD= 23 ± 1.9). Depression was evaluated with a brief scale adapted to demented patients (9). Scores range from 0 (no depression) to 15 (severe depression). Control and SDAT patients were rated for depression by 3 different physicians (PD, MR, YL) and the final score was the mean value of the 3 evaluations. SDAT patients mean score (± SD) was 4.7 ± 2.1 versus 4.6 ± 2 in control patients.

The dexamethasone suppression test was performed by administering 1 mg of oral dexamethasone at 11 pm. Blood samples for cortisol determination were drawn at 4 pm the following day. Serum cortisol levels were measured with a specific radioimmunoassay (Gammacoat 125 I). The technique has a sensitivity of 0.70 µg/dl. According to Carroll (1), a cortisolemic value over 5 µg/dl after dexamethasone administration was considered as abnormal DST i.e. lack of suppression. The data were analyzed with Student's t test, Mann and Whitney U test and Pearson r for correlation.

RESULTS

An abnormal DST was observed in 5/8 controls and 7/27 SDAT patients. There was no significant difference between suppressors and non suppressors with respect to their depression score. Depression scores were nor correlated to cortisolemic values in controls and SDAT patients taken as a whole (r=.403, r=.309, respectively). Cortisolemic values of SDAT patients were lower than values in control patients (4.84 ± 0.9 vs 7.67 ± 1.17) but were not significantly different. There was no correlation between cortisolemic values and age (r=-.027).

SDAT patients were subdivided in 2 subgroups with similar mean age and sex ratio, on the basis of their dementia rating (Table I)

Table I: DST results related to the severity of mental impairment in SDAT patients

	I.Severe Dementia (MMS Score 0-9)	II.Mild to Moderate Dementia (MMS Score 10-19)
Patients (N)	16	11
Abnormal DST (N)	7	0
AGE	82.6 ± 3.7	86 ± 7
MMS Score	4.2 ± 3.6	12.5 ± 3.2
Depression Score	5 + 2.3	4.2 + 1.8
Cortisol (µg/dl)	6.5 ± 5.6	2.3 ± 1.3 *

Values are means ± SD * $p < .05$, Mann and Whitney U test

Group I (N = 16) patients had a MMS score of 0 to 9. Group II (N = 11) patients had a MMS score of 10 to 19. 7/16 (43%) patients in group I were non suppressors. All the patients of group II were DST suppressors. The most severely impaired patients (group I) had significantly higher cortisolemic values than less affected patients (group II) ($p < .05$). Nevertheless, MMS scores and cortisolemic levels were not significantly correlated in SDAT patients taken as a whole ($r = -.127$). Depression scores in groups I and II were not significantly different. To test the relative sensitivity of DST, the proportion of abnormal results was also assessed with a cut-off level of 6 µg/dl plasma cortisol. The number of suppressors and non suppressors patients was not modified by this procedure.

DISCUSSION

Of the 27 SDAT patients, 25% were non suppressors. This percentage is much lower than that observed in other studies of SDAT patients (2-5). These studies showed 45-57% of non suppressors. An exception is the study of Jenike and Albert (6) who observed a proportion of non suppressors similar to ours (27%). They also noticed that non suppression was positively correlated with the severity of the dementia. In our sample, non suppression was found only in the group of most impaired patients. The percentage of non suppressors in this group is similar to that observed by other authors. In contrast, moderately impaired patients had a normal DST. Thus, dexamethasone non suppression seems to be related to the severity of the dementia rather than to age (mean age was the same in groups I and II).

The high frequency of abnormal DST in control patients is surprising since they had low depression scores. To our knowledge, such a high frequency of non suppressors has never been reported previously in the elderly free of depression. Many authors suggested that DST abnormal results could be related to age (10-14) but this has not been confirmed in an healthy elderly population study (15). Nevertheless the mean age in that study was lower than in ours (75.3) and the one subject who failed to suppress normally was the oldest, 87 year old. In fact, there is only one study of dexamethasone suppression in an age group similar to ours and it showed normal suppression (16). These discrepancies emphasized the need for a more extensive investigation of the DST in normal elderly above the age of 70.

If DST is not related to age, high frequency of abnormal results in control patients might be related to weight loss or systemic diseases (12). This was not the case in our population. Of the two patients with congestive heart failure, only one was DST non suppressor. Another explanation could be that some of these patients were somewhat depressed and that the scale used in the study for depression rating was not sensitive enough.

Lack of suppression was related to the severity of dementia but there was no significant correlation between cortisolemic values and MMS scores. This suggests that abnormal DST in SDAT might be related to an impairment in the hypothalamic-pituitary-adrenal (HPA) axis more than to cortical lesions.

The HPA axis is sensitive to adrenergic (17-18) and cholinergic (19-20) mechanisms, both impaired in SDAT. Since the former is inhibitory and the latter excitatory, it is likely that DST non suppression in SDAT could be related to norepinephrine loss rather than to a cholinergic deficit. Such an hypothesis is presently under investigation.

REFERENCES

1. B.J. Carroll, The Dexamethasone Suppression Test for Melancholia, Brit.J.Psychiat. 140, 292-304 (1982).
2. M. Raskind, E. Peskind, M.F. Rivard, R. Veith, R.Barnes, Dexamethasone suppression test and cortisol circadian rhythm in primary degenerative dementia, Am.J.Psychiatry. 139, 1468-1471 (1982).
3. J.E. Spar, R. Gerner, Does the dexamethasone suppression test distinguish dementia from depression ? Am.J.Psychiatry. 139, 238-240 (1982)
4. J. Balldin, C.G. Gottfries, I. Karlsson, G. Lindstedt, G. Langstrom, J.Walinder, Dexamethasone Suppression Test and serum prolactin in dementia disorders, Brit.J.Psychiat. 143, 277-281 (1983)
5. A. Coppen, M. Abou-Saleh, P. Milln, M. Metcalfe, J. Harwood; J. Bailey, Dexamethasone suppression test in depression and other psychiatric illness, Brit.J.Psychiat. 142, 498-504 (1983)
6. M.A. Jenike, M.S. Albert, The Dexamethasone suppression test in patients with presenile and senile dementia of the Alzheimer type, J.Am.Geriat.Soc. 32, 441-444 (1984)
7. American Psychiatric Association, Diagnostic and Statistical Manual of Mental Disorders. DSM III, Third Ed. Washington (1980)
8. M.F. Folstein, S.E. Folstein, P.R. Mc Hugh, Mini Mental State. A practical method for grading the cognitive state of patients for the clinician, J.Psychiat.Res. 12, 189-198 (1975)
9. L.Covi, R.S. Lipman, D.M. Mc Nan, T. Czerlinsky, Symptomatic volunteers in multicenter drug trials, Prog.Neuropsychopharmacol. 3, 521-533 (1979)
10. M.A. Schlesser, G. Winokur, B.M. Sherman, Genetic subtypes of unipolar primary depressive illness distinguished by hypothalamic pituitary adrenal axis activity, Lancet, 1, 739-741 (1979)
11. G.M. Asnis, E.J. Sachar, U. Halbreich, R.S. Nathan, H. Novacenko, L.C. Ostrow, Cortisol secretion in relation to age in major depression, Psychosom.Med. 43, 235-242 (1981)
12. B.J. Carroll, M. Feinberg, J.F. Greden, J. Tarika, A.A. Albala, R.F. Haskett, N. Mc James, Z.Kronfol, N. Lohr, M. Steiner, J.P. de Vigne, E. Young, A specific laboratory test for the diagnosis of melancholia, Arch.Gen.Psychiatry, 38,15-22 (1981)
13. G.F. Oxenkrug, N.Pomara, I.M. Mc Intyre, R.J. Branconnier, M. Stanley, S. Gershon, Aging and cortisol resistance to suppression by dexamethasone: a positive correlation, Psychiatry Research, 10, 125-130 (1983)
14. K.L. Davis, B.M. Davis, A.A. Mathé, R.C. Mohs, A.B. Rothpearl, M.I. Levy, L.K. Gorman, P. Berger, Age and the dexamethasone suppression test in depression, Am.J.Psychiatry, 141, 872-874 (1984)
15. M.F. Tourigny-Rivard, M.Raskind, D. Rivard, The dexamethasone suppression test in an elderly population, Biological Psychiatry, 16, 1177-1184 (1981)

16. M. Friedman, M.F. Green, D.E. Sharland, Assessment of hypothalamic-pituitary-adrenal function in the geriatric age group, J.Gerontol. 24, 292-297 (1969)
17. M.T. Jones, E. Hillhouse, J. Burden, Secretion of corticotropin releasing hormone in vitro, in:Frontiers in Neuroendocrinology, L. Martini and W.F.Ganong Eds, Raven, New York, vol 4, 195-226 (1976)
18. E.J. Sachar, G.M. Asnis, R.S. Nathan, U. Halbreich, M.A. Tabrizi, Dextroamphetamine and cortisol in depression, Arch. Gen.Psychiatry, 37, 755-757 (1980)
19. B.M. Davis, K.L. Davis, Cholinergic mechanisms and anterior pituitary hormone secretion, Biol. Psychiat. 15, 303-310 (1980)
20. S.C. Risch, R.M. Cohen, D.S. Janowsky, N.H. Kalin, D.L. Murphy, Mood and behavioral effects of physostigmine in humans are accompanied by elevations in plasma beta endorphin and cortisol, Science, 209, 1545-1546 (1980)

HORMONE-STIMULATED ADENYLATE CYCLASE ACTIVITY IN MAN:

STUDIES WITH PERIPHERAL MODELS

R.P. Ebstein, D. Selinger, J. Mintzer, G. Oppenheim, L.R. Goldin, B.S. Ebstein, O. Brawman, Z. Shemesh, and J. Stessman

Department of Geriatric Research, Ezrath Nashim Hospital
Jerusalem, P.O.B. 140, Israel

Cyclic AMP, the so-called "second messenger" mediates the effects of a number of hormones including catecholamines on a plethora of cell processes (1). The hormone-stimulated adenylate cyclase complex consists of three principal components. The receptor spans the plasma membrane and its external side provides a site for binding circulating hormones. The Ns and Ni proteins, or guanine-nucleotide binding regulatory subunits, link the receptor to the catalytic subunit of the enzyme. The activated or inhibited (in the case of Ni coupling) catalytic subunit converts ATP to cyclic AMP. The various components of the hormone-sensitive adenylate cyclase complex can to some extent be separately measured and a number of studies have demonstrated the functional independence of these subunits (2).

Studies in man of this important enzyme are limited by the suitability of ethically permissible protocols for human subjects. Nevertheless, in spite of these limitations a number of methods are available for studying adenylate cyclase in man including: perfusion studies (3,4), biopsy (5), parotid secretion (6), lumbar puncture (7), lymphocytes (8,9), platelets (10), fibroblasts (11) and Epstein-Barr virus transformed lymphoblasts (12). As discussed below our laboratory has extended and developed procedures for evaluating hormone-stimulated adenylate cyclase activity in man. In our investigations of hormone-stimulated adenylate cyclase activity we have considered the various effects that endogenous hormone levels, sex, heredity, drugs, disease, and age have on the activity of this important enzyme (3,4,8,9,13-15).

PERIPHERAL PERFUSION STUDIES

The usefulness of the peripheral perfusion technique is convincingly demonstrated in evaluating age-associated changes in the function of the beta-adrenergic sensitive adenylate cyclase in man (3). Biochemical response to salbutamol in a group of aged and younger individuals was determined by measurement of time-dependent changes in plasma cyclic AMP levels after salbutamol infusion. In the younger group salbutamol induced a three fold rise in plasma cyclic AMP levels between 20 and 30 min after drug administration (Fig. 1). In the older participants the maximum rise after salbutamol was only one and one-half fold. In addition to the reduced cyclic AMP response to salbutamol infusion in the elderly group,

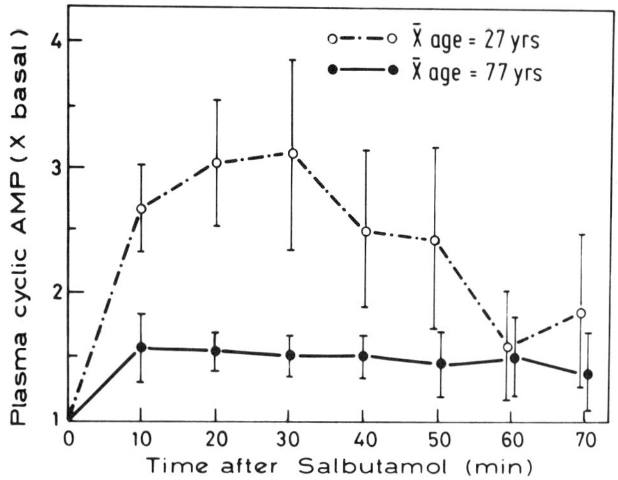

Fig. 1. The effect of salbutamol on plasma cyclic AMP levels in two age groups (3)

the clinical response to the drug infusion in the aged participants was also markedly blunted. Both pulse rate and systolic blood pressure response to salbutamol infusion was significantly reduced in the older individuals. The salbutamol-induced rise in plasma cyclic AMP derives from peripheral beta-receptors as does the epinephrine- and isoproterenol-induced rise in plasma cyclic AMP (16). The reduced response in the elderly individuals to salbutamol therefore suggests an age-related deterioration of peripheral beta-receptor-linked adenylate cyclase function in man.

Administration of glucagon in humans causes a profound hyperglycemic effect and leads to a marked rise in plasma cyclic AMP levels due to activation of glucagon-sensitive adenylate cyclase. The rise in plasma cyclic AMP that originates from intracellular cyclic AMP can be used as an in vivo measure of cyclase activity in man (17). Measurements of plasma cyclic AMP levels after intravenous glucagon administration were used to determine glucagon-stimulated adenylate cyclase activity in a group of young and elderly individuals (4). Parallel measurements of plasma glucose levels after hormone administration were also made. In both age groups, glucagon induced a similar increase in plasma cyclic AMP levels. In addition, no difference was observed between the old and young individuals in the rise in plasma glucose levels after glucagon administration.

Aging at the tissue and organ level in higher organisms is not a uniform process and in some tissues age-related changes are more prominent than in others. The glucagon study (4) was designed to detect a possible decline in activity of a second hormone-sensitive adenylate cyclase complex in aged man. However, the similar increase in plasma cyclic AMP and plasma glucose levels after glucagon infusion between a group of young and old subjects suggests that the blunted response of the beta-adrenergic adenylate cyclase to agonist stimulation (3) represents a specific loss of function and does not reflect a general decline in all hormone-stimulated adenylate cyclase function in aged man.

PAROTID GLAND

The parotid gland is particularly attractive for studies of beta-adrenergic function in man since the neurochemical control of parotid secretion has been well-defined in a number of animal studies (18). Parotid secretion can easily be collected by suction application of a small plastic collecting disk over the opening of Stensen's duct (19). We have extended the usefulness of the peripheral perfusion technique by examining the effect of salbutamol infusion on amylase and cyclic AMP concentrations in parotid secretion from ten young volunteers. Salbutamol induced a significant rise in both amylase (Fig. 2) and cyclic AMP (Fig. 3) levels which reached a maximum value 30 min after the start of the

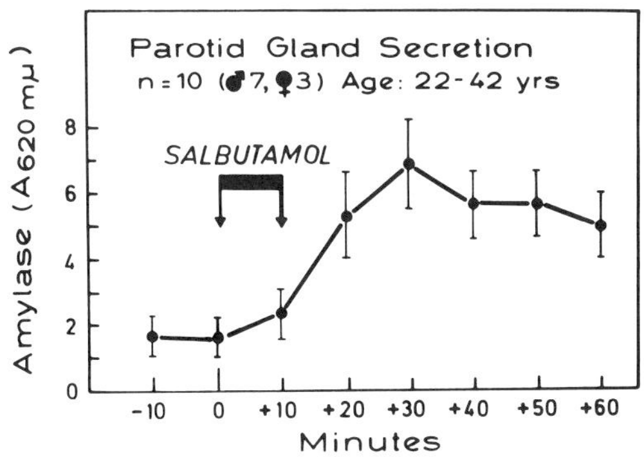

Fig. 2. The effect of salbutamol on parotid amylase levels (6)

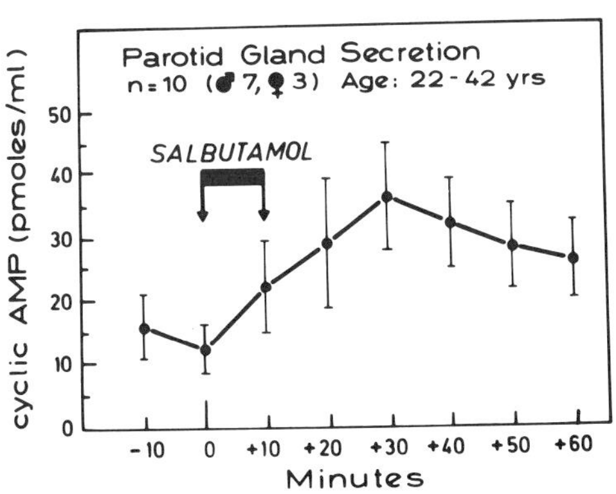

Fig. 3. The effect of salbutamol on parotid cyclic AMP levels (6)

infusion. These findings suggest that salbutamol-induced rises in parotid amylase and cyclic AMP levels will prove to be a worthwhile index of sympathetic function in man. Studies are now in progress to evaluate the effect of age, disease and drug treatment on beta-2 agonist induced changes in parotid gland secretion.

LYMPHOCYTES: BACKGROUND STUDIES

The easy accessiblity of lymphocytes and the non-invasive procedures required for their isolation from human subjects makes this tissue an attractive model for studying hormone-stimulated adenylate cyclase activity in man. Widespread use of this tissue in human investigations suggests that studies of the effect of sex and heredity on cyclic AMP accumulation in individual subjects is worthwhile. After these parameters are established in a general population sample, it will be possible to examine more meaningful variations of lymphocyte adenylate cyclase activity within and between patient and normal population groups.

We have investigated changes in hormone-stimulated cyclic AMP accumulation in lymphocytes obtained from women in different stages of the menstrual cycle (15). Blood samples were taken from 10 women at three different stages in the menstrual cycle and basal, forskolin, isoproterenol and PGE_1-stimulated cyclic AMP accumulation was determined. As shown in Fig. 4 a significant reduction in isoproterenol-stimulated cyclic AMP synthesis was observed in the luteal phase of the cycle (t=2.49;DF=20;p=0.021). No other significant differences were observed. The lowest level of isoproterenol-sensitive activity corresponds to the highest levels of hormone levels in the blood suggesting that reduction in beta-adrenergic function is due to the development of subsensitivity.

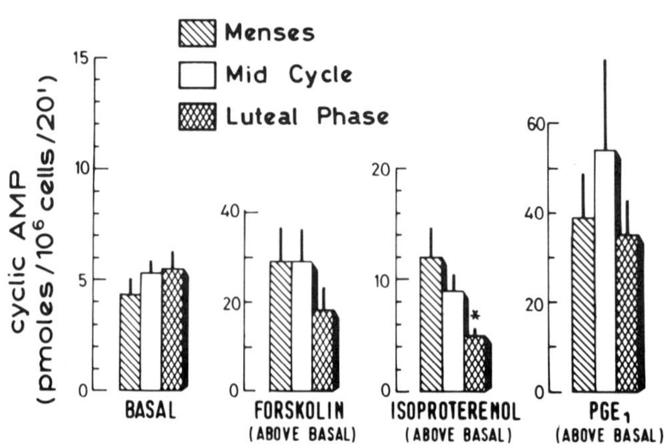

Fig. 4. Lymphocyte cyclic AMP synthesis at different stages of the menstrual cycle

The effect of heredity on hormone-stimulated adenylate cyclase activity in intact human lymphocytes was also examined (14). Isoproterenol, prostaglandin E_1 and forskolin-stimulated cyclic AMP accumulation were compared in intact lymphocytes obtained from nine monozygotic and nine sib pairs matched for age and sex. Heritability was calculated by three different methods, two based on the intraclass correlation coefficients and one based directly on the variances. Only for forskolin is a significant percentage of variance (0.68-0.91) attributable to genetic factors, suggesting that forskolin-stimulated activity may prove to be a valuable genetic marker in studies of human pathology. Neither basal nor isoproterenol and prostaglandin E_1-stimulated activity show significant heritability in intact human lymphocytes. The individual differences observed in levels of beta-adrenergic and prostaglandin stimulated receptor activity in human lymphocytes are, therefore, most likely due to environmental factors.

LYMPHOCYTES: OLD AGE AND SDAT

The use of peripheral blood elements such as lymphocytes and platelets as model systems that may reflect central neuronal function is based on the conservation in higher organisms of basic molecular structures and mechanisms in different tissues. Although various organs and tissues obviously differ in expression of specific function, certain basic mechanisms are maintained in the course of cellular differentiation, and where possible many molecular structures and pathways appear to be similar if not identical in different tissues. Considering the existence of many similar molecular structures in peripheral tissues and brain it is not unreasonable to suppose that in certain disease states or during the aging process, some of these mechanisms will be affected in parallel fashion. These considerations provide a rationale for studying adenylate cyclase activity in lymphocytes from normal, old subjects and SDAT patients.

We compared both isoproterenol and prostaglandin E_1 (PGE_1)-stimulated cyclic AMP accumulation in intact lymphocytes obtained from 10 SDAT patients, from 10 old subjects with no significant cognitive impairment, and from 10 young subjects (8). The effect of increasing concentrations of isoproterenol on lymphocyte cyclic AMP levels in the three subject groups is shown in Fig. 5(a). Cyclic AMP accumulation was significantly reduced both in SDAT patients ($F=8.15$, $p<.01$, 2-way ANOVA comparing SDAT patients to young subjects at all concentrations of isoproterenol) and in old subjects ($F=12.34, p<.01$, in comparison to the young subjects). No difference was observed between SDAT patients and old subjects. No significant difference between males and females was observed in any of the groups.

The effect of increasing concentrations of PGE_1 on lymphocyte cyclic AMP accumulation is shown in Fig. 5(b). Old subjects showed a significant decline in PGE_1-stimulated cyclic AMP accumulation in comparison to young subjects ($F=5.55, p<.05$, 2-way ANOVA). No significant difference between males and females was observed. However, lymphocyte PGE_1-stimulated cyclic AMP accumulation in SDAT patients showed no such decline, and no difference was observed between SDAT patients and young subjects. Moreover, a significant difference was seen between old subjects and SDAT patients ($F=6.03$, $p<.05$, 2-way ANOVA) who showed abnormally high PGE_1-stimulated cyclic AMP accumulation for their age.

Marked individual differences were observed for hormone-stimulated cyclic AMP accumulation in all three subject groups examined. Ratings of severity of cognitive decline in the SDAT patients using the global

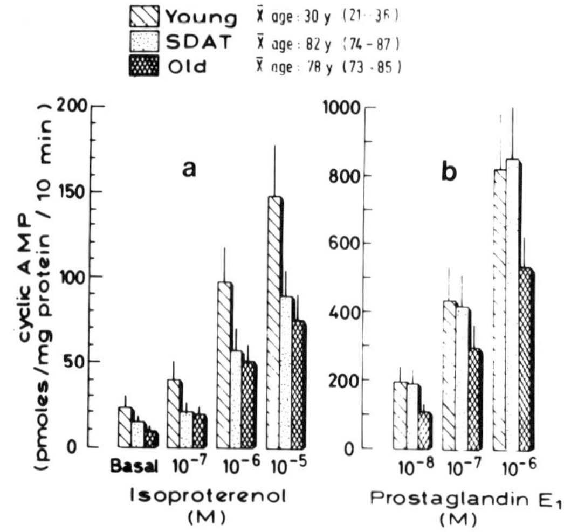

Fig. 5. Effect of L-isoproterenol (a) and PGE_1 (b) on lymphocyte cyclic AMP accumulation in young, old and SDAT subjects (8)

deterioration scale (GDS) showed a significant positive correlation with PGE_1-stimulated cyclic AMP accumulation (r=.752, p<.01, Pearson correlation). No correlation was observed between the GDS score and isoproterenol-stimulated cyclic AMP accumulation (r=.19, NS). None of the old subjects received a GDS score greater than 2.

Strategies aimed at potentiating central cholinergic function have so far proved disappointing in the treatment of Alzheimer's disease, and attempts to rectify additional neurotransmitter deficits may be in order. Our demonstration of a decline in peripheral beta-adrenergic responsiveness in SDAT provides a rationale for the use of adrenergic agonist therapy in this disease; attempts at correcting the specific cholinergic deficit of SDAT may remain unsuccessful as long as this background, age-related adrenergic hypofunction remains uncorrected. Moreover, since not all SDAT patients showed significant decline in beta-adrenergic function, a drug intervention tailored to individual biochemical profiles may be indicated.

Prostaglandins of the E series inhibit the lymphocyte cellular immune response in vitro both in experimental animals and in man (20). Reports have appeared of both an increased frequency of autoimmune disease with age and of the occurrence of brain specific antibodies in pathological conditions of brain damage (21). Although in the initial stages of SDAT immunoglobins IgG and IgM are reported to be increased, in the later stages a state of relative immunodeficiency is described (22). Our results demonstrating an increased PGE_1 receptor sensitivity in SDAT patients lend support to the concept that involvement of the immunological systems may be important in the pathogenesis of Alzheimer's disease.

An important characteristic of the beta-adrenergic adenylate cyclase complex is self-regulation. Catecholamines modulate both the number of receptors available for ligand binding and the activity of adenylate cyclase. Exposure of target cells to beta-adrenergic agonist induces rapid loss of receptors from the cell surface and a parallel reduction in adenylate cyclase activity. Acute desensitization of adenylate cyclase and down-regulation of beta-receptor number has been described in many tissues including lymphocytes (23).

Our studies of hormone-stimulated adenylate cyclase activity in man suggested that an additional characteristic of the beta-adrenergic complex, self-regulation, was worth investigating in aged subjects and in SDAT patients. Acute desensitization of lymphocyte adenylate cyclase was studied in vitro in intact lymphocytes obtained from 3 groups of subjects (9): young, aged and SDAT patients. In all three groups previous exposure of cells to isoproterenol resulted in a significant reduction in cyclic AMP accumulation upon subsequent incubation with isoproterenol. On the other hand, there was no significant reduction in PGE_1-stimulated cyclic AMP accumulation in lymphocytes previously exposed to isoproterenol, demonstrating the specificity of the desensitization response.

Although an important characteristic of the beta-receptor adenylate cyclase complex, self-regulation, was intact in lymphocytes obtained from both aged and SDAT subjects, other studies suggested age-associated deterioration in adenylate cyclase function. Just as we have shown not all hormone-stimulated adenylate cyclases are equally affected by the aging process (glucagon-activated cyclase), we have now demonstrated that not all properties (desensitization) of the beta-adrenergic complex show an age or disease-associated loss of function.

CONCLUSION

We are studying adenylate cyclase in man using peripheral perfusion techniques (3,4), lymphocytes (8,9,13,14), EBV-transformed lymphocytes (12), and platelets (10). All of these studies suggest an age-associated decline in man of peripheral hormone-stimulated adenylate cyclase activity. Morever, this decline in enzyme activity is functionally significant: we have shown that decreased synthesis of cyclic AMP underlies the blunted clinical response to adrenergic stimulation (3). Although in both lymphocytes (8) and platelets (10) a decline in PGE_1 receptor activity in normal aging was also significant, not every hormone-sensitive adenylate cyclase activity deteriorates with age. No significant deterioration in glucagon-stimulated adenylate cyclase activity could be detected (4). In addition, not all functions associated with adenylate cyclase activity appear to be equally affected by aging. We could not demonstrate any deterioration in the ability of the beta-adrenergic adenylate cyclase complex in lymphocytes to down-regulate after <u>in vitro</u> incubation with isoproterenol (9).

Our studies of SDAT patients demonstrate a deterioration in lymphocyte beta-adrenergic stimulated adenylate cyclase function that has also been observed in normal, old subjects. These results are not surprising since SDAT patients in addition to their disease-specific pathology are also burdened with the physiological consequences of normal aging. We presented evidence that alpha-adrenergic function deteriorates with age both in cognitively intact and in SDAT subjects (10). Our findings of a decline in both beta- and alpha-adrenergic in SDAT suggest that therapeutic use of more than one pharmacological agent may be justified in treatment of senile dementia; clinical trials that attempt to only treat the cholinergic deficit may not be successful as long as other age-associated biochemical dysfunctions are not corrected.

This work was supported in part by grants from the Herman Goldman Foundation, New York and the United Jewish Endowment Fund of Greater Washington-Pollinger Foundation.

REFERENCES

1. E.W. Sutherland, I. Oye, and R.W. Butcher, Rec. Prog. Hormone Res. 21:623 (1965).
2. G.L. Giles, M.G. Caron and R.J. Lefkowitz, Physiol. Rev. 64:661 (1984)
3. J. Stessman, R. Eliakim, C. Cahan, and R.P. Ebstein, J. Gerontol. 39: 667 (1984).
4. J. Stessman, R. Eliakim, and R.P. Ebstein, Age, 7:71 (1984).
5. M. Newman, E. Klein, B. Birmaher, M. Feinsod, and R.H. Belmaker, Brain Res. 278:380 (1983).
6. D. Selinger, D. Waksman, J. Stessman, and R.P. Ebstein, Salbutamol-induced rise in cyclic AMP and amylase levels in human parotid secretion, submitted.
7. R.P. Ebstein, J.Biederman, R. Rimon, J. Zohar, and R.H. Belmaker, Psychopharmacol. 51:71 (1976).
8. R.P. Ebstein, G. Oppenheim, and J. Stessman, Life Sci. 34:2239 (1984).
9. Oppenheim, G., J. Mintzer, I. Halperin, R. Eliakim, J. Stessman and R.P. Ebstein, Life Sci. 35:1795 (1984).
10. R.P. Ebstein, G. Oppenheim, M.S. Tropper, A. Yagur, and J. Stessman, Clin. Neuropharmacol. 7(Suppl.1):S23 (1984).
11. N.S. Nadi, J.I. Nurnberger, Jr., and E.S. Gershon, New Engl. J. Med. 311:225 (1984).
12. R.P. Ebstein, M. Steinitz, J. Mintzer, J., I. Lipshitz, and J. Stessman, Beta-adrenergic stimulated adenylate cyclase activity in normal and EBV-transformed lymphocytes, submitted.
13. J. Mintzer, O. Brawman, I. Lipshitz, Z. Shemesh, J. Stessman, and R.P. Ebstein, Hormone and forskolin-stimulated cyclic AMP accumulation in human lymphocytes: Reliability of longitudinal measurements, submitted.
14. R.P. Ebstein, J. Mintzer, Y. Lipschitz, Z. Shemesh, L.R. Goldin, and J. Stessman, Heritability of forskolin and hormone-stimulated adenylate cyclase activity in human lymphocytes, submitted.
15. R.P. Ebstein, O. Brawman, J. Mintzer, B.S. Ebstein and J. Stessman, Hormone-stimulated cyclic AMP synthesis in human lymphocytes during the menstrual cycle, submitted.
16. J.H. Ball, N.I. Kaminsky, J.G. Hardman, A.E. Broadus, E.W. Sutherland, and G.W. Liddle, J. Clin. Invest. 51:2124 (1972).
17. R.P. Ebstein, T. Kara, and R.H. Belmaker, Acta Pharmacol. Toxicol. 41: 80 (1977).
18. I.D. Mandel and R.L. Katz, J. Oral Ther. Pharmacol. 4:260 (1968).
19. D. Selinger, D.J. Cohen, S. Ort, G.M. Anderson, K.A. Caruso and J.F. Leckman, J. Am. Acad. Child Psychiatry, 23:392 (1984).
20. C.S. Henney, H.R. Bourne, and L.M. Lichtenstein, J. Immunol. 108:1526 (1972).
21. R.L. Walford, J. Gerontol. 17:281 (1962).
22. D. Cohen and C. Eisdorfer, Br. J. Psychiat. 136:33 (1980).
23. J.F. Krall, M. Connelly, and M.L. Tuck, J. Pharmacol. Exp. Ther. 214: 554 (1980).

ANTI-HALOPERIDOL ANTIBODIES AND THEIR AUTO-ANTI-IDIOTYPES: TOOLS IN THE STUDY OF NEUROLOGICAL DISORDERS

M. Schreiber, I. Sekler, D. Noff, M. Assael[1], D. Moscovich[2], I. Aberbuch[2] and S. Fuchs

Department of Chemical Immunology, The Weizmann Institute of Science, Rehovot 76100, Israel and Psychiatric Departments Kaplan Hospital[1] and Ezrat Nashim Hospital[2]

INTRODUCTION

Dopaminergic pathways appear to be involved in many brain functions including mental and emotional states (1). There is clinical and pharmacological evidence which indicates the involvement of dopaminergic mechanisms in neurological disorders of the central nervous system (2-4). Antibodies to dopamine receptors and to dopaminergic ligands may provide appropriate tools for the investigation of dopamine receptors. In addition, this may be especially attractive in view of the possibility that autoimmune mechanisms might also play a role in neurological disorders (5-7).

One approach to elicit antibodies against the dopamine receptor is to immunize animals with preparations containing the receptor, and isolating or selecting for the specific anti-receptor antibodies. This approach has been rather difficult for the dopamine receptor as it is present in very minute amounts even in tissues where it is present in relatively high concentrations, e.g. corpus striatum. Another, indirect approach for the preparation of anti-receptor antibodies is by the application of an anti-idiotypic route. By this approach, anti-ligand antibodies are first prepared and used later to produce anti-idiotypic antibodies directed against the variable region of the anti-ligand antibodies. Some of these anti-idiotypic antibodies can be considered as anti-receptor antibodies if they resemble in their binding specificity to that of the ligand to the receptor, thus comprising an "internal image" of the original ligand (Fig. 1). Indeed we have shown that anti-idiotypic antibodies elicited against anti-spiroperidol antibodies bind specifically to brain striatal membranes (8). Similar receptor recognition by anti-idiotypes against anti-ligand antibodies was demonstrated for several other receptor systems (9-13).

In this report we describe the production and characterization of specific polyclonal and monoclonal anti-haloperidol antibodies and their application in the determination of haloperidol levels in samples of sera of haloperidol-treated patients. We also describe the production of anti-idiotypic antibodies against anti-haloperidol antibodies and demonstrate the potential of some of them to bind to dopamine receptors.

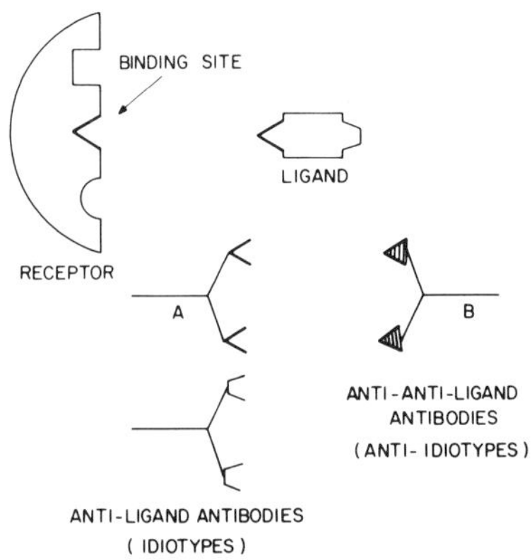

Fig. 1. Anti-ligand antibodies and their anti-idiotypes in relation to the receptor (schematic description).

RESULTS

Polyclonal Anti-haloperidol antibodies

Haloperidol is a butyrophenone derivative and is a strong dopaminergic antagonist which binds with high affinity to dopamine receptors (14). Polyclonal anti-haloperidol antibodies were elicited in rabbits following repeated immunizations with a conjugate of haloperidol and bovine serum albumin (BSA). Conjugation was performed either via the keto group (Halo(CO)-BSA) in a procedure similar to the conjugation of spiroperidol to BSA (8) or via the hydroxy group of haloperidol (Halo(OH)-BSA) prepared as described by Wurzburger et al. (15). Anti-haloperidol antibodies were determined by a radioimmunoassay (8) with (^{3}H)-haloperidol and their specificity was analyzed by competition experiments with unlabelled haloperidol and additional drugs of the butyrophenone family. Some differences in the specificity between antibodies elicited by the two conjugates were observed (Figs. 2,3).

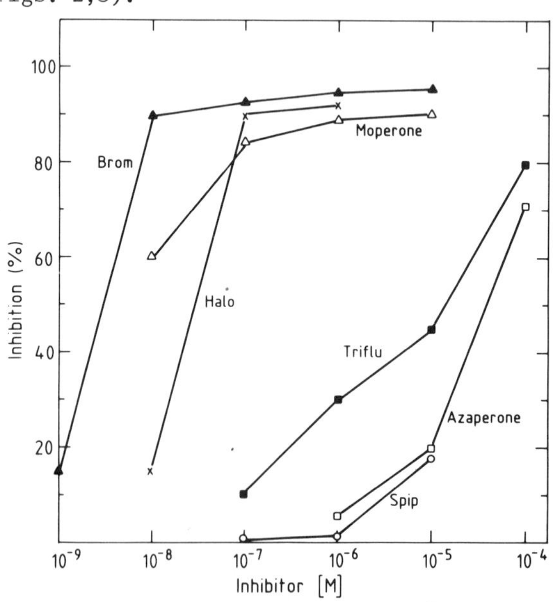

Fig. 2. Inhibition of the binding of (^{3}H)-haloperidol to polyclonal anti-Halo(CO)-BSA antibodies.

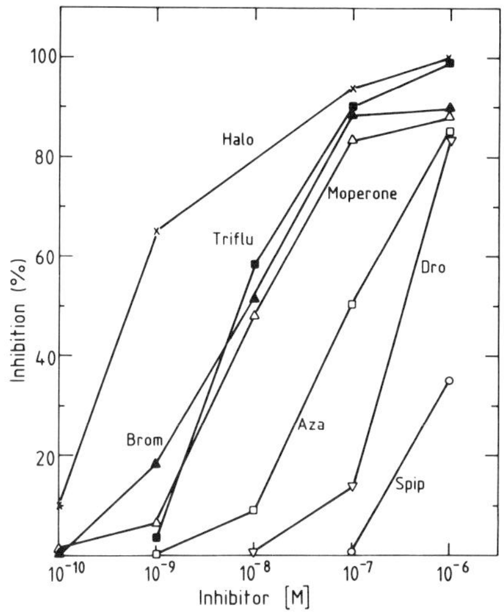

Fig. 3. Inhibition of the binding of (^{3}H)-haloperidol to polyclonal anti-Halo(OH)-BSA antibodies.

Monoclonal anti-haloperidol antibodies

Monoclonal anti-haloperidol antibodies were produced in a hybridoma obtained by fusion of NSO myeloma cells and spleen cells from mice immunized with Halo(CO)-BSA. The hybrid lines having anti-haloperidol activity (tested by radioimmunoassay with (^{3}H)-haloperidol) were cloned on agar and further propagated in vitro and in vivo as ascitic tumors. The monoclonal anti-haloperidol antibodies displayed a high affinity for haloperidol and cross reacted with other butyrophenone derivatives (Fig. 4).

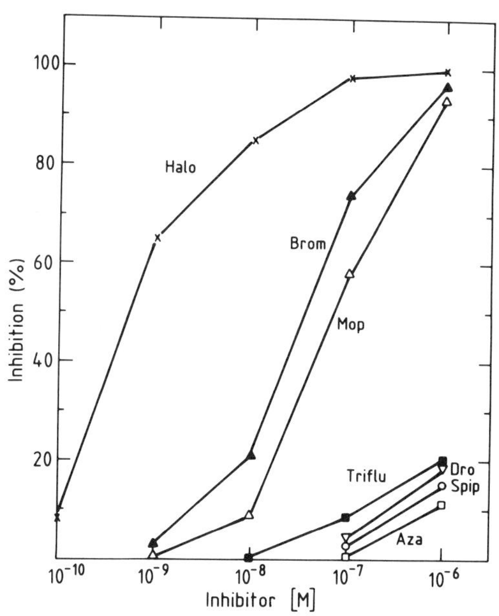

Fig. 4. Inhibition of the binding of (^{3}H)-haloperidol to monoclonal anti-Halo(CO)-BSA antibodies.

Determination of Haloperidol in Schizophrenic Patients

Monitoring of drug therapy by measurement of the drug concentration in plasma is a valuable procedure in clinical management. The most commonly used techniques for determination of neuroleptic drugs in serum and plasma have been gas chromatography (16), radioreceptor assay (17) and more recently radioimmunoassay using polyclonal anti-haloperidol antibodies (15,18). We have used monoclonal anti-haloperidol antibodies for determination of haloperidol levels in samples of sera of haloperidol-treated patients. The inhibition curve of the binding of (^{3}H)-haloperidol to anti-haloperidol monoclonal antibodies, by unlabelled haloperidol was used as a standard curve in these experiments.

Due to the high sensitivity of the assay only minute volumes (microliter quantities) of sera were employed and no extraction of drugs was required. Haloperidol levels as low as 2 ng/ml could be easily determined. The haloperidol levels in sera of schizophrenic patients, expressed as the average of duplicate determinations, in comparison with the daily dose of the drug are depicted in Table 1. There was a positive correlation between the two variables, although individual patients showed big differences in haloperidol levels, following a given dose. This suggests the need of adjusting the dose of haloperidol according to the serum level of the drug.

The main advantages of employing monoclonal antibodies for drug determination are their homogeneity and defined specificity and the ability to obtain practically unlimited quantities of the same antibody in a reproducible manner.

Anti-anti-haloperidol antibodies (anti-idiotypes)

According to the network theory of Jerne (19) anti-idiotypic antibodies may be a normal event in the regulation of the immune response and develop in the same animal producing the idiotype. Thus in animals producing anti-ligand antibodies one may look for antibodies (auto-anti-idiotypes) against the anti-ligand antibodies. The hybridoma methodology

Table 1. Haloperidol levels in sera of patients receiving haloperidol.

Subject	Age (years)	Dose (mg/day)	Duration of treatment (months)	Haloperidol levels (ng/ml)
1	29	100	2	88.0
2	37	80	3	0
3	45	60	8	12.1
4	48	30	3	25.6
5	62	40	5	15.8
6	51	20	4	17.0
7	38	80	2	34.7
8	51	25	48	51.0
9	41	60	1	17.0
10	28	30	5	15.0

enabled us to differentiate easily between the idiotype (anti-haloperidol) and the auto-anti-idiotype (anti-anti-haloperidol), and to specifically select for the auto-anti-idiotypic antibodies. This methodology has been recently employed in the acetylcholine receptor system (20).

The cell lines obtained from the hybridization of haloperidol sensitized spleen cells (described above) were also screened for auto-anti-idiotypic antibodies by binding experiments to purified anti-haloperidol antibodies and to membranes of bovine corpus striatum. Two out of 125 cell lines propagated in this fusion bound anti-haloperidol antibodies as well as membranes of corpus striatum (Fig. 5). Moreover, the binding of the auto-anti-idiotypic antibodies to dopamine receptor could be inhibited by anti-haloperidol antibodies (Fig. 6). Such anti-idiotypes should prove a useful tool for following the dopamine receptor and possibly auto-antibodies against this receptor in neurological disorders such as schizophrenia and Parkinson's disease.

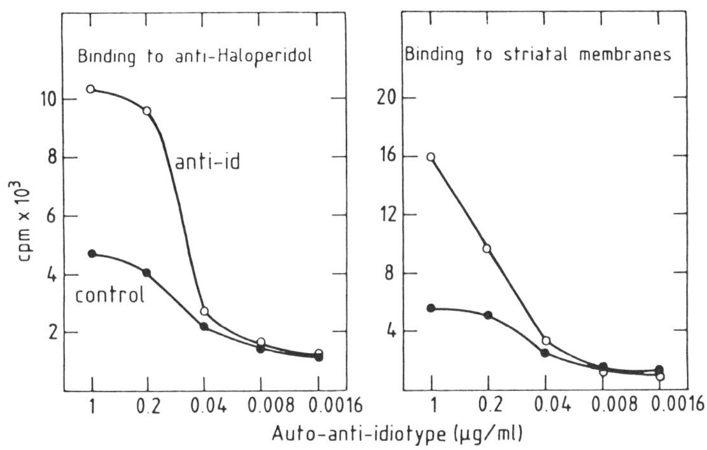

Fig. 5. Specificity of a monoclonal anti-anti-haloperidol antibody (auto-anti-idiotype)

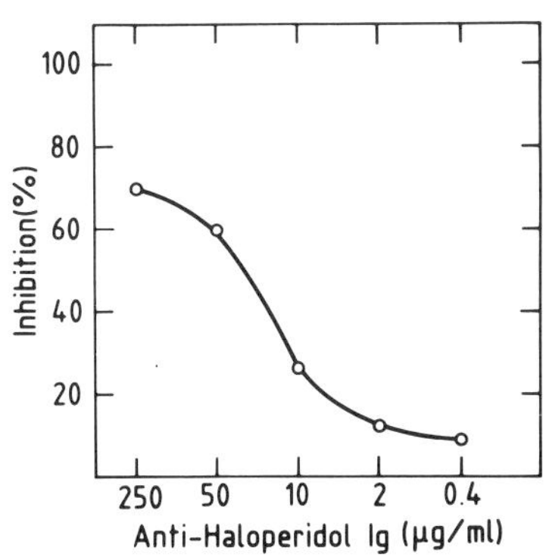

Fig. 6. Inhibition of the binding of monoclonal anti-anti-haloperidol antibodies (auto-anti-idiotypes) to dopamine receptor by anti-haloperidol antibodies.

REFERENCES

1. D.H. York, Amine receptors in CNS. II. Dopamine in Handbook of Psychopharmacology, L.L. Iversen, S.D. Iversen and S.H. Snyder, eds., Plenum Press, New York, pp. 23-61 (1975).
2. A.R. Cools and J. M. Van Rossum, Excitation mediating and inhibition mediating dopamine receptors: A new concept towards a better understanding of electrophysiological, biochemical, pharmacological, functional and clinical data. Psychopharmacologica 45: 243 (1976).
3. P. Seeman, Brain dopamine receptors. Pharmacol. Rev. 32:229 (1980).
4. I. Creese, D.R. Sibley, M.W. Hamblin and S.E. Leff, The classification of dopamine receptor: Relationship to radioligand binding. Ann. Rev. Neurosci. 6:43 (1983).
5. W.J. Fessel, Autoimmunity and mental illness, Arch. General Psychiatry 6: 320 (1962).
6. D. Abramsky and Y. Litvin, Autoimmune response to dopamine-receptor as a possible mechanism in the pathogenesis of Parkinson's disease and schizophrenia. Perspectives in Biology and Medicine 104 (1978).
7. J.G. Knight, Dopamine receptor-stimulating autoantibodies: A possible cause of schizophrenia. Lancet ii:1073 (1982).
8. M. Schreiber, L. Fogelfeld, M.C. Souroujon, F. Kohen and S. Fuchs, Antibodies to spiroperidol and their anti-idiotypes as probes for studying dopamine receptors. Life Sci. 33:1519 (1983).
9. A.B. Schreiber, P.O. Couraud, C. Andre, B. Uray and A.D. Strosberg, Anti-alprenolol anti-idiotypic antibodies bind to β-adrenergic receptors and modulate cathecolamine-sensitive adenylate cyclase. Proc. Natl. Acad. Sci. USA 77:7385 (1980).
10. C.J. Homcy, S.G. Rockson and E. Haber, An anti-idiotypic antibody that recognizes the beta-adrenergic receptor. J. Clin. Invest. 69:1147 (1982).
11. N.H. Wassermann, A.S. Penn, P.I. Freimuth, N. Treptow, S. Wentzel, W.L. Cleveland and B.F. Erlanger, Anti-idiotypic route to anti-acetylcholine receptor antibodies and experimental myasthenia gravis. Proc. Natl. Acad. Sci. USA 79:4810 (1982).
12. W.A. Marasco and E.L. Becker, Anti-idiotype as antibody against the formyl peptide chemotaxis receptor of neutrophil. J. Immunol. 128:963 (1982).
13. S. Ng David, C.C. Si Erwin and E. Gary, Binding of antimorphine anti-idiotypic antibodies to opiate receptors. Analgesics and Antagonists II. (1971-1976). Fed. Proc. 629 (1983).
14. P. Seeman, Brain Dopamine receptors. Pharmacol. Rev. 32:229 (1980).
15. R.W. Wurzburger, L.M. Russel, A.M. Eugene, A.C. Wayne and S. Sydney, A new radioimmunoassay for haloperidol: Direct measurement of serum and striatal concentrations. J. Pharmacol. Exp. Ther. 217:757 (1981).
16. A. Forsman, E. Martensson, G. Nyberg and R. Ohman, A gas chromatographic method for determining haloperidol. Arch. Pharmacol. 286: 113 (1974).
17. S.R. Lader, A radioreceptor assay for neurolaptic drugs in plasma. J. Immunoassay 1:57 (1980).
18. R.T. Rubin, A. Forsman, J. Heykants, B. Tower and M. Michiels, Serum haloperidol determinations in psychiatric patients. Arch. Gen. Psychiatry 37:1069 (1980).
19. N.K. Jerne, The immune system. Sci. Amer. 229:52 (1973).
20. W.L. Cleveland, N.H. Wassermann, R. Sarangarajan, A.S. Penn and B.F. Erlanger, Monoclonal antibodies to the acetylcholine receptor by a normally functioning auto-idiotypic mechanism. Nature 305:56 (1983).

PHARMACOLOGICAL PROTECTION AGAINST MEMORY RETRIEVAL DEFICITS AS A METHOD OF DISCOVERING NEW THERAPEUTIC AGENTS

Elkan Gamzu[1], George Vincent, Anthony Verderese,
Ed Boff, Linda Lee, Arnold B. Davidson
Hoffmann-La Roche Inc.
340 Kingsland Street
Nutley, NJ 07110

GENERAL INTRODUCTION

The material in this chapter represents one component of a more global approach to the discovery of drugs to treat a variety of cognitive disorders. The broader plan, which is described in greater detail elsewhere (1), is based on a pragmatic behavioral approach to the search for agents to treat cognitive disease states that may range from attention deficit disorders (or hyperkinesis) and dyslexia in children to forgetfulness and Alzheimer's disease in the aged. This overall broad-based approach requires examination of many types of behaviors representing a number of processes and is functional in nature. Although such a behavioral program can exist on its own, it is usually employed in conjunction with one or more specific biochemical or chemical hypotheses.

In brief, this pragmatic approach employs two types of tactics. The first is to attempt to pharmacologically improve the learning and memory of normal animals. The second and more common strategy is to pharmacologically overcome or alleviate a naturally occurring or experimentally-induced deficit in learning and/or memory. In implementing these strategies it is necessary to employ several types of behavior that differ in their motivation, require distinctly different motor patterns, and reflect different mnemonic processes. The experiments described in this paper reflect the portion of this overall strategy that focuses on protection against experimentally induced disruptions of memory retrieval.

RETRIEVAL DEFICITS

Retrieval deficit is the major memory problem in the elderly (2,3) and one of the two major memory problems in Alzheimer's disease (4). The nature of such problems may be captured by the so-called "tip of the tongue" phenomenon, in which an individual, aware of the information to-be-remembered, simply cannot retrieve it for articulation; however, when the information is provided, it is instantly recognized. While most

---

[1]Requests for reprints should be sent to Dr. Elkan Gamzu, Clinical Research Department, Warner-Lambert Company, 2800 Plymouth Road, Ann Arbor, MI 48105

people encounter this problem to a limited degree, the magnitude of retrieval problems in individuals with genuine cognitive disorders is such that it can prevent normal functioning in everyday life.

In the development of these experiments we had certain goals in mind. One was to demonstrate a phenomenon that could reasonably be attributed to memory retrieval problems. Another was to devise a test that would be sufficiently simple and rapid to allow for the evaluation of a relatively large number of compounds. This screening approach is necessary in the early stages of discovery of therapeutic drugs. In addition to volume considerations, it is of course crucial to have a test system that minimizes both the false positives (compounds known to lack therapeutic effects, but active in the screen) and the false negatives (compounds known to be therapeutically effective or active in learning and memory processes, but found to be inactive in the testing procedure). The absence of universally accepted standard agents for cognitive therapy renders the determination of false negatives the more complex of the issues.

Previously (1), we identified a variety of compounds with claimed clinical efficacy, or which are described as being active in other animal models of learning and memory. The major class of compounds in this area is the so-called nootropics (see 5,6 for reviews of the origins and definitions of this concept). Briefly, such compounds are inactive in virtually all other behavioral testing situations not specifically designed to evaluate learning and memory function. However, they can improve learning and memory function, or protect against learning impairment or brain insult, and have low toxicity. The most common exemplars of the class are the 2-pyrrolidinone containing moieties such as piracetam (5), aniracetam (7), and pramiracetam (8). Other important clinically used compounds include centrophenoxine (9), pemoline (10), and naftidrofuryl (11).

We have employed three different experimental manipulations to induce the memory retrieval deficits: a subconvulsive electrobrain shock (EBS), hypercapnic hypoxia, and scopolamine. The vast majority of the work reported here focuses on the EBS. Since the early 1930's it has been known that application of electroconvulsive shock produces beneficial effects in depressed patients, while also producing amnesia (12). In animals, an analogous procedure has also been used for some time to produce a pronounced retrograde amnesia. In some animal experiments (13), it has been possible to produce this brainshock-induced retrograde amnesic effect in the absence of gross whole-body motor convulsions. Indeed, it has been shown that measurable brainwave seizure activity is not absolutely necessary to produce retrograde amnesia (14). With this information in hand, and through the use of parametric manipulations, we have been able to establish a level of non-convulsant pulsatile electric shock that when applied transcorneally will reliably produce a transient memory retrieval deficit.

Hypoxia similarly has been known to disrupt cognitive function in humans (15). In fact, Gibson and his co-authors (see 16 for a review) have demonstrated that hypoxia produces biochemical effects that are similar in nature to those occuring in normal aging. Thus, a brief period of hypoxia was also a logical possibility to produce this type of memory deficit. Finally, scopolamine produces amnesia in humans (17) and has been widely studied in animals. Indeed, the work with scopolamine and other anticholinergics played a major role in the development of the so-called cholinergic hypothesis of Alzheimer's disease (18,19).

Behavioral Task: Shuttle Avoidance

The first behavioral task that we employed involved the learning of a simple one-way shuttle avoidance response. Each mouse was placed into one of two identical adjacent compartments that were linked to each other by a small aperture in the separating wall. When the animal was placed in the "start" box, a stimulus configuration was presented. This was to "warn" the animal of the fact that in 10 seconds a 1 mA shock would be applied to the floor of that compartment. The animal could either avoid or escape the shock by running into the "safe" compartment before or during the shock, whereupon the mouse was removed from the apparatus and placed in a holding cage.

On the first day of the experiment all mice received ten trials spaced one minute apart. On the second day of the experiment, the potential therapeutic agents were administered by varying routes and at appropriate pre-treatment times prior to the application of the experimental disruption. The application of the EBS was accomplished by holding the animal so that its eyes made contact with a pair of saline-moistened cotton pads which were attached to the electrodes. The shock parameters were as follows: 200 msec train of square-wave unipolar DC pulses (10 msecs of 10mA constant current at 60 Hz). We describe the effect of EBS colloquially as producing a "stunned state". The animals exhibit Straub tail for a few seconds and are very quiescent, standing immobile wherever placed. However, if touched the animals will move. We saw clonic convulsions rarely, and tonic convulsions even less frequently. When hypoxia was employed, the animals were placed in an enclosure and exposed to eight seconds of a pure carbon dioxide environment that resulted in brief (50-60 second) loss of righting reflex. Testing occurred five minutes after either the EBS or the hypoxia and consisted of an additional ten trials as described above.

The effects of EBS or hypoxia on this behavior were compared to sham shock or normoxia, (in which the animals were treated identically as above, except that electrical stimulation or carbon dioxide were not given) respectively, and are shown in Figure 1. Both EBS and hypoxia disrupted the animals' ability to retrieve the information that was available to animals given control treatment. It is also obvious that after EBS or CO_2, the pattern of recovery looks like a re-learning curve. This phenomenon is only seen if the animals are tested within five minutes of the disruptive procedure. When testing is delayed by 30 minutes, the behavior of control and experimentally treated mice is indistinguishable. This indicates that the information necessary to make the avoidance response is intact, and that the deficit seen when EBS or CO_2 precedes testing by five minutes is clearly one of retrieval.

In additional control experiments, we have taken animals that have received the EBS treatment and tested them for analgesic effects using the D'Amour-Smith tailflick procedure (20), since it is well known that convulsant brain shock definitely effects the opiate system (see 21 for a review). However, there were no differences between control and sham treated animals on this measure of analgesia when they were tested at the same time interval used in the behavioral assay. Similarly, at that same time point, no differences on rotarod performance were found between mice given hypoxic or normoxic treatments. Thus, the animals are motorically and motivationally intact at the point of testing. This is borne out by the fact that after EBS or hypoxia the mice respond appropriately to the onset of shock and they escape very rapidly and efficiently. In additional experiments we tried increasing the shock level to see whether the deficit was simply a motivational problem. While an increase in shock level increases the number of avoidances in EBS-treated mice, at no point

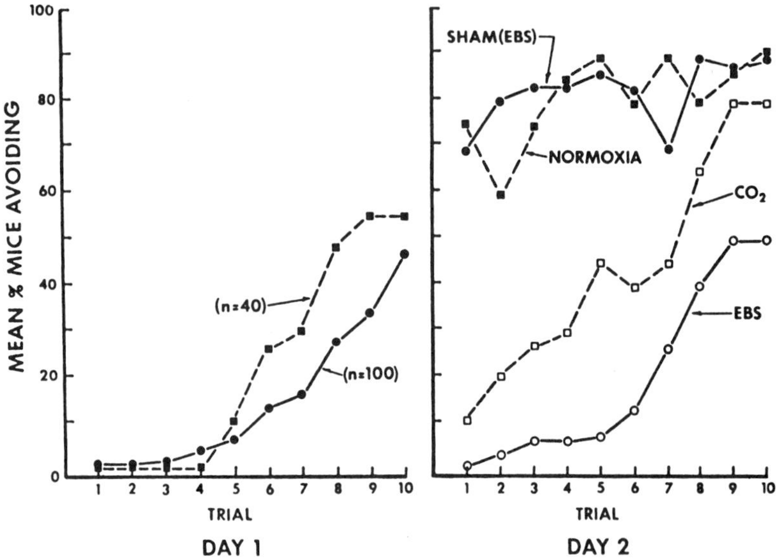

Fig. 1. The effects of EBS or hypoxia (CO_2) on retrieval of one-way shuttle avoidance in mice. Mean percent of mice avoiding shock during training (Day 1) is shown in the left panel. Performance for testing (Day 2) session starting 5 minutes following EBS or hypoxia (circles or squares respectively) administration are compared to the performance of sham shock or normoxia treated mice in the right panel.

does it elevate behavior more than slightly above the level obtained using our standard parameters.

If EBS produces a memory retrieval deficit, then it should do so regardless of how well the task has been learned. To test this, we varied the degree of training prior to the experimental manipulation. The first group of mice received EBS prior to testing on the second day as described above, while the second and third groups received the EBS after two or three days of training prior to testing on the third or fourth day, respectively. The results are shown in Figure 2. Control (sham) subjects rapidly reached asymptote by the third day and were avoiding on all trials. EBS always produced a significant disruption, although the magnitude of this effect was slightly smaller after additional training experience. Certainly, EBS-disruption is not dependent on its application only at a maximally labile point in the acquisition of avoidance.

In summary, non-consulvant EBS of the type employed here (and in all probability, also hypercapnic hypoxia) produces marked effects on behavior that are most reasonably characterized as disrupting memory retrieval for a brief period of time and in a reversible fashion.

Pharmacological Evaluation

A number of nootropic compounds protected against both EBS and CO_2 exposure in a dose-dependent fashion. This is shown in Figure 3 for piracetam. The bars on the left-hand side of the figure represent the mean number of avoidances for two control groups, both receiving vehicle.

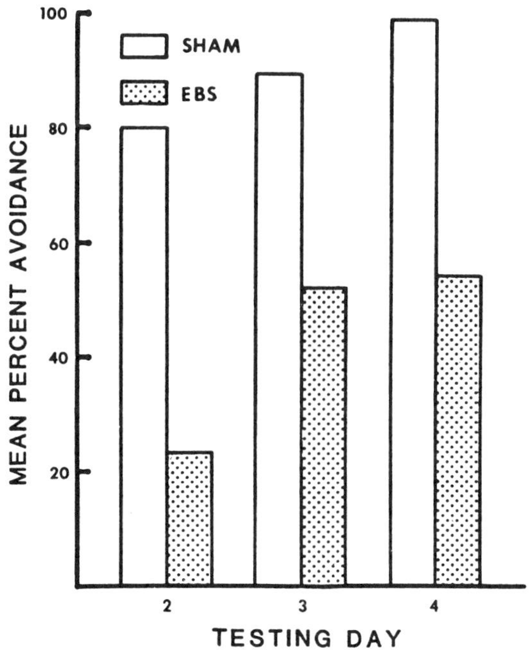

Fig. 2. Avoidance performance of groups of mice receiving EBS or SHAM treatment prior to testing on the day following one, two or three days of one-way shuttle avoidance training.

One pair of bars represents the mean number of avoidances for sham-shock and normoxia control groups; the other pair represents the vehicle treated groups receiving the experimental manipulations. All of the drug-treated groups received either hypoxia or EBS. Piracetam protected against both of these disruptions, with the restoration of behavior being approximately equivalent to control levels at the dose of 1000 mg/kg p.o. In order to facilitate cross-compound evaluation, we also computed a percent recovery of function (%RF) which is based on the ratio of the difference between the mean number of avoidances of the sham-control-treated and the drug-treated groups divided by the difference in mean number of avoidances between the two control groups. This ratio is then converted into a percentage by multiplying by 100. In the case of piracetam, the %RF at 1000 mg was 89 and 92 against EBS and CO_2 respectively. We have also shown that other compounds such as aniracetam and magnesium pemoline are equally effective in protecting against EBS and CO_2 in this test. Subsequently, we have concentrated on the EBS disruption, since it was easier to work with and appeared to be a less severe manipulation; hypercapnic hypoxic disruption being reserved for special studies.

Table 1 presents a list of putative learning and memory agents and their effects in protecting against EBS in the shuttle avoidance paradigm. It is immediately obvious that most of the 2-pyrrolidinone containing moieties (with the exception of oxiracetam) are active at one or more doses. In the case of aniracetam and piracetam, the %RF is high. Also

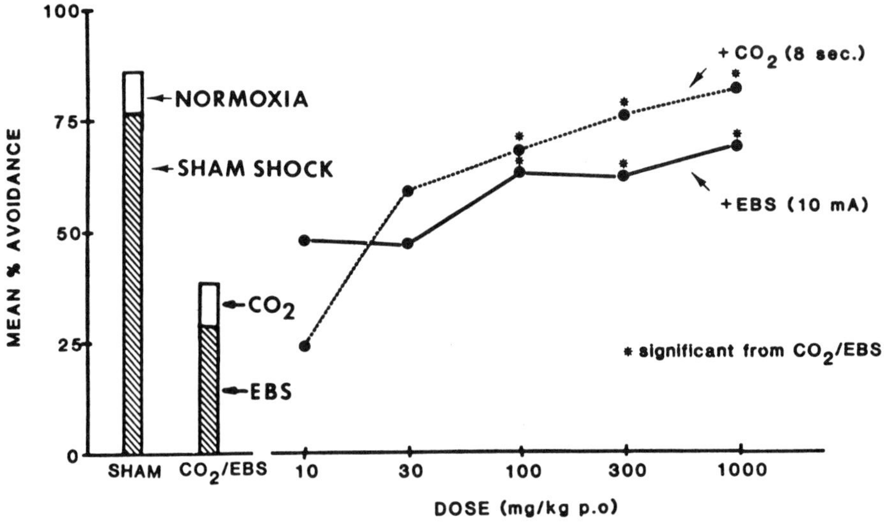

Fig. 3. The activity of piracetam in protecting against EBS and hypoxia (CO_2) disruption of memory retrieval in one-way shuttle avoidance.

active in the test are such diverse agents as centrophenoxine, naftidrofuryl, and the vinca alkaloid vincamine. Of the two agents that are approved in the U.S. for indications related to cognitive dysfunction, pemoline is highly effective, but Hydergine is inactive. This latter finding is not so surprising since the efficacy of Hydergine has been questioned (22,23), and there has been speculation that, when effective, this mixture of ergot alkaloids is acting to elevate mood rather than through any direct effect on cognitive ability (24). By and large, the vast majority of the putative clinically effective agents in Table 1 were active at one or more dose levels constituting suggestive evidence of relatively few false negatives. It should also be noted that the behavioral task enables distinctions to be made among these agents in terms of efficacy (%RF) and the number of active doses, as well as potency. Indeed, there is considerable variation in all three measures. The other aspect of pharmacological validation of the test is shown in Table 2 which demonstrates that a number of standard agents with psychotropic activity are inactive in this test. The lone exception was clonidine which has recently been reported to improve the learning and memory of older primates (25).

A potential artifact in any behavioral study in which the end point is an elevated rate of responding is non-specific psychomotor stimulation. Most of the compounds that protect against EBS disruption do not elevate responding over control level in an independent rodent test of motor activity (26). Moreover, amphetamine is inactive in protecting against EBS disruption of memory retrieval. Nonetheless, we decided to evaluate some of the compounds during the training session to see whether they would elevate the avoidance responding that constitutes the baseline behavior of this test. We chose the training rather than the testing period, since the level of performance in the latter would have been confounded by a ceiling effect. In contrast, the number of avoidances in

Table 1

PROTECTION AGAINST EBS-DISRUPTION OF MOUSE ONE-WAY SHUTTLE AVOIDANCE RETRIEVAL BY PUTATIVE PERFORMANCE ENHANCERS

Compound	Route	Pretreatment Time (Min.)	Dose Range Tested (mg/kg)	Active Doses (mg/kg)	Peak % Recovery of Function
ACTH 4-10	s.c.	30	0.1-3	0.3-1	57
Aniracetam	p.o.	30	10-100	30-100	93
Centrophenoxine	p.o.	60	3-1000	100-1000	61
CI 844	p.o.	60	3-100	Inactive	20
Diphenylhydantoin	p.o.	60	1-100	3-100	122
Etiracetam	p.o.	60	1-300	30Δ	36
Hydergine	p.o.	60	10-300	Inactive	5
Magnesium Pemoline	p.o.	30	0.3-30	1-30	91
Naftidrofuryl	p.o.	60	30-300	100	46
Naloxone	s.c.	15	0.3-10	1,3	54
Oxiracetam	p.o.	60	0.1-100	Inactive	20
Physostigmine	i.p.	15	0.003-0.3	0.03	56
Piracetam	p.o.	60	3-1000	10-1000	89
Pramiracetam	p.o.	60	1-10	3	47
Strychnine	p.o.	60	0.1-3	1-3	58
Vincamine	p.o.	60	3-100	30	43

Δ $p < 0.1$, all other active doses $p < .05$ two-tailed Dunnett t-test

the training session is low (but the variance is high). Consequently, there is room for a considerable elevation, but the effect has to be fairly uniform to produce a statistically significant effect. Of compounds active in protecting against EBS, only magnesium pemoline significantly elevated avoidance responding when given prior to the training session. This compound also increases motor activity in rats, and its ability to protect against EBS disruption could conceivably be attributed to a low-grade stimulant effect. On the other hand, since amphetamine does not significantly protect against EBS it appears that stimulation *per se* is not sufficient to protect against EBS-disruption of retrieval. Aniracetam, piracetam, and vincamine, all of which significantly protect against EBS disruption of memory retrieval, had no effects on avoidance responding in the training session. For these compounds (and probably the vast majority of the other compounds we have evaluated), the protection against EBS disruption is not attributable to a simple stimulatory effect on motor activity.

Thus, within the constraints of this limited study, protection against EBS-disruption of avoidance appears to be a reasonably valid pharmacological test for putative learning and memory enhancing drugs.

Table 2

EFFECTS OF AGENTS NOT CONSIDERED TO BE COGNITIVE PERFORMANCE ENHANCERS ON MOUSE ONE-WAY SHUTTLE AVOIDANCE RETRIEVAL*

Compound	Dose Range (mg/kg) p.o.	Active Doses (mg/kg) p.o.	Peak % Recovery of Function
Amphetamine	0.3-10	Inactive	15
Chlorpromazine	0.3-3	Inactive	3
Clonidine	0.03-0.3	0.1	44
Diazepam	0.3-30	Inactive	5
Dantrium	3-300	Inactive	37
Glucose	300	Inactive	36
Imipramine	10-100	Inactive	0
Pyruvate	300	Inactive	10

* All compounds were administered p.o. 60 minutes prior to testing.

Behavioral Task: Platform Avoidance

Although the validity and utility of the shuttle avoidance test appeared to have been confirmed, the non-automated aspects of the test left it open to experimenter bias and limited the number of agents that could be evaluated at any given time. Consequently, we designed an avoidance test which the animals could learn with similar rapidity and which produced a similar level of performance, but which could be automated both in terms of the handling of the animals and the recording of the data. This paradigm involved the use of a small elevated platform positioned above a grid floor. The equipment, the initial exposure, and the definition of a trial are shown in Figure 4. Initially the mouse is placed on the platform for a one minute adaptation period, at the end of which the first trial begins. Initiation of a trial is signaled by a tone and the release of the platform, which drops the mouse onto the grid floor. This signalled portion of the trial lasts for 15 seconds and is followed by the application of footshock (1.3 mA for 30 seconds) through the grid floor. The mouse can either avoid or escape the shock by jumping on to the platform prior to shock onset or during the shock presentation. When the animal safely reaches the platform, the tone is terminated, however, the shock remains on (in order to ensure that if the animal steps off the platform, it will return to it). Each trial concludes with a brief safety period of ten seconds. Training sessions involve a five-trial session in the morning and a five-trial session in the afternoon. Animals that fail to make any escape responses in the morning are not included in the experiment. [We have subsequently identified these mice as "poor learners" and have studied them independently. They are particularly sensitive to aniracetam's ability to enhance consolidation (27).] For the other animals, EBS is applied five minutes prior to a ten-trial session given the next day. Pharmacological manipulations occur prior to the application of EBS. The operation of all equipment was programmed via computer, making it possible to run at least three animals simultaneously, and eliminating any experimenter bias in the implementation or scoring of the results.

One of our first concerns was the behavioral and pharmacological equivalence between the two procedures. Figure 5 shows a comparison of the effects of pemoline, piracetam, and aniracetam in both procedures. It is clear that the compounds are effective in both, and that there is very

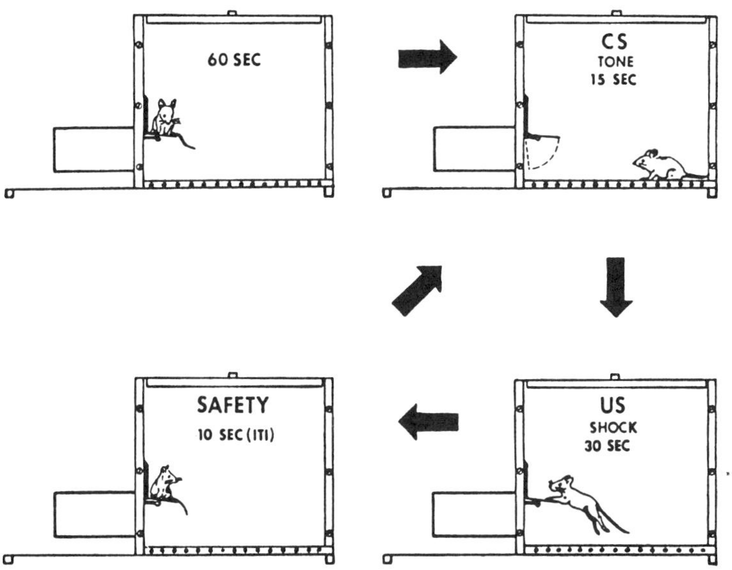

Fig. 4. The equipment and the various components of a testing trial for the platform jump avoidance procedure.

little difference between them. In the case of aniracetam, the dose response curve may be slightly shifted to the left in the platform avoidance procedure. Indeed, in comparing a variety of other standard agents, we have found that the platform procedure tends to be slightly more sensitive. Another feature that is immediately obvious in Figure 5 is the inverted U-shaped dose response function. It seems to be universally the case that agents that improve learning and/or memory show increasing effects with larger doses but only up to a certain point. Continued elevation of the dose beyond the optimal point invariably leads to a decrease back to control levels. This has been true for almost all of the compounds we have studied, and similar findings have been reported by other investigators in a variety of procedures (e.g. 28). From a clinical perspective, it makes the choice of doses to study in humans a particularly perplexing problem, since the choice of the wrong dose may produce a

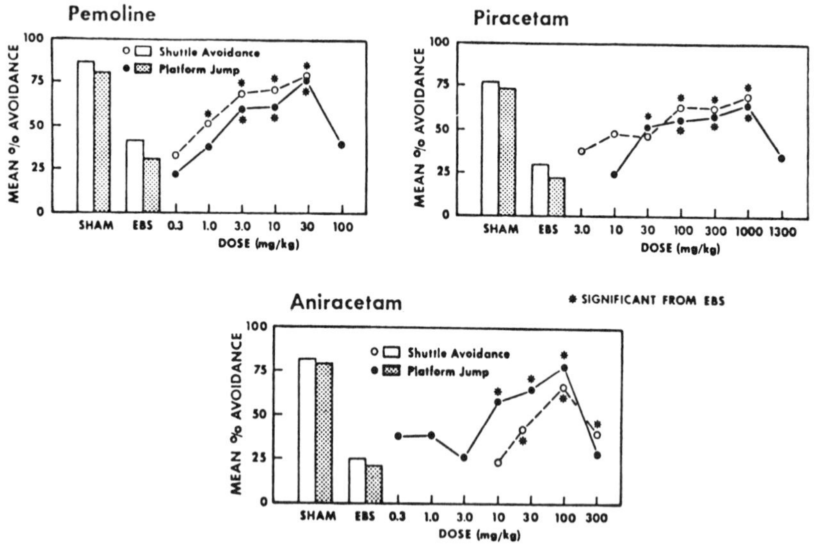

Fig. 5. The memory protective effects of pemoline, piracetam, and aniracetam in mice for both shuttle and platform jump avoidance procedures.

"false negative" response. Clearly, one of the needs in this area is for therapeutic agents that have a wide "window of activity".

We have now evaluated a large number of agents with purported effects in learning and memory in this version of the test; a summary of the results obtained is shown in Table 3. Once again, it is obvious that with some exceptions, the vast majority of these agents protect against EBS-induced disruption of memory retrieval in this task. As mentioned above, this task seems to be somewhat more sensitive to some of these agents than the shuttle avoidance task. Thus, for example, in this version of the EBS test we find pramiracetam to produce a wider dose response curve, similar to those of aniracetam and piracetam, and clearly shifted to the left. This is shown in terms of the %RF in Figure 6. In addition, CI-844 (3-phenoxypiridine; 29), which was inactive in the shuttle avoidance test, protected against disruption of memory retrieval in the platform avoidance test over a wide range of doses. As was the case for the shuttle avoidance test, most psychotropic agents of other classes did not protect against the disruption of memory produced by EBS.

Physiological and Mechanism of Action Studies

Having demonstrated the utility of the EBS test to our satisfaction, we were interested in some of the potential mechanisms of action. To this end, we have conducted a number of experiments, most of which have been successful only in eliminating certain possibilities rather than in defining mechanisms, either for the EBS effect, or for the pharmacological protection.

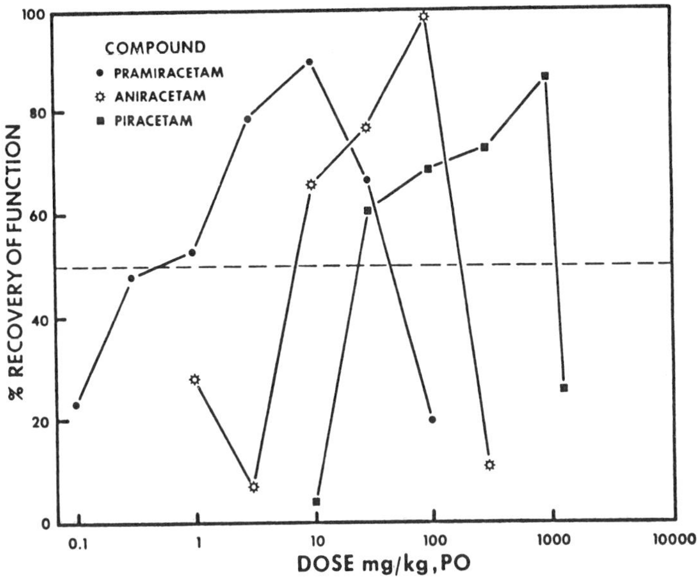

Fig. 6. Comparison of the effects of three standard pyrrolidinones in protecting against EBS-disruption of memory retrieval in mice.

The first series of studies examined electrical activity in the hippocampus. The hippocampus plays a major role in numerous representations of memory systems (30). Lesions of the hippocampus produce severe disruptions of learning and memory (31) as, indeed, will direct electrical stimulation of the hippocampus (32). In the first of this series of experiments (all of which were conducted in collaboration with Drs. Stwertka and MacNeil (33), we implanted hippocampal electrodes in mice and monitored the electrical activity before and after EBS of various milliamperages (mA) was applied in exactly the same fashion as described for the behavioral studies. With the appropriate current level, pronounced hippocampal afterdischarge activity followed the application of EBS. This was not seen at current levels below those that were behaviorally effective in disrupting avoidance retrieval. Indeed, there was a high correlation between seizure activity and behavioral outcome when the current (mA) of EBS was manipulated. There were no effects of transcorneally applied EBS on the electrical activity measured through an electrode whose tip was located one millimeter above the hippocampus. The hippocampal electrical effects were obtained in both anesthetized and unanesthetized mice.

Because of the close correlation between the hippocampal afterdischarge and behavioral disruption of EBS, we chose to study aniracetam (because of its clear activity in protecting against EBS), and diphenylhydantoin and phenobarbital (because of their anticonvulsant effect) in greater detail. Electrodes were implanted bilaterally in both hippocampii of rats. Stimulation was applied at one site, while electrical activity was recorded from both sites. As was expected, phenobarbital elevated seizure threshold, shortened seizure duration, and prevented the spread of the seizure. In contrast, as reported by previous investigators, diphenylhydantoin had little effect on seizure threshold, but also shortened duration of the seizure, and prevented its spread to the contralateral hippocampus. Aniracetam had no effect whatsoever on seizure threshold as measured by this technique. The behavioral effects of these compounds

Table 3
THE EFFECTS OF STANDARD PSYCHOTROPIC AGENTS ON THE EBS-DISRUPTION OF RETRIEVAL IN THE PLATFORM JUMP AVOIDANCE PROCEDURE

Compound	Route	Pretreatment Time (Min.)	Dose Range Tested (mg/kg)	Active Doses (mg/kg)	Peak % Recovery of Function
ACTH4-9 (Analog)	p.o.	30	.01-3.0	.3	67
Almitrine	p.o.	60	1.0-100	-	38
Aniracetam	p.o.	60	.3-300	10-100	99
Aregoline	i.p.	30	.03-3.0	-	25
Arg^8 Vasopressin	s.c.	30	.0003-1000	.003,.03,0.1	69
CI-844	p.o.	60	.0003-10	.001,.003,.01 .03,.1,.3,1.0,3,10	60
CI-911	p.o.	60	.03-30	-	17
	p.o.	30	.1-1.0	.3	68
3-4 DAP	p.o.	60	.00003-.03	-	39
DGLVP	s.c.	30	.01-3.0	.03,.1,.3,1.0	46
Fluoxetine	p.o.	60	1-100	10	54
HOE 175	i.p.	30	.1-100	10	51
	p.o.	60	1-100	-	35
HR 001	p.o.	60	1.0-100	30	76
Lergotrile	p.o.	60	.003-30	.03,.1,.3,1.0, 3.0,10.0	72
MK 771	p.o.	60	.1-30	-	48
	i.p.	30	.003-100	.03,.1,1.0,3.0,10	66
Nicergoline	i.p.	30	.03-3.0	-	25
Nimodipine	p.o.	60	.3-100	-	28
Pemoline	p.o.	30	.3-100	3,10,30	91
Pentoxifylline	i.p.	30	1-100	-	26
Phenobarbital	p.o.	30	.01-30	-	37
Piracetam	p.o.	60	10-1300	30,100,300,1000	87
Pramiracetam	p.o.	60	.1-100	.3,1,3.0,10,30	90
Pyritinol	p.o.	60	1-300	-	34
Somatostatin	s.c.	30	.0003-.1	.003	43
TRH	i.p.	30	.03-100	.1,.3,1.0,3.0,10,30	
	p.o.	60	1.0-100	-	40
Valproate	p.o.	60	1-100	-	52
Zimeldine	p.o.	60	.01-1000	.1,.3,1.0,10,30	52

protecting against EBS in mice are shown in Figure 7. In addition to the already documented finding of aniracetam's ability to protect against memory retrieval disruption, the figure shows a similar effect for diphenylhydantoin but demonstrates the lack of any protective effect after phenobarbital administration. Phenobarbital is definitely inactive in the platform avoidance test but has potent effects on electrical excitability of the hippocampus. A diametrically opposite profile was obtained for aniracetam, which was highly potent in the behavioral task but inactive electrophysiologically. Diphenylhydantoin is active in both, but diphenylhydantoin has also been shown to protect against memory disruption produced by puromycin (34), hypothermia (35), α-amino-isobutyrate (36), and cycloheximide (37), and may have effects on memory processes that are independent of its anticonvulsant potential. Interestingly, the biotransformation from pyrrolidinones to hydantoins has been reported (38). It is worth noting that carbamazepine also protected against EBS-disruption of memory retrieval. Because of their well-documented anticonvulsant effects, we evaluated both diphenylhydantoin and carbamazepine against CO_2 disruption of avoidance retrieval. Both compounds protected against CO_2 in a fashion equivalent to their protective effects against EBS. (The data are not shown here.)

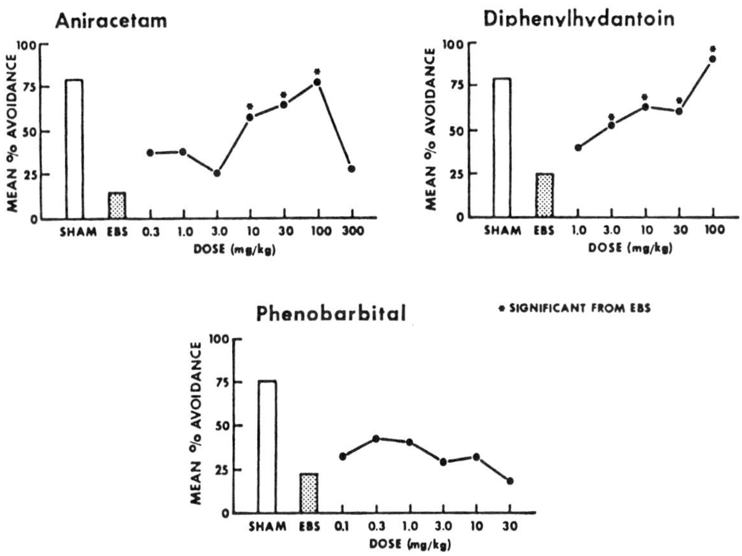

Fig. 7. The effects of aniracetam, diphenylhydantoin, and phenobarbital in protecting against EBS-disruption of memory retrieval in mice.

For obvious reasons one draws conclusions from these studies with some care. Especially since the behavioral studies were conducted in mice with globally applied shock, while the electrophysiological studies were conducted in rats with electrical stimulation applied directly to the hippocampus. Although electrical activity in the hippocampus seems to be correlated with the disruption of memory retrieval, pharmacological protection against hippocampal stimulation does not seem to be sufficient to protect against EBS-disruption (phenobarbital). Moreover, it is possible to protect against a retrieval deficit with a compound that has no direct effects on hippocampal excitability (aniracetam). Clearly additional work is necessary to delineate the role of hippocampal excitability in this phenomenon as well as the potential mechanisms by which one can protect against EBS disruption.

The fact that hippocampal afterdischarge is associated with EBS-disruption of avoidance behavior poses the possibility that some of the pharmacological protection is mediated by an anticonvulsant effect. Consequently, active memory protective agents are also independently evaluated for this effect. The same type of stimulation is used but with 25 mA current. With some exceptions (diphenylhydantoin and carbamazepine), the vast majority of compounds that protect against EBS-disruption of retrieval have no effect on electrically induced clonic-tonic convulsions. Moreover, compounds like diazepam which are effective anticonvulsants are inactive against EBS-disruption of memory retrieval.

Because of the positive effects obtained with various peptides shown in Tables 1 and 3, we have been interested in the possible role of certain endocrine organs in mediating the memory disruption caused by EBS. Recently, there has been a considerable interest in the role of peripheral mediation of apparent memory enhancing effects by certain peptides (39), and other agents (40). In order to better characterize the protective effects of TRH against EBS-disruption of memory retrieval, we have investigated the role of thyroid hormones in attenuating this form of memory disruption. These results will be reported in detail elsewhere (Stwertka et al. In preparation). Briefly, we have been able to show that the EBS-disruption of memory retrieval in this test can be demonstrated in both normal and hypophysectomized mice. Moreover, the memory protective effects of TRH are clearly unrelated to that compound's ability to elevate plasma levels of the thyroid hormones, triiodothyridine (T3) and thyroxine (T4).

In an effort to elucidate the mechanism by which ACTH and its analogs are active in this test, we measured plasma corticosterone levels in three groups of mice. The first group of mice was sacrificed 15 minutes after receiving transcorneal EBS and a second group was sacrificed 15 minutes after receiving sham shock, while a third group served as non-handled controls. The mean values were 34, 22, and 4 micrograms of corticosterone per 100 ml. Thus, both the EBS and the sham shocked groups had significantly higher plasma corticosterone levels than the non-handled controls. In addition, EBS animals had a significantly greater corticosterone level than the sham shocked animals. Although both groups of animals were undergoing considerable stress compared to non-handled controls, it seems unlikely that the additional elevation in the EBS group will be able to account for the pronounced behavioral effects of that manipulation. Indeed in a subsequent set of experiments, we have compared the effects of EBS and sham shock in adrenalectomized (ADX) and sham operated control mice. There are essentially no differences between these groups either in control behavior, nor in the ability of EBS to disrupt the memory retrieval for the avoidance response. Future experiments will evaluate the ability of various peptides to protect against EBS in ADX mice.

Both of these series of experiments suggest that EBS is exerting its effect at a central level that is independent of hormonal influences. A comparison of the effects of scopolamine and methylscopolamine confirms that disruption of avoidance behavior in this task can occur centrally with minimal peripheral involvement. In this series of experiments, either scopolamine or methylscopolamine was given prior to testing (no EBS was applied). While scopolamine was able to produce a dose-dependent decrease in the number of avoidances, methylscopolamine was essentially without effect across the same dose range. Although we have not attempted to protect against this effect of scopolamine in this test, it is of interest to note that nootropics do block scopolamine anterograde amnesia (7,41).

Summary and Conclusions

The work described in this paper represents the development of different ways of evaluating potential therapeutic agents for their ability to protect against memory disruption. We have shown that simple models can capture memory retrieval dysfunction, a phenomenon that is of primary importance in the cognitive difficulties experienced by the elderly and people suffering from Alzheimer's disease. Moreover, we have demonstrated the disruption of memory retrieval in at least two different fashions, and shown that it can be demonstrated with behaviors that require distinctly different motor patterns. Importantly, many compounds with putative effects on learning and memory protected against one or both memory disrupting manipulations. Although the mechanisms of action by which the disruption or the pharmacological protection against it occur are not known, these behavioral techniques are clearly of considerable utility in the discovery of new psychotherapeutic agents. The fact that a compound is active in this test is no guarantee that it will have general effects on learning and memory. Rather, it is crucial that this particular type of study be seen in a more global context which stresses broader strategies. Using this approach, aniracetam has been shown to protect against memory disruption caused by protein synthesis inhibitors, scopolamine, electroconvulsant shock, and hypoxia (7); to enhance consolidation in poor learners (42); to enhance memory under long delays in primates (42,43); and to have electroencephalographic characteristics that are predictive of a nootropic effect (44). Early clinical findings seem to indicate some measure of clinical efficacy (45,46,47). Thus, the application of research strategies and tactics of the type described in this paper in conjunction with a better understanding of learning and memory processes holds forth the promise of new therapeutic agents for the treatment of cognitive disorders.

Acknowledgements

We are particularly indebted to Domenica Iannicelli for typing and organizing the manuscript. We also thank John W. Sullivan for his editorial comments.

Bibliography

1. Gamzu, E. Animal models in the discovery of compounds to treat memory dsyfunction. In: Memory Dsyfunction: An Integration of Animal and Human Research From Clinical and Preclinical Perspectives. D. Olton, E. Gamzu, and S. Corkin, (eds.) Annals of the New York Academy of Sciences, New York, NY, 444:370-393, 1985.
2. Burke, D.M. and Light, L.L. Memory and aging: The role of retrieval processes. Psychological Bulletin, 90:513-546, 1981.
3. Branconnier, R.J. and DeVitt, D.R. Early detection of incipient Alzheimer's disease: some methodological considerations on computerized diagnosis. In: Alzheimer's Disease. B. Reisberg, (ed.) Free Press. New York, NY, 214-227, 1983.
4. Corkin, S., Growdon, J.H., Nissen, M.J., Huff, F.J., Freed, D.M., and Sagar, H.J. Recent advances in the neuropsychological study of Alzheimer's disease. In: Alzheimer's Disease: Advances in Basic Research and Therapies. R.J. Wurtman, S.H. Corkin, and J.H. Growdon. (eds.) Center for Brain Sciences and Metabolism. Cambridge, Mass, 1984.

5. Giurgea, C. Piracetam: Nootropic pharmacology of neurointegrative activity. Curr. Devs. Psychopharmac., 3:221-273, 1976.
6. Giurgea, C. and Salama, M. Nootropic drugs. Prog. Neuropsychopharmacol., 1:235-247, 1977.
7. Cumin, R., Bandle, E., Gamzu, E., and Haefely, W.E. Effects of the novel compound (Ro 13-5057) upon impaired learning and memory in rodents. Psychopharmacology. 78:104-111, 1982.
8. Poschel, B.P.H., Marriott, J.G., Gluckman, M.I. Pharmacology of the cognition activator pramiracetam (CI-879). Drugs Exptl. Clin. Res. IX:853-871, 1983.
9. Martindale The Extra Pharmacopoeia, Twenty-Eighth Edition. The Pharmaceutical Press, London, 1982.
10. Plotnikoff, N.P. Pemoline: Enhancement of maze performance in young rats. Behavioral Biology, 8:117-121, 1973.
11. Cox, J.R. Double-blind evaluation of naftidrofuryl in treating elderly confused hospitalised patients. Geront. Clin., 17:160-167, 1975.
12. Squire, L.R. ECT and memory dysfunction. In: ECT: Basic Mechanisms. B. Lerer, R.D. Weiner, and R.H. Belmaker, (eds.) Libbey, London, 1984.
13. Zornetzer, S. and McGaugh, J.L. Retrograde amnesia and brain seizures in mice. Physiology and Behavior, 7:401-408, 1971.
14. Zornetzer, S. and McGaugh, J.L. Retrograde amnesia and brain seizures in mice: A further analysis. Physiology and Behavior, 7:841-845, 1971.
15. Siesjo, B.K., Johannsson, H., Ljunggren, B., and Norberg, K. Brain dysfunction in cerebral hypoxia and ischemia. In: Brain Dysfunction in Metabolic Disorders. F. Plum. (ed.) Res. Proc. Assoc. Res. Nerv. Ment. Dis. 53:75-112, 1974.
16. Gibson, G.E. and Peterson, C. Pharmacologic models of age-related deficits. In: Assessment in Geriatric Psychopharmacology, T. Crook, S. Ferris, R. Bartus, (eds.) Mark Powley Associates, Inc., New Canaan, Connecticut, 323-343, 1983.
17. Drachman, D.A. Memory and cognitive function in man: Does the cholinergic system have a specific role? Neurology, 27:283-299, 1977.
18. Bartus, R.T., Dean, R.L., Beer, B., and Lippa, A.S. The cholinergic hypothesis of geriatric memory dysfunction. Science, 217:408-417, 1982.
19. Bartus, R.T., Dean, R.L., Pontecorvo, M.J., and Flicker, C. The cholinergic hypothesis: A historical overview, current perspective, and future directions. In: Memory Dysfunction: An Integration of Animal and Human Research From Preclinical and Clinical Perspectives. D. Olton, E. Gamzu, and S. Corkin, (eds.) New York Academy of Sciences. New York, NY, 444:332-358, 1985.
20. D'Amour, F. and Smith, D. A method for determining loss of pain sensation. J. Pharmacol. Exp. Ther., 72:74-79, 1981.
21. Tortella, F.C., Cowan, A., Belenky, G.L., and Holaday, J.W. Opiate-like electroencephalographic and behavioral effects of electroconvulsive shock in rats. European Journal of Pharmacology, 76:121-128, 1981.
22. McDonald, R.J. Hydergine: A review of 26 clinical studies. Pharmacopsychiatr., 12:407-422, 1979.
23. Hollister, L.E. and Yesavage, J. Ergolide mesylate for senile dementia: Unanswered questions. Ann. Intern. Med., 100:894-898, 1984.
24. Poschel, B.P.H. and Ninteman, F.W. Excitatory effects of hydergine on intracranial self-stimulation. Drug Development Research, 1:163-166, 1981.

25. Arnsten, A.F.T. and Goldman-Rakic, P.S. Catecholamine and cognitive decline in aged nonhuman primates. In: Memory Dysfunction: An Integration of Animal and Human Research From Preclinical and Clinical Perspectives. D. Olton, E. Gamzu, and S. Corkin, (eds.) New York Academy of Sciences. New York, NY, 444:218-234, 1985.
26. Boff, E., Gamzu, E., Poonian, D., and Zolcinski, M. Effects of cognitive performance enhancement reference compounds in a rat avoidance acquisition procedure. Soc. Neurosci. Abstr., 8:320, 1982.
27. Vincent, G., Verderese, A., and Gamzu, E. The effects of aniracetam (Ro 13-5057) and piracetam on the enhancement of memory in mice. Soc. Neurosci. Abstr., 10:258, 1984.
28. Schindler, U., Rush, D.K., and Fielding, S. Nootropic drugs: Animal models for studying effects on cognition. Drug Development Research. 4:567-576, 1984.
29. Butler, D.E., Poschel, B.P.H., and Marriott, J.G. Cognition-activating properties of 3-(Aryloxy) pyridines. J. Med. Chem. 24:346-356, 1981.
30. O'Keefe, J. and Nadel, L. The Hippocampus as a Cognitive Map, Oxford: Oxford University Press, 1978.
31. Olton, D., Becker, J., and Handelmann, G. Hippocampus, space, and memory. The Behavioral and Brain Sciences, 2:313-365, 1979.
32. Olton, D.S. and Wolf, W.A. Hippocampal seizures produce retrograde amnesia without a temporal gradient when they reset working memory. Behavioral and Neural Biology. 33:437-454., 1981.
33. Stwertka, S.A., MacNeil, D.A., and Gamzu, E. Effects of aniracetam (Ro 13-5057) and diphenylhydantoin on hippocampal afterdischarge in rats. Soc. Neurosci. Abstr., 9:824, 1983.
34. Cohen, H.C. and Barondes, S.H. Puromycin effect on memory may be due to occult seizures. Science, 157:333-334, 1967.
35. Gehres, L.D., Randall, C.L., Riccio, D.C., and Vandaris, R.M. Attenuation of hypothermic retrograde amnesia produced by pharmacological blockage of brain seizures. Physiol. & Behav., 10:1011-1017, 1973.
36. Gibbs, M.E. and Ng, K.T. Diphenylhydantoin facilitation of labile, protein-independent memory. Brain Research Bulletin, 1:203-208, 1976.
37. Gibbs, M.E. and Ng, K.T. Diphenylhydantoin extension of short-term and intermediate stages of memory. Behavioural Brain Research, 11:103-108, 1984.
38. Dell, H.-D., Jacobi, H., Kamp, R., Kurz, J., and Wunsche, C. 1-Methylhydantoin, ein unerwarteter metabolit der nootropen substanz dupracetam. Arch. Pharm., 314:697-702, 1981.
39. Ettenberg, A., Van der Kooy, D., LeMoal, M., Koob, G.F., Bloom, F.E. Can aversive properties of peripherally injected vasopressin account for its putative role in memory? Behavioral Brain Research, 7:331-350, 1983.
40. McGaugh, J.L. Peripheral and central adrenergic influences on brain systems involved in the modulation of memory storage. In: Memory Dsyfunction: An Integration of Animal and Human Research from Clinical and Preclinical Perspectives. D. Olton, E. Gamzu, and S. Corkin, (eds.) Annals of the New York Academy of Sciences. New York, NY, 444:150-161, 1985.
41. Schwam, E., Keim, K., Cumin, R., Gamzu, E., and Sepinwall, J. The effects of aniracetam in primate behavior and EEG. In: Memory Dysfunction: An Integration of Animal and Human Research from Clinical and Preclinical Perspectives. D. Olton, E. Gamzu, and S. Corkin, (eds.) Annals of the New York Academy of Sciences. New York, NY, 444:482-484, 1985.

42. Vincent, G., Verderese, A., and Gamzu, E. The effects of aniracetam (Ro 13-5057) on the enhancement and protection of memory in mice. In: Memory Dsyfunction: An Integration of Animal and Human Research from Clinical and Preclinical Perspectives. D. Olton, E. Gamzu, and S. Corkin (eds.) Annals of the New York Academy of Sciences. New York, NY, 444:489-491, 1985.
43. Pontecorvo, M.J. and Evans, H.L. Effects of aniracetam on delayed match-to-sample performance of monkeys and pigeons. Pharmacology, Biochemistry, and Behavior. 22:745-752, 1985.
44. Keim, K.L. and Gamzu, E.R. MSH/ACTH 1-10, MSH/ACTH 4-9 analog, vasopressin: Peptides protective against disrupted memory in mice and electroencephalotropic in monkey. XIV International Congress of the International Society of Psychoneuroendocrinology, New York, 1983.
45. Saletu, B., Grunberger, B.J., and Lunzmoger, C. Quantitative EEG and psychometric analysis in assessing CNS-activity of Ro 13-5057 - a cerebral insufficiency improver. Meth. Find. Expt. Clin. Pharm., 2:269-285, 1980.
46. Foltyn, V.P., Lucker, P.W., Schnitker, J., and Wetzelsberger, N. A test model for cerebrally active drugs demonstrated by the example of the new compound aniracetam. Arzneim-Forsch/Drug Res., 33:865-867, 1983.
47. Saletu, B. and Grunberger, J. Memory dysfunctions and vigilance: Neurophysiological and psychopharmacological aspects. In: Memory Dsyfunction: An Integration of Animal and Human Research from Clinical and Preclinical Perspectives. D. Olton, E. Gamzu, and S. Corkin, (eds.) Annals of the New York Academy of Sciences. New York, NY, 444:406-427, 1985.

NEUROCHEMICAL AND BEHAVIORAL ALTERATIONS IN AGING AND IN ANIMAL MODELS OF ALZHEIMER'S DISEASE

E. Friedman, M.J. Brennan, B.E. Lerer, K.A. Sherman, J.W. Schweitzer, and J. Kuster

New York University School of Medicine
Dept. of Psychiatry and Pharmacology
550 First Ave., New York, N.Y. 10016

INTRODUCTION

Central cholinergic neurons appear to play a critical role in cognitive function (Hington and Aprison, 1976; Deutsch and Rogers, 1979). Furthermore, it has been suggested that impaired cholinergic transmission may be at least partly responsible for the memory deficits occurring during aging (Drachman and Leavitt, 1974; Bartus et al., 1982; Davis and Yesavage, 1979). Much of the support for this hypothesis derives from pharmacological studies. For example, when scopolamine, a muscarinic receptor antagonist, was administered to yound adult humans and monkeys, decrements in cognitive task performance resulted which mimic those deficits found in aged subjects (Safer and Allen, 1971; Drachman and Leavitt, 1974; Bartus and Johnson, 1976). The scopolamine-induced cognitive dysfunction is selectively reversed by drugs which enhance cholinergic transmission (Drachman, 1977; Bartus, 1978a). Cholinomimetic drugs, such as physostigmine or arecoline or other pharmacologic cholinergic enhancement result in improved performance on memory tasks (Davies et al., 1978; Sitaram et al., 1978; Bartus, 1979) and also reverse the memory impairments due to age.

The nature of the cholinergic dysfunction in normal aging may be related to the decreases in brain choline acetyltransferase (CAT) activity (McGeer and McGeer, 1976 and; Perry et al., 1977b), or to the small decline in cortical muscarinic receptor binding which has been demonstrated in normal subjects who were over 60 years old (White et al., 1977; Perry, 1980). While these data must be interpreted cautiously, the occurrence of small reduction in CAT activity and in muscarinic cholinergic binding may combine to produce a cholinergic deficit which is responsible for a cognitive deficit.

In rodents, age-related changes in the performance of experimental tasks have been demonstrated. These may parallel the cognitive deficits observed in the elderly (Elias and Elias, 1976; Barnes, 1979). For example, retention after a single-trial passive avoidance training session was markedly impaired in senescent rats and mice (Bartus et al., 1982). In addition, deficits in exploration induced by novel stimuli were found in aged mice (Brennan et al., 1981). Pharmacological evidence indicates that ACh is one of the neurotransmitters which plays a critical role in both the retention of aversive conditioning (Buresova et al., 1964; Rosic and Bignani, 1970; Glick et al., 1973) and response to novel stimuli (Carlton and Markiewicz, 1968; Kokkindis and Anisman, 1976). Thus, there appears to be a generalizability across species both in the appearance of cognitive deficits during aging and in the role of ACh neurons in cognitive performance.

The greatest support for the role of ACh neurons in cognition has been provided by studies of Alzheimer's disease (AD). Alzheimer's patients suffer memory losses which are qualitatively similar to, but much more severe than, those normally associated with aging. It has been shown that the activity of CAT, the synthetic enzyme for ACh, is markedly reduced in several brain regions of Alzheimer's patients (Davies and Maloney, 1976; Perry et al., 1977a; White et al., 1977; Reisine et al., 1978). Moreover, the loss of CAT correlates closely with the extent of histological signs of AD, such as senile plaques and with the degree of documented memory impairment (Perry et al., 1978; Davies, 1979). A dramatic reduction in ACh esterase (AChE) has also been found in AD (Davies and Maloney, 1976; Perry et al., 1978). This decline in cholinergic metabolic enzyme correlates with the number of senile plaques in cortex (Perry et al., 1978). The decrease in CAT and AChE may indicate degeneration of cholinergic innervation to several brain regions in AD. Histochemical techniques confirm a loss of AChE-staining afferent fibers in hippocampus and cortex. On the other hand, muscarinic receptor binding appears to be unaffected in several brain regions, including cortical tissue obtained from Alzheimer's patients (Perry et al., 1977a; White et al., 1977; Davies and Verth, 1978; Perry, 1980).

The nucleus basalis of Meynert (nbM) in the substantia innominata gives rise to cholinergic neurons which project diffusely to neocortex (Parant et al., 1979). A substantial reduction in nbM neurons was documented in patients with AD thus raising the possibility that the degenerations of these neurons may be related at least in part to the cognitive changes in this disease. It is in light of this information and with the goal of developing information which may facilitate our understanding of the role of the cholinergic system in aging and in AD that we have undertaken to (1) investigate the neurochemistry of the cholinergic system in senescent animals, (2) test the relation between cholinergic deficiency, as elicited by a low-choline diet, and aged animals. Since these approaches may be more suited to the understanding of physiologic aging we have also attempted to (3) develop animal models which hopefully will aid in the understanding of AD and in the development of new therapeutic strategies for this disease. This latter goal was undertaken with a great deal of caution, since we realize fully the problems associated with any attempt to propose an animal model for a human neuropsychiatric disorder.

RESULTS AND DISCUSSION

Effect of Age on Brain Cholinergic Mechanisms in C57 BL/6NNia Mice

The effect of age on CAT activity in various brain regions was examined. Enzyme activity showed an age-related increased in the hippocampus, a significant increase in 28-32 mo old animals as compared to the 3-4 mo old animals and no change in enzyme activity was observed in the striatum.

Sodium-dependent high affinity choline uptake was diminished in synaptosomes obtained from aged animals. An age-related decrease in uptake was observed in the striatum, hippocampus and cortex. We have previously shown that a similar deficit in choline uptake exists in rat hippocampal tissue obtained from aged animals. This age effect was not found in synaptosomes which had previously been exposed to K^{+}- depolarization, indicating that the capacity to transport choline can be increased in both adult and aged

Table 1. Effect of Age on Sodium-Dependent High Affinity Choline Uptake

Age	Striatum	Hippocampus	Cortex
		p mole choline/mg p./2 min	
3-4 mo	469.4 ± 19.8 (7)	126.1 ± 11.0 (6)	125.7 ± 8.0 (7)
10-12 mo	422.5 ± 29.5 (5)	110.7 ± 10.7 (5)	102.0 ± 10.2 (5)
28-32 mo	333.1 ± 32.8 (6)*	99.1 ± 6.0 (6)*	95.0 ± 8.3 (6)*

$P < .05$

rodents (Sherman et al., 1981).

Binding of ^{3}H-QNB to brain membranes was found to be decreased in the striatum but not in cortex or hippocampus (Table 2). The decrease in striatal muscarinic binding was accompanied by an alteration in the distribution of agonist binding sites as determined by carbachol displacement of ^{3}H-QNB binding. Aged mice exhibited a significant shift in the relative number of high to low affinity binding sites. This decrease in high affinity sites and increase in low affinity sites was not observed in cortical muscarinic receptors (Table 3).

Strain Dependent Changes in Behavior and Striatal Receptor Binding with Age

The study of behavioral and neurochemical consequences of aging in animal models has typically involved the use of single inbred strains of mice or rats. While use of inbred strains allows for enhanced control over genotype of the subject population, restricted attention to a single genotype can obscure an important source of individual variation in the effects of aging. Genetic differences in aging are most apparent in terms of the longevity differences which have been observed between inbred mouse strains (e.g. Goodrick,1975). Further, strain differences also have been reported in terms of age-related changes in open-field behavior (e.g., Elias, Elias, and Eleftheriou, 1975), auditory sensitivity (Henry, 1982), and adrenal-pituitary responsivity to mild stress (Eleftheriou, 1974). Recently Waller et al (1983) have reported strain specific changes in brain acetylcholinesterase activity with age. In the present study, we have compared two parental strains, Balb/cNNia and C57BL/6NNia, and the CB6F1 hybrid. In an effort to establish strain specific and general effects of aging on behavior, we evaluated the performance of adult (8 month old) and aged (26-28 month old) mice from each of the strains in a number of different behavioral paradigms, including tests of exploratory behavior, spontaneous alternation, and three commonly used psychomotor tests.

Since we had previously observed differences in the effects of aging on stimulus-directed exploratory behavior and more general locomotor activity (Brennan et al., 1981), the frequency of stimulus directed head dip responses and general (horizontal) locomotor activity were recorded and tabulated for consecutive five minute periods within each test session.

As summarized in Table 4, significant age ($F_{1,96}$=7.96, P<0.01) and age x strain ($F_{2,96}$=7.23, P<0.01) differences in the frequency of head dip

Table 2. Muscarinic Binding in Mouse Hippocampus and Cortex

Age	Hippocampus	Cortex	Striatum
		pmole/mg protein	
3-4 mo	1.608 ± .055 (6)	1.837 ± .048 (13)	2.678 ± .102 (6)
10-12 mo	1.480 ± .044 (4)	1.832 ± .068 (11)	2.331 ± .069 (4)**
28-32 mo	1.470 ± .060 (6)	1.769 ± .034 (12)	2.198 ± .069 (6)*

*P<.005; *P<.05

Table 3. Cholinergic Agonist Binding Sites in Striatum and Cortex of Adult and Aged C57 Mice

	Adult	Aged
	Striatum	
%H	20.672 ± .713	17.391 ± 1.279+
$I_{c}50H$	.658 ± .0883	.418 ± .1019
% L	69.22 ± .574	72.658 ± 1.007++
$I_{c}50L$	83.299 ± 3.7333	84.033 ± 5.9455
%H	25.72 ± 2.814	26.66 ± 2.509
$I_{c}50H$	.4287 ± .05776	.3831 ± .0997
% L	67.30 ± 2.232	65.809 ± 1.368
$I_{c}50L$	60.10 ± 13.186	62.682 ± 4.227

+P < .05; ++P < .025

Table 4. Mean Frequency of Head Dip Responses

	Adult	Aged
Balb/cNNia	40.8 (± 5.02)	48.9 (± 8.66)
CB6F1	54.0 (± 3.72)	41.4 (± 2.72)*
C57BL/6NNia	63.6 (± 3.69)	32.8 (± 4.59)*

*P < 0.01

responding were noted during the first test session. While aged C57BL/6NNia and CB6F1 mice made significantly fewer head dip responses than adult mice, no significant differences in exploration were noted between adult and aged Balb/cNNia mice. In addition to differences in the overall frequency of exploration, differences were also noted between strains and age groups in terms of within-session habituation. During the first test session, the clearest indication of a within-session decrease in exploration was observed in adult CB6F1 mice. Balb/cNNia mice showed no within-session changes in exploration, while aged C57BL/6NNia mice exhibited a significant within-session increase in exploration. With the exception of aged C57BL/6NNia mice, adult and aged mice showed significant between-session habituation. Aged C57BL/6NNia mice exhibited a significant between-session increase in the frequency of head dip responses.

For the third test session, novel stimulus objects were placed beneath the floor holes to determine age and strain differences in responsivity to stimulus change. With the introduction of novel stimuli, age differences in exploration were once again evident. C57BL/6NNia and CB6F1 mice showed enhanced exploration during the third test session. The response to stimulus change tended to be greater for the adult mice in each strain. Neither adult nor aged Balb/cNNia mice exhibited any significant changes in exploration following the introduction of novel stimuli in the third test session.

We have used this paradigm because it appears to provide a means of distinguishing between the effects of aging on stimulus-directed exploration and age-related changes in more general locomotor activity. As was noted for the head dip response, Balb/cNNia mice were less active than CB6F1 or C57BL/6NNia mice and, with the exception of the Balb/cNNia strain, aged mice were found to be significantly less active than adult mice. Marked qualitative differences, however, were apparent between patterns of exploratory behavior and general locomotor (horizontal) activity. First, within-session habituation of locomotor activity was observed in each age and strain grouping during the first test session and in subsequent test sessions. Second, between-session habituation was observed in each group. Third, the introduction of novel stimuli did not result in any increase in the level of locomotor activity during the third test session.

One week following hole board testing, the mice were given two daily 30 sec adaptations to a modified T-maze and were then given four consecutive days of spontaneous alternation testing. As shown in Table 5, in each of the three strains, the probability of alternation decreased significantly with age in each of the strains.

One week following spontaneous alternation testing the mice underwent three different motor tests: the elevated path test, roto-rod test, and balance rod test. The elevated path test involved placing the subject in the center of 70 cm long x 2.54 cm wide clear plexiglas strip which was placed between two supports which raised the strip 17 cm above a table top. Each animal was given three 120 second trials. The trials were terminated when either the animal fell from the elevated path, remained on the elevated path for 120 seconds, or escaped to cages placed at either end of the elevated path. Total time scores were adjusted for escapes; the maximum score was 720. For the roto-rod test, the subjects were given three 60 second trials on wooden rod (2.54 cm dia) which was raised 25 cm above a bed of hardwood shavings. The maximum score for this test was 180. The balance rod is a narrow (0.64 cm dia) 70 cm long wooden dowel which is placed between two support stands which raised the rod 40 cm above a bed of hardwood shavings. Each subject was given three 120 sec trials on the balance rod, with a 30 sec inter-trial interval. A trial was terminated when either the subject fell from the rod, remained on the rod for 120 sec, or escaped

Table 5. Rates of Spontaneous Alternation by Adult and Aged Balb/cNNia, CB6F1, and C57BL/6NNia Mice

	Adult	Aged
Balb/cNNia	75.0%	62.5%
CB6F1	77.5	66.8
C57BL/6NNia	69.8	55.8

Table 6. Motor Test Performance of Adult and Aged Balb/cNNia CB6F1, and C57BL/6NNia Mice

(a) Elevated Path Test:

	Adult	Aged
Balb/cNNia	475.6 (±31.036)	399.6 (±31.694)
CB6F1	479.6 (±24.452)	411.4 (±30.642)
C57BL/6NNia	539.6 (±32.554)	408.5 (±48.276)*

(b) Roto-Rod Test:

	Adult	Aged
Balb/cNNia	102.7 (±10.118)	77.1 (±12.049)
CB6F1	149.1 (± 8.521)	84.7 (±13.143)*
C57BL/6NNia	166.0 (± 4.696)	100.5 (±16.444)*

(c) Balance Rod Test:

	Adult	Aged
Balb/cNNia	436.7 (±21.059)	344.1 (±30.114) *
CB6F1	481.1 (±22.310)	344.9 (±43.662) **
C57BL/6NNia	503.0 (±39.886)	119.4 (±23.911) ***

*Adult vs Aged $P < .05$; ** $P < .01$; *** $P < .001$

to two platforms placed on either end of the rod. Total times scores were adjusted for escapes. The maximum score was 720.

The results are summarized in Table 6. Though aged mice in each strain showed declines in motor performance, the magnitude of the decline differed between strains and between tests. Aged C57BL/6NNia mice showed significant declines in performance on all three tests. The magnitude of the decline differed between tests, with the greatest decline noted in the balance rod test. Significant age-related reductions in motor performance were observed in CB6F1 mice in the roto-rod and balance rod tests. The only significant motor decline noted for aged Balb/cNNia mice, was the 21.2% decline in balance rod performance.

These findings indicate strain and task dependent changes in behavior with age. In contrast to more generalized behavioral declines observed in aged C57BL/6NNia mice, significant age-related declines in performance by Balb/cNNia mice were only noted for spontaneous alternation and balance rod test. While similar to our findings in C57BL/6NNia mice, the magnitude of the behavioral declines in aged CB6F1 mice were not as pronounced as those noted for C57BL/6NNia mice.

A decrease in striatal dopamine binding (Severson and Finch, 1980) and striatal muscarinic receptor binding (Strong et al., 1980) have been observed in the C57BL/6J strain with age. Significant strain differences in striatal spiroperidol binding have been noted in adult mice (Michaluk et al., 1982; Severson et al., 1981). In the present study we examined the genotypic specificity of the effects of aging on striatal spiroperidol and QNB binding. The strain dependent changes, particularly, in spiroperidol binding, parallel our behavioral findings.

As shown in Table 7, significant age ($\underline{F}$ 1,23=12.874, P<0.010) and strain ($\underline{F}$ 2,23=5.634, P<0.025) differences in striatal spiroperidol binding were observed. Consistent with previous findings, a significant decline in spiroperidol binding was noted in aged C57BL/6NNia mice. In contrast to the 41% decline noted in C57BL/6NNia mice, Balb/cNNia mice showed a slight nonsignificant (7%) decline in striatal spiroperidol binding. While 17% decline in binding was observed in aged CB6F1 mice (P=0.097).

As summarized in Table 8, significant age ($\underline{F}$ 1,23=18.58, P<0.001) and strain ($\underline{F}$ 2,23=8.386, P<0.010) differences were also observed in terms of striatal QNB binding. Consistent with previous findings, a significant decline in QNB binding was noted in aged C57BL/6NNia mice. A marginally significant decline in QNB binding was noted for aged Balb/cNNia mice. No significant age-related change in striatal QNB binding was indicated for CB6F1 mice.

These behavioral and neurochemical findings indicate strain specific changes with age and, as such, contribute to a growing body of literature which indicates marked genotypic differences in the effects of chronological age. These types of findings do point to the limited generality of findings in single genotypes. Particularly in view of the parallels noted here between strain specific changes in behavior and striatal dopamine binding with age, these initial findings indicate the specific utility of a genetic approach to the investigation of the neurobiological mechanisms underlying behavioral change with age.

Effect of Choline-Deficient Diet on Mice Behavior and Brain Acetylcholine Levels

Dietary manipulations of choline availability have been shown to affect regional brain concentrations of acetylcholine (e.g. Cohn and

Table 7. Age and Strain Differences in Striatal ^{3}H-Spiroperidol Binding

	(pmole/mg protein)		
	Adult	Aged	
Balb/cNNia	0.770 (± 0.0659)	0.713 (± 0.0751)	P=0.5898
CB6F1	0.725 (± 0.0618)	0.603 (± 0.0219)	P=0.0936
C57BL/6NNia	0.708 (± 0.0325)	0.419 (± 0.0231)	P=0.0021

Table 8. Age and Strain Differences in Striatal ^{3}H-QNB Binding

	pmole/mg protein		
	Adult	Aged	
Balb/cNNia	2.453 (± 0.0703)	2.079 (± 0.1509)	P=0.0535
CB6F1	2.387 (± 0.1453)	2.048 (± 0.1405)	P=0.1297
C57BL/6NNia	2.118 (± 0.1549)	1.427 (± 0.0907)	P=0.0090

Wurtman, 1978) and to attenuate age-related changes in passive avoidance (Bartus, et al., 1982). To further explore the cholinergic involvement in age related changes in behavior which we have noted, we studied the hole board exploratory behavior of adult Swiss Webster mice after a 6 week exposure to a choline deficient diet.

Exposure of Swiss-Webster mice to a synthetic diet deficient in choline for 6 weeks resulted in no significant differences in body weight. This treatment produced a 17% decrease in striatal acetylcholine concentrations without a change in hippocampal or cortical transmitter levels. The characteristic habituation in frequency of head dip response seen during a testing session in adult mice was impaired in the choline deficient animals. This pattern is similar to the behavior of aged mice in this paradigm (see above). However, the age-related decrease in total head dip responses which is observed in senescent animals was not observed in the choline deficient animals. Furthermore, the locomotor activity which decreases during a 20 min testing period was not altered by choline deficiency, thus paralleling the effect of age (as seen above). These behavioral impairments induced by prolonged exposure to a choline-poor diet may mimic certain behavioral effects seen in aged animals and may provide a useful animal model for enhancing our understanding of the changes seen during normal aging.

The Effect of Loss of Neocortical or Hippocampal Cholinergic Afferents on Memory Processes in the Rat

Loss of cognitive function in AD is correlated with reductions in CAT activity. The reduction in this presynaptic marker is not accompanied by changes in postsynaptic cholinergic receptors. It has been suggested that

Table 9. Percentage of Alternations in an Unbaited Y-Maze

	Lesion	Control
Pre-operative	.67	.63
Post-operative	.23*	.55

*P< 0.025

cholinergic deficits in cortex are due to loss of afferents rather than to loss of intrinsic cholinergic neurons (Perry, 1980). This hypothesis is substantiated by a study of aged monkeys which suggested that cortical neuritic plaques partly consist of presynaptic cholinergic axons, as indicated by AChE staining techniques, and furthermore, many of these axons originate in the nucleus basalis of Meynert in the substantia innominata (Struble et al., 1982). Moreover, neuronal loss and morphological degeneration of the nucleus basalis have been documented in a postmortem examination of an AD patient. There was a 90% loss of the large neurons of this nucleus and the remaining cells showed granulovacuolar degeneration and neurofibrillary tangles (Whitehouse et al., 1982).

In experiments performed in rats, we have obtained reductions in CAT activity of about 40% in parietal cortex and up to 71% in frontal cortex after application of the neurotoxic agent, kainic acid, into the basalis. Direct application of the neurotoxin to fronto-parietal cortex did not reduce CAT nor did it result in behavioral impairment. This suggests that a large percentage of cortical cholinergic innervation may arise from the basalis pathway, with the rest derived from intrinsic neurons. Behavioral tests showed that lesioned rats had impaired retention over 24 hr in a step-through passive avoidance task, impaired habituation with prolonged exposure to novel stimuli and significant perseveration in a spontaneous alternation task (Friedman et al., 1982; Lerer and Friedman, 1982; Friedman et al., 1983).

In the test of hole poke exploratory behavior, unoperated control rats showed a 70% decrease in number of hole pokes over a 20 min period. Basalis lesioned rats showed only a 41% decrease in responding. This suggests that the rate of habituation in basalis rats was not as rapid as that noted in controls. This behavioral impairment was comparable to that which we noted in mice maintained on a choline deficient diet.

Young normal rats given two weeks of daily trials alternated in choosing left-versus-right arms of a Y-maze on about 65% of trials (Table 9). Following basalis lesions, subjects alternated on only 23% of trials and on the remainder of the trials they perseverated in their choice of the same arm on both the initial choice and re-entry choice (Lerer and Friedman, 1983). If one postulates solely a memory deficit as underlying the post-operative drop in alternation, one would expect random alternation from trial to trial. Thus one would expect a post-operative rate of alternation of about 50%. But the lesioned rats alternate at much less than chance level. In fact, the post-operative control rate of alternation resembled random alternation, while the lesioned rats seem to be actively perseverating in their choice of the same arm on initial and re-entry choices. A systematic manipulation of the delay between initial and choice trial is necessary to determine the nature and scope of this perseverative behavior. For passive avoidance testing, rats were placed in the lighted compartment of a 2-compartment shuttlebox and the subjects latency to enter the dark/shock compartment was recorded. Animals were trained on day 1 and tested 24 hr later. Control and lesioned animals did not differ with respect to the initial latency to enter the dark compartment on the training day. No differences between groups were noted in the number of shocks obtained on the training day. However, during the retention test, a memory impairment was indicated in lesioned animals. The mean latency to enter the dark compartment was significantly shorter (by more than 50%) in the lesioned groups than in the control animals.

In AD, the hippocampal formation is densely populated by neuritic plaques and neurofibrillary tangles, and the severe CAT losses are pronounced in the hippocampus and temporal cortex. The hippocampus is innervated by cholinergic (and other) fibers that originate in the medial septal nucleus (Lewis et al., 1967). This structure has long been implicated in learning and memory in both animals and humans (O'Keefe and Nadel, 1978; Olton et al., 1980; Scoville and Milner, 1957). Recent data gathered in our laboratory confirm that electrolytic fimbria-fornix damage to the pre- and post-commissural hippocampal connections produces deficits in radial arm maze learning. We furthermore found that CAT reductions in the hippocampus correlated (r=-0.89) very well with functional deficit after lesion (Hughey and Friedman, 1983). These data are consistent with the hypothesis that cholinergic innervation of hippocampus is critical to cognitive function.

CONCLUSION

The results presented support the idea that brain cholinergic systems play a role in memory processes. They furthermore suggest that some age-related functional deficits are associated with an impairment in this neurotransmitter system. The relationship between the cholinergic system, memory and aging is strengthened by the comparability, across a number of behavioral paradigms, of the performance deficits which are elicited in adult animals by various experimental manipulations of the central cholinergic system. In addition, the results emphasize the limited generality of findings obtained in aged animals of a single genotype.

The present results also suggest that animal models which attempt to mimic some of the landmarks of AD may lead to the efficient testing of new drugs for the treatment of age-related states of cognitive decline.

REFERENCES

Barnes, C.A., 1979, Memory deficits associated with senescence: A neurophysiological and behavioral study in the rat, J. Comp. Physiol. psychol., 93:74.

Bartus, R.T., 1978, Evidence for a direct cholinergic involvement in the scopolamine-induced amnesia in monkeys: Effects of concurrent administration of physostigmine and methylpheridate with scopolamine, Pharmacol. Biochem. Behav., 9:833.

Bartus, R.T., 1979, Physostigmine and recent memory: Effects in young and aged non-human primates, Sci., 206:1087.

Bartus, R.T., Dean, R.L., Beer, B., Lippa, A.S., 1982, The cholinergic hypothesis of geriatric memory dysfunction, Sci., 217:408.

Bartus, R.T. and Johnson, H.R., 1976, Short term memory in the rhesus monkey: Disruption from the anticholinergic scopolamine, Pharmacol. Biochem. Behav., 5:39.

Brennan, M.J., Allen, D., Alleman, D., Azmezia, E.C., Quartermain, D, 1984, Age differences in within-session habituation of exploratory behavior: effects of stimulus complexity, Behav. Neurobiol., 42: 61.

Brennan, M.J., Dallob, A., Friedman, E., 1981, Involvement of hippocampal serotonergic activity in age-related changes in exploratory behavior, Neurobiol. Aging, 2:199.

Buresova, O., Bures, J., Bohdanecky, Z., and Weiss, T., 1964, Effect of atropine on learning, extinction, retention and retrieval in rats, Psychopharmacol., 5:255.

Carlton, P.L., and Markiewicz, B., 1973, Behavioral effects of atropine and scopolamine, in: "Pharmacological and Biophysical Agents and Behavior," E. Furchtgott, ed., Academic Press, N.Y.

Cohn, E.L., and Wurtman, R.J., 1976, Brain acetylcholine: control by dietary choline, Sci., 191:561.

Davies, P., 1980, Biochemical changes in Alzheimer's disease senile dementia: Neurotransmitters in senile dementia of the Alzheimer's type, in: "Congenital and Acquired Cognitive Disorder," R. Katzman, ed., Raven Press, N.Y.

Davies, P. and Maloney, A.J.F., 1976, Selective loss of central cholinergic neurons in Alzheimer's disease, Lancet II:1403.

Davies, P., and Verth, A.H., 1977, Regional distributions of muscarinic acetylcholine receptor in normal and Alzheimer's-type dementia brains, Br. Res., 158:385.

Davis, K.L., Mohs, R.C., Tinklenberg, A., Pfefferbaum, A., Hollister, L.E., and Kopell, B.S., 1978, Physostigmine: Improvement of long-term memory processes in normal humans. Sci., 20:272.

Davis, K.L., and Yesavage, J.A., 1979, Brain acetylcholine and disorders of memory, in: "Brain Acetylcholine and Neuropsychiatric Disease," K.L. Davis and P.A. Berger, eds., Plenum Press, N.Y.

Deutsch, J.A., and Rogers, J.B., 1979, Cholinergic excitability and memory: animal studies and their clinical implications, in: "Brain Acetylcholine and Neuropsychiatric Disease," K.L. Davis and P.A. Berger, eds., Plenum Press, N.Y.

Drachman, D.A., 1977, Memory and cognitive function in man: Does the cholinergic system have a specific role, Neurol., 27:783.

Drachman, D.A., and Leavitt, J., 1974, Human memory and the cholinergic system: A relationship to aging?, Arch. Neurol., 30:113.

Eleftheriou, B.E., 1974, Changes with age in pituitary-adrenal responsiveness and reactivity to mild stress in mice, Gerontol., 20:224.

Elias, P.K., Elias, M.F., and Eleftheriou, B.E., 1975, Emotionality, exploratory behaviors and locomotion in aging inbred strain of mice, Gerontal., 21:46.

Friedman, E., Lerer, B., Kuster, J., 1983, Loss of cholinergic neurons in the rat neocortex produces deficits in passive avoidance learning, Pharmacol. Biochem. Behav., 19:309.

Friedman, E., Sherman, K.A., Brennan, M.J., Lerer, B., 1982, Neurochemical and behavioral alterations in aging. Paper presented at Aging of the Brain, Mantua, Italy.

Glick, S.D., Mittag, T.W., Green, J.P., 1973, Central cholinergic correlates of impaired learning, Neuropharmacol., 12:291.

Goodrick, C.L., 1975, Life span and the inheritance of longivity of inbred mice, J. of Gerontol., 30:257.

Henry, K.R., 1982, Age-related auditory loss and genetics: An electrochocleographic comparison of six inbred strain of mice, J. Gerontol., 37:275.

Hington, B.A., and Aprison, M.H., 1976, Behavioral and environmental aspects of the cholinergic system, in: "Biology of Cholinergic Function," A.M. Goldberg and I. Hanin, eds., Raven Press, New York.

Hughey, D., and Friedman, E., 1983, Correlation between working memory and level of hippocampal choline acetyltransferase in rats, Soc. Neurosci. Abs., 9:648.

Kokkindis, L., and Anisman, H., 1976, Interaction between cholinergic and catecholaminergic agents in a spontaneous alternation task, Psychopharmacol., 48:261.

Lerer, B., and Friedman, E., 1982, Neocortical cholinergic deficit and behavioral impairment produced by subcortical neurotoxic lesions, Soc. Neurosci. Abs., 8:838.

Lerer, B., and Friedman, E., 1983, Neurochemical lesion models of Alzheimer's disease, in: "Alzheimer's Disease," B. Reisberg, ed., The Free Press, N.Y.

Lewis, P.R., Shute, C.C.D., and Silver, A., 1967, Confirmation from choline acetylase of a massive cholinergic innervation to the rat hippocampus. J. Physiol., 191:215.

McGeer, E.B., and McGeer, P.L., 1976, Neurotransmitter metabolism in the aging brain, in: "Neurobiology of Aging," R.D. Terry and S. Gershon, eds., Raven Press, New York.

O'Keefe, J., and Nadel, L., 1978, The hippocampus as a cognitive map, Oxford University Press, Oxford, England.

Olton, D.S., Becker, J.T., and Handelmann, G.E., 1980, Hippocampal function: Working memory or cognitive mapping?, Physiol. Psychol., 8:239.

Parent, A., Gravel, A., Olivier, A., 1979, The extrapyramidal and limbic systems relationship at the Globus Pallidus level: A comparative histochemical study in the rat, cat and monkey, Adv. Neurol., 24:1.

Perry, E.K., 1980, The cholinergic system in old age and Alzheimer's disease, Age Aging, 9:1.

Perry, E.K., Perry, R.H., Blessed, B., and Tomlinson, B.E., 1977, Necropsy evidence of central cholinergic deficits in senile dementia, Lancet I:189.

Perry, E.K., Perry, R.H., Gibson, R.H., Blessed, G., and Tomlinson, B.E., 1977, Acholinergic connection between normal aging and senile dementia in the human hippocampus, Neurosci. Lett., 6:85.

Perry, E.K., Tomlinson, B.E., Blessed, G., Bergman, K., Gibson, P.H., and Perry, R.H., 1978, Correlation of cholinergic abnormalities with senile plaques and mental test scores in senile dementia, Br. Med. J., 52:1457.

Reisine, T., Yamamura, H.I., Bird, E.D., Spokes, E., and Enna, S.J., 1978, Pre and post-synaptic neurochemical alteration in Alzheimer's disease, Brain Res., 159:477.

Rosic, N., and Bignani, G., 1970, Depression of two-way avoidance learning and enhancement of passive avoidance learning by small doses of physostigmine, Neuropharmacol., 9:311.

Safer, D.J., and Allen, R.P., 1971, The central effects of scopolamine in man, Biol. Psychiat., 3:347.

Scoville, W.B., and Milner, B., 1957, Loss of recent memory after bilateral hippocampal lesion, J. Neurology, Neurosurgery and Psychiatry, 20:11.

Severson, J.A., and Finch, C.E., 1980, Reduced dopaminergic binding during aging in the rodent striatum, Br. Res., 192:147.

Sitaram, N., Weingartner, H., and Gillin, J.C., 1978, Human serial learning: Enhancement with arecoline and choline and impairment with scopolamine, Sci., 201:274.

Sherman, K.A., Kuster, J.E., Dean, R.L., Bartus, R.T., Friedman, E., 1981, Presynaptic cholinergic mechanism in brain of aged rats with memory impairment, Neurobiol. Aging, 2:99.

Strong, R., Hicks, P., Hsu, L., Bartus, R.T., Enna, S.J., 1980, Age-related alterations in the rodent brain cholinergic system and behavior, Neurobiol. Aging, 1:89.

Struble, R.G., Cork, L.C., Whitehouse, P.J., and Price, D.L., 1982, Cholinergic innervation in neuritic plaques, Sci., 216:413.

Waller, S.B., Ingram, D.K., Renolds, M.A., London, E.D., 1983, Age and strain comparison of neurotransmitter synthetic enzyme activities in the mouse, J. Neurochem., 41:1421.

White, P., Goodhardt, M.J., Keet, J.P., Hiley, C.R., Carrasco, L.H., Williams, F.E.I., Bowen, D.M., 1977, Neocotical neurons in elderly people, Lancet I:668.

Whitehouse, P.J., Price, D.L., Clark, A.W., Coyle, J.T., and Delong, M.R., 1982, Alzheimer's disease and senile dementia: Loss of neurons in the basal forebrain, Sci., 215:1237.

REVERSAL OF CEREBRAL METABOLIC DEFICITS IN RODENT MODELS FOR AGING AND ALZHEIMER'S DISEASE

Edythe D. London

Neuropharmacology Laboratory, Addiction Research Center
National Institute on Drug Abuse
Baltimore, MD

INTRODUCTION

The brain is one of the most highly metabolic organs in the human body, accounting for 20% of the resting total body oxygen consumption (Sokoloff, 1972). Inasmuch as glucose is the major substrate for oxidative metabolism in the adult brain (Sokoloff, 1972), cerebral glucose utilization is a measure of oxygen consumption and thereby of local function. Because of the close relation between energy metabolism and brain function, measures of cerebral metabolism have been used to assess cerebral functional activity in aging and dementia. This chapter deals with pharmacological approaches to reverse cerebral metabolic defects in these conditions, as assessed by measurement of the regional cerebral metabolic rate for glucose (rCMRglu) in rodent models.

CEREBRAL METABOLISM IN HUMAN AGING AND ALZHEIMER'S DISEASE

A pivotal advance in cerebral metabolic measurements was the development of the inert gas method to measure cerebral blood flow (CBF) in unanesthetized human subjects (Kety and Schmidt, 1945, 1948). The procedure involves the inhalation by the subject of a low concentration of nitrous oxide, and the measurement of nitrous oxide concentrations in arterial and cerebral venous blood, sampled from an internal jugular vein over a 10-min period. Application of the Fick principle to the resultant arterial and venous nitrous oxide concentration curves provides an average value of blood flow per minute per unit weight of the whole brain. Given the value for CBF, one can estimate the utilization by the brain of any substrate which can be measured in arterial and venous blood (Kety and Schmidt, 1948). Thus, the products of CBF and the arterio-venous differences for oxygen and glucose yield the cerebral metabolic rates for oxygen ($CMRO_2$) and glucose (CMRglu), respectively.

Numerous studies have measured these indices of global cerebral metabolism in relation to age and dementia. CBF, which usually is coupled to oxidative metabolism (Kety, 1956), was reduced with age in some studies (Fazekas et al., 1952; Scheinberg et al., 1953), but not in others (Shenkin et al., 1953). Similarly some studies suggested age-related declines in $CMRO_2$ (Fazekas et al., 1952; Lassen et al., 1960); whereas, others did not (Shenkin et al., 1953; Scheinberg et al., 1953).

Some of these early studies involved hospitalized patients (Kety, 1956), and the variability in findings partially may have reflected the medical status of the subjects. Therefore, Dastur et al. (1971) made comparisons between healthy young subjects and elderly men who were carefully screened for cardiovascular and other diseases. They found that CBF and $CMRO_2$ did not differ between the groups, but that CMRglu was significantly lower by 23% in the elderly. The authors minimized their positive finding by stating that blood glucose determinations in their laboratory were less accurate than blood oxygen measurements. Lying-Tunnell et al. (1980) subsequently showed no difference in CMRglu between two groups consisting of ten subjects each, with age ranges of 21-24 years and 55-65 years. They also noted no age differences in CBF and $CMRO_2$.

More recently, positron emission tomography (PET) has allowed measurement of rCMRglu using 2-deoxy-2-[^{18}F]fluoro-D-glucose (FDG), which serves as a tracer for the exchange of glucose between plasma and brain and its phosphorylation by hexokinase (Reivich et al., 1979). Kuhl et al. (1982) used the FDG method to study rCMRglu in forty normal resting volunteers aged 18 to 78 years. They reported that overall and regional CMRglu demonstrated a gradual decline when plotted as a function of age. In a later report, they provided an analysis of these data, indicating that the decline in rCMRglu with age was statistically significant ($p < 0.05$) (Hawkins et al., 1983). Duara et al. (1983) found that in twenty-one subjects between the ages of 21 and 83 years, neither mean hemispheric CMRglu nor rCMRglu in thirty-one brain regions was correlated significantly with age. This finding was maintained in an extension of the study to include forty men in the same age range (Duara, 1984). A similar lack of decline in rCMRglu with normal aging was reported by de Leon et al. (1984), who compared fifteen young normal subjects with twenty-two elderly normal subjects. In all of these studies, the subjects were healthy volunteers. However, the physiological state of the subjects was not equivalent. In the studies by Kuhl et al. (1982) and de Leon et al. (1984), subjects had their eyes open and ears unplugged; whereas, subjects in the study by Duara et al. (1983) had their eyes closed and ears plugged. Although it is possible that visual and auditory input may influence age effects on rCMRglu, inconsistent findings were obtained in the two studies in which subjects had their eyes open and ears unplugged.

In contrast with the conflicting results in FDG studies of normal aging, applications of the FDG technique to localize neuronal dysfunction in Alzheimer's disease have demonstrated regional metabolic decrements and suggest a potential diagnostic use of the procedure. Benson et al. (1983) reported that in a group of eight patients diagnosed as having Alzheimer's disease and three subjects with multi-infarct dementia, global CMRglu was reduced as compared with metabolism in sixteen age-matched controls. Although these authors reported equally severe changes in the frontal and temporal cortices, Friedland et al. (1983) presented evidence that the metabolic decrements of Alzheimer's disease were most concentrated in the temporoparietal cortex. These authors found strong negative correlations for both the Mattis Dementia Rating score and verbal IQ with the right/left frontal ratio, suggesting that these tests may reflect left frontal impairment. A high correlation between the performance IQ and the right/left temporoparietal ratio indicated the sensitivity of this measure to right posterior hemisphere impairment. These results agreed with those of Foster et al. (1983), who observed that patients, diagnosed as having Alzheimer's disease and showing a disproportionate failure of language function, had markedly reduced rCMRglu in the left frontal, temporal and parietal regions, as compared with corresponding areas of the right hemisphere. In the same study, patients with predominant constructional apraxia showed hypometabolism in the right temporal and parietal regions. Furthermore, scores on tests of verbal competency generally correlated with rCMRglu in the left frontal and temporal lobes; whereas, scores on tests of the ability to deal with two-dimensional designs and three-dimensional objects correlated with right parietal rCMRglu. Glucose utilization in the right posterior cerebral cortex was highly correlated with performance on visuoconstructive tests.

RODENT MODELS FOR HUMAN AGING AND ALZHEIMER'S DISEASE: PHARMACOLOGICAL APPROACHES TO REVERSE rCMRglu DECREMENTS

Age Differences in Regional Cerebral Metabolic Rates for Glucose in the Rat Brain

The FDG procedure is an extension of the 2-deoxy-D-[1-^{14}C]glucose (DG) method, which first was used to measure rCMRglu in rats (Sokoloff et al., 1977). Two laboratories used this method to demonstrate declines in rCMRglu by midlife in Sprague-Dawley and Fischer-344 rats, respectively (Smith et al., 1980; London et al. 1981). Results obtained by London et al. (1981) are shown in Table 1. In this study, rates of glucose utilization were lower at 12 months than at 3 months. Brain regions which showed apparent decrements of 25%-31% were the striatum, inferior colliculus and pons. These findings agreed generally with those of Smith et al. (1980). One difference was the observation of a significantly lower rCMRglu in the frontal cortices of 12 month old Fischer-344, but not Sprague-Dawley rats, as compared with younger animals. No age differences in rCMRglu were observed when comparing 12-, 24-, and 34 month old Fischer-344 rats, in agreement with the lack of a decrement in in rCMRglu in senescent Sprague-Dawley rats compared with middle-aged rats.

TABLE 1. REGIONAL CEREBRAL METABOLIC RATES FOR GLUCOSE IN FISCHER-344 RATS OF DIFFERENT AGES

Brain Region	Months of Age 3	12	24	34
	Glucose Utilization (μmol/100 g/min)			
Frontal cortex	77 ± 4	59 ± 2*	61 ± 4	63 ± 5
Sensory-motor cortex	74 ± 4	60 ± 3*	59 ± 3	61 ± 5
Hypothalamus & thalamus	53 ± 4	41 ± 3	42 ± 4	39 ± 3
Striatum	73 ± 4	55 ± 3*	52 ± 4	58 ± 4
Hippocampus	56 ± 3	46 ± 3*	43 ± 3	46 ± 4
Inferior colliculus	94 ± 5	68 ± 3*	57 ± 4	56 ± 4
Superior colliculus	64 ± 3	50 ± 3*	47 ± 4	46 ± 4
Midbrain basis & tegmentum	56 ± 3	43 ± 2*	39 ± 3	40 ± 4
Medulla	46 ± 2	36 ± 3*	34 ± 3	32 ± 3
Pons	48 ± 3	33 ± 2*	33 ± 2	33 ± 2

Data obtained from London et al. (1981). Each value is the mean ± S.E.M. for 7-10 rats.
*Significant difference from rCMRglu at previous age, $p \leq 0.05$, by one-way analysis of variance, with multiple comparisons performed using Duncan's multiple range test.

Effects of Co-dergocrine on rCMRglu

One approach to pharmacotherapy for cerebral deficits in aging has been the use of "metabolic enhancers," such as co-dergocrine mesylate (dihydroergotoxine, Hydergine ®). Co-dergocrine consists of four mesylated ergopeptines (dihydroergocornine, dihydroergocristine, dihydroergo-β-criptine and dihydroergo-α-criptine) in a ratio of 3:3:2:1, and has a high affinity for cerebral dopamine, serotonin, α_1-, and α_2-noradrenergic receptors (Loew et al., 1979). Whereas co-dergocrine acts as a dopamine and serotonin agonist, its effects on norepinephrine receptors appear to be inhibitory (Loew et al., 1979). Co-dergocrine's α-noradrenergic blocking properties have attracted attention because they were assumed to cause cerebral vasodilation (Rothlin, 1946/1947). However, co-dergocrine and other α-adrenolytic agents were shown to contract isolated cerebrovascular smooth muscle (Young et al., 1981). Whereas co-dergocrine and other α-adrenergic blockers produce anti-ischemic effects in animal models of cerebrovascular insufficiency (MacKenzie et al., 1984; Kovách et al., 1975), papaverine, a vasodilator, is not beneficial (Gygax et al., 1978; and Cahn and Borzeix, 1978). Therefore, the positive effects of co-dergocrine in models of cerebrovascular insufficiency, which account in part for its classification as a metabolic enhancer, seem to involve an action other than vasodilation.

Chronic co-dergocrine administration (1 mg/kg, intraperitoneally for 25 days) counteracts the age-associated decline in hexokinase and increase in lactate dehydrogenase seen in homogenates of rat forebrain tissue (12 months vs. 2.5 months; Djuričić and Mršulja, 1980). This finding suggests that co-dergocrine may increase the capacity for cerebral glucose oxidation. Therefore, it was of interest to determine if co-dergocrine could enhance cerebral glucose utilization <u>in vivo</u> as well. Middle-aged (12-15 month old) virgin male Fischer-344 rats were subjected to the autoradiographic DG procedure 35 min after the intraperitoneal injection of co-dergocrine (10 mg/kg) or the vehicle (propylene glycol).

Effects of co-dergocrine on rCMRglu are shown in Table 2. Co-dergocrine increased glucose utilization in many subcortical regions. Glucose utilization was increased by up to 30% throughout the extrapyramidal motor system and in the hippocampal formation. Increases of 20-25% were significant in the dorsal CA1 area of Ammon's horn, the dentate gyrus, and in subicular areas. Other areas of the brain related to learning and memory, such as components of the Papez circuit, the anterior thalamus, and mammillary body, also showed increases.

The locus ceruleus and its efferent pathway, the dorsal noradrenergic bundle, have been implicated in motivational states (see review by Mason, 1979). It is noteworthy that co-dergocrine stimulated rCMRglu in the locus ceruleus and the medial forebrain bundle, which contains the dorsal noradrenergic bundle. In contrast, no rCMRglu stimulation was observed in the cerebral cortex. Most cortical areas (pyriform, medial, sensory-motor and retrosplenial) showed no significant drug effect; however, co-dergocrine reduced rCMRglu in the frontal cortex.

TABLE 2. CO-DERGOCRINE EFFECTS ON REGIONAL CEREBRAL METABOLIC RATES FOR GLUCOSE

Brain Region	Vehicle	Co-dergocrine (10 mg/kg)
	Glucose Utilization (μmol/100 g/min)	
Sensory-motor cortex	80 $\pm$ 5	87 $\pm$ 4
Frontal cortex	87 $\pm$ 2	79 $\pm$ 2*
Retrosplenial medial cortex	76 $\pm$ 5	79 $\pm$ 4
Caudate-putamen	69 $\pm$ 5	83 $\pm$ 4*
Globus pallidus	46 $\pm$ 3	60 $\pm$ 3*
Substantia nigra (reticulata)	39 $\pm$ 2	59 $\pm$ 4*
Zona incerta	73 $\pm$ 5	81 $\pm$ 1
Anterodorsal thalamus	70 $\pm$ 4	92 $\pm$ 6*
Medial mammillary nucleus	82 $\pm$ 5	102 $\pm$ 5*
Medial forebrain bundle	47 $\pm$ 6	66 $\pm$ 4*
Locus ceruleus	58 $\pm$ 5	77 $\pm$ 4*
Dorsal hippocampus, CA1	42 $\pm$ 3	54 $\pm$ 3*
CA2-CA3	48 $\pm$ 3	59 $\pm$ 4
Dentate gyrus	47 $\pm$ 4	62 $\pm$ 5*
Subiculum	63 $\pm$ 3	73 $\pm$ 1*

Each value is the mean $\pm$ SEM for 7 rats.
* Significant difference from the value in vehicle-injected rats, $p \leq 0.05$ by Student's *t* test.

Some of co-dergocrine's effects on rCMRglu can be explained by interactions of the drug with specific neurotransmitter systems. For example, stimulation of rCMRglu in the extrapyramidal motor system may reflect a dopaminergic action, which has been implicated in co-dergocrine's stimulation of locomotor activity (Copeland et al., 1981; Vigouret et al., 1978); whereas, the decline in rCMRglu of the frontal cortex may be due to α-adrenergic blocking effects. Decreases in cortical glucose utilization also have been observed after treatment of rats with other α-adrenergic blocking agents (phenoxybenzamine, phentolamine and yohimbine) (Savaki et al., 1982). In the same study, α-adrenergic blockers also stimulated rCMRglu in the locus ceruleus, medial forebrain bundle and some nuclei related to cardiovascular control.

Thus, acute treatment with co-dergocrine counteracts the decline in rCMRglu which occurs in rats by midlife. The fact that co-dergocrine stimulates rCMRglu in the hippocampal formation and components of the Papez circuit, coupled with reports of improved performance in learning and memory paradigms (Loew et al., 1979), suggests a neuroanatomic basis for behavioral effects of co-dergocrine. However, despite possible correlations between rCMRglu and cognitive performance in patients with Alzheimer's disease (Friedland et al., 1983; Foster et al., 1983), it has not been shown than an increase in rCMRglu *per se* reflects a meaningful enhancement of cerebral function.

Effect of Oxotremorine on rCMRglu in Ibotenate-Lesioned Rats

Another major direction in pharmacotherapy for cerebral deficits in aging and Alzheimer's disease is treatment with cholinomimetics. This approach has resulted largely from the fact that the most consistent neurochemical finding in the brains of people who died with Alzheimer's disease is a loss of choline acetyltransferase in the neocortex and hippocampal formation (Bowen et al., 1976; Davies and Maloney, 1976; Perry et al., 1977; White et al., 1977; Davies, 1979; Rossor et al., 1980). Brains of individuals affected with Alzheimer's disease also show a loss of cholinergic neurons in the nucleus basalis of Meynert (Whitehouse et al., 1982), which innervates the cerebral cortex (Divac, 1975; Kievit and Kuypers, 1975; Mesulam and Van Hoesen, 1976).

Whereas cortical rCMRglu is reduced in Alzheimer's disease, biopsy samples obtained from cortices of patients with the disease exhibit enhanced glucose consumption when incubated _in vitro_ (Sims et al., 1981). This discrepancy raised the question of whether the reductions in cerebral metabolic activity observed in patients with Alzheimer's disease might result from the functional degeneration of cortical cholinergic afferent systems. To test this hypothesis, the DG method was used to examine the effects on rCMRglu of disrupting the cholinergic projection from the basal forebrain to the rat cerebral cortex (London et al., 1984). Lesions were produced by unilateral injections of ibotenic acid into the ventromedial globus pallidus. This area of the rat brain contains the nucleus basalis magnocellularis (Gorry, 1963), a sheet of cells which is believed to be homologous to the nucleus basalis of Meynert in the primate brain (Johnston et al., 1979; Lehmann et al., 1980). Stereotaxic injections of ibotenic acid, a neurotoxic analogue of L-glutamic acid (Schwarcz et al., 1979) into this nucleus in the rat produces selective reductions in presynaptic cholinergic markers of the ipsilateral cerebral cortex (Johnston et al., 1979).

Because of the suggestion that directly acting cholinomimetic agents might ameliorate cognitive deficits such as those seen in Alzheimer's disease (Sitaram et al., 1978), the effects of oxotremorine, a cholinergic muscarinic receptor agonist (Lévy and Michel-Ber, 1965), also were assessed on the neocortical rCMRglu of rats with ibotenate lesions in the ventromedial globus pallidus (London et al., 1984). Previous studies have indicated that oxotremorine produces a dose-dependent stimulation of neocortical rCMRglu in young rats (Dam et al., 1982). Furthermore, it stimulates rCMRglu in middle-aged and senescent rats to levels measured in young rats (Dam et al., 1984).

Ibotenate lesions of the nucleus basalis produced an ipsilateral decrease in cortical rCMRglu 3 days later. The decrement, which had a magnitude of approximately 25%, could be observed in autoradiograms of brain sections from rats subjected to the DG procedure (Fig. 1). The corpus striatum and nucleus accumbens in the lesioned hemisphere showed decreased rCMRglu as well. The striatal decrements may reflect decreased activity in corticostriatal afferents as well as some direct damage to the rostral striatum by the ibotenate injection. Treatment with oxotremorine (0.1 mg/kg, intraperitoneally) did not diminish the asymmetry in cortical glucose utilization, as evidenced by the fact that the ratio of lesioned to contralateral cortical rCMRglu was not altered by the drug (Table 3). However, oxotremorine stimulated rCMRglu in areas of the frontal and frontoparietal cortex. Oxotremorine's effect was statistically significant in the frontoparietal cortex. The mean rate of glucose utilization in the lesioned frontoparietal cortex was at the same level as cortical rCMRglu in the unlesioned hemisphere in rats which received no oxotremorine.

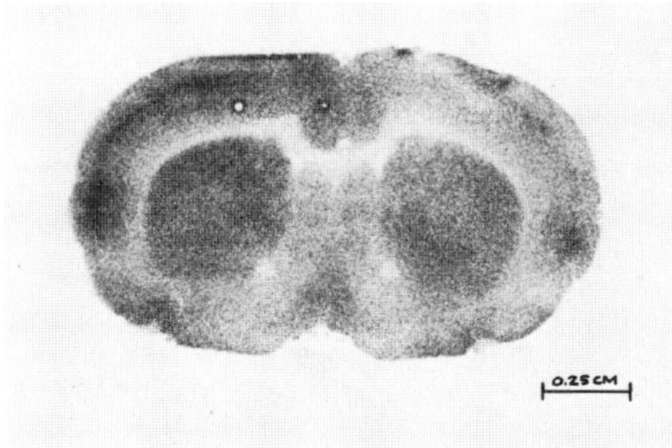

Fig. 1. Autoradiogram of a brain section from a representative rat lesioned with ibotenic acid (12 μg) 3 days prior to the DG procedure. Note the reduction in grain density, representing decreased rCMRglu, in portions of the autoradiogram corresponding with the frontoparietal cortex and striatum of the lesioned hemisphere.

TABLE 3. EFFECTS OF OXOTREMORINE ON CORTICAL GLUCOSE UTILIZATION AFTER IBOTENATE LESION OF THE VENTRAL GLOBUS PALLIDUS

		Lesioned side	Contralateral	
		rCMRglu (μmol/100 g/min)		Ratio
Frontal Cortex	Saline	55 ± 9 (3)	76 ± 8	0.72
	Oxotremorine	63 ± 5 (4)	86 ± 9	0.73
Frontoparietal Cortex	Saline	56 ± 16	82 ± 7	0.68
	Oxotremorine	77 ± 11*	110 ± 18*	0.70

Data from London et al. (1984).
Oxotremorine dose was 0.1 mg/kg, intraperitoneally, 2 min before DG.
Values of rCMRglu are means ± SEM for the number of rats indicated in parentheses.
*Significant effect of oxotremorine to increase rCMRglu, $F(1, 25) = 9.6$, $p \leq 0.01$, by 4-way analysis of variance (London et al., 1984).

Cortical rCMRglu decrements that occur after ibotenate injections reflect functional deficits inasmuch as rCMRglu is an index of oxidative metabolism. Decreases in cortical rCMRglu in lesioned rats indicate that the integrity of the subcortical cholinergic innervation is essential to maintaining normal levels of cortical metabolism. The present observations, therefore, support the hypothesis that neuronal loss or changes in the nucleus basalis of Meynert could be responsible, at least in part, for neocortical rCMRglu decrements in Alzheimer's disease.

The fact that oxotremorine produced a recovery of cortical rCMRglu in ibotenate-lesioned rats indicates that treatments with direct muscarinic receptor agonists may reverse some of the metabolic deficits in Alzheimer's disease. Postmortem studies of brains from victims who died with Alzheimer's disease indicate that despite marked presynaptic cholinergic losses, muscarinic receptors remain relatively unaffected (Davies and Verth, 1978; Nordberg et al., 1982). Therefore, pharmacotherapy which involves postsynaptic cholinergic sites may be more successful in enhancing cholinergic transmission than treatments which act primarily through presynaptic mechanisms. Nonetheless, the effects on behavior of tonic muscarinic receptor activation without an intact cortical cholinergic innervation are not established. Such treatments might not restore function because they do not adequately mimic normal phasic transmitter release.

CONCLUSION

In vivo studies in rats have shown decrements in rCMRglu associated with aging and disruption of the cholinergic innervation to the cerebral cortex by lesion of the nucleus basalis magnocellularis. These decrements can be reversed pharmacologically by treatment with co-dergocrine or oxotremorine. However, it has not been established that stimulation of rCMRglu *per se* can improve cognitive performance. Thus, the effects of drug-stimulated rCMRglu on behavioral performance require further elucidation.

REFERENCES

Benson, D. F., Kuhl, D. E., Hawkins, R. A., Phelps, M. E., Cummings, J. L., and Tsai, S. Y., 1983, The fluorodeoxyglucose ^{18}F scan in Alzheimer's disease and multi-infarct dementia, *Arch. Neurol.*, 40:711.

Bowen, D. M., Smith, C. B., White, P., and Davison, A. N., 1976, Neurotransmitter-related enzymes and indices of hypoxia in senile dementia and other abiotrophies, *Brain*, 99:459.

Cahn, J. and Borzeix, M. G., 1978, Comparative effects of dihydroergotoxine (DHET) on CBF and metabolism changes produced by experimental cerebral edema, hypoxia and hypertension, *Gerontology*, 24 (Suppl. 1):34.

Copeland, R. L., Jr., Bhattacharyya, A. K., Aulakh, C. S., and Pradhan, S. N., 1981, Behavioral and neurochemical effects of Hydergine in rats, *Arch. Int. Pharmacodyn. Ther.*, 252:113.

Dam, M., Wamsley, J. K., Rapoport, S. I., and London, E. D., 1982, Effects of oxotremorine on local glucose utilization in the rat cerebral cortex, *J. Neurosci.*, 2:1072.

Dam, M., Rapoport, S. I., and London, E. D., 1984, Aging and cholinergic system: A 2-deoxyglucose study in the rat brain, *in*: "Monographs in Neural Sciences," M. M. Cohen, ed., S. Karger, Basel.

Dastur, D. K., Lane, M. H., Hansen, D. B., Kety, S. S., Butler, R. N., Perlin, S., and Sokoloff, L., 1971, Effects of aging or cerebral circulation and metabolism in man, *in*: "Human Aging I: A Biological and Behavioral Study," J. E. Birren, R. N. Butler, S. W. Greenhouse, L. Sokoloff, and M. R. Yarrow, eds., DHEW Publication No. (ADM) 77-122, U.S. Government Printing Office, Washington, D. C.

Davies, P., 1979, Neurotransmitter-related enzymes in senile dementia of the Alzheimer type, *Brain Res.*, 171:319.

Davies, P. and Maloney, A. J., 1976, Selective loss of central cholinergic neurons in Alzheimer's disease, *Lancet*, 2:1403.

Davies, P. and Verth, A. H., 1978, Regional distribution of muscarinic acetylcholine receptor in normal and Alzheimer's-type dementia brains, *Brain Res.*, 138:385.

de Leon, M. J., George, A. E., Ferris, S. H., Christman, D. R., Fowler, J. S., Gentes, C. I., Brodie, J., Reisberg, B., and Wolf, A. P., 1984, Positron emission tomography and computed tomography assessments of the aging human brain, J. Comput. Assist. Tomog., 8:88.
Divac, I., 1975, Magnocellular nuclei of the basal forebrain project to neocortex, brain stem and olfactory bulb. Review of some functional correlates, Brain Res., 93:385.
Djuričić, B. M., and Mršulja, B. B., 1980, Key enzymes of glycolysis in rat brain: Effects of single and repetitive treatment with dihydroergotoxine (Redergin®), Gerontology, 26:99.
Duara, R., 1984, Cerebral metabolism during normal aging, in: Cutler, N.R., moderator. Brain imaging: Aging and dementia, Ann. Intern. Med., 101:355.
Duara, R., Margolin, R. A., Robertson-Tchabo, E. A., London, E. D., Schwartz, M., Renfrew, J. W., Koziarz, B. J., Sundaram, M., Grady, C., Moore, A. M., Ingvar, D. H., Sokoloff, L., Weingartner, H., Kessler, R. M., Manning, R. G., Channing, M. A., Cutler, N. R., and Rapoport, S. I., 1983, Cerebral glucose utilization, as measured with positron emission tomography in 21 resting healthy men between the ages of 21 and 83 years, Brain, 106:761.
Fazekas, J. F., Alman, R. W., and Bessman, A. N., 1952, Cerebral physiology of the aged, Am. J. Med. Sci., 223:245.
Foster, N. L., Chase, T. H., Fedio, P., Patronas, N. J., Brooks, R. A., and Di Chiro, G., 1983, Alzheimer's disease: Focal cortical changes shown by positron emission tomography, Neurology, 33:961.
Friedland, R. P., Budinger, T. F., Ganz, E., Yano, Y., Mathis, C. A., Koss, B., Ober, B. A., Huesman, R. H., and Derenzo, S. E., 1983, Regional cerebral metabolic alterations in dementia of the Alzheimer type: Positron emission tomography with [^{18}F]fluorodeoxyglucose, J. Comput. Assist. Tomogr., 7:590.
Gorry, J. D., 1963, Studies on the comparative anatomy of the ganglion basale of Meynert, Acta Anat. (Basel), 55:51.
Gygax, P., Wiernsperger, N., Meier-Ruge, W., and Baumann, T., 1978, Effect of papaverine and dihydroergotoxine mesylate on cerebral microflow, EEG, and pO_2 in oligemic hypotension, Gerontology, 24 (Suppl. 1):14.
Hawkins, R. A., Mazziotta, J. C., Phelps, M. E., Huang, S.-C., Kuhl, D. E., Carson, R. E., Metter, E. J., and Riege, W. H., 1983, Cerebral glucose metabolism as a function of age in man: Influence of the rate constants in the fluorodeoxyglucose method, J. Cereb. Blood Flow Metab. 3:250.
Johnston, M. V., McKinney, M., and Coyle, J. T., 1981, Neocortical cholinergic innervation: A description of extrinsic and intrinsic components in the rat, Exp. Brain Res., 43:159.
Kety, S. S., 1956, Human cerebral blood flow and oxygen consumption as related to aging, Research Publications of the Association for Research in Nervous and Mental Disorders, 35:31.
Kety, S. S. and Schmidt, C. F., 1945, The determination of cerebral blood flow in man by the use of nitrous oxide in low concentrations, Am. J. Physiol., 143:53.
Kety, S. S. and Schmidt, C. F., 1948, The nitrous oxide method for the quantitative determination of cerebral blood flow in man: Theory, procedure and normal values, J. Clin. Invest., 27:476.
Kievet, J. and Kuypers, H. G. J. M., 1975, Basal forebrain and hypothalamic connection to frontal and parietal cortex in the rhesus monkey, Science, 187:660.
Kovách, A. G., Hamar, J., Nyáry, I., Sándor, P., Reivich, M., Dóra, E., Gyulai, L.., and Eka, A., 1975, Cerebral blood flow and metabolism in hemorrhagic shock in the baboon, in: "Blood Flow and Metabolism in the Brain," M. Harper, B. Jehrett, D. Miller, and J. Rowan, eds., Churchill-Livingstone, Edinburgh.

Kuhl, D. E., Metter, E. J., Reige, W. H., and Phelps, M. E., 1982, Effects of human aging on patterns of local cerebral glucose utilization determined by the [18F]fluorodeoxyglucose method, J. Cereb. Blood Flow Metab., 2:163.

Lassen, N. A., Feinberg, I., and Lane, M. H., 1960, Bilateral studies of cerebral oxygen uptake in aged normal subjects and in patients with organic dementia, J. Clin. Invest., 39:491.

Lehmann, J., Nagy, J. I., Atmadia, S., Fibiger, H. C., 1980, The nucleus basalis magnocellularis: The origin of a cholinergic projection to the neocortex of the rat, Neuroscience, 5:1161.

Lévy, J. and Michel-Ber, E., 1965, Sur le metabolite de la tremorine, l'oxotremorine, Therapie, 20:265.

Loew, D. M., Vigouret, J. M., and Jaton, A. L., 1979, Neuropharmacology of ergot derivatives, in: "Dopaminergic Ergot Derivatives and Motor Function," Proceedings of International Symposium, K. Fuxe and D. B. Calne, eds., Pergamon Press, Oxford.

London, E. D., McKinney, M., Dam, M., Ellis, A., and Coyle, J. T., 1984, Decreased cortical glucose utilization after ibotenate lesion of the rat ventromedial globus pallidus, J. Cereb. Blood Flow Metab., 4:381.

London, E. D., Nespor, S. M., Ohata, M., and Rapoport, S. I., 1981, Local cerebral glucose utilization during development and aging of the Fischer-344 rat, J. Neurochem., 37:217.

Lying-Tunell, U., Lindblad, B. S., Malmlund, H. O., and Persson, B., 1980, Cerebral blood flow and metabolic rate of oxygen, glucose, lactate, ketone bodies and amino acids. I. Young and old normal subjects, Acta Neurol. Scand., 62:265.

MacKenzie, E. T., Goth, B., Nowicki, J. P., and Young, A. R., 1984, Adrenergic blockers as cerebral antiischaemic agents, in: L.E.R.S., Vol. 2, E. T. MacKenzie, J. Seylaz and A. Bes, eds., Raven Press, New York.

Mason, S. T., 1979, Noradrenaline and behavior, T.I.N.S. 2:82.

Mesulam, M. M. and Van Hoesen, G. W., 1976, Acetylcholinesterase-rich projections from the basal forebrain of the rhesus monkey to neocortex, Brain Res., 109:152.

Nordberg, A., Adolfsson, R., Marcusson, J., and Winblad, B., 1982, Cholinergic receptors in the hippocampus in normal aging and dementia of Alzheimer type, in: Aging, Vol. 20, "The Aging Brain: Cellular and Molecular Mechanisms of Aging in the Nervous System," E. Giacobini, G. Filogamo, G. Giacobini, and A. Vernadakis, eds., Raven Press, New York.

Perry, E. K., Perry, R. H., Blessed, G., and Tomlinson, B. E., 1977, Necropsy evidence of central cholinergic deficits in senile dementia, Lancet, 1:189.

Reivich, M., Kuhl, D., Wolf, A., Greenberg, J., Phelps, M., Ido, T., Casella, V., Fowler, J., Hoffman, E., Alavi, A., Som, P.,and Sokoloff, L., 1979, The [18F]Fluorodeoxyglucose method for the measurement of local cerebral glucose utilization in man, Circ. Res., 44:127.

Rossor, M., Fahrenkrug, J., Emson, P., Mountjoy, C., Iversen, L., and Roth, M., 1980, Reduced cortical choline acetyltransferase activity in senile dementia of Alzheimer type is not accompanied by changes in vasoactive instestinal polypeptide, Brain Res., 201:249.

Rothlin, E., 1946/1947, The pharmacology of the natural and dehydrogenated alkaloids of ergot, Bull. Schweiz. Akad. Med. Wiss. 2:249.

Savaki, H. E., Kadekaro, M., McCulloch, J., and Sokoloff, L., 1982, The central noradrenergic system in the rat: A metabolic mapping study with α-adrenergic blocking agents, Brain Res. 234:65.

Scheinberg, P., Blackburn, I., Rich, M., and Saslaw, M., 1953, Effects of aging on cerebral circulation and metabolism, Arch. Neurol. Psychiatry (Chicago), 70:77.

Schwarcz, R., Hökfelt, T., Fuxe, K., Jonsson, G., Goldstein, M., Terenius, L., 1979, Ibotenic acid-induced neuronal degeneration: A morphological and neurochemical study, Exp. Brain Res. 37:199.

Shenkin, H. A., Novak, P., Goluboff, B., Soffe, A. M., and Bortin, L., 1953, The effects of aging, arteriosclerosis, and hypertension upon the cerebral circulation, J. Clin. Invest., 32:459.

Sims, N. R., Bowen, D. M., and Davison, A. N., 1981, [^{14}C]Acetylcholine synthesis and [^{14}C]carbon dioxide production from [U-^{14}C]glucose by tissue prisms from human neocortex, Biochem. J., 196:867.

Sitaram, N., Weingartner, H., and Gillin, J. C., 1978, Human serial learning. Enhancement with arecholine and choline and impairment with scopolamine, Science, 201:274.

Smith, C. B., Goochee, C., Rapoport, S. I., and Sokoloff, L., 1980, Effects of aging on local rates of cerebral glucose utilization in the rat, Brain, 103:351.

Sokoloff, L., 1972, Circulation and energy metabolism of the brain, in "Basic Neurochemistry," 2nd edition, G. J. Siegel, R. W. Albers, R. Katzman, and B. W. Agranoff, Little, Brown and Company, Boston.

Sokoloff, L., Reivich, M., Kennedy, C., Des Rosiers, M. H., Patlak, C. S., Pettigrew, K., Sakurada, O., and Shinohara, M., 1977, The ^{14}C-deoxyglucose method for the measurement of local cerebral glucose utilization: Theory, procedure, and normal values in the conscious and anestheized albino rat, J. Neurochem., 28:897.

Vigouret, J. M., Burki, H. R., Jaton, A. L., Zuger, P. E., and Loew, D. M., 1978, Neurochemical and neuropharmacological investigations with four ergot derivatives: Bromocriptine, dihydroergotoxine, CF 25-397 and CM 29-712, Pharmacology, 16, Suppl. 1:156.

White, P., Hiley, C. R., Goodhardt, M. J., Carrasco, L. H., Keet, J. P., Williams, I. E. I., and Bowen, D. M., 1977, Neocortical cholinergic neurons in elderly people, Lancet, 1:668.

Whitehouse, P. J., Price, D. L., Struble, R. G., Clark, A. W., and Coyle, J. T., Delong, M. R., 1982, Alzheimer's disease and senile dementia: Loss of neurons in the basal forebrain, Science, 215:1237.

Young, A. R., Bouloy, M., Boussard, J. F., Edvinsson, L., and MacKenzie, E. T., 1981, Direct vascular effects of agents used in the pharmacotherapy of cerebrovascular disease on isolated cerebral vessels, J. Cereb. Blood Flow Metab., 1:117.

RADIAL MAZE PERFORMANCE DEFICITS FOLLOWING LESIONS OF RAT BASAL FOREBRAIN

B. E. Lerer[1] and John Warner[2]

[1]CNS Diseases Research, Du Pont Pharmaceuticals
Wilmington, DE, USA, 19898 and [2]Department of Psychology
Busch Campus, Rutgers University, New Brunswick, NJ, USA, 08903

INTRODUCTION

In humans and animals, intact central cholinergic transmission is critical for normal learning and memory (1,6); clinical data from Alzheimer's Disease (AD) patients indicate that dementia severity correlates with degree of cortical cholinergic deficit (24). It is likely that cortical cholinergic neurons, arising from the nucleus basalis of Meynert, mediate many cognitive functions that are impaired in AD. In the rat, neurotoxic lesions of the magnocellular basal forebrain (MNBF) cell bodies, which comprise the homologue of the human nucleus basalis, decrease cholinergic innervation selectively in cortex and impair acquisition and retention of aversively- and appetitively-motivated behavior (8,9,14,15,17). Young rats with bilateral MNBF lesions display several important features common to AD, thus, the lesion may provide an animal model useful for studying AD.

Common features of AD and the MNBF model

AD patients and rats with MNBF lesions suffer significant losses of presynaptic cholinergic innervation of frontal and parietal cortex, as measured by decreased acetylcholine release (18,26) and decreased activity of choline acetyltransferase (ChAT), the enzyme marker for cholinergic neurons (4,13). These losses correlate with cognitive dysfunction in AD and impaired memory in MNBF rats. Postsynaptic cortical receptors are relatively spared (5,20), and physostigmine temporarily ameliorates perseverative errors in AD (27) and impaired behavior in MNBF rats (7).

Histologically, post-mortem AD brains have severe nucleus basalis cell loss and neuronal degeneration (29,30) that match the effects of the MNBF lesion. Although the characteristic senile plaques and neurofibrillary tangles of AD cortex and hippocampus are not found in MNBF rats, a recent study of temporal cortex biopsies showed that AD dementia was always accompanied by cholinergic deficit but not always by plaques and tangles (2).

Using the MNBF lesion to research the cholinergic aspect of cognition does not imply that only a cholinergic deficit is relevant to AD dementia. There is growing evidence that several neurotransmitters (somatostatin, substance P, serotonin) are significantly depleted in AD (4,25,26), although the functional properties of these deficits are unclear at present. MNBF lesions, which do not directly impair monoamine systems, may cause serotonin to decrease in frontal cortex as a result of reduced cortical cholinergic innervation (16); striatal dopamine may be indirectly affected in a similar fashion.

MNBF lesions and the radial maze

In AD, the initial deficit is in short-term memory, or memory of recent events; long-term memory remains relatively intact until the latest stages of the disease. Short-term memory temporarily holds a limited number of items of information that are easily displaced by new, interfering items. Long-term memory, by contrast, keeps a virtually unlimited, permanent store of information enabling us to speak and understand speech, recall names and faces, and perform mathematical calculations. Multi-stage memory theories maintain that these are disciminably different types of memory which are differentially affected by disease, drugs, alcohol and experimental variables.

MNBF and sham-operated control rats were trained to enter each arm of an 8-arm radial maze (21) to find sunflower seeds. Error-free performance entailed entering each maze arm once to find the seed hidden in the food well. This task differentiates short-term and long-term processes: Short-term memory remembers, or stores, a list of already-entered arms which the rat continually updates throughout a trial. If list-memory is impaired, the rat will have difficulty obtaining 8 seeds without re-entering a previously chosen arm. Long-term memory stores the constant maze features and task requirements that do not change from trial to trial. For instance, the maze has 8 arms; in any arm, there is only one seed, and it is at the distal end of the arm; once a seed is eaten, there will be no more in that arm in that trial. Thus, short-term (or "working") memory holds those items of information, obtained in a single trial, that are useful only for that trial; long-term memory holds those items useful for all trials (23).

Because the task requires that a rat remember a list of visited arms, it measures the development of serial list learning and, as such, provides an obvious parallel to a human skill impaired at an early stage of AD. AD patients, during free recall of serial lists, typically make perseverative errors that are probably cholinergically-mediated as they are alleviated by physostigmine (27).

METHOD

Male Sprague-Dawley rats (n = 6) were injected bilaterally with 1 ug kainic acid in 1 ul 0.2M sodium-phosphate buffer (pH 7.19) at the following coordinates: 0.7 mm posterior to bregma, 2.7 mm lateral to the midsagittal suture and 7.0 mm below the dura; bregma and lambda were horizontal. Control subjects (n = 6) had similar operations without injections. The mean preoperative weight was 270 g.

An 8 arm radial maze, constructed of wood coated with polyurethane, was mounted on a pivoting base 71 cm high. The center platform was 24 cm diameter; each arm was 69 cm long with a shallow food well at its end. Arms were baited with hulled sunflower seeds; extra-maze visual cues and an auditory stimulus allowed spatial orientation.

Behavioral training began 29 - 38 days after surgery, as subjects recovered from post-operative aphagia and locomotor abnormalities (9,17). When subjects weighed at least 20 g more than their preoperative weights, they were acclimated to a controlled feeding schedule of 15 - 20 g/day for several days prior to training. On two training days, subjects were habituated to the maze and trained to find seeds in the food wells with trails of seeds placed along each arm. Testing began the next day. Each arm was baited with one seed in its food well. A trial began when a subject was placed on the central platform of the maze; the trial ended when the rat had collected and eaten all 8 seeds (maximum trial duration = 10 min). An arm choice was defined "entered arm with four paws", a correct choice was "entered arm containing a seed" and "entered a previously chosen arm" was an error. A rat met task criterion after the fifth consecutive trial criterion of at least 7 correct in the first 8 choices. Rats had one trial per day for a minimum of 10 trials. Testing stopped when a rat met task criterion or after 30 trials.

Statistical Analysis: Parametric data were analyzed by two-tailed Student's *t*-test.

RESULTS

The MNBF group did not differ from controls in the number of trials needed to find all 8 seeds within 10 min (controls = 2.67 ± 0.5 mean ± SEM trials; MNBF = 4.2 ± 0.6; $p < .20$). Throughout the experiment, they completed trials as quickly as the controls. However, controls first met trial criterion in 2.1 ± 0.5 trials while MNBF rats took 9.7 ± 2.8 trials ($p < .05$). Controls all reached trial criterion in 12 trials (median = 10), while no MNBF rat reached criterion in less than 24 trials and only 3 of 6 MNBF rats met criterion in 30 trials (median = 29.5, $p < .01$, two-tailed Mann-Whitney test). Figure 1 shows the mean number of correct choices made within the first 8 choices of a trial.

Because of the different numbers of trials for each subject, we based our subsequent statistical comparisons of a rat's performance on its last 5 trials. During these last 5 trials, MNBF rats made significantly more errors than controls (5.5 ± 1.0 vs 1.8 ± 0.5, $p < .02$).

The probability of a correct choice changed as a function of the number of correct choices already made. For example, an error after two choices (when six correct choices were available) had greater magnitude than an error after seven choices (when only one correct choice remained). To account for the changing probability of a correct choice, we calculated transformed maze scores (22) and found that MNBF rats scored better than chance level but worse than controls on arm choices 3, 5, 6 and 8 ($p < .05$; see Figure 2).

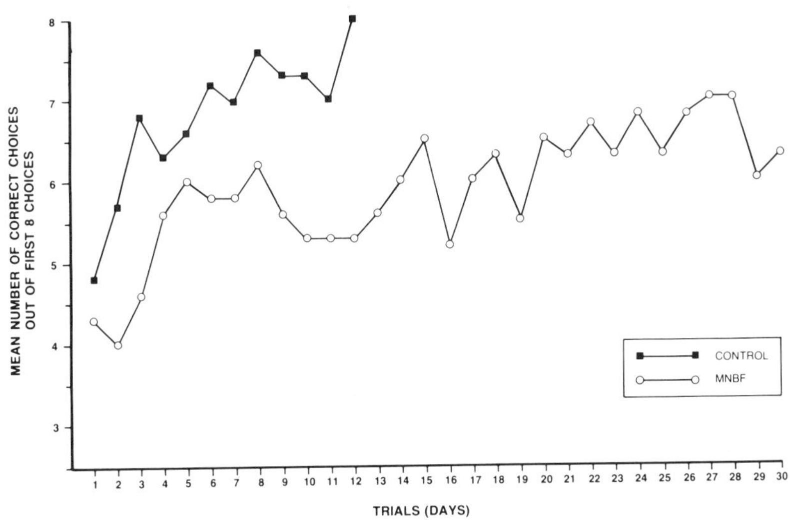

Fig. 1. Mean number of correct (i.e., different) choices made during the first eight choices of a trial.

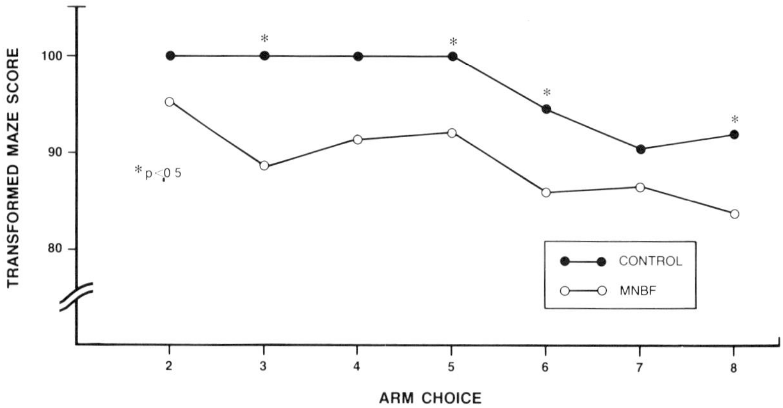

Fig. 2. Transformed maze performance scores for MNBF and control rats (see text for explanation of transformation). These data were taken from the last 5 trials for each rat. The MNBF group scored significantly lower than controls on arm choices 3, 5, 6 and 8.

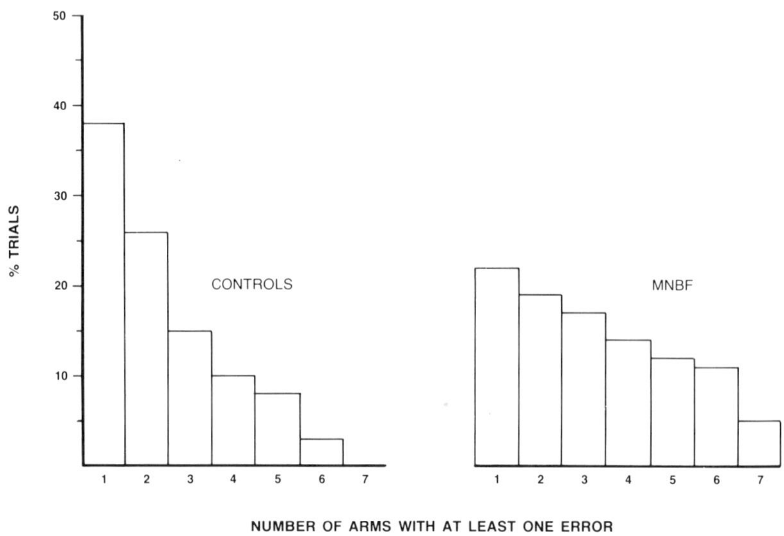

Fig. 3. The distribution of arm repetitions according to the serial position of correct choices, that is, the order in which the arms were originally chosen. The highest number on the abscissa is 7 because the eighth choice terminated a trial and, therefore, could not be repeated.

The distribution of errors by serial position of correct choices showed that controls made 40% of their errors by repeating their first choice and were less likely to err to more recent choices; that is, errors were made most often to remote choices and recently chosen arms were remembered best. The MNBF rats randomly distributed their errors and were only slightly less likely to repeat a recently chosen arm over an arm chosen earlier in the trial (see Figure 3).

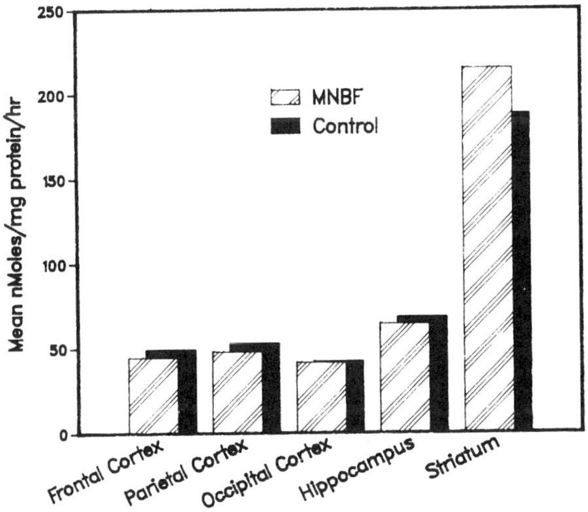

Fig. 4. Choline acetyltransferase (ChAT) activity was the index of regional brain cholinergic content. ChAT activity was measured under saturating conditions for choline and ^{14}C-Acetylcoenzyme A, and expressed in nMoles/mg protein/hr (16).

Although MNBF rats were behaviorally impaired, their regional ChAT activity levels were not significantly decreased (see Figure 4). ChAT activity, measured under saturating conditions for both choline and ^{14}C-Acetylcoenzyme A (16), was decreased about 10% in frontal and parietal areas of MNBF cortex (MNBF frontal cortex = 44.67 ± 2.3 nMoles/mg protein/hr vs control = 49.03 ± 1.9; MNBF parietal cortex = 47.98 ± 1.1 vs control = 52.61 ± 2.4). ChAT activity also did not change in occipital cortex (MNBF = 41.44 ± 0.1 vs control = 41.85 ± 1.1), striatum (MNBF = 215.1 ± 9.2 vs control = 187.8 ± 12.9), or hippocampus (MNBF = 66.47 ± 1.1 vs control = 68.05 ± 1.2, $p < .10$ n.s.).

In two MNBF rats, frontal cortex ChAT was decreased 21%, but there was no correlation between ChAT activity and maze performance, and these rats did no worse on the maze than an MNBF rat with no frontal cortex ChAT deficit. For MNBF rats, the correlation between ChAT and transformed maze score was $r = .145$ for frontal cortex and $r = .379$ for hippocampus. Across both groups of rats, the correlation between ChAT and "days to task criterion" was $r = -0.536$ for frontal cortex and $r = -0.553$ for hippocampus (critical r value = 0.576, $p < .05$, two-tailed), which suggests a trend for ChAT to be inversely related to "days to criterion"

DISCUSSION

MNBF rats made many more errors than controls and frequently repeated the same errors several times; that is, they persisted in re-entering arms even after they saw the arms no longer contained seeds. This pattern of repeated irrelevant errors, or perseverations, was observed in other spatial discrimination tests of MNBF rats (14,16). Perseveration is also common in AD serial recall performance, and it is sensitive to cholinergic pharmacological agents (27).

Controls erred only once or twice a trial, usually by repeating arms chosen at the very beginning of a trial (see Figure 3). This pattern, resembling the "recency" effect in serial position data of human list-learning, suggests maze behavior was mediated by short-term memory. To run the maze efficiently, rats may keep track of arm choices with a list of locations held in short-term memory (it would be counterproductive to keep the list in long-term memory because a new list is generated each trial). As the list is updated after each choice, older list items may get displaced by newer ones because short-term memory has a limited storage capacity.

Controls reached task criterion in 12 trials while the MNBF group failed to meet criterion in 30 trials. MNBF rats learned to run the maze and find 8 seeds, but they made many errors right from the start of a trial (see Figure 1). They were much less efficient than controls probably because short-term memory storage of previous choices was defective. Long-term memory appeared to be relatively intact given that MNBF rats learned to find seeds in about the same number of trials as controls, and scored higher in maze performance than would be expected if they were randomly choosing arms. Also, their latencies to choose arms, running speeds and trial completion times were not different from controls, which suggests they remembered the task reqirements and that trial-independent memory was spared.

Because rats must be appetitively motivated to learn the maze, we worried that a slight residual feeding deficit had persisted from the post-operative aphagia (15,16,17) and was a non-cognitive source of impairment. But MNBF rats ate all their seeds and completed their trials as fast as controls, so we were satisfied that lack of motivation was not the prime source of impairment.

Although MNBF lesions did not significantly decrease ChAT activity, we saw a trend for days to task criterion to be related to ChAT. Perhaps the ChAT decrease was not significant because we failed to assay cortical areas most affected by the lesion. Our previous kainate lesions depleted cortical ChAT 30-40% (15,16,17), and we used the same rat strain, sex, and injection coordinates that were successful previously. But the mortality rate in this experiment was very high; we lesioned a dozen rats that did not survive post-operative seizures and aphagia. Kainic acid is extremely toxic and perhaps only those rats with minimal damage could survive. There are several less toxic excitatory amino acids that produce significant neuronal damage and they are preferred for future lesions.

We worried that hippocampal damage might have impaired behavior because the maze task is particularly sensitive to damage of the septo-hippocampal system or its extrinsic connections (23). Combined MNBF and medial septal lesions impaired learning more severely than either lesion alone (10): MNBF lesions impaired short-term memory in an appetitive spatial discrimination task (11), but adding a hippocampal deficit added a long-term memory impairment (which is characteristic of AD dementia in its later stages). We did not observe a significant decrease in hippocampal ChAT activity, so cholinergic hippocampal damage was not the source of impairment; however, kainic acid may have damaged CA3 cells (19) and this non-cholinergic hippocampal damage would impair maze behavior. Histological examination did not reveal any gross hippocampal abnormalities, and kainic acid injected directly into CA3 did not impair radial maze performance (12). Similarly, accidental lesioning of the striatum might impair maze learning, but the absence of a striatal ChAT decrease suggests that the cholinergic intrinsic neurons were intact.

We attempted to selectively lesion the cholinergic basal forebrain because we were interested in the cognitive functions mediated by this system; we used kainic acid to destroy the MNBF cell bodies and spare nearby monoamine tracts (e.g., the medial forebrain bundle). But the kainic acid could have damaged these tracts with its non-specific toxicity (19). Damaging these systems, which modulate appetitive reward, would interfere with the motivation for learning the maze. Alternatively, disrupting the MNBF innervation of cortex may have, in turn, disrupted the output of a corticofugal system (such as the glutamate pathway to striatum) mediating a subcortical system critical to normal cognition. Regional monoamine biochemical assays are needed before we can substantiate these possibilities.

A recent report described cortical ChAT recovery several weeks after unilateral lesions (28). Our MNBF rats may have had cholinergic deficits sufficient to impair learning at the time of the maze test, but perhaps they recovered before ChAT was assayed 10 weeks after surgery. Had we continued testing, we may have observed concomittant behavioral recovery, although after 30 days of testing this did not seem imminent; the MNBF rats not at criterion were not close to meeting it.

We believe the MNBF lesion produces a valid animal model of AD. Even though these lesions lacked a significant ChAT effect, other MNBF lesions, made in our and other laboratories, have selectively reduced cortical ChAT and impaired behavior (8,9,10,16,17). Certainly we need more reliable lesions with consistent cortical ChAT reductions. But the severely impaired behavior we observed encourages us to pursue this research and manipulate pharmacological variables to improve learning.

Currently there are no therapeutic agents available to slow cognitive decline or reverse dementia. The MNBF model will have its greatest utility in evaluating compounds with cognition-enhancing properties useful for treating AD.

REFERENCES

1. Bartus, R. T., Dean, R. L., Beer, B. & Lippa, A. S. (1982): Science 217: 408-417.
2. Bowen, D. M., Francis, P. T. & Palmer, A. M. (1985): Paper presented at 30th OHOLO Biological Conference, Eilat, Israel.
3. Coyle, J. T., Price, D. & DeLong, M. (1983): Science 219: 1184-1190.
4. Davies, P. (1983). In: The Dementias (eds) R. Mayeux & W. F. Rosen, Raven Press, New York, pp. 75-86.
5. Davies, P. & Verth, A. H. (1977): Brain Res. 138: 385-392.
6. Drachman, D. (1977): Neurology 27: 783-790.
7. Fibiger, H. C., Murray, C. L. & Phillips, A. G. (1983): Soc. Neurosci. Abstr. 9: 332.
8. Flicker, C. et al. (1983): Pharm. Biochem. Behav. 18: 973-981.
9. Friedman, E., Lerer, B. E., & Kuster, J. (1983): Pharmacol. Biochem. Behav. 19: 309-312.
10. Hepler, D. J. et al. (1985): J. Neurosci. 5: 866-873.
11. Hepler, D. J. et al. Brain Res. (in press).
12. Jarrard, L. (1983): Behav. Neurosci. 97: 873-889.
13. Johnston, M. V., McKinney, M. & Coyle, J. T. (1981): Exp. Brain Res. 43: 159-172.
14. Lerer, B. E. & Friedman, E. (1983). In: Alzheimer's Disease (ed) B. Reisberg, Macmillan, New York, pp 421-427.
15. Lerer, B. E., Gamzu, E. & Friedman, E., (in press). In: Dynamics of Cholinergic Function (ed) I. Hanin, Plenum Press, New York.
16. Lerer, B. E., Warner, J., Friedman, E., Vincent, G. & Gamzu, E. Behav. Neurosci. (in press).
17. Lerer, B. E. et al. (1983): Soc. Neurosci. Abstr. 9: 97.
18. LoConte, G. et al. (1982): Pharmacol. Biochem. Behav. 17: 933-937.
19. Mason, S. T. & Fibiger, H. C. (1979): Science 204: 1339-1341.

20. McKinney, M. & Coyle, J. T. (1982): J. Neurosci. 2: 97-105.
21. Olton, D. S. (1977): Scientific Amer. 236 (b): 82-98.
22. Olton, D. S. & Samuelson, J. (1976): J. Exp. Psychol. 2: 97-116.
23. Olton, D. S., Walker, J. A. & Gage, F. H. (1978): Brain Res. 139: 295-308.
24. Perry, E. K. et al. (1978): Br. Med. J. 52: 1457-1459.
25. Reynolds, G. P. et al. (1984): Neurosci. Lett. 44: 47-51.
26. Sims, N. R., Bowen, D. M. & Davison, A. N. (1981): J. Biochem. 196: 867-876.
27. Thal, L. J., Fuld, P. A., Masur, D. M. & Sharpless, N. S. (1983): Ann. Neurol. 13: 491-496.
28. Wenk, G. & Olton, D. (1984): Brain Res. 293: 184-186.
29. Whitehouse, P. J. et al. (1981): Ann. Neurol. 10: 122-126.
30. Whitehouse, P. J. et al. (1982): Science 215: 1237-1239.

THE AF64A-TREATED RAT AS AN EXPERIMENTAL MODEL FOR ALZHEIMER'S DISEASE: A CRITICAL EVALUATION

A. Fisher and I. Hanin
Israel Institute for Biological Research
P.O.Box 19, Ness-Ziona, 70450, Israel; and
Loyola University Stritch School of Medicine
Chicago, Illinois

INTRODUCTION

Alzheimer's Disease or Senile Dementia of Alzheimer's Type (SDAT) is characterized clinically by a progressive chronic cognitive impairment; severe for memory of recent events, whereas memory for the past remains relatively intact (1). Histopathological studies on brains of SDAT patients revealed characteristic abnormalities such as senile plaques, neurofibrillary tangles and granulovacuolar degeneration in select brain areas (2-5).

Neurochemical and histological studies of SDAT brains have indicated a loss of specific populations of cholinergic cell bodies in the basal forebrain [the nucleus basalis of Meynert (nbM), medial septum (MS) and diagonal band of Brocca (dbB)] which project to the cerebral cortex and hippocampus. In addition, marked reductions in presynaptic cholinergic markers were found in the cerebral cortex and hippocampus. These include decreases in choline acetyltransferase (ChAT) and acetylcholinesterase (AChE) activity, impaired acetylcholine (ACh) synthesis and reduced choline (Ch) uptake (1-8). On the other hand, no significant change in muscarinic receptors (mAChR) has been reported in a large number of studies (review 4), although recently alteration in mAChR binding in SDAT has been shown in a few laboratories (9, 10).

In SDAT the decrease in ChAT activity is paralleled by morphological changes probably due to cholinergic nerve terminal degeneration, which in turn correlate with the severity of cognitive loss (11, 13). These findings, coupled with pharmacological investigations in humans and animals indicating a major role of the cholinergic system in learning and memory, are consistent with the cholinergic hypothesis in SDAT. Other neurotransmitter systems appear to be relatively unaffected in this disorder (2,4,11-13).

Research and development in SDAT was hampered until recently by lack of adequate animal models that can mimic all aspects of this neuropsychiatric disease. Since the etiology of SDAT is unknown, no homologous animal model for this disorder has been developed as yet. At the same time, attempts have been made to develop animal models that can mimic certain facets of this disease (14). In this regard, ethylcholine aziridinium ion (AF64A) can be a potential tool in developing an animal model of a number of neuropsychiatric disorders (including SDAT) in which a central cholinergic hypofunction has been implicated (15-38).

In the following sections we will review briefly such critical points as: AF64A-induced cholinotoxicity in rats from the neurochemical, behavioral and histological aspects; care that should be taken when performing experiments with AF64A, and potential errors in interpretation of data; comparison with other well-known neurotoxins (e.g. catecholaminergic neurotoxins and excitotoxins); comparison with other animal models for SDAT. Finally, some future strategies for research and development will be discussed.

INTRACEREBROVENTRICULAR AND INTRACEREBRAL INJECTIONS OF AF64A NEUROCHEMISTRY

A number of studies have shown that intracerebroventricular (icv) or intracerebral (ic) administration of AF64A in rats produces a persistent reduction in presynaptic cholinergic markers without concomitant atterations in other neurotransmitters studied. Table 1 represents a collection of data from various experiments performed by us and others. These studies examining dose- and time-dependent effects showed, in general, that low doses of AF64A, usually in the nmolar range, caused a long-lasting selective cholinergic hypofunction. Thus, high-affinity choline uptake (HAChT), ChAT activity, ACh levels and synthesis were reduced whereas catecholamines, indoleamines, their metabolites, Ch levels, uptake of norepinephrine (NE), dopamine (DA) and γ-aminobutyric acid (GABA), activity of glutamic acid decarboxylase (GAD) and tyrosine hydroxylase (TH), and mAChR binding were unaffected.

From icv injections of AF64A one can conclude that the cholinergic hypofunction obtained is confined to certain brain areas, the hippocampus being the most vulnerable followed by the frontal cortex. The striatum on the other hand is not affected (Table 1).

Ic administration of low doses of AF64A showed the same specific biochemical cholinergic characteristics as for icv injections (Table 1).

BEHAVIOR

The behavioral effects following administration of AF64A icv or ic in rats have been reviewed recently (23,37,38). Therefore only the findings with immediate relevance to this chapter are summarized here. In general, low doses of AF64A (3 nmol/side, icv) are sufficient to induce cognitive dysfunctions in rats in several behavioral paradigms. These learning and memory impairments are long-lasting (months) and can be ameliorated by means of drugs known to increase the cholinergic activity. Thus a cholinesterase inhibitor (physostigmine) or a specific direct muscarinic agonist (AF30) are capable of restoring memory impairments induced by AF64A in the passive avoidance test (23, 39). These are the first reports of reversal of AF64A-induced cognitive dysfunctions by means of central cholinotonic drugs, thus emphasizing the potential use of this experimental animal model in research and development of drugs for SDAT. Interestingly, very few studies have been conducted with cholinergic drugs such as physostigmine in another animal model for SDAT, e.g. in rats injected into the Nucleus basalis Magnocellularis (NbM) with ibotenic acid (40, 41).

TABLE 1: SPECIFIC CHOLINOTOXICITY INDUCED BY AF64A IN RAT BRAINS IN VIVO (PERCENT OF CONTROL)

DOSE/TIME nmol/side /days	PARAMETER	icv CORTEX	icv HIPPOCAMPUS	icv STRIATUM	ic HIPPOCAMPUS	ic STRIATUM	ic nbM-CORTEX	References
	CHOLINERGIC							
3/ 7&21	ChAT	NS	42 - 42	NS				24
3/ 10&94		NS	32 - 75	130 - 80				23
2/ 5					42			32
4/ 120					61			35
8/ 7						54		33
02/ 7&14							83	21
3/ 10&62	AChE	NS - 80	32 - 70	NS - 115				23
3/ 7&21	HAChT	NS	32 - 52	NS				24
2/ 5					33			32
2/ 5	LAChT				NS			32
3/ 7&21	mAChR	NS	NS - 89	NS				24
5/ 7	ACh	NS	35	NS				28
7.5/ 120		NS	38	NS				47
15/ 120		38	57	NS				47
2/ 5					43			32
8/ 7						75		33
7.5, 15/120	Ch	NS	NS	NS				47
2/ 5					NS			32
3/ 7&21	KAChR	NS	76 - 65	NS				24
5-10/7	OUABAIN-AChRelease		65					28
	DOPAMINERGIC NORADRENERGIC SEROTONERGIC GABA-ERGIC							
7.5/120	DA, HVA, NE, 5HT	NS	NS	NS				47
5/7	DA, NE, 5HT	NS	NS	NS				28
4/ 120	DA, HVA, NE, 5HT				NS			35
2/ 5	NE, 5HT-UPTAKE				NS			32
8/ 7	TH, DA-UPTAKE, GAD GABA, GABA-UPTAKE					NS		33
02/ 7&14	DA, 5HT						NS	21

Abbreviations not mentioned in the text: KAChR - potassium-stimulated ACh release; Ouabain-ACh Release - Ouabain stimulated ACh release; HVA - homovanillic acid; 5HT - 5-hydroxy tryptamine;

COMPARISON WITH OTHER NEUROTOXINS; SPECIFICITY, HISTOLOGY AND HISTOCHEMISTRY

"Experience has shown that the blind acceptance of the degenerative action of a used neurotoxin as being restricted exclusively to structures in accord with the theory is unwarranted" (Jonsson, 42). No neurotoxin, including AF64A, is absolutely specific and under certain experimental conditions, it could produce irreversible damage to all nerve cells; however, at the same time a concentration can be achieved at the extra-neuronal milieu that might limit most of the damage to very specific cells.

When one has to decide whether the effects produced by AF64A are specific or non-specific to cholinergic neurons there is a need to review the pertinent literature on other well-known neurotoxins:

A. 6-Hydroxydopamine (6OHDA)

Although 6OHDA is the most studied neurotoxin for the dopaminergic system, some varying and sometimes contradictory results have been reported from various laboratories with respect to specific versus non-specific action. Thus, at least two groups (43-46) concluded that 6OHDA given by ic injection produces lesions which are no more selective than those seen after electrolytic, mechanical or chemical treatment. However, 6OHDA is still the neurotoxin of choice for the catecholaminergic nervous system since it denervates this system with less nonspecific damage than is possible by any other currently available technique.

One "imperfection" which appears to be inherent in use of 6OHDA (and for this matter in other neurotoxins as well) is the appearance of a region of nonspecific damage at the tip of the cannula tract (43-49). The extent of the damage increases with increasing doses of 6OHDA. The difference among the studies are in the size of the reported necrosis (large or small), its description, as well as interpretation of the data following these lesions. It was clear from these studies that among the factors which can influence the extent of non-specific damage are the parameters of 6OHDA injection such as the amount, concentration and injection rate of the 6OHDA solution (50, 51).

B. 5,6-and 5,7-Dihydroxytryptamine (5,6-DHT and 5,7-DHT, respectively)

These are the neurotoxins of choice for the serotonin neurons (42). 5,6-DHT causes a substantial degree of non-specific damage to non-monoamine-containing nerve cells. 5,7-DHT is a better tool then 5,6-DHT because it has a higher neurotoxic potency for serotonin neurons and more limited non-specific cytotoxic effects for non-monoamine neurons. Nevertheless, local microinjection of 5,7-DHT into the CNS causes greater non-specific damage than injection of the solvent alone, although the lesion in this case is smaller than that produced by electrolytic lesion (52).

C. Kainic Acid and other excitotoxins

The actions of kainic and other excitotoxins (including ibotenic acid) appear to be mediated by receptors localized to neuronal perikarya, and dendrites. Kainic acid, however, is not specific to one neurotransmitter substance. It has been shown to exert a degenerative effect on the cell bodies of a variety of neurotransmitter-containing nerve terminals in the brain, including ACh.

As in the case with 6OHDA, 5,6-DHT or 5,7-DHT local microinjection of kainic acid can cause extensive neuronal necrosis at the needle tract (53-55). Ic injection of kainic acid is followed by tissue shrinkage, ventricular dilatation and a significant reduction in mass and protein content (56-59). This phenomenon is most probably a result of death of cell bodies in the injected brain areas, and extensive gliosis following the neuronal perikarya destruction.

D. AF64A

AF64A is one of the most potent synthetic neurotoxins when injected icv or ic, and at least as potent as kainic acid. In addition, certain brain areas are more vulnerable to the cytotoxic activity of this agent than others.

Therefore, certain precautions should be taken in order to avoid nonspecific effects. In the literature there are descriptions of studies with AF64A that showed specific effects and a few studies that have showed non-specific effects at the injection site around the tip of the needle (review 29 and 37). The differences among these studies are: the size of this possible necrosis - large, small or nonsignificant; interpretation of data; use of various batches of AF64A; and, of course, variations in experimental conditions.

The extent of specific cholinergic damage induced by AF64A will depend on several factors, some of which may be regarded as constant, and some can be manipulated experimentally in an advantageous way. The following main factors can affect the cholinotoxicity of AF64A after icv or ic injections:

1. Synthesis and purity of AF64A;

2. Dose injected and concentration at the extraneuronal milieu;

3. Injection technique (rate of injection, total time of injection, injection volume, cannula used);

4. Diffusion conditions and ionic strength of the solution;

5. Membrane uptake mechanism; area of injection;

6. Anesthetics used;

7. Age and sex of the animals;

8. Circadian variation.

Some problems with AF64A can arise because of insufficient attention to factors 1-8. Other problems might arise because of misinterpretation of the data.

D.1. Synthesis and purity of AF64A. The relative purity of AF64A might dictate whether the lesions obtained are specific to cholinergic neurons or are unwanted non-specific cytotoxic effects. The synthesis of the precursor of AF64A, compound 3, is according to the following scheme:

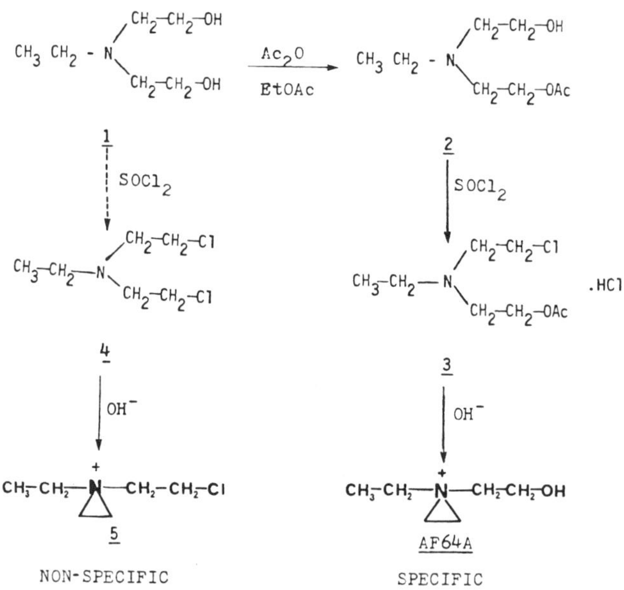

It is absolutely imperative to purify 2 from any residual of compound 1, before preparing compound 3. Otherwise, a two-armed mustard will be obtained (as an impurity), compound 4.

Compound 4 is a well-known mustard that is extremely cytotoxic and affects all type of cells. Therefore, even minor impurities of 4 in 3 might cause nonspecific cytotoxic effect. Quality control of 3 (HCl) should be done in a most comprehensive way. In this regard the compound sold by RBI fulfills the most rigorous quality control criteria defined by us, including: high resolution NMR, high resolution GC-MS, TLC, IR and melting point.

It should be emphasized that the preparation of AF64A from 3 should be done carefully according to the method described by us (32). The aziridinium ion concentration (AF64A) can be analyzed by titration with sodium thiosulpate. However, by no means is this method satisfactory to indicate formation of AF64A only, if 3 contains some residual quantities of 4.

In fact, an impurity of 5 in AF64A might increase the toxicity of AF64A, rather than decrease it, leading eventually to a misinterpretation of the data obtained and possible non-specific cytotoxic effects. It is, therefore, not surprising that different data, sometimes contradictory, have been published from different laboratories regarding AF64A, employing different batches of the precursor 3 (60-63). In this regard, the precursor sold so far by RBI is the most recommended by us, since we have performed the most extensive quality control on this product.

D.2. Dose injected and concentration at the extraneuronal milieu. It is possible that in sufficiently high concentration, AF64A could produce irreversible damage to different nerve cells. However, since the compound is interacting selectively with cholinergic neurons, it is possible to limit most of the damage primarily to these cells.

Depending on the experimental technique used, one should work-out the most appropriate dose-cholinotoxic response. It is reasonable to assume that regardless of the brain area injected, a more selective cholinergic lesion could be achieved if, at every given time during administration of AF64A, its concentration in the extraneuronal milieu is kept as low as possible. We can also assume that this concentration should be in the uMolar range in the synaptic milieu, in order not to saturate the HAChT[#].

If this condition could be fulfilled an avid accumulation of the cholinotoxin from the extraneuronal milieu might occur. At the same time it appears that a critical level of AF64A has to be attained intraneuronally, before degenerative events occur.

The dose injected into each brain area (ic injection) should also depend on the relative size of that brain area. This is not surprising when one considers that the concentration attained in each brain area injected is inversely proportional to the relative volume of that particular site. Therefore very low doses of AF64A (0.02 nmol) are needed for selective cytotoxic effects in the NbM when compared with 100 times higher doses in the dorsal hippocampus (2nmol) (21, 32). An alternative explanation for this very potent action of AF64A in the NbM region would be the following: a) the cholinotoxin would lesion a population of cholinergic nerve terminals from an unknown origin (or cholinergic interneurons) but projecting on inhibitory neurons such as: GABA-ergic, glycinergic or amino acidergic neurons; or b) a degeneration of these cholinergic nerve terminals would induce an uncontrolled release of one of these amino acids, resulting in a very prolonged depolarization of the postsynaptic receptor(s) to this amino acid. The neurons eventually would die due to this irreversible or prolonged excitation.

This last mechanism appears to be very attractive since it can explain why the "end-product" of excitotoxins lesions (e.g. kainic or ibotenic acid) and AF64Ainduced lesions is qualitatively, at least, the same. Of course, other reasons, as well, could be also responsible for the extreme vulnerability of the NbM to AF64A.

D.3. Injection technique (rate of injection, total time of injection, injection volume, needle or cannula used). The injection technique is extremely important when one intends to inject a neurotoxin icv or ic. Since AF64A is very potent, the rate of injection should be as slow as possible. It is advisable to use an infusion pump that will deliver the effective dose of the cholinotoxin during a few minutes. A small injection volume and a slow injection rate might avoid possible mechanical damage. For kainic acid, for example 28 nmol were delivered at 0.02 ul/min, ic (64). So far, AF64A was not reported to be injected at such low rates of infusion, but we believe that this is a very useful way to avoid mechanical and unwanted nonspecific damage.

A Kopf Instruments Microinjection Unit (Model 5000) which is attached to a stereotaxic instrument and is manually operated, has been used successfully in one lab at least, for AF64A infusion icv or ic (Walsh, T., personal communication).

The cannula or needle used is very important when one wants to minimize, as much as possible, necrosis at the tip of the needle and to diminish the size of the needle tract. Therefore, a needle with a very

---

[#] IC_{50} of AF64A on HAChT is 0.9-3.5 uM depending on the brain area studied.

small diameter should be preferred. Specific cholinotoxic effects, without non-specific tissue damage were obtained when: a) AF64A (total dose 15 or 30 nmol, bilaterally) was infused icv through a 34 gauge needle (22); b) ic in the striatum AF64A (8 nmol), through a 0.3 mm needle (33); c) ic in the dorsal hippocampus, AF64A (2 nmol), through a 31 gauge needle (32). For ic or icv injections we can recommend also the use of a glass micropipette with a tip diameter of 0.1 mm, attached to a 10 ul Hamilton syringe as described for kainic acid (54).

An alternative way to avoid nonspecific cytotoxicity would be to inject divided doses of AF64A that should be only slightly cholinotoxic, but their chronic injection 2 or 3 times at a few hours interval could produce the same degree of ACh depletion as a single large dose of AF64A. This method could be used also to induce maximal depletion of ACh without unwanted nonspecific effects. Interestingly, this technique is employed successfully with 6OHDA (65).

D.4. Diffusion conditions and ionic strength of the solution. When anatomical specificity is not required, non-specific damage can be minimized if one injects a selective neurotoxin like 6OHDA into the cerebrospinal fluid by way of the lateral ventricle (66). The same technique could be applied for AF64A. In this case, the ionic strength of the solution is important in order to minimize any possible non-specific effects. Therefore, an isotonic saline or freshly prepared artificial cerebrospinal fluid (CSF) are recommended as the vehicle of choice (see also 26). The same precaution should be applied for intra-cerebral injections in different brain areas. In both cases the injection techniques described in D.3. should be the most appropriate approach.

By icv injection the diffusion of the cholinotoxin is regulated mainly by the CSF in the ventricle so that the agent is diluted, and diffuses relatively rapidly to brain areas adjacent to the ventricle. However, by nature of the intracerebral injection, diffusion and, therefore, dilution of the cholinotoxin, is a relatively slow process depending entirely on the morphology of the brain area injected. It is not surprising, therefore, that in this case very careful injections such as those described in D.3. should be employed in order to minimize possible necrosis at the needle tract.

D.5. Membrane uptake mechanism and area of injection. These two factors are dealt together since they are interrelated. In case of 6OHDA, since the high-affinity uptake system by which 6OHDA is concentrated resides primarily in the terminal region, specific effects are more easily produced there than in the area of the cell body where little specific uptake takes place. The same situation is not necessarily applicable to AF64A. Although we tend to believe that AF64A acts primarily in the nerve terminal region, we cannot ignore the findings that very low doses of this neurotoxin are needed in order to lesion the cholinergic cell bodies in the NbM (21, 67; see also section D.2.). Since a HAChT in this brain region was not reported, we do not know as yet how AF64A exerts its cholinotoxic effect in this region. It is possible that some high-affinity uptake sites for Ch do exist in this area, and this could be enough to accumulate AF64A and eventually cause cholinotoxicity. Accumulation of AF64A by the low affinity transport of Ch (LAChT) found in cell bodies cannot be excluded as a possible explanation for this cholinotoxicity in the NbM, although this explanation appears to be the least plausible due to the very low doses of AF64A needed to induce cholinotoxicity (at least 100 times lower than for the dorsal hippocampus; 21, 32, 67). The relative vulnerability of different brain areas to AF64A-induced cholinotoxicity was described above (for possible explanation see review 37).

In order to manipulate the membrane uptake mechanism we can employ drugs that can increase ACh turnover in the brain. For example, atropine will increase Vmax of HAChT in the cortex and hippocampus and not in the striatum (68). This approach should accumulate AF64A faster in the cholinergic neurons, and in fact, we have preliminary data indicating that atropine potentiates AF64A-induced cholinotoxicity (69). Thus, by pretreatment with atropine we can suggest a way to increase HAChT activity and therefore a more avid and selective accumulation of AF64A given by icv or ic injection.

Another alternative could be to inject AF64A icv or ic under depolarizing conditions (high K+ included in the vehicle) when the Vmax of HAChT is known to be increased (see review 68).

D.6. Anesthetics used. Pentobarbital was found to reduce HAChT in the cortex and hippocampus (68). Therefore this might affect the balance between specific (mainly on the HAChT) and non-specific effects (LAChT and other systems, as well) of AF64A. To our knowledge, a careful study on this topic has not yet been conducted, therefore, it is not clear how important this factor is in AF64Ainduced cholinotoxicity. Interestingly, various anesthetic agents such as pentobarbital were found to reduce the NE depleting action of 6OHDA while ether anesthesia during a similar procedure resulted in a higher reduction of NE (65).

At this point we cannot recommend the anesthetic of choice to be used with AF64A (icv or ic injections). We have obtained selective cytotoxic effects with AF64A (icv or ic) after ether, equitensin or pentobarbital anesthesia.

D.7.-D.8. Age, sex, strain and specie of the animals; circadian variations. Since the sensitivity of neurons varies widely, the dose-response curve of AF64A should be determined for each brain area examined. It must be remembered that for a given brain area, the dose response curve may vary depending upon age, sex, strain and specie of the animals as well as possible circadian variations. All these factors have not been evaluated rigorously, as yet. From a careful examination of the literature it appears that there is no uniform sensitivity of different strains of rats towards AF64A icv-induced lethality and cholinotoxicity.

Although a comparative study under the same experimental conditions has not yet been conducted, it appears that certain strains of rats are able to tolerate higher doses of icv AF64A without increased toxicity. These strains are: Fischer 344 (22); Wistar (25, 28); CFY (26). On the other hand the SpragueDawley strain appears to be more sensitive towards AF64A icv-induced lethality and cholinotoxicity (32, 70).

Finally, it is recommended that comprehensive histological as well as neurochemical evalutions of AF64A-induced neurotoxicity be conducted, in order to obtain a reliable interpretation of the data. Only if by both these methods nonspecific effects could be revealed at a certain dose, this dose should be lowered in order to obtain specific cholinotoxic effects.

In this regard, a comprehensive histochemical and electromicroscopic study described in this volume (26) showed that in general for icv and ic injections the proper dose of AF64A should be less than 5 nmol and 0.25 nmol respectively, in order to obtain selective cholinotoxicity. Interestingly in two other studies selective cholinotoxicity with AF64A, ic in the NbM, was obtained in the dose range of 0.02-0.1 nmol and 0.02-0.5 nmol, respectively (21, 67).

TABLE 2: CHOLINERGIC ALTERATIONS IN SDAT VERSUS THE AF64A-TREATED RAT

PARAMETER	PERCENT OF CONTROL								Refs for	
	CORTEX		HIPPOCAMPUS		STRIATUM		NbM			
	SDAT	AF64A	SDAT	AF64A	SDAT	AF64A	SDAT	AF64A	SDAT	AF64A
ChAT		NS		42 ; 42		NS NS				24
	10-48	NS	10-30	32 75	40-80	130 80			6,8	23
							10		2	
				61				*		35,21
				42						32
HAChT	56	NS	NR	32 52	NR	NS			6	24
							NR	NR		
	50		20	33	NR				7	32
AChE	10-50		10-50		30-60				2	21
								**		
		NS-80		32 70		NS 115				23
mAChR	NS	NS	NS	NS 89	NS	NS			4	24
			50						9	
			>100						10	
ACh	51	NS,38	NR	38;57;	NS	NS			70	47
		NS		35		NS				28
				43						32
ACh-SYNTHESIS	59	NR	NR	71 51	NR	NR			6	24
Ch	NS	NS	NR	NS	NS	NS			70	47

NR - NOT REPORTED; NS - NOT SIGNIFICANT; ND - NOT DETERMINED
*ChAT ACTIVITY WAS REDUCED IN FRONTAL CORTEX BY 17%; **AChE - STAINING WAS REDUCED (21)

AF64A-INDUCED CHOLINOTOXICITY: COMPARISON WITH OTHER EXPERIMENTAL ANIMAL MODELS FOR SDAT

The data obtained following AF64A administration in experimental animals (mainly rats) show remarkable similarity to the neurochemical and behavioral deficits observed in SDAT (Tables 1 and 2). Thus the AF64A-treated rat may consequently be an excellent candidate for a suitable animal model for SDAT based on the collection of data shown in these tables as well as the following considerations:

a) AF64A mimics, at least qualitively, the profound reductions of presynaptic cholinergic parameters in the forebrain of SDAT patients.

b) This cholinergic hypofunction following AF64A (icv) is paralleled by long term impairment of memory and learning in affected rats; in SDAT the persistent reduction of cholinergic markers is paralleled by cognitive dyfunctions.

c) The AF64A-treated rat mimics to some extent the short-term memory impairment in SDAT (shown in the 8-arm radial maze test) as well as spatial orientation dysfunction in SDAT (shown in the Morris swimming maze).

In Table 3 a comparison was made among the reported animal models for SDAT. No animal model shown in this Table is perfect and each one was developed in order to mimic certain characteristics of SDAT. In this regard the AF64Atreated rat can be best compared to the excitotoxin-induced lesioned animal in the NbM (kainic or ibotenic acid). At the same time, it should be pointed out that the excitotoxin induced lesions damage contiguous noncholinergic neurons at the injection site (71,72). Thus for example, rats with ibotenic acid-induced lesions in the dorsolateral globus pallidus suffered also passive avoidance deficits even though their cortical ChAT activity was not decreased (73). This later limitation might be avoided by using AF64A, which by its nature is a selective cholinotoxin. In this regard, the AF64A-induced lesions can be considered a "conceptual" experimental model for SDAT superior to the excitotoxin-induced degenerations.

However, the AF64A-animal model is still imperfect since it has not yet been shown that it can mimic the histopathological characteristics of SDAT, nor has it been shown whether it can mimic deficits in somatostatin which have been reported to be reduced in SDAT (1,2,13).

IMPLICATION OF THE AF64A-INDUCED LESION ON THE CHOLINERGIC DYSFUNCTION IN SDAT: A VERY SPECULATIVE TREATISE

Although a number of hypotheses have been published to explain the etiology of SDAT, the cause of neuronal death in SDAT is still an enigma. In this regard, AF64A is a synthetic cholinotoxin, most probably not found *in vivo*, but it can offer some mechanistic clues about the etiology of SDAT.

AF64A exerts its cholinotoxic effects by interacting mainly with cholinergic neurons where it can be accumulated via the HAChT system. The relative brain area selectivity and vulnerabity to this agent (icv injection) follows the order: hippocampus > cortex > striatum. In addition the NbM region appears to be extremely vulnerable to the cytotoxic activity of this cholinotoxin since very low doses of AF64A are effective in this area (0.02-0.1 nmol, 21) compared for example

TABLE 3: POTENTIAL ANIMAL MODELS FOR SDAT

CRITERIA	AGED RODENTS	AGED MONKEYS	ANOXIA/ HYPOXIA (RATS)	SCOPOLAMINE/ HEMICHOLINIUM-3 (RODENTS)	ALUMINUM (EXPTL. ANIMALS)	EXCITOTOXINS (RATS)	AF64A (RATS)	SDAT
CHOLINERGIC HYPOFINCTION								
A. Specific	NO	NO	NO	YES	NO	NO	YES	PRIMARY
B. Pre-synaptic	YES	YES	YES	YES (HC-3)	NO	YES	YES	YES
C. Post-synaptic	YES	YES	YES	YES (SCOPOLAMINE)	NO	NO	NO	NO
D. Persistent	YES	YES	NO	NO	NO	YES	YES	YES
In:								
E. Frontal cortex	YES	YES	YES	YES	NO	YES	YES	YES
F. Hippocampus	YES	YES	YES	YES	NO	YES	YES	YES
G. Nucleus Basalis						YES	YES	YES
COGNITIVE IMPAIRMENTS								
A. Persistent	YES	YES	NO	NO	YES	YES	YES	YES
B. Reversible	NO	NO	YES	YES	NO	NO	NO	NO
CHOLINERGIC DRUGS REVERSE COGNITIVE IMPAIRMENTS	YES	YES	YES	YES	Not reported	YES	YES	YES
HISTOPATHOLOGY								
A. Plaques	NO	YES	NO	NO	NO	NO	NO	YES
B. Tangles	NO	NO	NO	NO	YES	NO	? (Not clear yet)	YES

with the dose required in the hippocampus (2 nmol) or with kainic acid (4 nmol in the NbM, 71).

As a speculative working hypothesis let us presume that AF64A can model an endogenous neurotoxin that at sufficient and chronic accumulation could induce SDAT in humans. How would one look for such a natural neurotoxin? One assumption would be that such an endogenous agent can be a toxic analog of the neurotransmitter ACh (1).

Since cholinergic neurons do not take-up their neurotransmitter, ACh, but they do take up Ch, one may seek a potentially endogenous cytotoxic analog of Ch that could induce similar cholinotoxicity to AF64A, since Ch is metabolized according to the following scheme:

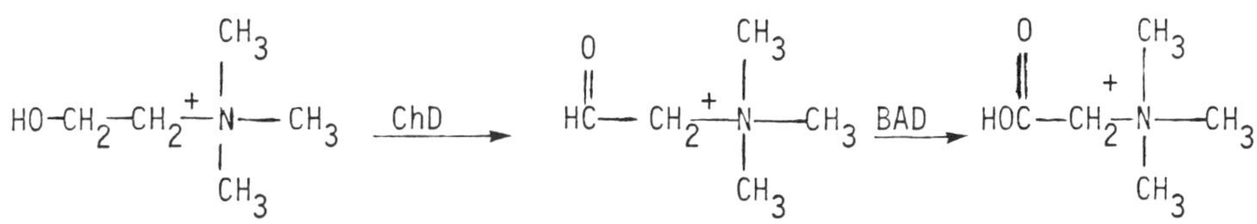

Ch Betaine aldehyde Betaine

The oxidation of Ch to betaine aldehyde is catalyzed by the mitochondrial enzyme, choline dehydrogenase, ChD, (EC1.1.99.1). The second enzyme, betaine aldehyde dehydrogenase, BAD, (EC 1.2.1.8) is a soluble enzyme that converts the aldehyde to betaine. ChD is found in tissues of various species; kidneys and liver of humans also contain significant amounts of this enzyme (74).

If betaine aldehyde could be stabilized _in vivo_, then it might become _cytotoxic_. Aluminum has been suggested as having an important role in the histopathology of SDAT in humans, but this issue is still controversial. We would like to suggest here that an exogenous toxic agent, such as aluminum, might form some complex with betaine aldehyde (a possible endogenous toxic compound). Such a complex (see below) might induce SDAT in humans if it could fulfill the following conditions:

a. The complex should be stable enough in order to exist _in vivo_; this would require that betaine aldehyde formed could be trapped by an exogenous toxic agent (e.g. aluminum) before it is transformed to betaine by BAD as it is formed.

b. Such a hypothetical complex could be transported into the brain through the blood-brain barrier.

c. Once in the CNS, the complex should be targeted to the cholinergic neurons, where it has to be accumulated intraneuronally _via_ the HAChT, for example (vide infra). At the same time it has to spare other neurotransmitter systems.

d. Inside the cholinergic neuron (mainly nerve terminals) the complex should decompose slowly to neurotoxic moieties such as betaine aldehyde and another aluminum complex. The betaine aldehyde by nature of its instability** could impair vital metabolic processes; Aluminum (in form of its complexes) can induce neurofibrillary

---

**that is, enhanced chemical reactivity due to the aldehyde group

tangles. Inside the cholinergic neuron a retrograde transport of the complex towards the neuronal perikarya could also occur so that tangles could originate in this region.

e. The steady-state concentration of the betaine aldehyde-aluminum complex should be very small so that only after a while (months or years) a critical cholinergic deficiency could be induced leading to the first behavioral symptoms of SDAT. This situation is reminiscent of the insidious appearance of SDAT in humans.

Clearly, such a hypothesis is very speculative. However, it links some unexplained questions about SDAT such as:

1) Why is SDAT associated with aging?

2) Why has SDAT sometimes genetic aspects?

3) What is the meaning of an increased blood-brain permeability in SDAT?

4) What is the importance of aluminum in SDAT?

5) Why is SDAT, in fact, primarily due to a cholinergic hypofunction?

A few hypothetical structures of complexes between aluminum and betaine aldehyde could be the following:

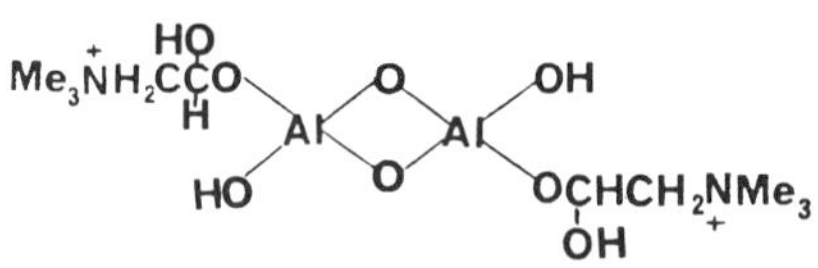

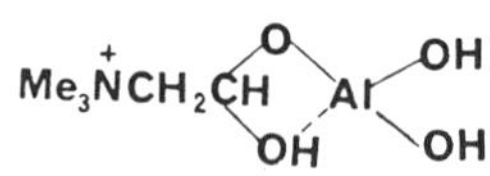

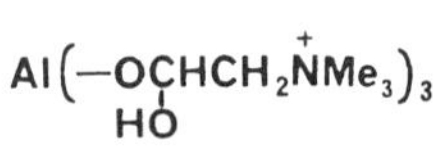

... and others

In all these structures a hemiacetal (of betaine aldehyde) forms a complex with aluminum. This hemiacetal structure is very similar to Ch and hemicholinium, therefore easily identified by the HAChT since it has the minimal requirements to interact with the Ch transport system (15).

Whether such complexes can be formed in aqueous solution is not clear as yet. However, it is known that aluminum alkoxides are stable to a sufficient degree, and that the aluminum-oxygen bond is almost covalent, and thus has little tendency to dissociate to give free alkoxide ions (75). If at least some types of the above mentioned structures could exist in the proper milieu they could easily cross the blood-brain barrier in a way similar to Ch or due to possible increased blood-brain permeability in aging. An increased permeability of blood-brain barrier was reported in SDAT (see review 76). The possible functional heterogeneity of HAChT system among the cortex, hyppocampus and striatum could dictate the selective impairment of the cholinergic activity in these brain areas, the cortex and hippocampus, in particular (77).

In summary, the above mentioned mechanism is at this stage only a speculation that tends to link findings from SDAT patients with the information accumulated so far on AF64A. In order to prove such a hypothesis ChD and BAD activity should first be evaluated in SDAT, in aging and in young human volunteers; also one should look for high levels of betaine aldehyde or low levels of betaine in SDAT patients when compared with aged matched controls. If such a hypothesis could be proved it would show a possible way for treatment and even for preventing SDAT.

Interestingly, Wurtman et al (76) have suggested, as a possible etiology for SDAT, a deficiency of normal supply of Ch in the cholinergic neurons; this leads to a breakdown of membrane phosphatidyl Ch in order to maintain the Ch concentration needed for ACh synthesis. The outcome of this process is an "autocannibalism" of cholinergic neurons.

Both hypothesis could be linked together in a scenario in which the above mentioned endogenous neurotoxin could impede access of Ch to the regular sites of synthesis of ACh, thus causing eventually a "cascade" effect in which membrane phosphatidyl Ch breaks down in order to supply more Ch for endogenous ACh synthesis.

REFERENCES

1. Terry, R.D. and Davies, P. Some morphologic and biochemical aspects of Alzheimer Disease, in: "Aging of the Brain". eds. Samuel, D. et al. Raven Press, New York, pp. 47-59 (1983).
2. Coyle, J.T., Price, D.L. and Delong, M.R. Alzheimer's disease: a disorder of cortical cholinergic innervation. Science. 219:1184-90 (1983).
3. Perry, E.K., Tomlinson, B.E., Blessed, G., Bergman, K., Gibson, P.H. and Perry, R.H. Correlation of cholinergic abnormalities with senile plaques and mental test scores in senile dementia. Br. Med. Journal 2:1457-59 (1978).
4. Bartus, R.T., Dean, R.L., Beer, B. and Lippa, A.S. The cholinergic hypothesis of geriatric memory dysfunction. Science 217:408-17 (1982)
5. Perry, E.K. The cholinergic system in old age and Alzheimer's disease. Age and Aging, 9:1-8 (1980).
6. Sims, N.R., Bowen, D.M., Allen, S.J., Smith, C.C.T., Neary, D., Thomas, J.J. and Davison, A.N. Presynaptic cholinergic dysfunction in patients with dementia. J. Neurochem. 40:503-9 (1983).
7. Rylett, R.J., Ball, M.Y., Colhoun, E.H. Evidence for high affinity choline transport in synaptosomes prepared from hippocampus and neocortex of patients with Alzheimer's disease. Brain Res. 289: 169-75 (1983).
8. Bowen, D.M., Francis, P.T. and Palmer. A.M. Cholinergic and non-cholinergic hypothesis for Alzheimer's disease: the biochemical evidence. This volume.
9. Reisine, T.D., Yamamura, H.I., Bird, E.E., Spokes, E. and Enna, S.J. Pre-and post-synaptic neurochmical alterations in Alzheimer's disease. Brain Res. 159:477-81. (1978).

10. Nordberg, A., Larsson, C., Adolfson, R., Alafuzoff, I. and Winbladt, B. Muscarinic receptor complusation in hippocampus of Alzheimer's patients. J. Neural Trans. 56:13-9 (1983).
11. Davies, P. Neurotransmitter-related enzymes in senile dementia of the Alzheimer type. Brain Res. 171:318-27 (1979).
12. Davis, K.L. and Yamamura, H.I. Minireview: Cholinergic under-activity in human memory disorders. Life Sci. 23:1729-34 (1978).
13. Davies, P. Neurotransmitters and neuropeptides in Alzheimer's disease, in: "Banbury Report 15: Biological Aspects of Alzheimer's Disease", ed. R. Katzman, Cold Spring Harbor Laboratory, pp. 255-265 (1983).
14. Bartus, R.T., Flicker, C. and Dean, R.L. Logical principles for the development of animal models of age-related memory impairments. In: Assessment in Geriatric Psychopharmacology. Eds. Grooh, T., Ferris, S. and Bartus, R.T. Mark Powley Associates, Inc. pp. 263-299 (1983).
15. Fisher, A. and Hanin, I. Minireview: Choline analogs as potential tools in developing selective animal models of central cholinergic hypofunction. Life Sci. 27:1615-34 (1980).
16. Mantione, C.R., Fisher, A., Hanin, I. The AF64A-treated mouse: possible model for central cholinergic hypofunction, Science, 213:579-80 (1981).
17. Hanin, I., Mantione, C.R. and Fisher, A. AF64A-induced neurotoxicity: A potential animal model in Alzheimer's disease, in: "Alzheimer's Disease: A Report of Progress in Research, (Aging, Volume 19)", eds. S. Corkin, K.L. Davis, J.H. Growdon, E. Usdin and R.J. Wurtman, New York, Raven Press, pp. 267-70 (1982).
18. Fisher, A., Mantione, C.R., Grauer, E., Levy, A. and Hanin, I. Manipulation of brain cholinergic mechanisms by ethylcholine aziridinium (AF64A), a promising animal model for Alzheimer's Disease. In: "Behavioral Models and The Analysis of Drug Action", eds. A. Levy and M.Y. Speigelstein pp. 333-42 (1983).
19. Hanin, I., Coyle, J.T., DeGroat, W.C., Fisher, A. and Mantione, C.R. 1983. Chemically induced cholinotoxicity in vivo: Studies utilizing ethylcholine aziridinium ion (AF64A), in: "Banbury Report: Biological Aspects of Alzheimer's Disease", ed. R. Katzman, Cold Spring Harbor Laboratory, pp.243-53 (1983).
20. Kozlowski, M.R. and Arbogast, R.E. Histochemical and biochemical effects of the injection of AF64A into the nucleus basalis of Meynert: relevance to animal models of senile dementia of Alzheimer's type. In: Dynamics of Cholinergic Function. Ed. I. Hanin, Plenum Press, New York. In press.
21. Arbogast, R.E. and Kozlowski, M.R. Reduction of cortical choline acetyltransferase activity following injections of ethylcholine mustard aziridinium ion (AF64A) into the nucleus basalis of Meynert. Soc. Neurosci. Abstr. 341.15 (1984).
22. Walsh, T.J., Tilson, H.A., DeHaven, D.L., Mailman, R.G., Fisher, A. and Hanin, I. AF64A, a cholinergic neurotoxin, selectively depletes acetylcholine in hippocampus and cortex, and produces long-term passive avoidance and radial-arm maze deficits in the rat. Brain Res. 321:91-102 (1984).
23. Brandeis, R., Fisher, A., Pittel, Z., Lachman, C., Heldman, E., Luz, S., Dahir, S., Levy, A. and Hanin, I. AF64A-induced cholinotoxicity: behavioral and biochemical correlates. This volume.
24. Leventer, S., McKeag, D., Clancy, M., Wulfert, E. and Hanin, I. Intracerebroventricular AF64A reduces ACh release from rat hippocampal slices. Neuropharmacol. 24: 453-459 (1985).
25. Kuhn, F.J., Lher, E. and Hinzen, D.H. AF64A neurotoxicity: behavioral and electrophysiological alterations in rats. Soc. Neurosci. Abst. 10: 224.11 (1984).

26. Kasa, P., Szerdahelyi, P., Fisher, A. and Hanin, I. Histochemical and electronmicroscopic study of the brain of the AF64A-treated rat. This volume.
27. Bailey, E. Overstreet, D.H. and Crocker, A.D. Effects of intra-hippocampal injections of the cholinergic neurotoxin AF64A on open field activity and avoidance learning in the rat. Personal cummunication; paper submitted to Behav. Neurobiol.
28. Potter, P.E., Harsing, L.G., Jr., Kakucska, I., Gaal, Gy., Vizi, E.S., Fisher, A. and Hanin, I. Effects of AF64A on hippocampal cholinergic and monoaminergic systems *in vivo*, *FASEB* April (1985).
29. Hanin, I. AF64A: a useful tool in cholinergic research. *In*: Neurobiology of Acetylcholine, ed. N. Dun, Plenum Press. In press.
30. Sandberg, K., Sanberg, P.R., Coyle, J.T. Effects of intrastriatal injections of the cholinergic neurotoxin AF64A on spontaneous nocturnal locomotor behavior in the rat. *Brain Res.* 299:339-43 (1984).
31. Sanberg, P.R. Neurobehavioral changes in some animal models of age-related neuropsychiatric disorders. This volume.
32. Mantione, C.R. Ethylcholine aziridinium a new cholinergic specific presynaptic toxin. Ph.D. Thesis. University of Pittsburgh, Pittsburgh, PA, U.S.A. (1983).
33. Sandberg, K., Hanin, I., Fisher, I. and Coyle, J.T. Selective cholinergic neurotoxin: AF64A's effects in rat striatum. *Brain Res.* 293:49-55 (1984).
34. Sandberg, K., Sanberg, P.R., Hanin, I., Fisher, A. and Coyle, J.T. Cholinergic lesion of the striatum impairs acquisition and retention of a passive avoidance response. *Behav. Neurosci.* 98:162-65 (1984).
35. Walsh, T.J., DeHaven, D.L., Tilson, H.A., Mailman, R.B., Fisher, A. and Hanin, I. Cholinergic lesions of the hippocampus produce long-term alterations of reactivity and cognitive function. *Soc. Neurosci. Abstr.* 10:75.4 (1984).
36. Fisher, A., Hanin, I. and Abraham, D.J. Novel tritium labelled N-mustard type compounds and a process for their production. *U.S. Patent Application*, filed on October 18. (1984).
37. Fisher, A. and Hanin, I. Animal models for senile dementia of Alzheimer's type, with particular emphasis on AF64A-induced cholinotoxicity. *Ann. Rev. Pharmacol. Toxicol.* In press.
38. Walsh, T.J. and Hanin, I. A review of the behavioral effects of AF64A, a cholinergic neurotoxin. This volume.
39. Levy, A., Brandeis, R., Dachir, S., Luz, S., Karton, Y., Heldman, E., Pittel, Z., Fisher, A. and Hanin, I. Reversal of AF64A-induced memory impairment by cholinergic compounds. *Soc. Neurosci.* Dallas, Texas (1985)
40. Murray, C.L. and Fibiger, H.C. Learning and memory deficits after lesions of the nucleus basalis magnocellularis: reversal by physostigmine. *Neurosci.* 14:1025-32 (1985).
41. Davidson, V., Haroutuninan, R.C., Mohs, B.M., Davies, T.B., Horvath and K.L. Davies. Human and animal studies with cholinergic agents: how clinically exploitable in the cholinergic deficiency in Alzheimer's Disease. This volume.
42. Jonsson, G. Chemical neurotoxins as denervation tools in neurobiology. *Ann. Rev. Neurosci.* 3:169-87 (1980).
43. Poirier, L.J., Langelier, P., Roberge, A., Boucher, R., Kitsikis, A. Non-specific histopathological changes induced by the intracerebral injection of 6-hydroxydopamine (6OHDA). *J. Neurol. Sci.* 16:401-16 (1972).
44. Butcher, L.L., Eastgate, S.M. and Hodge, G.K. Evidence that punctate intracerebral administration of 6-hydroxydopamine fails to produce

selective neuronal degeneration. N.S. Arch. Pharmacol. 285:31-70 (1974).
45. Butcher, L.L. Degenerative processes after punctate intracerebral administration of 6-hydroxydopamine. J. Neurol. Transmi. 37:189-208 (1975).
46. Butcher, L.L., Hodge, G.K. and Schaeffer, J.C. Degenerative processes after intraventricular infusion of 6-hydroxydopamine, in: "Chemical Tools in Catecholamine Research". Vol. 1, eds. Jonsson, G., Malmfors, T. and Sachs, CH. pp. 83-90 (1975).
47. Marshall, J.F. and Gotthelf, T. Sensory inattention in rats with 6-hydroxydopamine-induced degeneration of ascending dopaminergic neurons: apomorphine-induced reversal of deficits. Exptl. Neurol. 65:398-411 (1979).
48. Hokfelt, T. and Ungerstedt, U. Specificity of 6-hydroxydopamine-induced degeneration of central monoamine neuron. An electron and fluorescence microscopy study with special reference to intracerebral injection of the nigro-striatal dopamine system. Brain Res. 60:269-97 (1973).
49. Ungerstedt, U. Histochemical studies on the effect of intracerebral injections of 6-hydroxydopamine on monoamine neurons in the rat brain, in: "6-Hydroxydopamine and Catecholamine Neurons", eds. T. Malmfors and H. Thoenen, North-Holland, Amsterdam, pp. 101-128 (1971).
50. Sachs, C. and Jonsson, G. Mechanisms of action of 6-hydroxydopamine. Biochem. Pharmacol. 24:1-8 (1975).
51. Kelly, P.H., Joyce, E.M., Minneman, K.P. and Phillipson, O.T. 1977. Specificity of 6-hydroxydopamine-induced destruction of mesolimbic or nigrostriatal dopamine-containing terminal. Brain Res. 122:382-87 (1977).
52. Lorens, S.A., Guldberg, H.C., Hole, K., Kohler, C., Srebro, B. Activity avoidance learning and regional 5-hydroxytryptamine following intrabrainstem 5,7 dihydroxytryptamine and electrolytic midbrain raphe lesions in the rat. Brain Res. 108:97-113 (1976).
53. Meibach, R.C., Brown, L. and Brooks, F.H. Histofluorescence of kainic acidinduced striatal lesions. Brain Res. 148:219-23 (1978).
54. Herndon, R.M., Coyle, J.T. and Addics, E. Ultrastructural analysis of kainic acid lesion of cerebellar cortex. Neurosci. 5:1015-26 (1980).
55. Pisa, M. Kainic acid injections into the rat neostriatum: effects of learning and exploration, in: "Excitotoxins", eds. Fuxe, K., Roberts, P. and Schwarcz, R. McMillan Press, London, pp. 280-94 (1983).
56. Yamamura, H.I., Hruska, R.E., Schwarcz, R. and Coyle, J.T. Effect of striatal kainic acid lesions on muscarinic cholinergic receptor binding: Correlation with Huntington's Disease. In: Animal Models in Psychiatry and Neurology, Eds. Hanin, I. and Usdin, E. Pergamon Press, pp. 415-419 (1977).
57. Sanberg, P.R. and Fibiger, H.C. Body weight, feeding and drinking behaviors in rats with kainic acid-induced lesions of striatal neurons - with a note on body weight symptomatology in Huntington's Disease. Exptl. Neurol. 66:444-66 (1979).
58. Krammer, E.B., Lischka, M.F., Karobath, M. and Schonbeck. Is there a selectivity of neuronal degeneration induced by intrastriatal injection of kainic acid. Brain Res. 177:577-82 (1979).
59. Nagy, J.I., Vincent, S.R., Lehmann, J., Fibiger, H.C. and McGeer, E.G. The use of kainic acid in the localization of enzymes in the substantia nigra. Brain Res. 149:431-41 (1978).
60. Caulfield, M.P., May, P.J., Pedder, E.K. and Prince, A.K. Behavioral studies with ethylcholine mustard aziridinium (ECMA). Proceedings Brit. Pharmac. Soc. April 1983. 79:287p. (1983).

61. Casamenti, F., Bracco, L., Pedata, F. and Pepeu, G. Biochemical and behavioral effects of AF64A in the rat, in: "Dynamics of Cholinergic Function", ed. I. Hanin, Plenum Press, New York. In press.
62. Colhoun, E.H., Brajac, D.J. and Rylett, R.J. Observations on the toxicity and cholinergic dysfunction resulting from intracerebroventricular injections of choline mustard aziridinium ion. Soc. Neurosci. Abstr. 78.8 (1983).
63. Pope, C.N., Englert, L.F. and Ho, T.B. Passive avoidance deficits in mice following ethylcholine aziridinium chloride treatment. Pharmacol. Biochem. Behav. 22:297-299 (1985).
64. McGeer, P.L. and McGeer, E.G. Kainic acid: the neurotoxic breakthrough. CRC Critical Rev. Toxicol. March 1-26 (1982).
65. Kostrzewa, R.M. and Jacobowitz, D.M. Pharmacological actions of 6-hydroxydopamine. Pharmacol. Rev. 26:199-288 (1974).
66. Wolf, G., Stricker, E.M. and Zigmond, M.J. Brain lesions: induction, analysis and the problem of recovery of function, in: "Recovery of Function from Brain Damage", ed. S. Fingler, Plenum Press, New York, pp. 91-112 (1978).
67. McGurk, S.R. and Butcher, L.L. Neuropathology following intracerebral infusion of ethylcholine mustard aziridinium (AF64A). Fed. Proceed 44(4). Abst #2840 (1985).
68. Jope, R. High affinity choline transport and acetyl CoA production in brain and their roles in the regulation of acetylcholine synthesis. Brain Res. Rev. 1:313-44 (1979).
69. Fisher, A., Mantione, C.R. and Hanin, I. Atropine potentiates AF64A-induced pharmacological effects in mice in vivo, Fed. Proc. 40:269 (1981).
70. Richter, J.A., Perry, E.K. and Tomlinson, B.E. Acetylcholine and choline levels in post-mortem human brain tissue: Preliminary observations in Alzheimer's disease. Life Sci. 26:1683-89 (1980).
71. Coyle, J., McKinney, M., Johnston, M.V. and Hedreen, J.C. Synaptic neurochemistry of the basal forebrain cholinergic projection. Psychopharmacol. Bull. 19:441-47 (1983).
72. Salamone, J.D., Beart, P.M., Alpert, J.E. and Iversen, S.D. Impairment in T-maze reinforced alteration performance following nucleus basalis magnocellularis lesions in rats. Behav. Brain Res. B:63-70 (1984).
73. Flicker, C., Dean, R.L., Watkins, D.L., Fisher, S.K. and Bartus, R.T. Behavioral and neurochemical effects following neurotoxic lesions of a major cholinergic input to the cerebral cortex in the rat. Pharmacol. Biochem. Behav. 18:973-81 (1983).
74. Haubrich, D.R., Gerber, N.H. and Pflueger, A.B. Choline availability and the synthesis of acetylcholine, in: "Nutrition and the Brain. Vol 5", eds. A. Barbeau, J.H. Growdon and R.J. Wurtman. Raven Press, New York. pp. 57-71 (1979).
75. Cotton, F.A. and Wilkinson, G., in: "Advanced Inorganic Chemistry". Interscience Publishers, New York, London, Sydney. pp. 434-55 (1967).
76. Wurtman, R.J., Blausztajn, J.K. and Maire, J.-C. The "autocannibalism" of choline-containing membrane phospholipids in the pathogenesis of Alzheimer's Disease. This volume.
77. Mantione, C.R., Fisher, A. and Hanin, I. Biochemical heterogeneity of high affinity choline transport (HAChT) systems demonstrated in mouse brain using ethylcholine mustard aziridinium (AF64A), Trans. Am. Soc. Neurochem. 12:219 (1981).

HISTOCHEMICAL AND ELECTRONMICROSCOPIC STUDY OF THE BRAIN OF THE AF64A-TREATED RAT

Peter Kása, Peter Szerdahelyi, Abraham Fisher[x] and Israel Hanin[xx]

Central Research Laboratory, Medical University, Szeged Hungary, [x]Israel Institute for Biological Research, Ness-Ziona, Israel, [xx]Dept. of Pharmacology and Experimental Therapeutics Loyola University Stritch School of Medicine Chicago, Illinois

INTRODUCTION

It has recently been demonstrated by biochemical means (12,14,17) that ethylcholine aziridinium ion, AF64A (1,12,17), injected intracerebroventricularly (i.c.v.), (12), intrastriatally (i.s.) (18,19,20) or intrahippocampally (i.h.), (14) reduces high affinity choline transport (HAChT), choline acetyltransferase (ChAT) activity, and acetylcholine (ACh) levels in the hippocampus, and to a lesser extent in the striatum, but it does not affect the number of muscarinic acetylcholine-receptors (mAChR-s) (1,2). It has been suggested that AF64A is a neurotoxin which destroys the cholinergic axon terminals and can therefore be considered a "cholinotoxin". However, Levy et al. (11) and Jarrard et al. (6) injected AF64A into the substantia nigra or i.c.v., and concluded that AF64A affects other axons besides the cholinergic ones: They thus have cast doubt on the usefulness of AF64A for the specific destruction of cholinergic axon terminals. Since neither Fisher et al. (2) nor Levy et al. (11) presented detailed morphological evidence to support their views, we have decided to conduct our own histochemical and histological studies, including detailed electronmicroscopic investigations. In this paper evidence is given that AF64A is a neurotoxin, and that it can be used as a cholinotoxin if it is administered in the appropriate dose and concentration, at a suitable site of application. Some of these findings have been presented earlier (8,22).

MATERIALS AND METHODS

Animals

CFY rats weighing 200-300 g were used in the experiments. The amount of AF64A injected i.c.v. or i.s., and the length of the survival period are indicated in TABLE 1.

Surgical Manipulations

Three different kinds of operations were performed:

TABLE 1

Survival in days	Dose of AF64A (nmol)											
	intrastriatal					intracerebroventricular						
	0.25	0.5	1	2	8	2.5	5	8	10	20	40	65
1	b,d	b,d			b,d		b,d	b,d		e	a,b d	e
3	a,b c,d	b,d	b,d		b,c d		b,c d	b,d				e
4							a,c					
5		b,d					a					
6	c			a,c			c	a,e	c	e		
7	c	a,b d		a,c			b,d e	b,d				
8								a	e	e		
9							c	b,d				
10						a	a,b f		a,f			
12	a	a	a							a		
15		b,d				a	a,b d,e	b,d	a			
17									a			
21							b,d e	b,d	e		a	
28							e				b,d e	
33							b,d					

The methods used were: (a) AChE histochemistry; (b) Toluidine blue staining; (c) Silver impregnation; (d) Electron microscopy; (e) Timm's staining; (f) CAT immunocytochemistry.

One set of experiments was carried out to gain information on the effects of AF64A injected i.c.v. The animals were anesthetized with ether, and different amounts of AF64A (see TABLE 1) were administered (coordinates: A: 4.0, L: 1.5, V: 3.5 mm) (16). The AF64A was freshly prepared as described by Fisher et al. (2), but all dilutions were made in Krebs-Ringer solution, and the osmolality of the injected solution was 347.2 mOsmol. All injected solutions were sterilized via a membrane filter (Sartorius) with a pore size of 0.2 µm. The solution (1.0 nmol/µl) was injected at a rate of approximately 1.0 µl/min. The needle of the Hamilton syringe was left *in situ* for at least 1.0 min after the completion of each injection. The same procedure was used for injection of the vehicle, Krebs-Ringer solution. At the end of the experiments, some of the brains were fixed in formalin solution, then embedded in Histoplast and sectioned, and the samples were subjected to hematoxylin eosin or toluidine blue staining. In other brain samples, the neurotoxic effect of AF64A was studied with a silver impregnation technique (5). Changes in trace metal distribution in different cells or axon terminals were demonstrated with the Timm sulfide-silver technique, as described earlier (21).

In the second set of experiments, AF64A was injected (see TABLE 1) into the striatum. The coordinates for i.s. injections of AF64A were: anterior to bregma, 1.0 mm; L: 2.8 mm and V: 5.0 mm (16). After different survival periods, the animals were sacrificed. Brain samples were subjected to AChE histochemical (7) and ChAT immunocytochemical (25) staining. In some samples the degenerated nerve fibers were demonstrated with the Hjorth-Simonsen silver-impregnation technique (5). To discover finer structural changes caused by AF64A, samples were processed for ultrastructural studies using a routine procedure for embedding striatal samples.

The third set of experiments was designed to prove or disprove the specificity of the cholinotoxin AF64A on cholinergic axons and axon terminals. Rats were anesthetized and the fimbria-fornix complex was transected s surgically to destroy the septo-hippocampal cholinergic input to the dorsal hippocampus. After a 3-month survival period, 5 nmol AF64A was injected i.c.v., and 3 days later coronal sections of the brain from the region of the dorsal hippocampus were processed for fiber degeneration (5). Some animals were perfused with 4% formaldehyde and 2.5% glutaraldehyde solution (pH 7.4), and different parts of the dorsal hippocampus (CA3, CA4 and CA1) were processed for ultrastructural studies. Our working hypothesis in this experiment was that, if the cholinotoxin is specific for cholinergic fibers, then after fimbria-fornix transection the i.c.v. injected AF64A should not cause axon and axon terminals degeneration in those layers of the hippocampus where the cholinergic septo-hippocampal fibers terminate.

RESULTS

Only the most prominent effects and most characteristic changes will be described here; a detailed description of the changes in well-defined regions will appear in a series of papers elsewhere (9,10).

Histological investigations of AF64A-treated brain samples

It was shown in Nissl-stained samples that 2.5 and 5 nmol AF64A injected i.c.v. did not cause neuronal degeneration in the most sensitive part (CA3) of the dorsal hippocampus (Fig. 1a). However, 8 nmol AF64A did cause pyramidal cell degeneration in the CA3 region (Fig. 1b). If the dose was further increased (10, 20, 40 and 65 nmol), an even larger area was damaged, and in the center of the injected area the neurons were degenerated and glial cells accumulated instead. Intrastriatal injection of 0.25 nmol AF64A had a very damaging effect at the center of the injected area. The number of cells reduced (Fig. 1c). Here again, as the amount of the neurotoxin was raised, the normal cell bodies were affected and degenerated in an increasingly large area.

Histochemical investigation of AF64A-treated brain samples

(a) AChE histochemistry: The normal distribution of AChE activity in the hippocampus is depicted in Fig. 2a. Enzyme activity appears mainly in the infra- and suprapyramidal, and in the infra- and supragranular layers, as well as in the area dentata. 5 nmol AF64A (i.c.v.) reduced the staining intensity, to only a minor extent 4 days after injection. However, a dramatic reduction of AChE activity was revealed in all parts of the hippocampus after 10 nmol AF64A (i.c.v.), with a survival period of 17 days (Fig. 2b). Similarly, the AChE activity was reduced on the injected side, in the cortex (Fig. 2c), while no changes were observed on the contralateral side. A very characteristic staining pattern appeared in the septum and the fimbria hippocampi . As demonstrated in Fig. 2d,

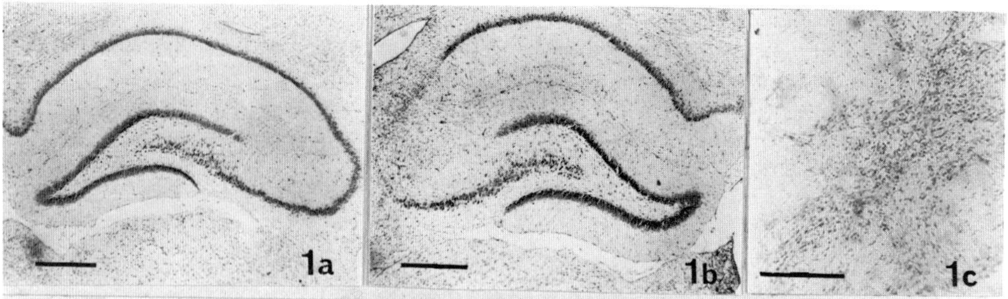
1a
1b
1c

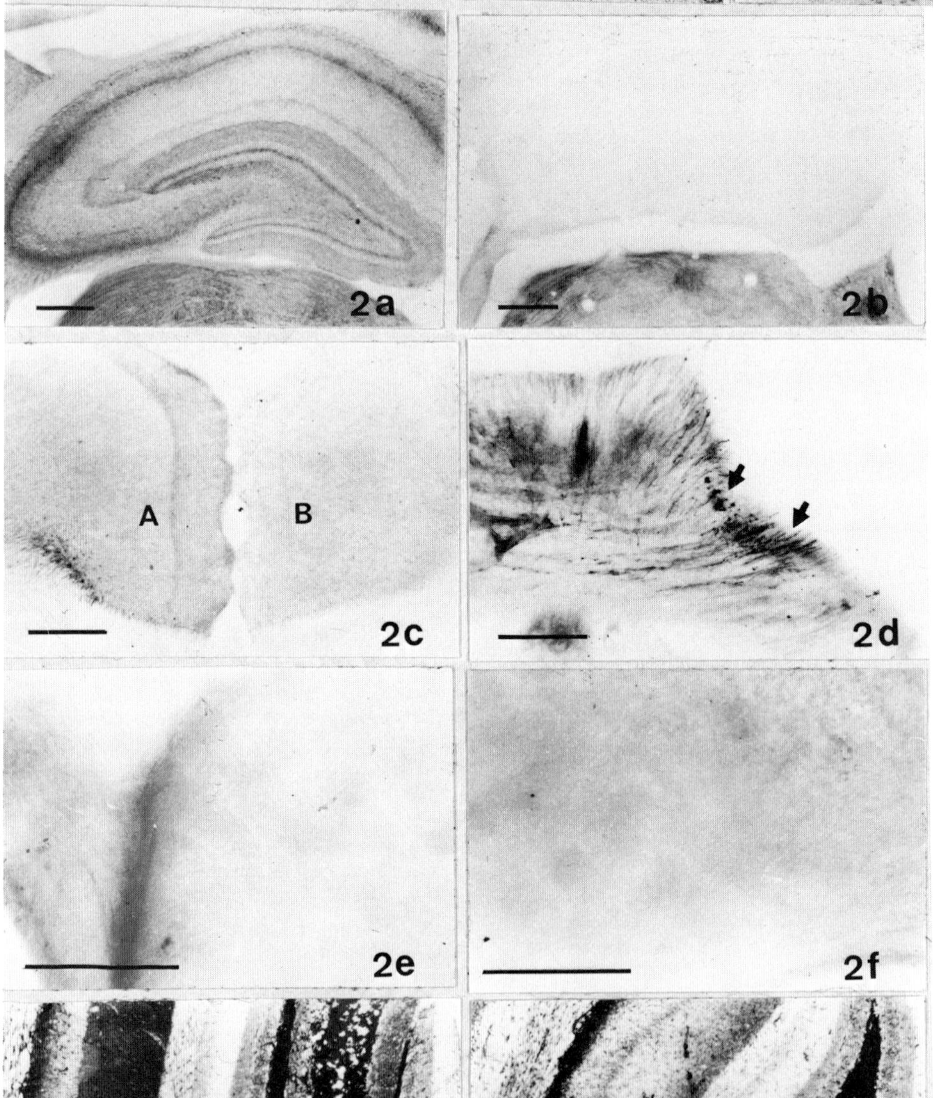
2a
2b
A
B
2c
2d
2e
2f
2h

Fig. 1. Nissl-stained samples. (a) Hippocampus from rat injected i.c.v. with 5 nmol AF64A; survival time 10 days. Note the well-preserved layers and pyramidal cells in all areas of the hippocampus. (b) Hippocampus; 8 nmol AF64A i.c.v.; survival time 3 days. The pyramidal cells have disappeared from areas CA3, CA2 and (partly) CA1 (arrows). (c) Striatum; injected i.s. with 0.25 nmol AF64A; survival time 3 days. Note the reduced number of neuronal cell bodies at the center of the injected area . Bar: 0.5 mm

Fig. 2. Histochemically stained brain samples after AF64A treatment. (a) AChE activity in the control hippocampus. Heavy end-product is present in the str. oriens, str. radiatum and str. infra- and supragranulare. (b) Hippocampus; 10 nmol AF64A i.c.v.; survival time 17 days. Note the disappearance of AChE staining from the different layers of the hppocampus. Some reaction end-product can be revealed at higher magnification in the area dentata, where AChE-positive neurons are present. (c) Cingulate cortex; 10 nmol AF64A i.c.v.; survival time 17 days. AChE activity is present on the non-treated side (A) while the reaction end-product is missing on the treated side (B). (d) Septum; 8 nmol AF64 i.c.v.; survival time 8 days. Heavy AChE staining can be revealed in fibers (arrows) originating from the medial part of the septum. (e) Hippocampus from control sample stained for ChAT (immunocytochemistry). Note the ChAT positivity in the str. oriens where AChE activity was found (compare with Fig. 2a). (f) Hippocampus; 5 nmol AF64A i.c.v.; survival time 10 days. ChAT immunohistochemistry. The ChAT staining disappeared and demonstrates the effectiveness of the cholinotoxin on cholinergic fibers. (g) Hippocampus stained for trace metals. Heavy reaction end-product appears in area CA3 (where the mossy fibers terminate), in the alveus and str. radiatum of area CA1 and in the area dentata. (h) Hippocampus stained for trace metals after i.c.v. injection of 20 nmol AF64A survival time 6 days. Note the disappearance of the stained material from the stratum radiatum of area CA1. Bar: 0.5 mm

the staining intensity in some fibers increased in the septum, probably as an indication of AChE accumulation in the septo-hippocampal cholinergic fibers due to the blockade of axonal transport by AF64A.

(b) ChAT immunocytochemistry: ChAT was demonstrated in the hippocampus using a monoclonal antibody (23). The reaction end-product appeared mainly in the str. oriens of the hippocampus where AChE activity can also be demonstrated (Fig. 2e).

After treatment with 5 or 10 nmol AF64A (i.c.v.), enzyme activity was not demonstrable in the hippocampus (Fig. 2f).

(c) Trace metal staining: with a technique (20) to demonstrate different trace metals in brain tissues, it was shown that Zn^{2+} and Cu^{2+} are present in different cells (pyramidal, Purkinje and Golgi cells) and axon terminals (mossy fibers in the hippocampus and cerebellum and some other axon terminals, as yet unidentified). Animals treated with 5, 8, 10, 20, 40 and 65 nmol AF64A (i.c.v.) showed a different staining pattern in the hippocampus on the treated side as compared to the contralateral one (Fig. 2g). This technique demonstrated that, above 8 nmol, AF64A caused a depletion of the trace metals from the CA3 region and from the strata radiatum and moleculare in the CA1 part of the hippocampus (Fig. 2h).

Degenerated fibers due to AF64A treatment, revealed by the silver-impregnation technique

No detectable changes in AChE activity were observed 4 or 6 days after AF64A treatment, either in the hippocampus or in the striatum. In the silver-impregnated samples, however, the pattern of degeneration was clearly evident in both structures. The degenerating toxic effect of AF64A was verified in both coronal (Fig. 3a) and horizontal (Fig. 3b) sections of the brain. In the Hjorth-Simonsen preparations, the i.c.v. injection of AF64A caused a diffuse pattern of degenerations in the ipsilateral cingulate cortex (Fig. 3c), hippocampus (Fig. 3d), habenula (Fig. 3e), striatum (Fig. 3f) and colliculus superior (Fig. 3h). Massive degeneration was found in the fimbria hippocampi and fibers originating from the nucleus basalis magnocellularis (Fig. 3g). A few degenerated axons were observed in the substantia nigra, the interpeduncular nuclei, the thalamus and the tegmental part of the mesencephalon. The only part of the ipsilateral brain region where no degenerated fibers were detected was the amygdala. If degeneration occurred on the contralateral side, it was revealed mainly in structures around the third ventricle and cerebral aqueduct.

Fimbria transection followed by AF64A treatment

To study the specificity of action of AF64A on cholinergic axons and axon terminals, the fimbria-fornix was surgically transected unilaterally. After a 3-month survival period, 5 nmol AF64A were injected i.c.v. ipsilaterally. Three days after cholinotoxin treatment, some of the brains were processed for silver impregnation to study the degeneration pattern (if any). From other similarly treated brains (fimbria transection + 5 nmol AF64A), different areas of the hippocampus (CA1, CA3 and CA4) were embedded for electronmicroscopic investigations.

The light microscopic results show that fimbria transection caused massive degeneration in different regions of the hippocampus (Fig. 4). Most of the silver grains indicative of degenerated fibers disappeared within 14 days, and no axon remnants were detected after one month. When the fimbria-transected and AF64A-treated brains were stained for degenerated fibers 3 days after i.c.v. AF64A injection, no silver particles were found in the ipsilateral hippocampus (Fig. 5). Similar results were obtained when the samples were analyzed under the electron microscope. The only exception was the area dentata (Fig. 6), where some electron-dense (dark degenerated) axon terminals could be revealed.

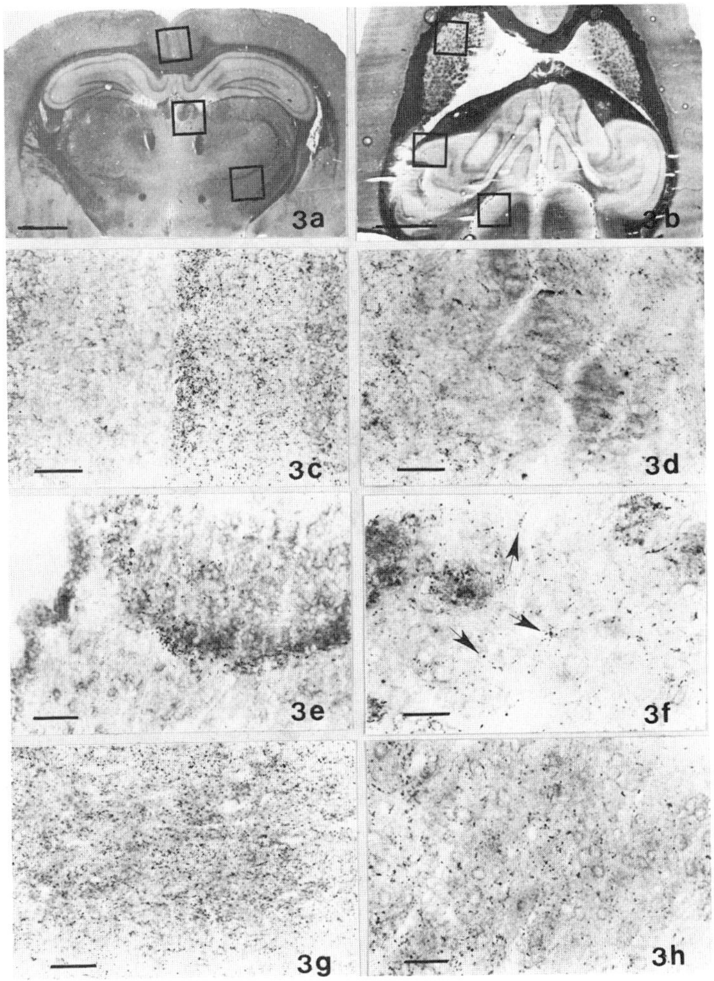

Fig. 3. Silver-impregnated samples revealing degenerated nerve fibers after AF64A treatment. (a) Coronal section of a brain at the level of the dorsal hippocampus. The animal was treated with 5 nmol AF64A; survival period 4 days. (b) Horizontal section of a brain, where the animal was treated with 5 nmol AF64A; survival period 6 days. Bar: 1.0 mm
The rectangles in Fig. 3a and Fig. 3b show the positions of the high-power magnification pictures. (c) Cingulate cortex; same section as in Fig. 3a. Silver particles indicate the fiber degeneration. No reaction is seen on the contralateral side. (d) Hippocampus, area CA3; same section as Fig. 3b. Considerable degeneration is seen in all layers, but most in the alveus. (e) Part of the habenula; same section as Fig. 3a. Degenerating fibers are seen mostly in the medial part. (f) Striatum; same section as in Fig. 3b. Note the silver particles (arrows) at the farthest area from the injection site. No reaction was seen on the contralateral side. (g) Fibers arising from the nucleus basalis magnocellularis; same section as in Fig. 3a. Heavy degeneration is present near the internal capsule and the lateral part of the thalamus. (h) Part of the superior colliculus; same section as in Fig. 3b. Many silver particles are present in the granular layer. No reaction can be seen on the contralateral side. Bar: 0.1 mm

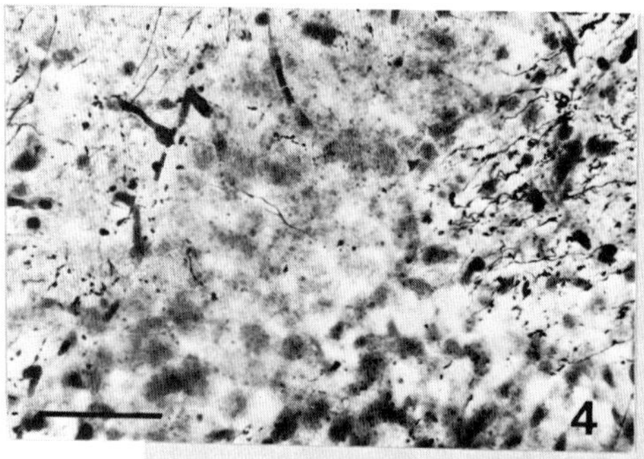

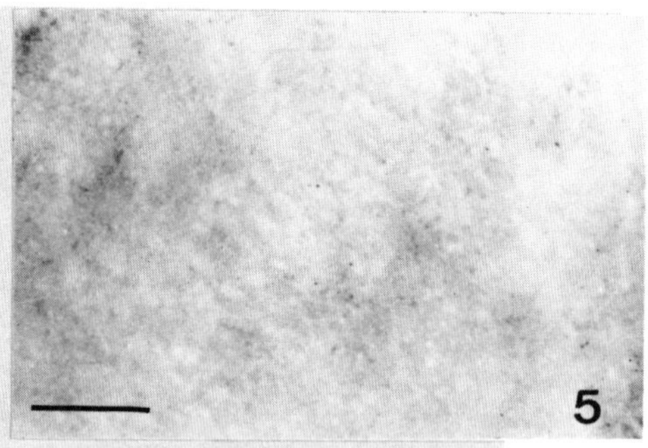

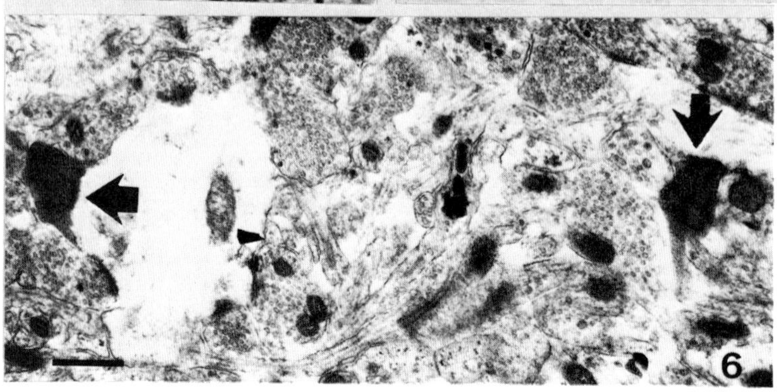

Fig. 4. Silver-impregnated sample revealing degenerated nerve fibers in the hippocampus 9 days after fimbria-fornix transection. Heavy reaction is present in the alveus and the str. radiatum of area CA3. No particles are seen on the contralateral side. Bar: 0.1 mm

Fig. 5. Silver- impregnated sample demonstrating degenerated nerve fibers in area CA3 of the hippocampus where the fimbria-fornix was surgically transected 3 months earlier, and 5 nmol AF64A was then given i.c.v. After survival period of 3 days, no degenerated fibers were revealed either on the transected + treated side or on the contralateral side. Bar: 0.1 mm

Fig. 6. Part of area dentata. Ultrastructurally, some axon terminals were affected (arrows) 3 months after fimbria-fornix transection and 3 days after 5 nmol AF64A treatment. Bar: 0.5 μm

Ultrastructural investigation of brain samples after AF64A treatment

Samples from the cingulate and the temporal cortex, the striatum, the hippocampus, the habenula and the septum were analyzed after different doses of AF64A and different time intervals (see TABLE 1). The ultrastructural studies led to the following generalizations:
(a) Above 5 nmol (i.c.v.) AF64A causes non-specific tissue damage in a dose-dependent manner. Not only the cholinergic axons and axon terminals are affected; the neuronal cell bodies are damaged as well. (b) As the dose of cholinotoxin is increased, the non-specific tissue damage increases accordingly. (c) The intrastriatal application of the drug causes non-specific tissue damage at a much lower dose (0.25 nmol) than does the i.c.v. injection. (d) The osmolality of the injection solution should always be controlled; otherwise the hypoosmotic solution itself will cause non-specific tissue damage. (e) When AF64A is injected either i.c.v. (5 nmol) or i.s. (0.25 nmol), various zones appear around the site of application: in the first zone (A), non-specific tissue damage occurs, not only to the cholinergic axon terminals, but also to the neuronal perikarya; in the second zone (B), the cholinergic axons and axon terminals are degenerated specifically, other axons remaining unaffected; in the third zone (C), no effect of AF64A can be revealed. (f) AF64A always affects those axon terminals that contain round synaptic vesicles, but not those where dense-core or flattened vesicles are present. However, not all the axon terminals with round vesicles are damaged.

Our ultrastructural studies have also demonstrated that, in zone B of the cingulate cortex (Fig. 7a), striatum (Fig. 7b), hippocampus (Fig. 7c) (in all layers in the CA3 region) and septum (Fig. 7d), dark degenerated axon terminals develop after AF64A treatment. As the time progresses, some of these terminals are encircled by glial processes (Fig. 7e), while others become atrophic. In the affected areas the glial cells proliferate; this is most prominent in zone A.

DISCUSSION

The most important finding emerging from these studies is that ethylcholine aziridinium ion can be used as a specific cholinotoxin, if it is applied in an appropriate manner (concentration, amount, osmolality, site and mode of application). We have found that the i.c.v. application of 5 nmol AF64A causes specific degeneration of cholinergic axons, without influencing the neuronal perikarya and non-cholinergic fibers. Similar results can be obtained with the i.s. application of AF64A, if the amount is reduced below 0.5 nmol and the concentration is 1 nmol/μl. Levy et al. (11) and Jarrard et al. (6) recently questioned the specificity of AF64A as a cholinotoxin. The difference in our results and theirs may be due to the fact that they used much higher concentrations of AF64A (3-12 nmol/μl) and diluted their samples in distilled water. We have found that a combination of both high concentration of AF64A and a low osmolality of the vehicle solution used in these experiments is most dangerous, and results in non-specific destruction of tissue.

Our histochemical results demonstrate that the i.c.v. injection of AF64A reduces not only the HAChT (2,11), ChAT activity (2,13,17,18) and ACh levels (2,13,17,25), but also AChE activity. The reduction in AChE activity may be due to the degeneration of presynaptic cholinergic axons, to the postsynaptic structures; or possibly to a combination of these. The ChAT disappearance revealed by neurochemical means or immunohistochemically (Vizi, personal communication) suggests a specific effect of AF64A on cholinergic fibers. The results of silver impregnation relating to degenerated axons show that AF64A injected i.c.v. has an effect not only locally, but at an appreciable distance, as well. Even the superior colliculus (8 mm from the injection site) can be affected. Our ultra-

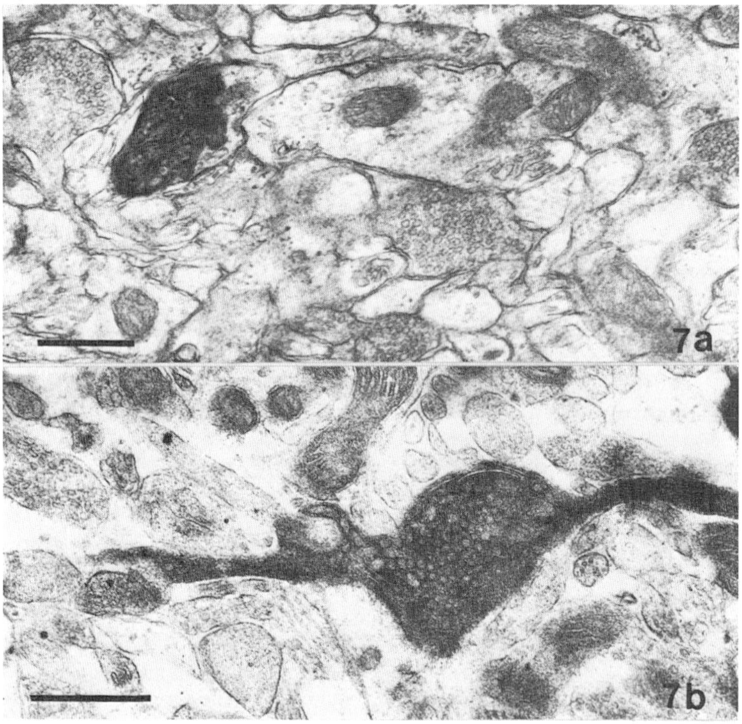

Fig. 7. Ultrastructural investigation of different areas of rat brain. Dark (degenerated) and normal axon terminals can be revealed in the same tissue section. (a) Cingulate cortex; 5 nmol AF64A i.c.v.; survival time 4 days. (b) Striatum;;8 nmol AF64A i.c.v. survival time 24 hours. (c) Hippocampus; area CA3; 5 nmol AF64A i.c.v.; survival time 7 days. (d) Septum; 8 nmol AF64A i.c.v.; survival time 2 days. (e) Hippocampus; area CA3; 5 nmol AF64A i.c.v.; survival time 9 days. The dark, atrophic axon terminals is encircled into a glial cell process. Bar: 0.5 μm

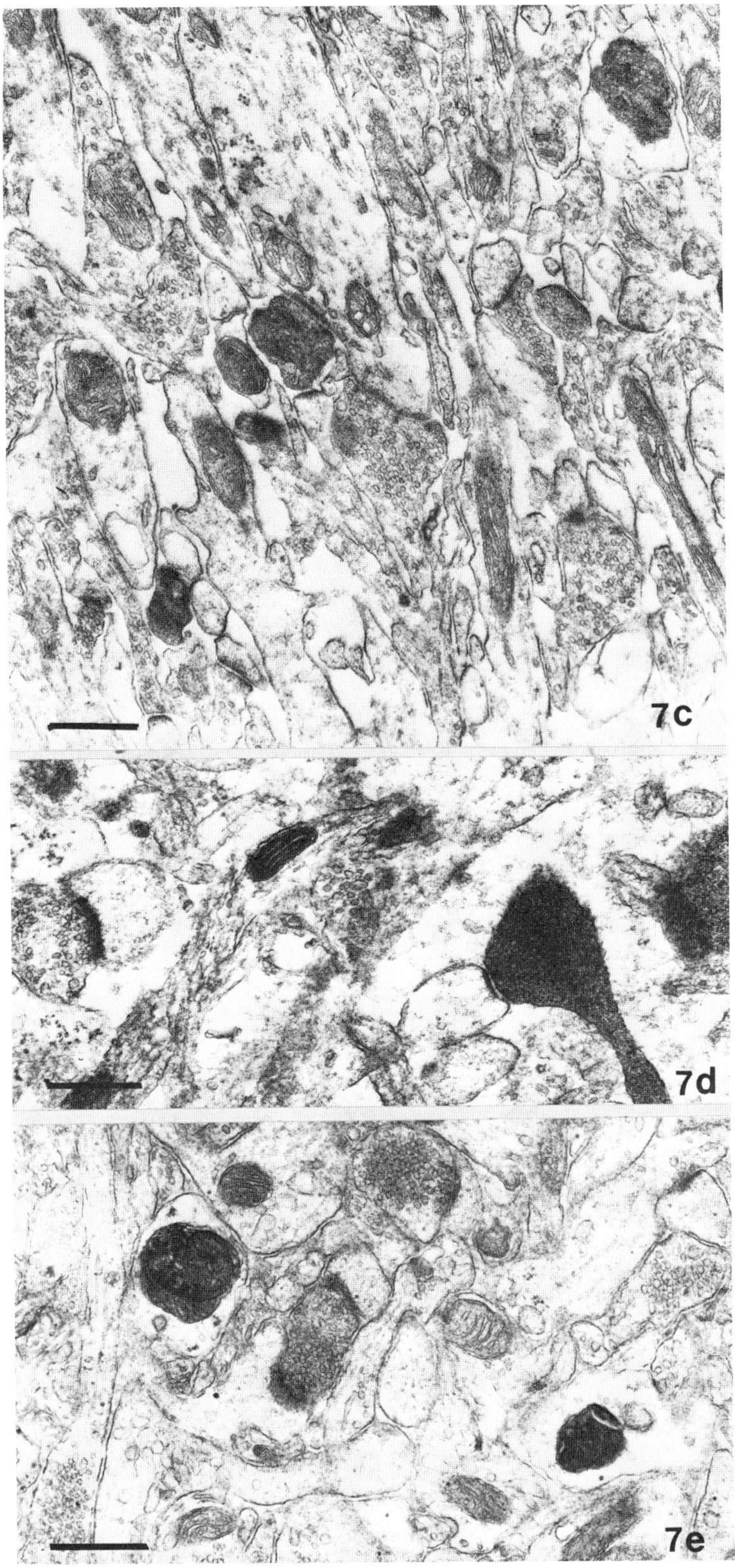
7c
7d
7e

structural studies demonstrate that the i.c.v. or i.s. injection of AF64A causes specific degeneration of one type of axon terminals in different parts of the rat brain (cingulate cortex, striatum, hippocampus, septum and habenula). The affected axonal boutons always contained spherical vesicles, but not all the nerve endings with round synaptic vesicles were affected. This type of degeneration matches that for ChAT activity (7). The electron immunohistochemical results on ChAT also revealed that the reaction end-product was present in terminals having spherical synaptic vesicles (10).

Our neurochemical, histological and ultrastructural (8) results support the view (4) that AF64A specifically affects the presynaptic cholinergic axon terminals. However we wish to underline the important suggestion made in 1981 by Mantione et al. (12): "The biological effect of AF64A is dependent on the degree of its exposure to the tissue, on the site of its administration, and on the dose/s used".
It is our experience that the proper dose should be less than 5 nmol in the case of i.c.v. injection, and less than 0.25 nmol on intracerebral injection; otherwise, a non-specific necrotic and perikaryon-damaging effect will occur. Also, one should be cautious not to dilute AF64A with distilled H_2O, since its osmolality is then reduced so much that one cannot differentiate between the effects of distilled H_2O and AF64A diluted with this soluent. We wish to emphasize, however, that more morphological and neurochemical work has to be done in different brain regions and the peripheral nervous system before the full specificity of the action of AF64A on the cholinergic neurons can be proved.

Acknowledgement: This work was supported by the Scientific Research Council, Ministry of Health, Hungary (06/4-20/457), and by NIMH grant no. MH 34893.

REFERENCES

1. Fisher A. and Hanin I. Choline analogs as potential tools in developing selective animal models of central cholinergic hypofunction. Life Sci. 27, 1615-1634 (1980).

2. Fisher A., Mantione C.R., Abraham D.J. and Hanin I. Long-term central cholinergic hypofunction induced in mice by ethylcholine aziridinium ion (AF64A) in vivo. J. Pharm. Exp. Ther. 22, 140-145 (1982).

3. Gaal Gy., Potter P.E., Harsing L.G.,Jr. Kakucska I., Fisher A., Hanin I. and Vizi E.S. Histological changes caused by AF64A in rat hippocampus. in: Regulation of Transmitter Function: Basic and Clinical Aspects. (eds.: Vizi E.S. and Magyar K.) pp. 295-300, Akademiai Kiado, Budapest (1984).

4. Hanin I., DeGroat W.C., Mantione C.R., Coyle J.T. and Fisher A. Chemically-induced cholintoxicity in vivo: Studies utilizing ethylcholine aziridinium ion (AF64A). in: Banbury Report 15: Biological aspects of Alzheimer's disease, 243-253 (1983).

5. Hjorth-Simonsen A. Fink-Heimer silver impregnation of degenerating axons and terminals in mounted cryostat sections of fresh and fixed brains. Stain Technol. 45, 199-204 (1970).

6. Jarrard L.E., Kant G.J., Meyerhoff J.L. and Levy A. Behavioral and neurochemical effects of intraventricular AF64A administration in rats. Pharm. Biochem. Behav. 21, 273-280 (1984).

7. Kasa P. Histochemistry of choline acetyltransferase. in: Cholinergic Mechanisms (eds.: P.G.Waser) pp. 271-281, Raven Press, New York, 1975.

8. Kasa P., Farkas Z., Szerdahelyi P., Rakonczay Z., Fisher A. and Hanin I. Effects of cholinotoxin (AF64A) in the central nervous system: Morphological and biochemical studies. in: Regulation of Transmitter Function: Basic and Clinical Aspects. (eds.: Vizi E.S. and Magyar K.) pp. 289-293, Akademiai Kiado, Budapest (1984).

9. Kasa P., Szerdahelyi P., Farkas Z., Fisher A. and Hanin I. Morphological analysis of the in vivo effects of cholinotoxin AF64A in the central nervous system of the rat: I. Light microscopic investigation. J. Neuropathol. Exp. Neurol. (submitted)

10. Kasa P., Farkas Z., Szerdahelyi P., Fisher A., Hanin I. Morphological analysis of the in vivo effects of cholinotoxin AF64A in the central nervous system of the rat: II. Electron microscopic investigation. J. Neuropathol. Exp. Neurol. (submitted)

11. Levy A., Kant G.J., Meyerhoff J.L. and Jarrard L.E. Non-cholinergic neurotoxic effects of AF64A in the substantia nigra. Brain Res. 305, 169-172 (1984)

12. Mantione C.R., Fisher A. and Hanin I. The AF64A-treated mouse: Possible model for central cholinergic hypofunction. Science 213, 579-580 (1981)

13. Mantione C.R., Fisher A. and Hanin I. Possible mechanisms involved in the presynaptic cholinotoxicity due to ethylcholine aziridinium (AF64A) in vivo. Life Sci. 35, 33-41 (1984)

14. Mantione C.R., Zigmond M.J., Fisher A. and Hanin I. Selective presynaptic cholinergic neurotoxicity following intrahippocampal AF64A injection in rats. J. Neurochem. 41, 251-255 (1983)

15. Mantione C.R., DeGroat W.C., Fisher A. and Hanin I. Selective inhibition of peripheral cholinergic transmission in the cat produced by AF64A. J. Pharm. Exp. Ther. 225,616-622 (1983)

16. Paxinos G. and Watson, Ch. The Rat Brain in Stereotaxic Coordinates. Academic Press, New York, 1982

17. Rylett R.J. and Colhoun E.H. An evaluation of irreversible inhibition of synaptosomal high-affinity choline transport by choline mustard aziridinium ion. J. Neurochem. 43, 787-794 (1984)

18. Sandberg K., Hanin I., Fisher A. and Coyle J.T. Selective cholinergic neurotoxin: AF64A's effects in rat striatum. Brain Res. 293, 49-55 (1984)

19. Sandberg K., Sandberg P.R. and Coyle J.T. Effects in intrastriatal injections of the cholinergic neurotoxin AF64A on spontaneous nocturnal locomotor behavior in the rat. Brain Res. 299, 339-343 (1984)

20. Sandberg K., Schnaar R.L., McKinney M., Hanin I., Fisher A. and Coyle J.T. AF64A: An active site directed irreversible inhibitor of choline acetyltransferase. J. Neurochem. 44, 439-445 (1985)

21. Szerdahelyi P., Kasa P., Fisher A. and Hanin I. Effects of the cholinotoxin, AF64A, on neuronal trace-metal distribution in the rat hippocampus and neocortex. Histochemistry 81, 497-500 (1984)

22. Szerdahelyi P. and Kasa P. Histochemistry of zinc and copper. Int. Rev. Cytol. 89, (eds.: Bourne G.H. and Danielli J.F.) Academic Press, New York, 1-33 (1984)

23. Vizi E.Sz. (personal communication)

24. Wainer B.H., Bolam J.P., Freund T.F., Henderson Z., Totterdell S. and Smith A.D. Cholinergic Synapses in the rat brain: a correlated light and electron microscopic immunohistochemical study employing a monoclonal antibody against choline acetyltransferase. Brain Res. 308, 69-76 (1984)

25. Wainer B.H., Levey A.I., Mufson E.J. and Mesulam M.-M. Cholinergic systems in mammalian brain identified with antibodies against choline acetyltransferase. Neurochem. Int. 6, 163-182 (1984)

26. Walsh T.J., Tilson H.A., DeHaven D.L., Mailman R.B., Fisher A. and Hanin I. AF64A, a cholinergic neurotoxin, selectively depletes acetylcholine in hippocampus and cortex, and produces long-term passive avoidance and radial-arm maze deficits in the rat. Brain Res. 321, 91-102 (1984)

A REVIEW OF THE BEHAVIORAL EFFECTS OF AF64A, A CHOLINERGIC NEUROTOXIN

Thomas J. Walsh and Israel Hanin

Laboratory of Behavioral and Neurological Toxicology
National Institute of Environmental Health Sciences
Research Triangle Park, NC 27709, and Loyola University
Stritch School of Medicine, Chicago, Illinois

INTRODUCTION

Acetylcholine (ACh) was the first substance shown to mediate synaptic transmission in the nervous system. Since those early studies the biochemical events involved in the metabolism of ACh and its' interaction with muscarinic and nicotinic receptors have been studied in great detail. Despite these efforts to unravel the molecular biology of ACh the functional properties of cholinergic systems and their involvement in neurological and psychiatric disorders remain undetermined. During the past five years however, there have been several important advances in our understanding of cholinergic biology. A general principle that has emerged from these efforts is the interdependent nature of discoveries in clinical and basic neuroscience. For example, delineating the structural, neurochemical and behavioral pathology of senile dementia of the Alzheimer's type (SDAT) contributed to a better understanding of cholinergic involvement in disease states and also provided fundamental information about the anatomical and functional organization of cholinergic neurons.

SDAT affects 4-6 % of the population over the age of 65 and is the most prevalent form of adult-onset dementia (27). This disorder is characterized by a progressive deterioration of cognitive and mnenomic ability. Morphological, neurochemical and behavioral studies suggest a primary involvment of the cholinergic system in SDAT (21). Histological analysis of clinical samples has revealed a select degeneration of cholinergic cell bodies in the basal forebrain which project to the cerebral cortex and hippocampus (HPC) (8,21). The neurochemical changes are consistent with the underlying cell loss and consist of decreases in all markers of presynaptic cholinergic function (11,19,22). Alterations of other transmitter systems might occur in subpopulations of SDAT patients or late in the course of the disease but they are not related to the prevailing cognitive impairment (13,14).

Several converging lines of evidence indicate that cholinergic dysfunction contributes to the clinical signs of SDAT. For example, a significant correlation between the cognitive loss observed in SDAT and decreases of (1) ChAT activity in cortex and HPC, (2) rate of ACh synthesis in the temporal lobe, and (3) ACh concentrations in the cerebrospinal fluid has been reported (4,13,19). In essence, the degree of dementia is proportional to the loss of cholinergic tone. The learning and memory deficits observed in SDAT can be reproduced in healthy young adults by the administration of scopolamine, a muscarinic antagonist (9). Furthermore, physostigmine, but not amphetamine, attenuates these drug-induced cognitive alterations. Considered together, these studies indicate that the memory impairments associated with SDAT are probably dependent upon the chronic disability of cholinergic processes subserving cognition. This hypothesis is consistent with the animal literature which also indicates the involvement of cholinergic mechanisms in neural and behavioral plasticity (3). In brief, the following observations support a role for ACh in learning and memory: (1) cholinergic activity is enhanced in the HPC subsequent to a learning experience, (2) inhibiting cholinergic tone with drugs or lesions of the cholinergic nuclei in the basal forebrain impair cognitive processes, and (3) cholinomimetics improve learning and retention (3,26,28,29,30,31).

The development of an animal model of SDAT has been hampered by the lack of long-acting cholinergic antagonists. Currently available drugs such as atropine and scopolamine exhibit a short duration of action, limited CNS specificity, and a high degree of toxicity. Biochemical studies however indicate that neurotoxic analogs of choline might be well suited for developing a model of chronic cholinergic hypofunction (10). Cytotoxic analogs of catecholamines and indoleamines have been valuable tools for exploring the physiology and plasticity of these systems. In a similar context, ethylcholine aziridinium ion (AF64A) is structurally similar to choline but it also contains a reactive aziridinium component. AF64A irreversibly inhibits high affinity choline uptake (HAChU) and produces a persistent reduction of presynaptic cholinergic markers including HAChU, choline acetyltransferase (ChAT) activity, and ACh concentrations in rodents (16,17). Thus, AF64A might be a useful tool for investigating the neurobiology of the cholinergic system and also for developing an animal model of SDAT (11). In the following sections we will review the behavioral effects of AF64A and discuss these findings in relation to the pathophysiology of SDAT and other age-related dementias.

INTRACEREBROVENTRICULAR INJECTION OF AF64A

A number of studies have shown that intracerebroventricular (icv) administration of AF64A produces a specific pattern of behavioral effects together with a long-term reduction of cholinergic markers in rats. Our experiments examined the dose- and time-dependent effects of AF64A according to the experimental protocol outlined in Table 1. Other relevant studies are discussed in the text.

Table 1
Experimental Design of AF64A Studies

1. Baseline Behavioral Measures: 7 Days Prior to Surgery
   (Locomotor Activity, Hot-Plate Latencies)

2. Surgery (Infusion of Artificial CSF or AF64A)

3. Behavioral Measures: 2, 7, 14, 21 and 28 Days After Surgery
   (Locomotor Activity, Hot-Plate Latencies)

4. Passive Avoidance: 35 Days After Surgery
   (24 Hour Retention Test)

5. Radial-Arm Maze Performance: 60-90 Days After Surgery

6. Regional Neurochemical Assessment: 120 Days After Surgery
   (ACh, Ch, ChAT, NE, DA, DOPAC, HVA, 5-HT, 5-HIAA)

In our first series of studies male Fischer rats were injected with 15 or 30 nmols of AF64A (7.5 or 15 nmol/side). Neurochemical assessment performed 120 days after dosing revealed that the concentration of ACh in the HPC was significantly reduced (44-62 %) in both AF64A groups, and the content of ACh in the frontal cortex was decreased (63 %) in the 30 nmol group. There was no effect of AF64A on levels of ACh in the striatum. Furthermore, the regional concentrations of catecholamines, indoleamines, their metabolites, or choline were not affected. Therefore, the behavioral effects discussed below are probably related to a selective loss of cholinergic function.

AF64A produced a delayed increase in both locomotor activity and reactivity on the hot-plate. The 15 nmol group was significantly more active than the control group 28 days after surgery. Both AF64A groups reacted faster than controls on the hot-plate 14 and 21 days following injection. Jarrard and colleagues (12) also reported a delayed increase in activity which became evident 6 days after icv injection of 6 nmols of AF64A and persisted through 21 days of testing.

Retention of a step-through passive avoidance response was impaired following administration of AF64A. During the training trial the step-through latencies of the three groups were similar and all rats reacted to footshock with a burst of motor activity and vocalization. The retention latencies of the 15 and 30 nmol groups were significantly shorter (27-42 %) during the 24 hour retention test. Therefore, AF64A impaired the acquisition or retention of an inhibitory avoidance task. Casamenti and coworkers (5) also reported impaired passive avoidance retention and decreased ChAT activity (41 %) in the HPC 20 days following injection of AF64A (32 nmol/icv).

Acquisition and performance of a radial-arm maze (RAM) task was also impaired by AF64A throughout the period of testing (60-90 days following treatment). The treated rats made fewer correct responses in the first eight choices and they required more choices to obtain all 8 pellets during a session. During the last block of three trails the control group made on the average 7.5 correct responses during their first eight choices while the AF64A groups made 5-6 correct responses. Since both doses of AF64A impaired RAM performance but only the higher dose (30 nmol) reduced the concentration of ACh in the cortex, it appears that the depletion of ACh in the HPC is sufficient to account for these behavioral deficits.

The AF64A-treated rats readily explored the maze and performed the motor responses to obtain and consume the food following a correct arm entry. Therefore, the deficits in performance were not secondary to changes in motivation or locomotor behavior. Rather, the data suggest that the AF64A groups were unable to inhibit responding to previously entered arms. One hypothesis which might account for their performance is that their "working memory" of which arms had or had not been chosen during a test session was impaired.

In a recent study (Walsh et al., in preparation) low doses of AF64A (3 nmol/side/icv) impaired performance in a delayed match-to non-sample task which required the explicit use of working memory. In this task 4 out of 8 arms of the RAM were baited with food while the other 4 arms were closed by guillotine doors. The rats retrieved food from the four baited arms and were returned to their home cages. Following a 2 hour delay they were returned to the maze in which all 8 arms were open and the previously closed arms were now baited. The rats had to "remember" where they obtained food from prior to the delay and avoid reentering those arms (win-shift). The spatial configuration of baited and non-baited arms varied randomly from day to day with the provision that not more than two adjacent arms were baited (96 possible combinations). The information acquired prior to the delay (i.e., which arms are baited) was useful only for that given day. This task prevents the use of response strategies and algorhythms and provides a cognitive task which corresponds to those used in studies of human learning and memory.

Rats were trained for 20 trials prior to surgery. Following training they were injected with AF64A (3 nmol/side/3 ul i.c.v.) or vehicle, allowed 21 days to recover, and then were reintroduced to the task. The performance of the controls recovered to pre-operative levels within 5 sessions. The performance of the AF64A group however remained at chance level (i.e., 2 correct in the first 4 post-delay choices) throughout the 20 post-operative trials (see Figure 1). Therefore, low doses of AF64A produce a persistent, and perhaps permanent, disruption of spatial working memory.

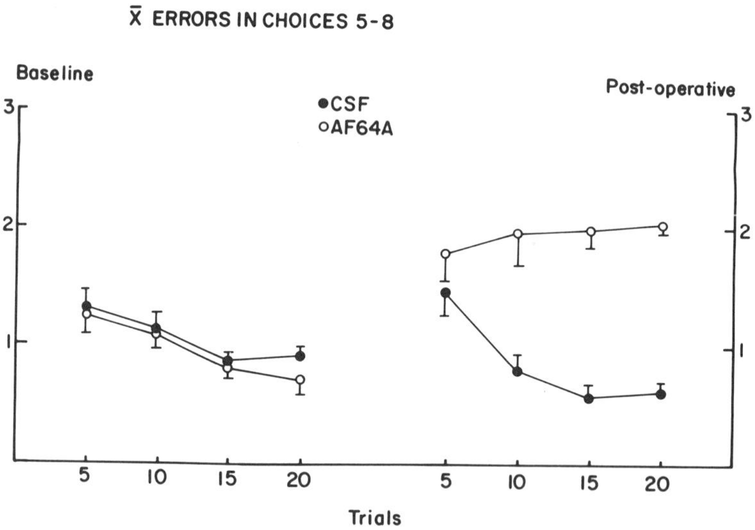

Fig. 1. Number of correct choices during the first 4 post-delay choices. Data are presented as mean $\pm$ SEM.

AF64A INJECTIONS INTO THE HIPPOCAMPUS

Mantione and coworkers (17) reported significant decreases in cholinergic markers following injection of AF64A into the HPC. To further clarify the role of hippocampal cholinergic mechanisms in the modulation of behavior we examined the consequences of injecting CSF or AF64A (0.25, 1.0 or 4.0 nmols/side/0.5 ul) directly into the dorsal HPC. The experimental design is presented in Table 1.

Motor activity was increased 40-50 % over control values in the 8 nmol group 7, 14 and 21 days following injection. The rate of within-session habituation however was not affected. Hot-plate latencies were decreased in all AF64A groups for up to 28 days following surgery. The magnitude and persistence of these changes suggest an important role for hippocampal cholinergic mechanisms in reactivity to aversive stimuli.

Acquisition of RAM task was significantly impaired in the 2.0 and

8.0 nmol groups. Both of these groups required 2 to 3 times as many trials as the control group to achieve a criterion of accurate performance (i.e., 3 consecutive days with a mean of 7 correct choices in the first 8 choices). Furthermore, the 8 nmol group exhibited impaired performance throughout the 20 days of testing.

AF64A produced a dose-related decrease of ChAT activity in the HPC. The 0.5 and 2.0 nmol AF64A groups exhibited a 12-16 % decrease of hippocampal ChAT activity while the 8 nmol group exhibited a 22 % decrease of ChAT activity 120 days after injection. Norepinephrine (NE), dopamine (DA), serotonin (5-HT) and their metabolites were not affected by AF64A. These data demonstrate that small perturbations of cholinergic tone in the HPC can have long-lasting behavioral consequences. In contrast, extensive depletion of forebrain NE following injection of 6-hydroxydopamine into the dorsal noradrenergic bundle or after systemic administration of DSP-4 had no effect on cognitive function or behavioral reactivity (6,30).

Bailey and coworkers (1) also reported increased motor activity and impaired acquisition and retention of both passive and 2-way active avoidance responses 7-14 days after injection of 10 nmols of AF64A into the HPC (5 nmol/side/2 ul). Damage to the HPC facilitates acquisition of 2-way active avoidance responding. Therefore, the behavioral changes induced by intrahippocampal AF64A are due to a disruption of cholinergic mechanisms and not to non-specific or incidental damage to the HPC.

AF64A INJECTIONS INTO THE STRIATUM

The preceding sections outlined how AF64A has been used to delineate the involvement of hippocampal and cortical cholinergic processes in the modulation of behavior. An inherent theme of these studies is that AF64A might be useful in developing an animal model of SDAT. In a similar context, AF64A might also be useful in evaluating the contribution of cholinergic mechanisms to other neurological and psychiatric disorders. For example, Sandberg and colleagues (23,24,25) have utilized intrastriatal injections of AF64A to indirectly examine the role of striatal cholinergic neurons in the pathophysiology and clinical course of Huntington's Disease.

Huntington's Disease (HD) is a progressive neurological disorder characterized by motor dyskinesias, emotional lability and cognitive impairments which culminate in dementia (15). The morphological and neurochemical alterations associated with HD include a loss of neurons in the neostriatum and reductions in presynaptic markers of both cholinergic and GABAergic function. In contrast, the concentration of transmitters which project to the striatum such as 5-HT, DA, NE, and their synthetic enzymes are not affected in HD.

Several investigators have suggested that intrastriatal injection of kainic acid might provide a useful model of HD in rats since it reproduces many of the neurochemical, behavioral and neuropathological changes observed in HD (7,18,20). While kainic acid destroys cell bodies in the striatum, sparing fibers of passage, both cholinergic and GABAergic neurons are affected to a similar extent. Therefore, the potential contribution of these different systems to the neurological deficits observed after kainic acid cannot be determined.

In an effort to determine the relative involvement of cholinergic hypofunction in the deficits induced by kainic acid Sandberg and colleagues examined the biochemical and behavioral consequences of injecting AF64A into the striatum. AF64A, in doses ranging from 2-26 nmols, produced a persistent dose-related decrease of ChAT activity, ACh concentrations and

HAChU without affecting biochemical indices of GABA or DA processes (24). Therefore, AF64A induced a selective presynaptic cholinergic deficit in the striatum.

The behavioral deficits produced by intrastriatal AF64A injections included alterations in motor behavior and avoidance learning. A micro-analysis of motor behavior performed 35 days following bilateral injection of 8 nmols of AF64A into the striatum revealed that nocturnal activity (1700-0800 hrs) was significantly increased by the treatment (23). Similar effects have been observed following injection of kainic acid into the striatum (20).

Acquisition and retention of a passive avoidance response was also disrupted by injection of AF64A (8 nmols/side) into the striatum (25). In this study, rats were injected with AF64A or vehicle and trained 35 days later in a step-down passive avoidance task. The AF64A group required more time to acquire the task (i.e., refraining from stepping off the platform for 300 sec) and they exhibited impaired retention of the task 7 days following training. Shock thresholds required to elicit a flinch, jump or vocalization were not affected by the treatment. Furthermore, motor activity recorded during the diurnal phase was not different. Therefore, the impaired acquisition and retention of the task was likely due to alterations in learning and memory processes rather than to changes in nonassociative factors. In this and the previously mentioned study neurochemical analyses revealed that ChAT activity was significantly decreased (25 %) by AF64A in the striatum but not in the HPC or cortex. Furthermore, GAD activity was not affected in any of the three regions.

Although several transmitters are affected in the kainic acid model of HD the data of Sandberg and coworkers implicate cholinergic neurons as being critically involved in the behavioral effects produced by this excitotoxin. Several systems might be comparably affected in HD but the cholinergic deficit might be more germane to the symptomatology associated with the disorder. Correcting the cholinergic deficit might therefore be the most efficacious pharmacological strategy for alleviating the symptoms of HD. In fact, several reports have found that augmenting cholinergic tone can produce temporary improvements of motor performance and cognitive function in HD patients (2).

SUMMARY

In conclusion, AF64A is a neurotoxic analog of choline which produces a chronic cholinergic hypofunction and cognitive impairments in the rat. Since AF64A reproduces many of the neurochemical and behavioral deficits characteristic of SDAT we believe it is an important tool for developing a useful animal model of the disorder. Furthermore, dietary, environmental and pharmacological strategies designed to attenuate age-related memory disorders are currently being evaluated in the AF64A-treated rat.

This work was supported in part by NIMH Grant MH 34893 to I.H.

REFERENCES

1. E.L. Bailey, D.H. Overstreet and A.D. Crocker. Neurosci. Lett. Suppl. 19:S37 (1985).
2. A. Barbeau. Can. J. Neurol. Sci. 5:157-160 (1978).
3. R.T. Bartus, R.L. Dean, B. Beer and A.S. Lippa. Science 217:408-417 (1982).
4. D.W. Bowen, D. Neary, N.R. Sims and J.S. Snowden. In: Dynamics of

Cholinergic Function. (Ed.) I. Hanin, Plenum Press (in press).
5. F. Casamenti, L. Bracco, F. Pedata and G. Pepeu. In: Dynamics of Cholinergic Function. (Ed.) I. Hanin, Plenum Press (in press).
6. J.C. Crobak, D.L. DeHaven and T.J. Walsh. Behav. Neural. Biol. (in press).
7. J.T. Coyle, E.D. London, K. Biziere and R. Zaczek. Adv. in Neurology 23:593-608 (1979).
8. J.T. Coyle, D.L. Price and M.R. DeLong. Science 219:1184-1190 (1983).
9. D.A. Drachman. Neurology 27:783-790 (1977).
10. A. Fisher and I. Hanin. Life Sci. 27:1615-1634 (1980)
11. A. Fisher, C.R. Mantione, E. Grauer, A. Levy and I. Hanin. In: Behavioral Models and the Analysis of Drug Action. M. Y. Speigelstein and A. Levy (Eds.), Elsevier Scientific Publishing Co., Amsterdam, The Netherlands, 1983, pp. 333-342.
12. L.E. Jarrad, G.J. Kant, J.L. Meyerhoff and A. Levy. Pharmacol. Biochem. Behav. 21:273-280 (1984)
13. C.A. Johns, V. Haroutunian, B.S. Greenwald, R.C. Mohs, B.M. Davis, P. Kanof, T.B. Horvath and K.L. Davis. Drug Devel Res. 5:77-96 (1985)
14. J.J. Mann, M. Stanley, A. Neophytides, M.J. DeLeon, S.H. Ferris and S. Gershon. Neurobiol. Aging 2:57-60 (1981)
15. J.B. Martin. Neurology 34:1059-1072 (1984)
16. C.R. Mantione, A. Fisher and I. Hanin. Science 213:579-580 (1981)
17. C.R. Mantione, M.J. Zigmond, A. Fisher and I. Hanin. J. Neurochem. 41:251-255 (1983)
18. P.L. McGeer and E.G. McGeer. CRC Crit, Rev. Toxicol. 1-26 (1982)
19. E.K. Perry, B.E.Tomlinson, G. Blessed, K. Bergman, P.H. Gibson and R.H. Perry. Brit. Med. J. 2:1457-1459 (1978).
20. M. Pisa, P.R. Sanberg and H.C. Fibiger. Physiol. Behav. 24:11-19 (1980)
21. D.L. Price, P.J. Whitehouse, R.G. Struble, A.W. Clark, J.T. Coyle, M.R. DeLong and J.C. Hedreen. Neurosci. Commentaries 1:84-92 (1982)
22. R.J. Rylett, M.J. Ball and E.H. Colhoun. Brain Res. (1983).
23. K. Sandberg, P.R. Sanberg and J.T.Coyle.Brain Res. 299:339-343 (1984)
24. K. Sandberg, I. Hanin, A. Fisher and J.T. Coyle. Brain Res. 293:49-55 (1984)
25. K. Sandberg, P.R. Sanberg, I. Hanin, A. Fisher and J.T. Coyle. Behav. Neurosci. 98:162-165 (1984)
26. N. Sitaram Drug Devel Res. 4:481-488 (1984)
27. R.D. Terry and R. Katzman. Ann. Neurol. 14:497-506 (1983)
28. T.J. Walsh, D.L. DeHaven, R.B. Mailman, A. Fisher and I. Hanin. Soc. Neurosci. Abstr. Vol 10, 257 1984.
29. T.J. Walsh, H.A. Tilson, D.L. DeHaven, R.B. Mailman, A. Fisher and I. Hanin. Brain Res. 321:91-102 (1984)
30. T.J. Walsh, J.C Crobak, H.A. Tilson, D.L. DeHaven and I. Hanin. Ann. N.Y. Acad. Sci. (in press)
31. G. Wenk, D. Hepler and D. Olton. Behav Brain Res. 13:129-138 (1984).

AF64A INDUCED CHOLINOTOXICITY: BEHAVIORAL AND BIOCHEMICAL CORRELATES

R. Brandeis, Z. Pittel, C. Lachman, E. Heldman, S. Luz,
S. Dachir, A. Levy, I. Hanin* and A. Fisher

Israel Institute for Biological Research
Ness-Ziona, 70450, Israel

*Loyola University Stritch School of Medicine
Chicago, Illinois

INTRODUCTION

The postulated involvement of the cholinergic system in Alzheimer's disease (AD) has highlighted the research and therapeutic approach of this affliction during the last decade (1). There is little doubt at the present stage that a clear hypofunction of the cholinergic system is in evidence in certain brain areas in AD patients. Other neurotransmitter systems seem to be relatively unaffected (1).

Therapeutic approaches based on the "cholinergic hypothesis in AD" have as yet yielded controversial results (2). There is no doubt that progress in this field could be furthered if a workable animal model, parallelling most of the morphological and functional deficits of AD, could be developed. So far this aim has had only partial success by the introduction of models based on lesions induced in brain areas of relevance (3). In this regard, ethylcholine aziridinium ion (AF64A), a new cholinotoxin synthesized by us, induces in selective areas of mice and rats a long-term cholinergic hypofunction following intracerebroventricular (icv) injection of doses in the nmol range. This cholinergic underactivity may mimic the hippocampal and cortical cholinergic deficiency reported in AD (3).

In the present study, apparent cognitive impairments induced by low icv doses of AF64A have been studied using behavioral paradigms in correlation with biochemically tested cholinergic hypofunction. The behavioral studies include: 1) one-trial passive avoidance (PA) test; 2) radial-arm maze (RAM); and 3) Morris water maze (MWM).

MATERIALS AND METHODS

AF64A Preparation and Injection

AF64A was freshly prepared from acetylethylcholine mustard (Acetoxy AF64A) as follows: 23 mg Acetoxy AF64A (hydrochloride salt) was dissolved in 9 ml H_2O. Under continuous pH measurement, the pH of the solution was raised to 11.5-11.7 by titration with 6N NaOH. The alkaline pH was maintained for 20 minutes by periodic addition of 3 ul 6N NaOH. The reaction was terminated by adding 6N HCl and adjusting the pH to 7.0. The final volume of the solution containing now AF64A was adjusted to 10 ml (10 mM), and then diluted in artificial cerebrospinal fluid (CSF) to the appropriate concentration, for icv injection. This solution was then kept on ice and used within 4 hours. Male Sprague-Dawley rats were anesthesized with Equithesin (0.3 ml/100 gr, i.p.). Bilateral injections were made by stereotaxic application of AF64A or vehicle into the lateral cerebroventricles (icv) (AP - 0.8 mm from bregma; L + 1.5 mm from bregma; DV-4.7 mm from skull surface. The rats were injected with either 3 or 5 nmoles in 0.5-2 ul (0.25 ul/min) on each side, with a 28 ga. injection cannula. Control rats were injected in the first passive-avoidance experiment with distilled water and in later experiments with artificial CSF in order to avoid nonspecific effects due to the hypo-osmotic vehicle (see also Kasa et al., this volume).

Apparatus and Procedure

PA Test. A conventional two-compartment box was used for the step-through passive avoidance test. The rats were individually placed in the small lighted front compartment and the latency to enter the large dark compartment was measured. Scrambled foot-shock (0.4-0.6 mA for 3 sec.) was administered immediately following entry into the dark compartment. In case of drug treatment, rats were injected with physostigmine salicylate (0.06 mg/kg i.p.) or saline 60 sec. after administration of the shock. Retention was tested 24 hours after training by measuring the latency to enter the dark compartment, with a cut-off point at 600 sec. The behavioral testing was conducted 27, 42 or 57 days after AF64A or vehicle injection.

RAM Test. An elevated eight-arm radial maze, made of transparent Plexiglass was used. The arms (8x45 cm) extended from an octagonal central arena (24 cm wide). A clear Plexiglass barrier (4.5 cm high) was installed in each arm, 5 cm from the point of attachment to the central arena. A procedure of baiting consistently 4 out of the 8 arms was used. This procedure has been shown to enable a distinction between working memory (WM) and reference memory (RM) impairments (5). Testing of AF64A-injected and control rats was conducted once a day. Elapsed time (with a cut-off of 5 min.) as well as correct (food containing) and incorrect (empty arms) responses were recorded. Rats were trained for a few weeks to a plateau level of performance, then injected with either AF64A or CSF, and tested following three weeks of recovery. 7-8 weeks following injection, the effect of a drug treatment (physostigmine 0.1 mg/kg i.p.) against saline control was studied on alternating days, when rats were tested 15 min. following injection.

MWM Test. A circular pool was used (diameter: 1.4 m; height 0.4 m (4) which was painted white and was filled to a height of 18 cm with water in which milk-powder had been dissolved. A white wooden platform (12x12 cm), was present inside the pool, 2 cm below the surface of the water. A trial consisted of placing a rat by hand into the water, at one of four starting locations and measuring the latency to find the platform with a cut-off point of 120 sec. The behavioral testing was conducted on two consecutive days, with each rat receiving 8 trials on each day. During trials 1-12 the platform was located in the center of the south-east quadrant and during trials 13-16 the platform was located in the center of the north-west quadrant. Immediately before testing, on each day, half of the AF64A and half of the CSF-injected rats were treated with physostigmine salicylate (0.1 mg/kg, i.p.) while the other half were treated with saline. The behavioral testing was conducted 3-3.5 months after AF64A injection and 2-2.5 months after passive avoidance testing.

Determination of choline acetyltransferase (ChAT) activity. A modification of the radiochemical method for the determination of ChAT activity (6) was used as follows: 10 ul of a homogenate of selected brain areas were incubated with 10 ul reaction mixture containing 600 mM NaCl, 40 mM $MgCl_2$, 2 mM eserine, 0.05% (w/v) bovine serum albumin, 0.87 mM [^{14}C]-acetyl-CoA (5 uCi/nmole) and 10 mM choline chloride. After 20 minutes incubation at 37°C the reaction was stopped by transferring the tubes to an ice bath and addition of tetraphenyl boron in heptanone (75 mg/ml, 150 ul). The newly synthesized [^{14}C]-ACh was extracted into the organic phase by vigorous shaking and 0.1 ml was removed for radioactivity measurement.

RESULTS AND DISCUSSION

PA. No significant difference was found between the initial step-through latencies of all the groups tested in the first experiment (Fig. 1). This seemed to indicate that, as far as motivation and motoric performance were concerned, all the groups responded similarly. However, retention of the step-through response was impaired in all the AF64A-injected groups, at all the time intervals tested, as shown by the significantly shorter latencies depicted in Fig. 2 [$F(3,102)=20.49$; $p<0.01$]. Initial latencies were also similar in the CSF and AF64A-injected groups tested in the second experiment (Fig. 3). However, while the step-through latency of the AF64Ainjected group (3 nmoles/2 ul per side) during retention-test was significantly shorter than that of the CSF group, [$F(1,36)=20.18$; $p<0.01$], physostigmine treatment (0.06 mg/kg i.p.) significantly prolonged this latency as compared to the saline-treated control group [$F(1,36)=4.08$; $p<0.05$].

RAM. As shown in Figure 4, significant impairment in performance was detected in the AF64A-injected group (3nmoles/2 ul per side) with no decrement in the CSF-injected groups, during the first week of testing following injection [$F(1,11)=5.99$; $p<0.05$]. However, the improvement under physostigmine treatment was not statistically significant (Fig. 5). It might be that careful optimization of the dose should be attempted in order to detect some beneficial effects of physostigmine in this test.

MWM. Escape-latency, in blocks of two trials, is presented in Fig. 6. The escape-latency measures of the AF64A-injected group (3 nmoles/2 ul per side) were significantly longer than that of the CSF-injected group [$F(1,34)= 14.88$; $p<0.001$]. However, while physostigmine treatment (0.1 mg/kg i.p.) showed a tendency to prolong this latency, the difference was not statistically significant.

ChAT Activity. After bilateral icv injection of AF64A, ChAT activity was decreased significantly in hippocampus but not in frontal cortex or striatum. The residual activities of the hippocampal ChAT after various doses of AF64A at three different periods after icv injection are shown in Table 1.

Fig. 7 shows the kinetics of the inhibition of ChAT activity after treatment with AF64A. Maximum inhibition was obtained 10 days post-AF64A injection. Slow but continuous recovery was observed up to 50 days post-injection. From 50 days post-injection and further on, ChAT activity stabilized at the level of 80% of control. We also found that doses of AF64A that produced greater inhibition of hippocampal ChAT activity, induced greater impairments in the passive avoidance acquisition (compare Table 1 and Fig. 7 with Fig. 2). In addition, when a certain treatment produced greater initial reduction in ChAT activity, the cognitive impairment was also greater. This can be demonstrated by comparing treatments with 3 nmoles in 0.5 ul/side with 3 nmoles in 2 ul/side (compare Fig. 2 with 7). However, our kinetic studies revealed that the relationships between the degree of the hippocampal ChAT inhibition and cognitive impairment were more complex. Thus the periods in which maximum cognitive impairment was observed (see Fig. 2) did not necessarily coincide with the period in which maximum inhibition of hippocampal ChAT occurred.

These results may be rationalized as follows: AF64A produces a progressive damage to cholinergic neurons, starting at their terminals and progressing toward the somata (see also Kasa et al., this volume). An indication for retrograde degeneration was obtained in experiments with cultured rat septum where damage to axons became apparent before we observed any damage to cell bodies (7). It is possible that only when destruction of the degenerating cholinergic neurons is complete, cognitive impairments show up. ChAT activity drops when the damage to the cholinergic terminals takes place. However, at a later stage, cholinergic neurons that survived the AF64A-induced lesion, could sprout, resulting in a partial recovery of ChAT activity. Alternatively, the remaining cells may increase their ChAT activity either by de novo synthesis of the enzyme, or through other activating mechanisms. Thus ChAT activity starts to recover after its initial inhibition. Nevertheless, it appears that the observed recovery was not sufficient to return normal neural activity to the critical sites that are responsible for the expression of the cognitive function which is examined in the PA test.

Still, recovery of ChAT activity may be of some relevance to the reversal of the cognitive impairment induced by physostigmine. Thus, when recovery of ChAT activity occurs, more ACh may be available at important target sites provided that it would not be degraded by AChE. Inhibition of AChE would

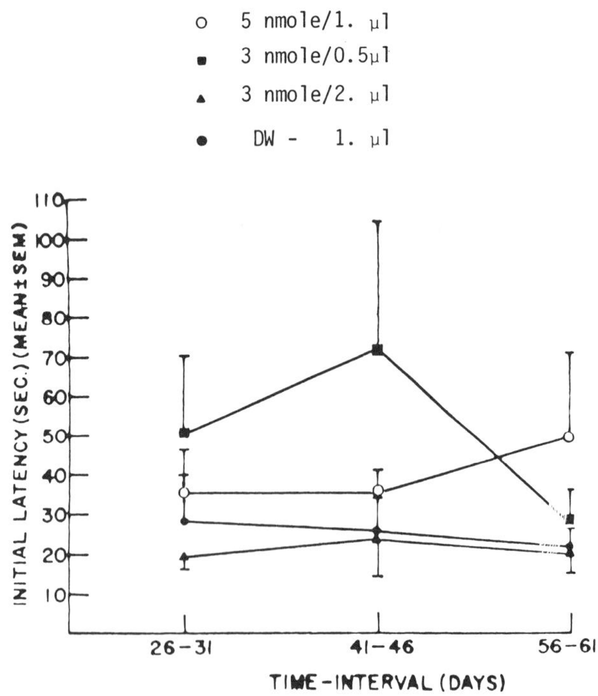

Fig. 1: Initial latency measures (sec.) as a function of dose/volume of AF64A and post-injection intervals of time.

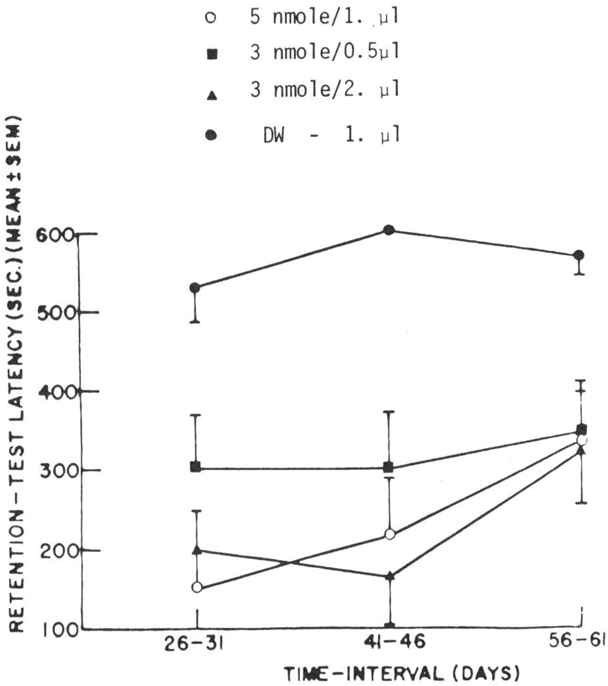

Fig. 2: Retention-test latency measures (sec.) as a function of dose/volume of AF64A and post-injection intervals of time.

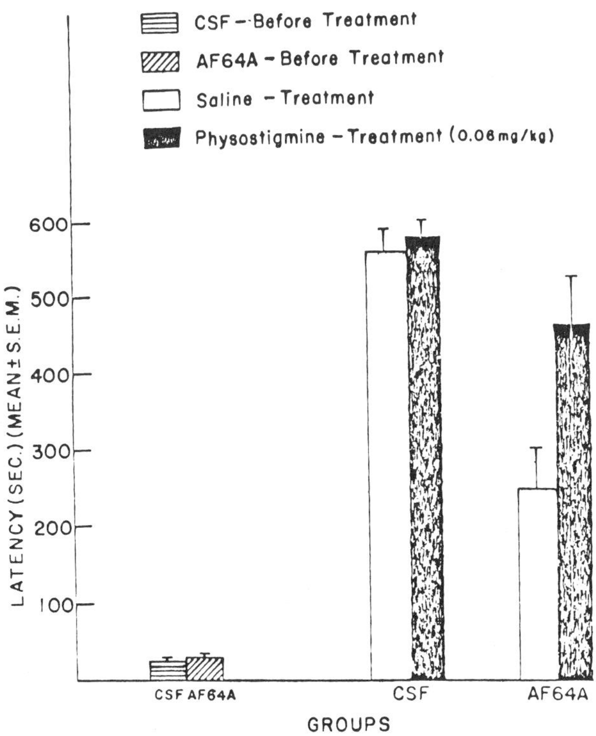

Fig. 3: Initial latency and retention-test latency measures (sec.) of the AF64A and CSF-injected groups, before and after physostigmine of saline administration.

therefore permit more ACh to reach the area of the target sites. Indeed, we could demonstrate that physostigmine, a central and peripheral reversible cholinesterase inhibitor, reversed memory impairments in the PA test in the AF64A-treated rats.

These data support the notion that cholinergic hypofunction is responsible for the cognitive impairments observed in AF64A treated rats.

Table 1: Hippocampal ChAT activity after various doses of AF64A injected icv to rats (% of control + standard deviations; n = number of animals in each group)

	Days after icv injection of AF64A		
Dose	13	52	95
1.5 nmoles/0.5 ul/side	96 + 34[a]	--	--
3.0 nmoles/0.5 ul/side	53 + 17[a]	80 + 14[b]	81 + 14[c]
3.0 nmoles/2 ul/side	--	71 + 3[c]	78 + 17[c]
5.0 nmoles/1 ul/side	--	69 + 18[b]	80 + 12[d]

[a]n=10; [b]n=6; [c]n=7; [d]n=3

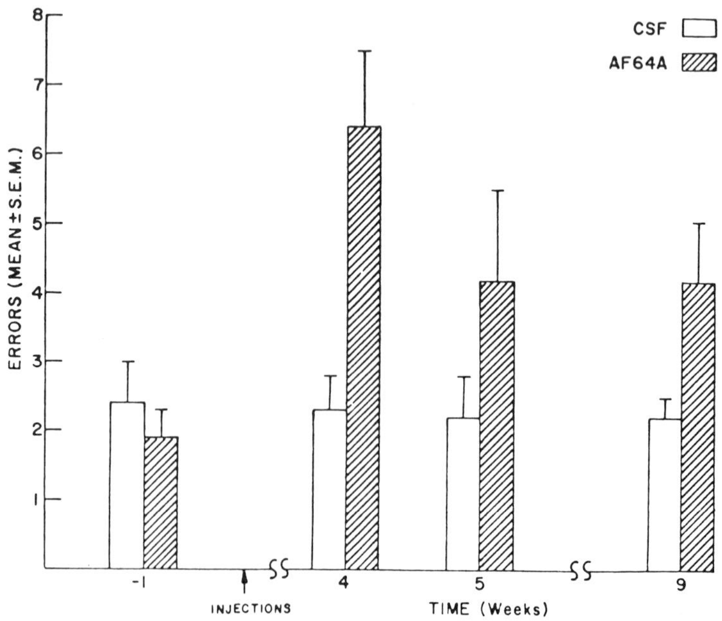

Fig. 4: The effect of icv injection of AF64A and CSF on the performance of rats in the RAM.

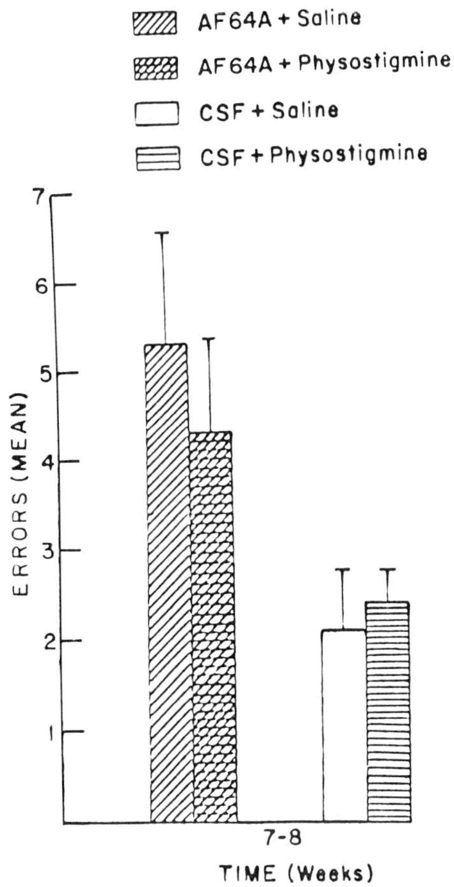

Fig. 5: The effect of physostigmine treatment (0.1 mg/kg i.p.) on AF64A and CSF-injected rats in RAM.

CONCLUSIONS

A) Cognitive impairments, induced by icv injection of AF64A to rats, were found in three different behavioral paradigms.

B) Reduction in ChAT activity was found after icv injection of AF64A. The reduction was confined to the hippocampus and was not manifested in the frontal cortex or the striatum.

C) Treatments with AF64A that caused greater inhibition of hippocampal ChAT activity also induced larger cognitive impairments.

D) Physostigmine at the doses tested partially reversed the AF64A-induced cognitive impairment as measured by PA, but not by RAM or MWM.

E) The above mentioned data are consistent with the view that these cognitive impairments are induced by a cholinergic deficit in hippocampus.

F) AF64A-induced cholinotoxicity may mimic the cholinergic hypofunction and certain cognitive impairments found in AD.

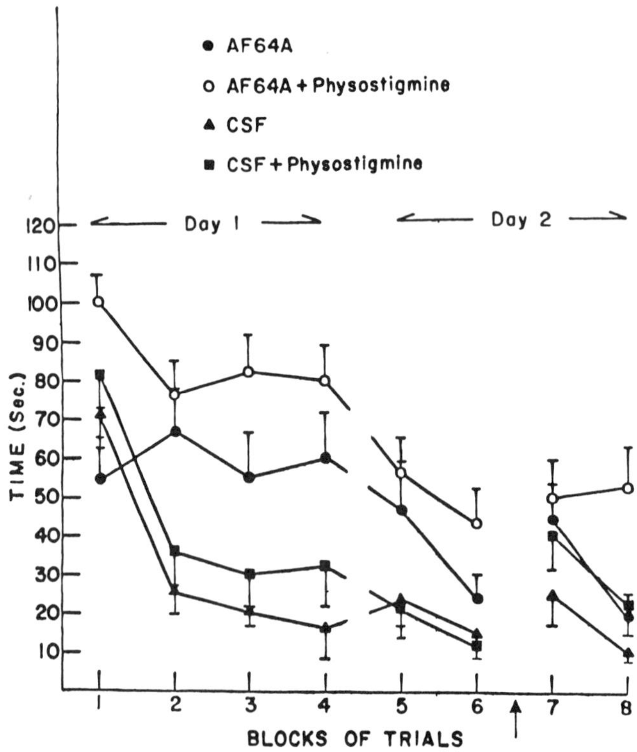

Fig. 6: Escape latency measures, in blocks of 2 trials, of the AF64A and CSFinjected groups, after physostigmine (0.1 mg/kg i.p.) administration.

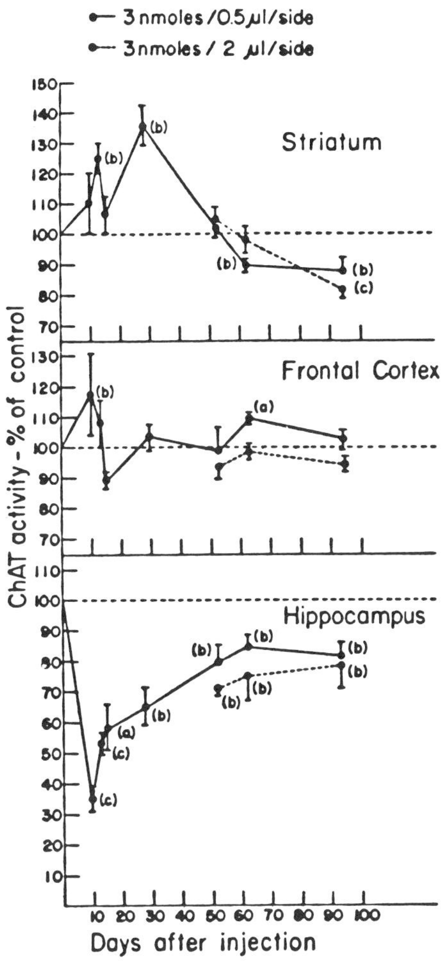

Fig. 7: ChAT activity in hippocampus, frontal cortex and striatum at various times after icv injection of AF64A

REFERENCES

1. Coyle, J.T., Price, D.L. and Delong, M.R. Alzheimer's disease: A disorder of cortical cholinergic innervation. Science 219: 1184-1190 (1983).
2. Bartus, R.T. Physostigmine and recent memory: Effects in young and aged non human primates. Science 206: 1087-1089 (1979).
3. Fisher, A. and Hanin, I. Animal models for senile dementia of Alzheimer's type with particular emphasis on AF64A-induced cholinotoxicity. Ann. Rev. Pharmacol. Toxicol. (1986).
4. Morris, R. Developments of a water maze procedure for studying spatial learning in the rat. J. Neurosci. Meth. 11: 47-60 (1984).
5. Jarrard, L.E., Kant, G.J., Meyerhoff, J.C. and Levy, A. Behavioral and Neurochemical effects of intraventricular AF64A administration rats. Pharmacol. Biochem. Behav. 21: 273-280 (1984).
6. Fonnum, F. A rapid radiochemical method for the determination of choline acetyltransferase. J. Neurochem. 24: 407-409 (1975).
7. Amir, A., Heldman, E., Pittel, Z., Fisher, A. and Schachar, A. Unpublished data.

NEUROBEHAVIORAL ASPECTS OF SOME ANIMAL MODELS OF AGE-RELATED NEUROPSYCHIATRIC DISORDERS

Paul R. Sanberg

Behavioral Neuroscience Laboratory
Department of Psychology
Ohio University
Athens, Ohio 45701

Animals have proven valuable as model systems to understand how the human brain degenerates in such age-related disorders as Huntington's disease, Parkinson's disease and Alzheimer's disease. Furthermore, animal models afford a technique whereby brain-behavior interrelations can be analysed under controlled conditions. Within these analyses there exists a degree of sophistication in determining many neuroanatomical and neurochemical correlates of brain degeneration. On the other hand, commonly employed behavioral techniques usually do not elucidate many differences between animal models of age-related neuropsychiatric disorders. Thompson (1978) demonstrated this most clearly in his "Behavioral Atlas of the Rat Brain." In this study, lesions in many different areas of the brain resulted in the same behavioral deficits. For example, there were no fewer than 50 different brain areas from the neocortex to the midbrain that resulted in a "Maze Deficit." In human neuropsychological evaluations of the dementia disorders there are clear distinctions between the pattern of mental deterioration that occurs in each disease. In many animal models, however, these distinctions can not be made. Thus, it is important to develop more precise behavioral analysis techniques that can be used effectively in determining the "abnormal" behaviors that occur in different animal models.

We have been evaluating various behavioral paradigms as potential tools for differentiating between neuropsychiatric animal models; primarily focusing on the movement abnormalities that result from extrapyramidal lesions in rats. Specifically, the research discussed here is concerned with analysing in detail the pattern of abnormal locomotion found in rats with various types of telencephalic lesions. These animal models are briefly presented in the next section.

The Animal Models

The Kainic Acid Model. At present, there exists no experimental animal model which has exactly the same genetic and neurological abnormalities seen in humans with Huntington's Disease (HD). According to McGeer and McGeer (1982), however, rats which receive bilateral injections of kainic acid (KA) into the striatum (KAL rats) provides the best animal model of HD yet achieved. Kainic acid is a neurotoxin that specifically destroys cell bodies. The resulting biochemical and histological sequela following KA-induced striatal damage has been found to be strikingly similar to that found in the striatum of patients with HD after post-mortem examination (Coyle et al, 1978; McGeer and McGeer, 1982; Sanberg and Coyle, 1984), although neuronal loss in KAL rats is typically more complete (Coyle et al, 1977). The neuropathological sequelae of intrastriatal KA injections have been reviewed extensively (see Coyle et al, 1978). Generally, consistent alterations in the neurochemical indices for cholinergic, GABAergic, monoaminergic, peptidergic and amino acid transmitter systems have been found in the striatum between the animal model and HD.

The AF64A Model. Recently, there has been a resurgence of interest in the role that acetylcholine may play in behavior. This has been kindled by the findings of a specific cholinergic deficit in the brains of people suffering from Alzheimer's disease (Whitehouse et al, 1982). Also, a selective neurotoxin for cholinergic neurons has become available. Recently, it was demonstrated that the choline mustard analog, AF64A, produced significant and persistent reductions in presynaptic markers for cholinergic neurons at concentrations that did not cause reductions in markers for GABAergic neurons and dopaminergic neurons within the striatum (Sandberg et al, 1985). Thus, this novel cholinergic neurotoxin allows for the characterization of selective striatal cholinergic lesions on behavior. Accordingly, we have been examining the role of the striatal cholinergic system after bilateral injections of AF64A into the striatum.

The MAM Model. The mitotic inhibitor methylazoxymethanol (MAM), is a potent alkylating agent that ablates actively dividing neuroblasts while sparing cells that have already divided. Thus, the injection of MAM into rats on Day 15 of pregnancy (a time when the striatum and cortex are developing) produces a severe and lasting hypoplasia of these areas in the offspring with a resulting hyperinnervation of ascending neurotransmitter systems to the forebrain (Beaulieu and Coyle, 1981; Johnson and Coyle, 1980). There are many biochemical and anatomical similarities between this animal model and several clinical disorders, such as schizophrenia and hyperkinesis. In addition, there is evidence of a "genuine hypoplasia, or dwarfism, of the corpus striatum as a consequence of failure of neuronal maturation of the interneuronal neuropil (in Tourette's Syndrome) so that the striatum remains arrested at a stage of development normally found in a young child" (Richardson, 1982). Similarly, Moran et al (1983) found that the MAM animals have a delayed maturation of inhibitory cortical processes on stimulation-induced behaviors. Thus, the MAM model may prove useful for studying underlying mechanisms of Tourette Snydrome.

The Cortical Suction Lesion Model. Experimental focal cortical injury has been employed as a model for studying the mechanisms underlying the behavioral changes which accompany stroke or brain trauma. As is the case with the human condition, in rats the magnitude and type of neurochemical and behavioral change depends in part upon both lesion site and lesion size (Robinson, 1979). Robinson and his co-workers have demonstrated that right hemisphere frontal suction lesions produced spontaneous hyperactivity and bilaterial depletions of norephinephine and dopamine while identical left lesions did not (Robinson, 1979; Moran et al, 1984b). This hyperkinetic response was of interest in the present investigations of discriminant locomotor analysis.

The Behavior Tests

Passive-Avoidance Behavior. Paramount among the behavioral tests used by neuroscientists to indicate possible alterations in learning and memory is the passive-avoidance paradigm. Its popularity stems from two major points. First, it is a simple paradigm requiring little training of the experimenter or animal subjects. Second, results can be obtained within a couple of days. Essentially, the task involves placing an animal in a "safe" place. Once the animal moves from this place it receives an electric shock; thereby, requiring the animal to return to the safe area. Thus, the successful "learning" of this task requires the animal to remain "passive."

Passive-avoidance has proven valuable as a screening test to determine if an experimental treatment can cause behavioral changes, which can be interpreted as a learning or memory impairment (Polgar et al, 1981). As can be seen from Table 1, when some of the models described above were tested in this task all of them showed deficits. While the magnitude of the differences are not depicted in this table, they did not yield sufficient information for discriminatory analysis (Sanberg et al, 1978; Sandberg et al, 1984a). This is supported by Thompson (1978) who reported that over 50 different brain areas along the full rostral-caudal extent of the brain produced deficits in avoidance acquisition.

Locomotor Behavior. If there is one behavioral test which can be considered a standard by neuroscientists, it is the measurement of activity. Yet by no means is this test standardized. Many devices are commonly employed for this purpose, including running wheels, "jiggle boxes," open-fields, and photocell-cages. Each test gives its own definition of what is measured as activity. The one aspect that most of these tests have in common is that they yield only one-dependent measure. This one measure, though, makes it practically impossible to use locomotor behavior for discriminatory analysis of different animal models. To substantiate this point further Thompson (1978) has demonstrated at least 100 brain areas in which a similar change in activity was measured following electrolytic lesions.

Another major problem in most locomotor studies is that the rodent models are usually tested during the wrong period of the day. Most patients with extrapyramidal movement disorders show greater abnormal movements during their awake period and when aroused (Shapiro et al, 1978; Shoulson & Chase, 1975). Thus, when examining the motor behavior of animal models as an analogue to human movement, it is important to take into account diurnal variations, especially nocturnal activity, in the rat model, since it is at this time that abnormal motion would be most apparent. Almost all previous studies in the rat have limited the behavioral testing to daytime periods. In addition, the paradigms have been contrived; and testing situations, in which only one "activity" variable was measured,

Table 1. Passive-Avoidance Behavior in Some Animal Models of Neuropsychiatric Disorders

Model	Acquisition	Retention	Shock Sensitivity	Daytime Activity
Kainate Striatal Lesions	Impaired	Impaired	Normal	Normal
AF64A Striatal Lesions	Impaired	Impaired	Normal	Normal
MAM Cortical Lesions	Impaired	Impaired	Normal	Normal

have been limited. It is not surprising, therefore, that, with only one such measure, many types of brain manipulations would produce the same result (i.e., increased nocturnal activity). Activity, per se, involves many aspects of movement, such as forward locomotion, velocity, rearings, stereotyped movements, rotational behavior, etc., and an increase in any one of these would produce increased machine counts, and by definition, increased activity. Furthermore, such a limited dependent measure would not allow us to define exactly what the locomotion abnormalities following experimental brain manipulations were.

Using recently developed computerised Digiscan Animal Activity Monitors (Omnitech, Inc.), which simultaneously measure over 20 aspects of locomotion, including many indices of horizontal, vertical, stereotypical, and rotational behavior, recent studies have found locomotor abnormalities that appear to be specific to various types of experimental manipulations (Sanberg, Hagenmeyer, and Henault, 1985).

Using this system, the topography of locomotion for the animal models described above was ascertained. Briefly, the rats were individually placed into one of four activity monitors (Omnitech). The animal activity monitors consist of an open field (16" x 16" x 12") with horizontal and vertical movement sensors. The apparatus utilizes a total of 24 infrared beams, spaced one inch apart. The horizontal movement sensors are located in four strips, with each strip directing either eight infrared beams from front to back or directing eight infrared beams from side to side. Interruption of any of these beams will lead to an increase in the horizontal activity count. There are also eight beams in each of the two vertical activity sensors. When any of these beams are interrupted the vertical activity counter is incremented by one.

The activity monitor accumulates data for a given time period which is specified by the investigator. At the end of the time period, it stores the accumulated data in an Apple IIe computer and starts gathering data for the next period. The measurements made by the activity counter include: (1) horizontal activity- the total number of beam interruptions which occurred in the horizontal sensors: (2) vertical activity- the total number of beam interruptions which occurred in the vertical sensors: (3) total distance- the distance travelled by an animal, in inches: (4) rest time- computed by the monitor by subtracting the total time spent moving from the investigator specified sampling period: (5) stereotypy time- the time spent breaking the same beam repeatedly (accumulated for various beams during the sampling interval): (6) vertical time- when the animal activates the vertical sensors by rearing this parameter starts incrementing and continues to do so until the animal goes below the level of the vertical sensor: (7) movement time- as long as the animal is moving (as measured by the interruption of different beams) this parameter is incremented; when the animal takes longer than one second to move, this parameter is stopped until the next beam is broken- thus, this measure corresponds to the amount of time the animal is in motion during a given sampling period: (8) number of stereotypic behaviors- the number of times the monitor records stereotypic behavior in the animal, as measured by repeated measures of the same infrared beam, with a break of one second or more separating one stereotypic movement from the next: (9) number of vertical movements- each time the animal rears, this parameter is increased by one; the animal must go below the level of the vertical sensor for at least one second before the next rear can be registered: (10) number of movements- each time a movement is registered by a beam interruption, separated by at least one second, this parameter is increased by one: (11) speed- the animal's speed is calculated in inches per second: (12) average distance- the average distance the animal moves (in inches) during a movement bout: (13) number of clockwise movements: and (14) number of counterclockwise movements. Finally, the

Table 2. Topography of Noctural Locomotion in Animal Models of Neuropsychiatric Disorders*

Model	Ambulation							Rearing			Stere-otypy		Revolu-tions	
	HA	TD	MT	RT	SP	NM	AD	VA	VT	VM	ST	NS	CL	AC
Kainate Striatal Lesions	+	+	+	−			+				+	+		
AF64A Striatal Lesions	+	+	+	−			+				+	+		
MAM Cortical Lesions	+	+			+		+	+	+	+			+	+
Cortical Suction Lesions	+	+			+		+	+						

* The +/- represent the direction of those variables that were significantly different from control animals. HA, horizontal activity; TD, total distance; MT, movement time; RT, rest time; SP, average speed of movement; NM, number of movements; AD, average distance; VA, vertical activity; VT, vertical time; VM, vertical movements; ST, stereotypy time; NS, number of stereotypies; CL, clockwise rotations; AC, anticlockwise rotations.

remaining nine measures indicate the amount of time the animal spent in any one of nine different zones within the open-field environment. A summary of the results for the animal models above is shown in Table 2.

Rats with bilateral striatal kainic acid or cholinergic lesions induced by AF64A were found to have increased spontaneous nocturnal locomotor activity. The topography of locomotion was characterized by an increase in the amount of time spent moving, the total distance travelled and the number of episodes and time of stereotypic behaviors. No significant differences between control and striatal rats were found in the actual velocities between the two groups indicating that the rats were simply spending more time moving rather than moving with greater speed. In addition, stereotypy was increased in striatal lesioned rats. The similarities between the two striatal lesioned groups may reflect that the destruction of cholinergic intrinsic neurons by kainic acid may account for the abnormal topographical pattern of locomotion seen in these rats (Sandberg et al, 1984b).

When the MAM animals were examined for spontaneous locomotion in the Digiscan Monitors there were no differences between MAM-treated and age-matched controls during the daytime. However, during the nocturnal period the MAM-treated rats demonstrated a pronounced hyperkinesis compared to controls as early as Day 10 of age. Although Day 10 animals showed hyperactivity only on distance travelled, during subsequent development the hyperactivity became apparent on more aspects of locomotion. While the adult MAM lesion rats travelled further than control animals there were no increases in the number of movement bouts or time spent moving. What these animals did do was move faster during each bout of activity. Rearing behavior was also markedly increased in MAM animals, as were their excursions around the perimeter of the test cage. On the other hand MAM animals showed no differences in stereotyped behaviors from controls. Thus, the MAM hyperkinesis was characterized by the animals running around the perimeter of the test cage more often and faster than controls, in addition to rearing more (Sanberg et al, 1984).

In agreement with previous results in running wheels by Dr. Robinson's laboratory (Moran et al, 1984), lesions of the right frontal cortex produced nocturnal hyperactivity. However, using the Digiscan apparatus it was found that this hyperactivity did not represent a generalized increase in activity, but only an increase in the horizontal indices, total distance travelled, average distance per movement and average speed of movement. Vertical, rotational and stereotypic measures were not changed. Thus, the topography of the lateralized hyperactivity was defined as increased length and speed of horizontal movement (Moran et al, 1984b).

All four of the above rat animal models resulted in increased spontaneous nocturnal locomotion and if measured solely by the dependent measure of number of photocells crossed (horizontal activity) there would have been no qualitative differences between the effects of the different lesions (i.e., they were all hyperactive). Evidently, this would have been a premature conclusion, since there were quite obvious differences induced by the various lesions on the topography of locomotion.

It is important to note that it is not the change in each separate variable which is important, but rather the pattern or topography of all the changes taken together that gives the power to determine the abnormal changes in animal models. The effects of experimental agents could then be studied in terms of whether they actually ameliorate the behavioral deficits (e.g., return the abnormal pattern to normal) or just produce modulatory effects (e.g., not actually changing the abnormal pattern but just causing a generalized change in the overall pattern).

Finally, it is apparent that the Digiscan locomotor analysis may prove useful in discriminating between different animal models. With the use of this multifactorial approach to animal locomotion, it should be possible to test experimental therapeutic agents on species-dependent abnormal behaviors in rodent models of age-related neuropsychiatric disorders that are mechanistically more analogous with the human condition.

Acknowledgement

Appreciation is extended to the following individuals who collaborated in the research reported here: J.T. Coyle, T.H. Moran, K. Sandberg, R. Robinson, K.L. Kubos, M.A. Henault, and S.H. Hagenmeyer. This work was supported by a Pratt Family and Friends HD Grant, the Hereditary Disease Foundation, the Huntington's Disease Foundation of America, the OURC, MH40127, and Omnitech Electronics, Inc.

References

Beaulieu, M. and Coyle, J.T., 1981, Effects of fetal methylazoxymethanol acetate lesion on the synaptic neurochemistry of the adult rat striatum. J. Neurochem. 37, 878-887.

Coyle, J.T., McGeer, E.G., McGeer, P.L., and Schwarcz, R., 1978, Neostriatal injections: A model for Huntington's chorea, in: "Kainic Acid as a Tool in Neurobiology," E. G. McGeer, J. W. Olney, and P. L. McGeer, eds., Raven Press, New York, pp. 139-159.

Coyle, J.T., Schwarcz, R., Bennett, J.P., and Campochiaro, P., 1977, Clinical, neuropathological and pharmacological aspects of Huntington's disease: Correlates with a new animal model, Prog. Neuro-Psychopharm., 1, 13-30.

Johnston, M.V. and Coyle, J.T., 1980, Ontogeny of neurochemical markers for noradrenergic, GABAergic, and cholinergic neurons in neocortex lesioned with methylazoxymethanol acetate, J. Neurochem., 34, 1429-1441.

McGeer, P.L. and McGeer, E.G., 1982, Kainic acid: The neurotoxic breakthrough, CRC Crit. Rev. Toxicol., 10, 1-26.

Moran, T.H., Sanberg, P.R., and Coyle, J.T., 1983, Stimulation induced behavior in normal and methylazoxymethanol (MAM) treated infant rats, Soc. Neurosci. Abst. 9, 978.

Moran, T.H., Kubos, K.L., Sanberg, P.R., and Robinson, R.G., 1984a, Marked behavioral and biochemical sensitivity to lesion size in the posterior cortex of the rat, Life Sci., 35, 1337-1342.

Moran, T.H., Sanberg, P.R., Kubos, K.L., Goldrich, M., and Robinson, R.G., 1984b, Asymmetrical effects of unilateral cortical suction lesions: Behavioral characterization, Behav. Neurosci., 98, 747-752.

Polgar, S., Sanberg, P.R., and Kirkby, R.J., 1981, Is the striatum involved in passive avoidance behavior? A commentary, Physiol. Psychol., 9, 354-358.

Richardson, E.P., Jr., 1982, Neuropathological studies of Tourette Syndrome, Adv. Neurol., 35, 83-87.

Robinson, R.G., 1979, Differential behavioral effects of right versus left cerebral infarction: Evidence for cerebral lateralization in the rat. Science, 205, 707-710.

Sanberg, P.R. and Coyle, J.T., 1984, Scientific approaches to Huntington's disease. CRC Crit. Rev. Clin. Neurobiol., 1, 1-44.

Sanberg, P.R., Hagenmeyer, S.H., and Henault, M.A., 1985, Automated measurement of multivariate locomotor behavior in rodents, Neurobehavioral Toxicology and Teratology, in press.

Sanberg, P.R., Lehmann, J., and Fibiger, H.C., 1978, Impaired learning and memory after kainic acid lesions of the striatum: A behavioral model of Huntington's disease, Brain Research, 149, 546-551.

Sanberg, P.R., Johnson, D.A., Moran, T.H., and Coyle, J.T., 1984, Investigating locomotion abnormalities in animal models of extrapyramidal disorders: A commentary, Physiological Psychology, 12, 48-50.

Sandberg, K., Sanberg, P.R., Hanin, I., Fisher, A., and Coyle, J.T., 1984a, Cholinergic lesion of the striatum impairs acquisition and retention of a passive avoidance response, Behavioral Neuroscience, 98, 162-165.

Sandberg, K., Sanberg, P.R., and Coyle, J.T., 1984b, Effects of intrastriatal injections of the cholinergic neurotoxin AF64A on spontaneous noctural locomotor behavior in the rat, Brain Research, 299, 339-343.

Sandberg, K., Schnaar, R.L., McKinney, M., Hanin, I., Fisher, A., and Coyle, J.T., 1985, AF64A: An active site directed irreversible inhibitor of choline acetyltransferase, J. Neurochem., 44, 439-445.

Shapiro, A.K., Shapiro, E.S., Brown, R.D., and Sweet, R.D., 1978, "Gilles de la Tourette Snydrome," Raven Press, New York.

Shoulson, I. and Chase, T.N., 1975, Huntington's disease, Ann. Rev. Med., 26, 419-426.

Thompson, R., 1978, "A Behavioral Atlas of the Rat Brain," Oxford University Press, New York.

Whitehouse, P.J., Price, D.L., Strueble, R.G., Clark, A.W., Coyle, J.T., and DeLong, M.R., 1982, Alzheimer's disease and senile dementia: Loss of neurons in the basal forebrain, Science, 215, 1237-1239.

DYSFUNCTION OF CENTRAL CHOLINERGIC SYSTEM IN HYPERKINETIC RATS, FOLLOWING POSTNATAL ANOXIA

Zipora Speiser, Chen Sharafan, Simon Gitter, Sasson Cohen, Baruch Gonen and Moshe Rehavi

Department of Physiology and Pharmacology
Tel Aviv University Sackler Faculty of Medicine
Tel Aviv, Israel 69978

INTRODUCTION

Rats exposed during the first 24 hours following birth to 100% nitrogen for 25 minutes, demonstrated increased motor activity in the open field between 10-40 days of age (1). At maturity, however, they still displayed deficits in 6-choice discrimination learning (2). Biochemical studies of the brain revealed an increase in the density of muscarinic cholinergic receptors in the hippocampus, which appeared early in life and before any changes in other brain receptors tested could be detected (dopaminergic in caudate and β adrenergic in hippocampus). The increased $[^3H]$ QNB binding in the hippocampus, demonstrated already at six days of life, reached peak values at 15-20 days, then decreased towards normal values at 40 days of life (2).

The cholinergic system is especially sensitive to hypoxia. Chemical or hypoxic hypoxia decreases acetylcholine synthesis (3,4). It has been shown that even mild hypoxia at a level that does not affect carbohydrate oxidation significantly decreases acetylcholine synthesis (3,4). We assumed, therefore, that postnatal anoxia could have caused damage, underdevelopment or even cholinergic nerve activity deficits. The increased density of muscarinic receptors found during the hyperactive stage could be a compensatory manifestation in face of reduced release of transmitter.

The role of the central cholinergic system in the control and modulation of motor activity (5,6) and in processes of memory and learning is well documented (5-8). The cholinergic system in the brain is inhibitory to the arousal and motor activity (6). The ontogenetic decrease in spontaneous motor activity of normal rats at 20-25 days of age is attributed, among other factors (9), to the lack of maturation of the cholinergic inhibitory system (6,10-12). Moreover, central or peripheral injection of cholinergic agonists to mature rats may cause decreased motor activity and catalepsy (13-16), which could be blocked by injection of anticholinergics (16). The cholinergic system in the brain is known also to affect memory and learning. Injection of cholinergic agonists, peripherally or centrally, improved memory (17) passive avoidance performance (18) and facilitated attention (8,19). Dysfunction of the cholinergic system underlies the etiology of senile dementia of the Alzheimer type (20,21).

The present work was dedicated to the study of the integrity of the central cholinergic muscarinic systems in rats following postnatal anoxia at various stages of development. Two biochemical parameters were studied: uptake of [^{3}H] choline into the nerve endings and choline acetyltransferase activity (ChAT). The purpose was to find whether both these correlate with behavioral parameters in rats following postnatal anoxia. More specifically, the following parameters were studied: 1) changes in presynaptic activity of cholinergic nerve endings; 2) density of postsynaptic muscarinic cholinergic receptors; 3) development of spontaneous motor activity throughout maturation; 4) motor response to acute administration of a muscarinic cholinergic antagonist. The main focus was on the hippocampus which is considered to be an inhibitory structure (7,22) influencing behavioral maturation (5,7) and modulating motor activity through its connections to areas controlling arousal and motor activity (23-27). Lesions to the hippocampus caused increased motor and exploratory activity in rats and lack of habituation at a novel situation (15,28-33). Lesion to the septum or interference with the synthesis of acetylcholine in the hippocampus, by use of hemicholinium, caused hyperreactivity in rats to external stimuli (34) and therefore distracted attention. Moreover, interruption of cholinergic input to the hippocampus can cause deficits in motivation learning, passive avoidance and storing of memory (5,7). In order to learn if the changes in the cholinergic system following anoxia are restricted mostly to the hippocampus or may affect the cholinergic system also in other brain regions, we also studied ChAT activity in the caudate.

RESULTS AND DISCUSSION

Correlation Between Increased Density of Muscarinic Receptors in the Hippocampus of Rats, Exposed Postnatally to Anoxia, and their Motor Response to Scopolamine

Dose response curves to injected scopolamine (0.5 - 10 mg/kg subcutaneously) were performed at various stages of development, namely, the 20th, 40th and 90th day of life. Twenty minutes after injections motor activity, expressed as numbers of crossings of infra red beam lights, was recorded for one hour, in a fully computerized activity cage. For each age group, different animals were used at different time periods. The aim of this experiment was to ascertain if rats, exposed postnatally to anoxia at the age when an increased number of muscarinic receptors were found, will respond with changes in motor activity to very small amounts of scopolamine, which do not affect significantly the activity of control rats. Fig. 1 shows that rats exposed to postnatal anoxia responded to scopolamine with increased motor activity at the age of 20 days, especially at doses of 0.5 - 1 mg/kg, which were ineffective in controls. The time schedule for the increased response of the anoxia group to scopolamine is well correlated with the period in which elevated [^{3}H] QNB binding was observed in their brains. This effect cannot be attributed to the general hyperactive response of these rats to drugs, since the anoxia rats did not respond to small doses of amphetamine which otherwise would cause pronouned hyperactivity in control rats of the same age (2). The difference of response to scopolamine between the two groups disappeared at the ages of 40 and 90 days. The increased motor response to scopolamine in the rats exposed postnatally to anoxia could result from blockade of postsynaptic receptors to an already diminished amount of inhibitory transmitter in the hippocampus or other brain areas related to modulation of motor activity.

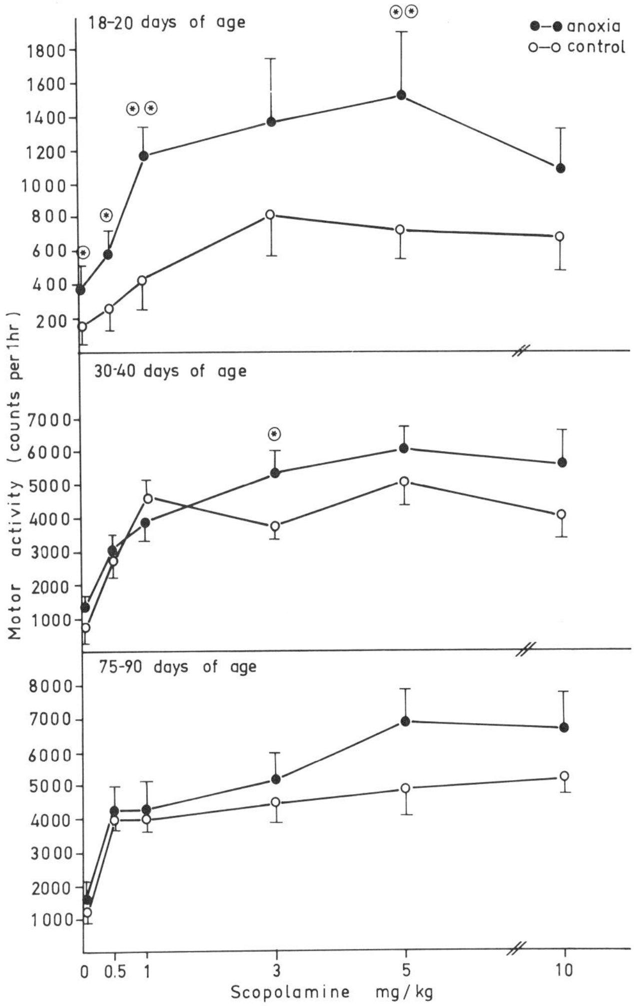

Fig. 1. The effect of scopolamine on motor activity in rats exposed to postnatal anoxia in comparison to controls, during development. Each point represents mean activity ± S.E.M. of at least 6-10 animals. Asterisks denote significant differences between groups calculated by a two tailed Student's t-test. *P<0.05; **P<0.01;***P<0.001.

ChAT Activity during Development

ChAT activity was investigated *in vitro* as described previously by Fonnum (35) in the brains of rats which were exposed to postnatal anoxia, on days 15,20,40, 90 and 180, in comparison to controls. Fig. 2 shows a gradual decline in the activity of ChAT in both the hippocampus and caudate, a tendency which became more pronounced with further development. The enzymatic decline in activity in the hippocampus was 6% below control at 15 days of life and 20% at 180 days of age. In contrast, and already at 15 days of age, a 20% reduction in enzymatic activity was found in the the caudate of the anoxia group, which further fell to 35% below control at 90 days of age. Generally speaking, a long lasting decline in ChAT activity, expressed as a lower rate of acetylcholine synthesis, could be demonstrated in two brain areas of rats exposed to postnatal anoxia. The more pronounced effect in the caudate could be explained on the basis of its earlier ontogenetic maturation (36-38) and therefore greater vulnerability to anoxia. We assume that decreased levels of released acetylcholine, during development and maturity, could cause a compensatory increase in postsynaptic receptors, hyperkinesis and learning deficits, all these being changes found in the anoxia rats during their development.

[^{3}H] Choline Uptake during Development

[^{3}H] Choline uptake into brain synaptosomes was carried out in vitro by the method of Yamamura and Snyder (39) in the hippocampus of rats exposed postnatally to anoxia at 10,15,20,30,40 and 60 days of age, in comparison to controls. In contrast to ChAT activity, we could demonstrate an increase in choline uptake in the anoxia group which reached peak values around 40 days of life [50% potentiation in relation to controls (Fig. 3)]. This tendency declined to 25% but still persisted up to 60 days of life. High affinity sodium-dependent choline uptake is known to be the rate limiting step in the synthesis of acetylcholine (40). It reflects the actual activity of cholinergic neurons (41) in adjusting to the demands for the rate of acetylcholine turnover (41). The rate of choline uptake is also very much affected by the actual amount of neurotransmitter in the nerve (42). We assume that low acetylcholine levels resulting from

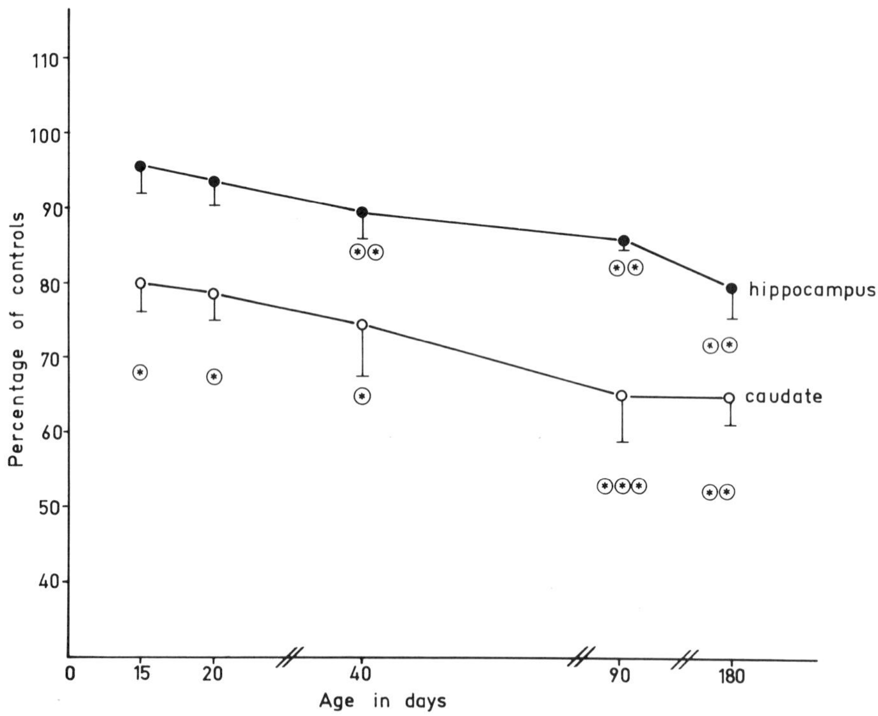

Fig. 2. ChAT activity during development in hippocampus and caudate of rats exposed to postnatal anoxia. The values presented are the relative ChAT activity in the anoxia group expressed as percent of control. Each point represents mean value ± S.E.M. of at least 15 animals. (*P< 0.05; **P<0.01; ***P<0.001; by two tailed Student's t-test).

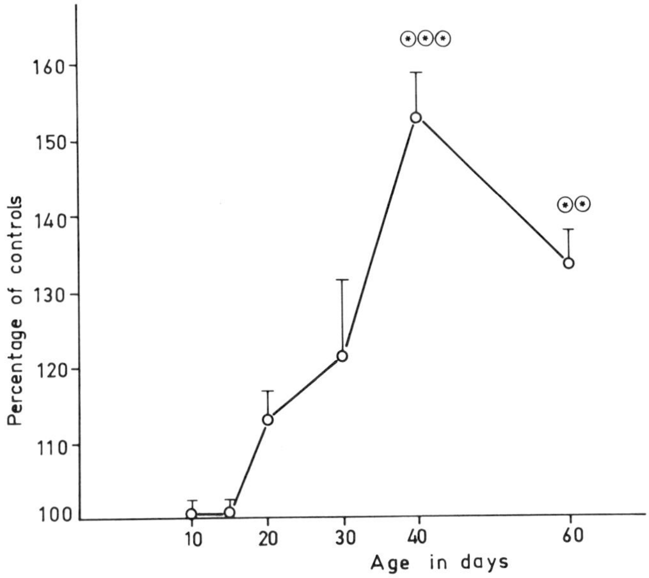

Fig. 3. $[^3H]$ Choline uptake during development in hippocampus of rats exposed to postnatal anoxia. The values presented are the relative uptake in the anoxia group expressed as percent of control. Each point represents mean values ± S.E.M. of at least 20 animals (**P<0.01; ***P<0.001; by two tailed Student's t-test).

low ChAT activity in the anoxia rats are compensated by an increase in $[^3H]$ choline uptake in order to maintain normal levels of neurotransmitter. This phenomenon could explain both the return to normal behavior, and the concomitant decrease in the density of postsynaptic receptors to normal levels, at the age of six weeks. It can be seen, however, that the compensatory increase in choline uptake decreases with time and therefore may not provide full balance to a declining ChAT activity with age, thus resulting in cholinergic deficit later in life.

CONCLUSIONS

1. Single exposure of rats to postnatal anoxia caused a long lasting dysfunction of the cholinergic system as expressed by a gradual decline in ChAT activity throughout development and maturity.

2. The decline in ChAT activity which is presently found in the hippocampus and caudate is probably not restricted to these two areas. We assume that other cholinergic areas in the brain are also affected by anoxia.

3. The first compensatory response to decreased levels of acetylcholine is the increase in density of postsynaptic muscarinic receptors, which maturate relatively earlier than the presynaptic enzymes. With further development, however, a compensatory increase in choline uptake was found with return to normal behavior and a decrease in postsynaptic receptor density to normal values.

4. One can assume that a lack of a compensatory increase in choline uptake in some brain areas other than the hippocampus, or its decline with age, can cause severe dysfunction of the cholinergic system, especially in old age.

5. Anoxia subjected rats may therefore serve as a model for Alzheimer disease in which there is a dysfunction of the central cholinergic system.

AKNOWLEDGEMENT

The investigation was supported by the Recanati Fund for Medical Research and the Andy Lebach Chair of Clinical Pharmacology and Toxicology provided to S.G.

REFERENCES

1. Z. Speiser, A.D. Korczyn, I. Teplitzky and S. Gitter, Hyperactivity in rats following postnatal anoxia, Beh. Brain Res. 7:379 (1983).
2. M. Hershkowitz, V.E. Grimm and Z. Speiser, The effects of postnatal anoxia on behavior and on the muscarinic and beta adrenergic receptors in the hippocampus of the developing rat, Develop. Brain Res. 7:147 (1983).
3. G.E. Gibson and J.P. Blass, Impaired synthesis of acetylcholine in brain accompanying mild hypoxia and hypoglycemia, J. Neurochem. 27:37 (1976).
4. G.E. Gibson and T.E. Duffy, Impaired synthesis of acetylcholine by mild hypoxic hypoxia or nitrous oxide, J. Neurochem. 36:28 (1981).
5. R.W. Russell, Cholinergic system in behavior: The search for mechanisms of action, Ann. Rev. Pharmacol. Toxicol. 22:435 (1982).
6. B.A. Campbell, L.D. Lyttle and H.C. Fibiger, Ontogeny of adrenergic arousal and cholinergic inhibitory mechanisms in the rat, Science 146:635 (1969).
7. J. Altman, R.I. Brunner and S.A. Bayer, The hippocampus and behavioral maturation, Behav. Biol. 8:557 (1973).
8. D.M. Warburton and K. Brown, The facilitation of discrimination performance by physostigmine sulphate, Psychopharmacologia 27:275 (1972).
9. P.D. Mabry and B.A. Campbell, Serotonergic inhibition of catecholamine induced behavioral arousal, Brain Res. 49:381 (1973).
10. H.C. Fibiger, L.D. Lyttle and B.A. Campbell, Cholinergic modulation of adrenergic arousal in the developing rat, J. Comp. Physiol. Phychol. 72:384 (1970).
11. B.A. Campbell and P.D. Mabry, The role of catecholamines in the behavioral arousal during ontogenesis, Psychopharmacologia 31:253 (1973).
12. W.H. Moorcraft, Ontogeny of forebrain inhibition of behavioral arousal, Brain Res. 35:513 (1971).
13. S.T. Mason and H.C. Fibiger, Interaction between noradrenergic and cholinergic systems in the rat brain: Behavioral function in locomotor activity, Neuroscience 4:517 (1979).
14. S.T. Mason, Pilocarpine: Noradrenergic mechanism of a cholinergic drug, Neuropharmacology 17:105 (1978).
15. R.N. Leaton and R.H. Rech, Locomotor activity increases produced by intrahippocampal and intraseptal atropine in rats, Physiol. Behav. 8:539 (1972).
16. S.L. Hartgrave and P.H. Kelly, Role of mesencephalic reticular formation in cholinergic-induced catalepsy and anticholinergic reversal of neuroleptic induced catalepsy, Brain Res. 307:47 (1984).

17. G.N.O. Brito, J.B. Davis, L.C. Stopp and M.E. Stanton, Memory and the septo-hippocampal cholinergic system in the rat, Psychopharmacology 81:315 (1983).
18. D. Blozovski and N. Hennocq, Effects of antimuscarinic cholinergic drugs injected systemically or into the hippocampus-entorhinal area upon passive avoidance learning in young rats, Psychopharmacology 76:351 (1982).
19. C.M. Baratti, P. Huygens, J. Mino, A. Marlo and J. Gardella, Memory facilitator with posttrial injection of oxotremorine and physostigmine in mice, Psychopharmacology 64:85 (1979).
20. A.C. Cuello and M.V. Sofroniew, The anatomy of the CNS cholinergic neurons, TINS 7:74 (1984).
21. B.T. Hyman, G.W. Van Hoesen, A.R. Damasio and C.L. Barnes, Alzheimer's Disease: Cell-specific pathology isolates the hippocampal formation, Science 225:1168 (1984).
22. D. Kimble, The effect of bilateral hippocampal lesions, J. Comp. Physiol. Psychol. 56:273 (1963).
23. G.S. Lynch, G. Rose and C.M. Gall, Anatomical aspects of the septo-hippocampal projections in functions of the septo-hippocampal system, Elsevier Exerpta Medica, Holland, (1978).
24. L.W. Swanson, The anatomical organization of septo-hippocampal formation (with a note on the connections to septum and hypothalamus) in functions of septo-hippocampal systems, Elsevier Exerpta Medica, Holland, (1978).
25. L.W. Swanson and M.W. Cowan, Hippocampo-hypothalamic connections: Origin in subicular cortex not Ammons's Horn, Science 189:303 (1975).
26. J.F. De France, J.E. Marchand, J.C. Stanley and R.W. Silzes, Convergence of excitatory amygdaloid and hippocampal input in the nucleus accumbens, Septi, Brain Res. 185:183 (1980).
27. J.F. De France, M. Yoshikara, Fimbria input to the nucleus accumbens, Septi. Brain Res. 90:159 (1975).
28. C. Kim, H. Choi, J.K. Kim, R.S. Park and I.Y. Kang, General behavioral activity and its component patterns in hippocampectomized rats, Brain Res. 19:379 (1970).
29. D.P. Kimble, The effect of bilateral hippocampal lesion in rats, J. Comp. Physiol. Psychol. 56:273 (1963).
30. C.B. Sengstake, Habituation and activity patterns of rats with large hippocampal lesions under various drive conditions, J. Comp. Physiol. Psychol. 65:504 (1968).
31. L.E. Jarrard, Behavior of hippocampal lesioned rats in home cage and novel situation, Physiol. Behav. 3:65 (1968).
32. P.N. Strong and W.Y. Jackson, Effect of hippocampal lesions in rats on three measures of activity, J. of Compar. Physiolog. Psychol. 70:60 (1975).
33. B.A. Campbell, P. Ballantine and G. Lynch, Hippocampal control of behavior arousal: Duration of lesion effects and possible interactions with recovery after frontal cortical damage, Exp. Neurol. 33:159 (1971).
34. R.W. Russell and J. Macri, Central cholinergic involvement in behavioral hyperreactivity, Pharmacol. Biochem. Behav. 10:43 (1979).
35. F. F. Fonnum, A rapid radiochemical method for the determination of choline acetyltransferase, J. Neurochemistry 24:407 (1975).
36. J.V. Nadler, D.A. Mathews, C.W. Cotman and G.S. Lynch, Development of cholinergic innervation in the hippocampal formation of the rat, Develop. Biol. 36:142 (1974).
37. M.J. Kuhar, N.J.M. Birdsall, A.S.V. Burgen and E.C. Hullme, Ontogeny of muscarinic receptors in rat brain, Brain Res. 184:375 (1980).
38. J.T. Coyle and H.I. Yamamura, Neurochemical aspects of the ontogenesis of cholinergic neurons in the rat brain, Brain Res. 118:429 (1976).

39. H. I. Yamamura and S.H. Snyder, High affinity uptake of choline into synaptosomes of rat brain, _J. Neurochem._ 21:1355 (1973).
40. M.J. Kuhar and L.Ch. Murrin, Sodium dependent high affinity choline uptake, _J. Neurochem._ 30:15 (1978).
41. S. Atweh, J.R. Simon and M.J. Kuhar, Utilization of sodium dependent high affinity choline uptake in vitro as a measure of the activity of cholinergic neurons in vitro, _Life Sci._ 17:1535 (1975).
42. D.R. Haubrich and Th.J. Chippendale, Regulation of acetylcholine synthesis in nervous tissue, _Life Sci._ 20:1465 (1977).

IMPLANTATION OF ALZHEIMER'S DISEASE BRAIN TISSUE IN YOUNG RAT BRAIN : PARENCHYMAL AND VASCULAR REACTIONS

Ph. van den Bosch de Aguilar[1], Ph. Janssens de Varebeke[2], F. De Paermentier[2]

1. Laboratoire de Biologie Cellulaire, Université Catholique de Louvain, Belgium
2. Continental Pharma Inc., Belgium

The loss of cerebral neurones is a significant feature of the aging process in man (1) macaques (2) and rodents (3). The extent and severity of this loss varies amongst species and from region to region in the brain.

In Alzheimer's-Type Dementia (AD) neuronal loss is exacerbated (4) with the loss mainly located in the frontal and temporal cortical lobes and the hippocampus (5). Currently, the causes of neuronal death in the aging brain of those with the pathological conditions of AD, are largely unknown. By its manifestations AD might appear to be a dramatic exaggeration of aging but the distinctions between "normal" and "pathological" aging are not precisely defined.

It has been suggested that the evolution of AD is associated with specific deficiencies in cortical and hippocampal cholinergic innervation, leading to losses of neurons in the septal nucleus and the nucleus basalis of Meynert (6, 7). Other factors may play a part in the disease, including unconventional infectious agents (8) and decreases or absences of specific neurotrophic activity (9).

Recently attempts have been made to establish the transmissibility of AD by inoculation of AD brain homogenates into monkey cortex (10).

In this study, two models have been investigated which could provide a new approach for the study of the inducing process responsible for aging and AD. The first model relied on the implantation of young, old and AD human brain tissue into cavities prepared in the cerebral cortex of young rats. The second model involved the injection of human brain homogenates into rat cerebral ventricles.

Under these conditions, it was considered that some factor(s) present in the implant or in the homogenate might act on the host brain tissue to induce changes resembling those of AD. In these models, both parenchymal and vascular reactions were analyzed. Additionally, the effects of suloctidil on cerebrovascular changes were examined. Suloctidil is an antispasmodic agent which has been shown to significantly improve subjective and objective indices of cognitive and other functions in AD patients (11).

MATERIALS AND METHODS

Ten week old male Wistar rats were used as host animals. Temporal cortex tissues were sampled post-mortem from brains of two AD patients (79 and 82 years old), two healthy aged individuals (65 and 84 years old), and two healthy young individuals (3 and 34 years old). "normal" subjects had died without any apparent neurological symptoms. The clinical diagnoses were confirmed post-mortem histopathologically. Senile plaques and tangles were identified in both old and AD brains, but with a higher incidence noted in the latter.

For implantation into the rat cortex, the brain samples were sliced into small fragments (1 mm3). These were inserted into a cavity (1.5 mm diameter) made by aspiration of tissue in the rat cortex occipital area (12). The same procedure without implantation was used for the sham-operated animals.

The brain samples pooled according to the donor's categories were homogenized and sonicated for 15 seconds. The homogenates were centrifuged (2 min at 3.000 x g) and the supernatant discarded from the pellet. Thirty microliters of the pellet were slowly injected (injection time : 10 min) through a stereotaxically fixed Hamilton syringe into the right ventricle. During the operation rats were anaesthetized by an i.m. injection of Hypnorm ®.

Following either procedure, rats were sacrificed under ether anaesthesia 7, 14, 21 and 28 days (n = 5 per time) after the operation by an intra-aortic perfusion of the Karnowsky fixative mixture (13). The brain was removed from the skull and selected area were routinely processed for light and electron microscopic studies. Cellular counts were made on semi-thin sections stained by toluidine blue. Sections of cortex and hippocampus from the ipsi-and contralateral side of the injection were taken at random among the serial sections made in these structures. Cells were counted on randomly chosen fields by two independent neurohistologists unaware of treatments administrated.

The microvascularisation that appeared around the prepared cavity after a few days was quantified. The vascular network was visualised by perfusion of Ilford L4 nuclear emulsion diluted 1/3 (V/V) in warm water (14). Serial sections (100 μm) of the brain performed with a vibratome were developed in D19 (Kodak) and fixed in 20 % Na thiosulfate. No counterstain was used. Morphometric study of the vascular network was made with using a planimeter (MOP - digiplan).

MATERIALS AND METHODS

For the drug studies, suloctidil (30 mg/kg, 2x daily) was administered 3 days before surgical aspiration of brain tissue and 4 days after, at which time the animals were sacrificed. Microvascularisation in the region adjacent to the lesion site was compared.

RESULTS AND DISCUSSION

1. Cavity without implantation

When a cavity was made by aspiration in the occipital cortex, the lesion induced a parenchymal and a vascular reaction.

The parenchymal reaction was characterized by some cellular necrosis at the vicinity of the cavity and the classically described astrocytic gliosis. Seven days after the lesion, astrocyte processes and dilated

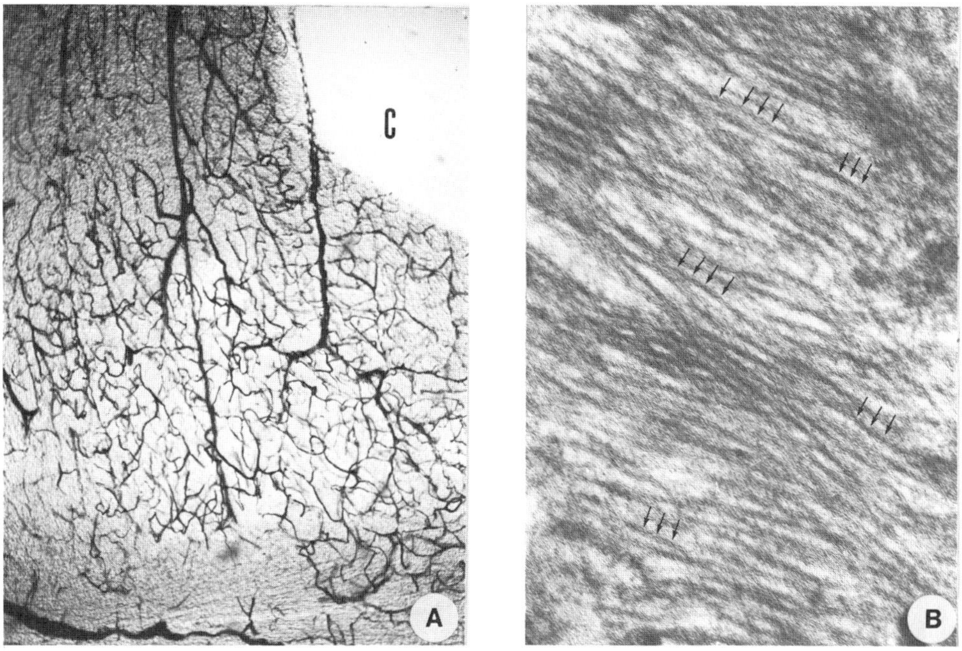

Fig. 1A : Nuclear emulsion perfused vascular network at the periphery of a cavity (C) in the rat occipital cortex (100 x).
Fig. 1B : Twisted filaments (arrows) in reactive astrocyte process after implantation of AD brain tissue (50,000 x).

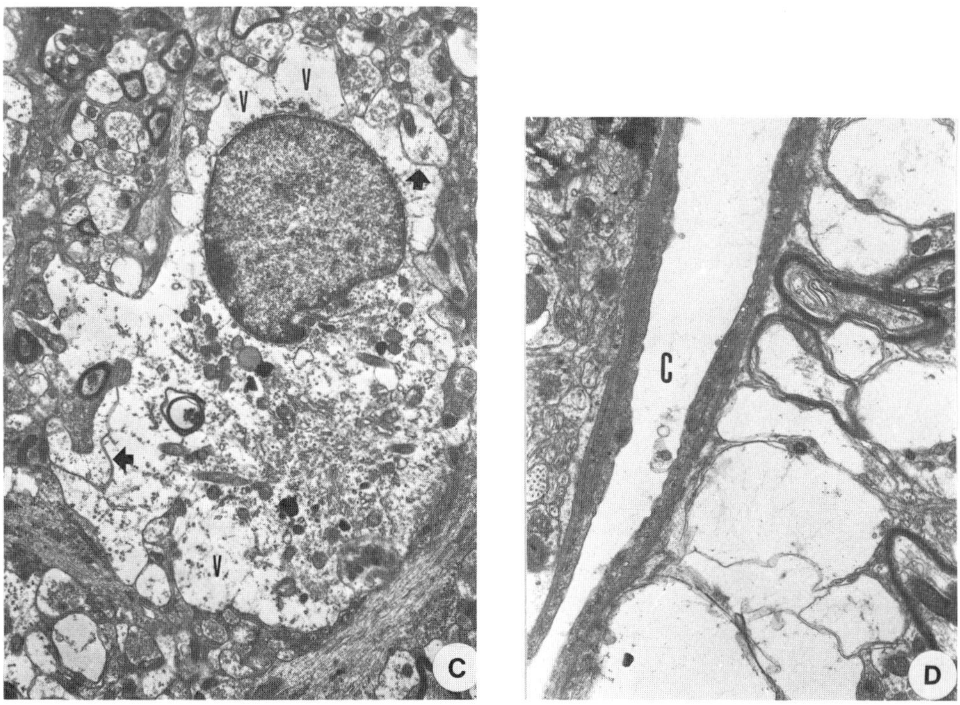

Fig. 1C : Spongiform necrotic neuron with extensive vacuolisation (V) and multilaminated membranes (arrows) (4,000 x).
Fig. 1D : Impaired astrocyte processes at the periphery of a capillary (C) (18,000 x).

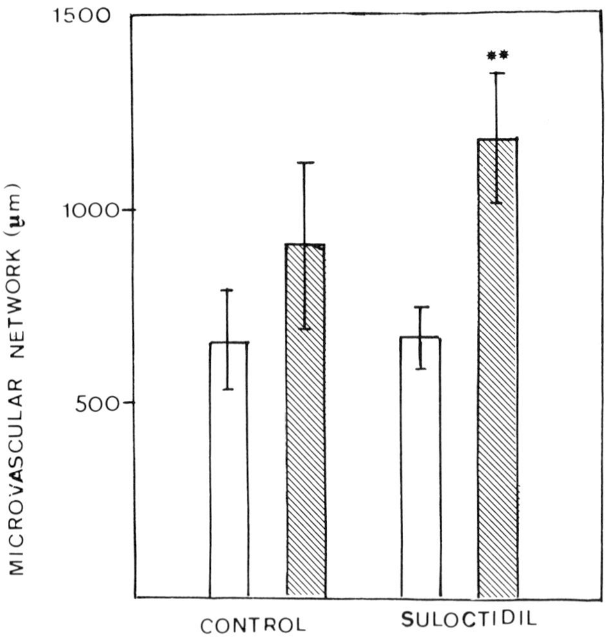

FIG. 2 Microvascular network around the cavity in the rat cerebral cortex (means ± SD, n=4) 4 days after the operation. The open columns correspond to the values obtained in the contralateral cerebral cortex and the dashed columns to those obtained in the cortex around the cavity. 30 mg/kg of suloctidil was administered twice a day for 7 days.** $p < 0.01$ when the two dashed columns were compared using the three ways ANOVA statistical analysis.

capillaries invaded the periphery of the cavity and formed a spongy tissue containing some macrophages. These reactions ended two weeks after the operation and the tissue restoration was completed by the phagocytotic action of the macrophages and astrocytes which eliminated the haemorrhage and cellular debris. Subsequently, the restored meninges closed the upper part of the cavity and the gliovascular reaction did not progress further, leaving a hole in the center of the cavity (16).

After vascular perfusion of the nuclear emulsion (L4) (Fig. 1A), morphometric studies indicated 37 % increase of the vascular network in the vicinity of the cavity compared to the contralateral side on the same slide (Fig. 2).

Suloctidil was shown to promote this cerebral vascular proliferation. Previously, chronic administration of suloctidil had been shown to produce an increase in the density of capillaries in skeletal muscle (17). In the current studies, suloctidil was administered to rat (30 mg/kg p.o. twice a day ; 3 days before the lesion and 4 days after, at which time the animals were sacrificed. The increase in the vascular density reached 41 % compared to the placebo group (Fig. 2). Moreover, treatment with suloctidil favored tissue repair (49 % increase) as indicated by the reduction of the cavity areas.

Two alternatives exist in order to explain the restoration process after lesion. First, it has been reported that brain injury caused an increase in the levels of neuron survival promoting factors close to the lesion area (18, 19). The second possibility is that the reaction to injury involved release of angiogenesic factors which could contribute to the tissue repair (20).

2. Implantations in the cavity

Implantation of small fragments of old and AD brain tissue into the rat host occipital cortex did not induce significant cellular necrosis up to 1 month after the operation. At this time, the implanted human brain was totally destroyed and, in the case of AD, only residual tangles could be identified in the cavity. The host cortical reaction was morphologically similar to that described above for the cavity alone. Nevertheless, some important variations were observed. A greater invasion of macrophages occured seven days after the operation. The astrocytic reaction was more intense and glial filament synthesis was obviously increased. Electron microscopy revealed in the case of AD but not "normal" tissue that some processes of astrocytes close to the cavity contained among their filament bundles numerous twisted filaments similar to the tangles associated with AD in man (16) (Fig. 1B).

3. Administration in the ventricles

Intraventricular injections of young, old and AD brain tissue homogenates induced cellular necrosis in the young rat cortex seven days after their administration. Two types of necrosis were identified. In the first type of necrotic cells, the cytoplasm became homogenous, and the cell membranes was shrinken. Mitochondria were swollen, and intracellular membrane systems had become distorted, containing often flocullent dense material. This type of necrosis essentially affected neurones.

The second type of cellular necrosis was characterized by severe vacuolisation of the cytoplasm and a deposit of tufty material between the vacuoles (Fig. 1C). Cell membranes were destroyed in numerous places opening communications between the cell and the extracellular space. One striking feature seen in these cells was the formation of multilaminated membranes, consisting of numerous parallel laminae over variable distances.

The presence of synaptic junctions allowed to identify neurons, and the large deposit of aggregated filaments characterized astrocytes. In the neuropile, empty destroyed cell processes appeared among well preserved processes. Impaired astrocyte processes were particularly abundant at the periphery of the capillaries (Fig. 1D). The extension of these alterations gave to the cerebral tissue a typical spongiform aspect.

In order to discrimate the action of the different homogenates used, a quantification of the cellular necrosis was performed on cortex and hippocampus semi-thin sections. As the injection procedure itself might induce necrosis, the necrotic cells were counted in the contralateral brain structures at the same level as that of the site of injection. Results in Figure 3 show that necrosis in the rat brain was induced by injection of human brain homogenates regardless of the age and the pathological condition of the donor. However the extend of the necrosis was significantly increased when old and AD brain samples are compared to the young. This was particularly true for the spongiform type of lesion. The degree of necrosis shows that the hippocampus was more susceptible to the alteration than the cortex.

Thus, using this model, we are able to induce in young rats some important characteristic alterations of the AD brain.

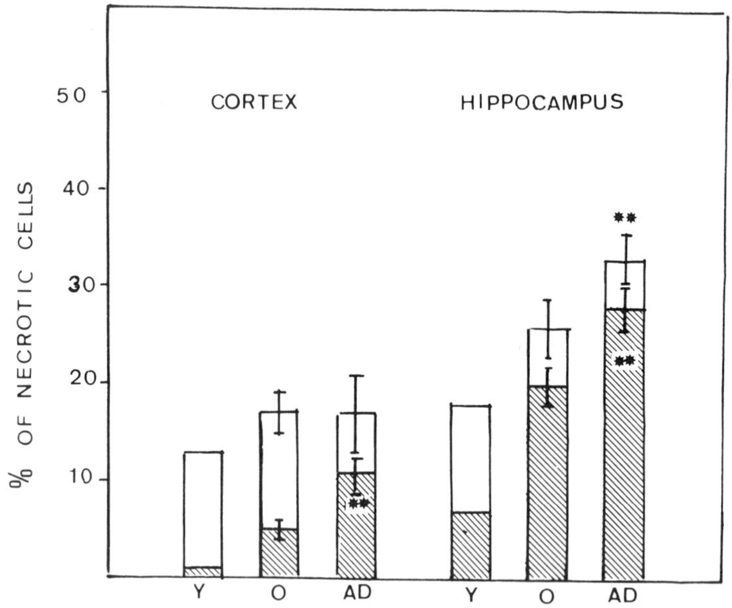

Fig. 3. Total cellular necrosis (whole columns) including spongiform necrosis (dashed columns) in the rat hippocampus and cortex seven days after intraventricular injection or homogenates from young (Y, n=2), old (O, n=5) and AD (n=4) human brain tissue. Results are expressed as mean ± S.D. of the number of necrotic cells in the total amount of cells counted over five microscopic fields for each cerebral area. Student's t test : AD vs. O (** = $p < 0.01$). Measurements of the necrotic cells were realized in the contralateral brain structures at the same level than the side of the injection.

CONCLUSIONS

A major problem in planning research into the pathogenesis and treatment of AD is the absence of a fully satisfactory animal model. In this study, we investigated the action of an implant on its host cortical environment. At the tissue level, three reactions are observed in the vicinity of the cavity : necrosis of lesioned neurons at the periphery of the cavity, gliosis of astrocytes and restoration of vascular network. The restoration phenomenon is sustained by the activity of one or more neurotrophic substances released at the periphery of the lesion by neurons, astrocytes and/or vessels (19). These substances are also probably the biological supports of the brain plasticity and the present model could provide a simple approach to study their actions under various experimental conditions and to identify their nature. The attempt made in this way using suloctidil shows that this substance enhances the cerebral tissue repair probably via its action on growing vessels.

It was observed that implantation of AD brain tissue in a cortical cavity stimulated the fibrous astrocyte glial reaction. This reaction may have been induced by the tangles, since it has been shown in humans that tangles appear to be a strong stimulus for astrocytes when they are not segregated from the environment by the neuronal cell membrane (21).

Implantation of AD brain tissue involves the presence in the host cortex not only of tangles but also probably of some abnormal precursors from which these tangles are built. The endocytosis and metabolisation of these precursors in the processes of the reactive astrocytes and their incorporation into the glial filaments bundles may be the origin of the twisted glial filaments observed. Another possibility is the presence in the implant of some substance responsible for the tangle formation which may interfere with the normal building of glial filaments.

It should be pointed out that implantations of old or AD human, as well as young or old rat nervous tissues, never induces an increase of necrosis in the surrounding cortex of young rats (VAN DEN BOSCH DE AGUILAR, unpublished results).

In the case of intraventricular injection, the lesion is very limited and gliovascular reaction does not occur. Cellular necrosis was abundant and its extent increased with the donor's age and the involvement of AD. The spongiform aspect of the brain is characteristic of old brain tissue. This was particularly marked in the AD case. Cellular vacuolisation has been reported in numerous cases of AD (22) in normal old rat brain (23), in old mice (24), and after intracerebrally inoculation of brain suspension from kuru patients in monkey brain and after experimental Creutzfeld-Jakob disease and scrapie in mice and hamsters (25).

According to BECK (25) the brain status spongiosus and the occurence of multilaminated membranes are very similar in all these cases of transmissibles encephalopathies. We observed the same pictures after administration of old and AD brain homogenates.

It is tempting to speculate that the same cytotoxic substance (or substances)exerts its actions during physiological aging, as well as during phathological aging and in the case of transmissible encephalopathies. The nature of this activity remains to be elucidated. A preliminary study in our laboratory showed that injection of homogenates of rat brain tissue that has been previously implanted with grafts from AD patients into young rat occipital cortexes induces the same alterations in the host that those observed previously in the donor. However, the time of "incubation" is longer (3 to 4 months) and can perhaps be attributable to the dilution of the cytotoxic substance. In the present model, the action of this substance seems to be non specific, destroying neuronal and glial cells, but some cerebral areas (hippocampus) appears to be more susceptible to its action.

The appearance of cellular necrosis depended on the mode of administration, implantation or injection of the human brain tissue. In both cases the implanted tissue is destroyed. However the same potentially cytotoxic substance was present in the human brain before the two procedures and was released in the cortex. After implantation, the activity of the cytotoxic substance could be antagonized by the phagocytic cells. Another possibility is that the activity of this substance was inhibited by the trophic substances released during the glio-vascular reaction induced by the lesion and was not inhibited after the injection, due to the lack of significant lesion.

In conclusion, the presented evidence supports further studies on brain aging and AD phenomenon in the light of a possible competitive action between neurotrophic substances, supporting the brain plasticity, and cytotoxic substances, reducing progressively the brain neuronal network. In this respect, our intraventricular injection model could provide a valuable tool for further investigations on the pathogenesis of AD.

SUMMARY

This study investigates two models which could provide a new insight for the analysis of the inducing process responsible for the physiological aging and the pathological condition of Alzheimer's disease. After implantation of AD patient's brain tissue in young rat cortex, some astrocyte processes in the vicinity of the implant contain twisted filaments. Injection of human brain homogenates in the ventricles induces cellular necrosis in the cortex and hippocampus. The importance of the necrosis increases with the donor's age. These experiments support the hypothesis that cytotoxic substances are released during aging. This release is enhanced in AD status. Moreover implantation methodology is validated by the study of cavities without implants. In this way the vascular reaction is analysed and the action of suloctidil is tested.

ACKNOWLEDGEMENTS

We are very grateful to Prof. Flament-Durand and Dr. J.P. Brion for the gift of samples of human brain used in this study. We are indebted to P. Heuschling and B. Knoops for the quantification of cellular necrosis. This study was supported in part by grant n° 2.4517-82 from the "Fonds de la Recherche Fondamentale Collective."

REFERENCES

1. Henderson, G., Tomlinson, B.E. and Gibson, P.H. (1980). J. Neurol. Sci., 46 : 113-136.
2. Brizzee, K.R., Ordy, J.M. and Bartus, R.T. (1980). Neurobiol. Aging, 1 : 45-52.
3. Johnson, H.A. and Erner, S. (1972). Exp. Gerontol., 7 : 111-117.
4. Terry, R.D. and Katzman, R. (1983). Am. Neurol., 14 : 497-506.
5. Hyman, B.M., Van Hoesen, G.W., Damasio, A.R. and Barnes, C.L. (1984). Science, 225 : 1168-1170.
6. Whitehouse, P.J., Price, D.L., Struble, R.G., Clark, W., Coyle, J.M. and De Long, M.R. (1982). Science, 215 : 1237-1239.
7. Coyle, J.M., Price, D.L. and De Long, M.R. (1983). Science, 219 : 1184-1190.
8. Prusiner, S.B. (1981). Science, 216 : 136-138.
9. Appel, S.M. (1981). Am. Neurol., 10 : 449-505.
10. Goudsmit, J., Morrow, C.H., Asher, D.M., Yamagihara, R.T., Masters, C.L., Gibbs, C.J., Gajdusek, D.C. (1980). Neurology, 30 : 945-950.
11. Itil, T.M., Mukherjee, S., Michael, S.T., Dayican, G., Shapiro, D.M., Kunitz, A. and Saerens, E. (1983). Psychopharmacol. Bull., 9 : 730-733.
12. Das, G.D., Hallas, B.H. and Das, K.G. (1979). Experientia, 35 : 143-153.
13. Descarries, L. and Schroder, J.M. (1975). J. Microscopie, 7 : 281-286.
14. Van Reempts, J., Hasedonckx, M. and Borgers, M. (1983). Microvascul. Res., 25 : 300-306.
15. Roba, J., Defreyn, G. and Biagi, G. (1983). Thromb. Res. Suppl. 4 : 53-58.
16. Van den Bosch de Aguilar, Ph., Langwendries-Weverbeers, Ch., Goemaere-Vanneste, J., Flament-Durand, J., Brior, J.P. and Couck, A.M. (1984). Experientia, 40 : 402-403.
17. Caddeu, R., Carta, M., Cherchi, R., Pinna, M., Savona, G. and Brotzu, G. (1981). G. Ital. Angiol., 1 : 77-81.

18. Neito-Sampedro, M., Manthorpe, M., Barbin, G., Varon, S. and Cotman, C.W. (1983). J. Neurosci., 3 : 2219-2229.
19. Nieto-Sampedro, M., Whittemore, S.R., Needels, D.L., Larson, J. and Cotman, C.W. (1984). Proc. Natl. Acad. Sci. U.S.A., 81 : 6250-6254.
20. Banda, M.J., Kinghton, D.R., Hunt, T.K. and Werb, F. (1982). Proc. Natl. Acad. Sci. USA, 79 : 7773-7777.
21. Probst, A., Ulrich, J. and Heitz Ph. V. (1982). Acta Neuropath., 57 : 75-79.
22. Flament-Durand, J. and Couck, A.M. (1979). Acta Neuropath., 46 : 159-162.
23. De Estable-Puig, R.F. and De Estable-Puig, J.F. (1975). Virchous Arch. B. Cell Path., 17 : 337-346.
24. Curcio, C.A. and Coleman, P.D. (1982). J. Comp. Neurol., 212 : 158-172.
25. Beck, E., Daniel, P.M., Davey, A.J., Gajdusek, D.C. and Gibbs, C.J. (1982), Brain, 105 : 755-786.

FUNCTIONAL PROPERTIES OF SEPTO-HIPPOCAMPAL NEURONS IN THE RAT

Y. Lamour, P. Dutar and A. Jobert

Unité de Recherches de Neurophysiologie Pharmacologique
INSERM (U. 161)
2 rue d'Alésia, 75014 Paris (France)

INTRODUCTION

The septo-hippocampal pathway is one of the best characterized central cholinergic pathways[1]. It provides a convenient preparation for studying the central cholinergic system. This pathway is probably not purely cholinergic. The proportion of cholinergic neurons among the septo-hippocampal neurons (SHNs) is of 30 to more than 80% depending on the techniques and the area investigated[2,3,4]. The purpose of the present series of experiments was to analyse the properties of the SHNs and to try to characterize various subpopulations among these neurons. We studied SHNs in the anaesthetized rat, using extra and intracellular techniques and microiontophoresis. These neurons were located in the vertical limb of the nucleus of the diagonal band of Broca and in the medial septum (MS-nDBB). They were identified by the electrical antidromic stimulation of their axons within the fimbria. Parts of the present results have already been published[5].

MATERIAL AND METHODS

Extracellular Recordings

Male Sprague-Dawley albino rats (200-300 gr) were anaesthetized with urethane (1.5 g/kg i.p.) or chloral hydrate (450 mg/kg i.p.). Two stimulating electrodes were positioned in the fimbria on each side of the midline. Antidromic responses to fimbria stimulation (square pulses of 0.2 msec, 40 to 800 uA) were identified using the collision test. Other criteria were also used (fixed latency and ability to follow high rates of stimulation). Conventional amplification methods were used to record neuronal activity from micropipettes filled with 1M NaCl and 2% pontamine sky blue.

Intracellular Recordings

In vivo intracellular recordings were obtained from SHNs, using glass micropipettes filled with KCl 3M in animals anaesthetized with either pentobarbital (40 mg/kg i.p. initially, supplemented i.v. during the experiment) or urethane (2 g/kg i.p.). Tips (< 1 um diameter) were bevelled immediately before use in order to obtain 20-60 MΩ resistances. Current injections were performed through the bridge circuit of a DC preamplifier (WPI M707).

Effect of Peripheral Stimulation

In this series of experiments, animals were anaesthetized with either urethane (1.5 g/kg or 2 g/kg i.p.) or fluothane (halothane 0.75% in a mixture of 1/3 O_2, 2/3 N_2O). Rats ventilated spontaneously under urethane anaesthesia whereas they were paralyzed with an i.v. infusion of gallamine triethiodide (Flaxedil) and artificially ventilated under fluothane. The level of anaesthesia was checked using an electrocorticogram.

When a SHN was identified, its response to peripheral somatic stimulation was investigated. The peripheral receptive field (RF) was defined, using non-noxious and noxious mechanical and thermal stimulation. When a SHN was excited by a noxious mechanical stimulus, its response to thermal stimulation was investigated using a hot water bath applied on the RF. Intraperitoneal bradykinin injections were also performed.

Microiontophoresis Experiments

Animals were anaesthetized with urethane (1.5 g/kg i.p.). For microiontophoresis the recording micropipette was rigidly attached to the side of a multibarreled pipette (tip diameter 8-10 µm) filled with solutions for testing by iontophoresis. Automatic current balancing was routinely used.

The final recording site of each penetration was marked with a dye deposit (20 µA for 20 min). At the end of the experiment, the animal was perfused through the heart with saline followed by a solution of 10% formaldehyde in saline. Frozen 100 µm thick sections of the whole brain were cut and stained with cresyl violet. Electrode penetrations were reconstructed on camera lucida drawings of these sections.

RESULTS

The present report is based on the study of 652 SHNs recorded under various conditions of anaesthesia. They were located in the medial region of the septum, including the medial septal nucleus (MS) and the nucleus of the diagonal band of Broca (nDBB), mostly its vertical limb.

Spontaneous Activity

The mean ($\pm$ SEM) spontaneous activity of the SHNs, under urethane anaesthesia, was 20.3 $\pm$ 1.2 impulses per second. Under these experimental conditions, 45% of the SHNs had a characteristic mode of discharge in rhythmic bursts. The burst frequency was 3-6 Hz (Fig. 1). Each burst lasted about 50-200 ms with 2 to 18 spikes. A few SHNs were able to switch from a non-bursting to a bursting mode of discharge, or vice-versa. Appearance of a rhythmic bursting activity was sometimes observed in a non-bursting SHN following strong mechanical peripheral stimulation.

Antidromic Latency and Conduction Velocity

The mean latency of antidromic activation following fimbria

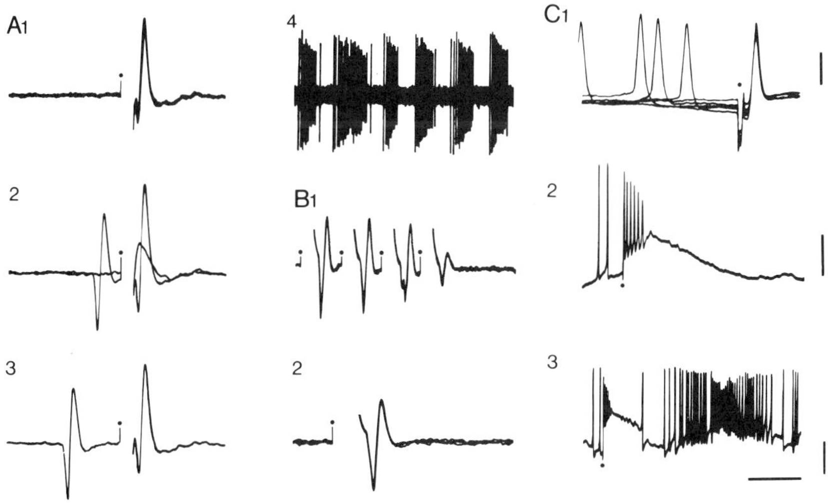

Fig. 1. Examples of septo-hippocampal neurons.
A. Antidromic response of a SHN to fimbria stimulation (latency : 0.6 msec). 1: 4 superimposed traces. Star indicates stimulus artifact. 2: 2 traces (one antidromic response and one trace with collision between a spontaneous orthodromic spike and the antidromic spike). 3: 2 traces. Lack of collision. 4: Spontaneous rhythmically bursting pattern of discharge at about 3 Hz.
B. Another SHN (Latency: 1.4 msec). 1: 1 trace. High frequency following (300 Hz). 2: 3 traces. Antidromic response.
C. Intracellular recording of a septo-hippocampal neuron (pentobarbital anaesthesia). Vertical calibration bar: 20 mV. 1: Antidromic response (latency: 0.6 msec, five superimposed traces). 2: Fimbria stimulation. Chloride dependent potential recorded a few minutes after cell penetration (KCl filled pipette). This potential was initially in the hyperpolarizing direction and reversed polarity. Notice the burst of spikes on the initial phase of this reversed IPSP. 3: Effect of fimbria stimulation photographed at slower sweep speeds. The depolarizing potential which follows the reversed IPSP is clearly visible. Time scale: A 1,2,3, 2.5 msec ; A4, 500 msec ; B1, 5 msec ; B2, 2.5 msec ; C1, 5 msec; C2, 50 msec ; C3, 125 msec.

stimulation under urethane anaesthesia, was 2.3 $\pm$ 0.2 ms (range 0.5 - 18 ms, n = 254) (Fig. 1). The vast majority of the SHNs were however driven from the fimbria at less than 2 ms. The mean conduction velocity was 1.5 m/s. If only SHNs driven at less than 2 ms are taken into account, then the mean conduction velocity would be between 2.5 and 3 m/s.

Intracellular Recordings

Intracellular recordings were obtained from 42 SHNs, with membrane potentials of -40 to -60 mV. Spontaneous synaptic activity mostly consisted in EPSPs of 1 to 4 mV and also in some hyperpolarizing potentials.

Electrical stimulation of the fimbria evoked, beside the antidromic response, a complex sequence of synaptic potentials. Initial depolarizing synaptic potentials (EPSPs) were present in most cases. These EPSPs rarely evoked spikes. They had a mean latency of 2 msec. Hyperpolarizing potentials following fimbria stimulation were observed in all SHNs with a mean latency of 6.3 msec. They were accompanied by an average 33% increase in membrane conductance. The hyperpolarizing potential reversed polarity in a few minutes following cell penetration. These potentials are likely to be IPSPs since they could be observed in the absence of a preceding spike, reversed polarity in a chloride-dependent fashion and were associated with a suppression of spontaneous firing. The IPSPs were, in some SHNs, followed by a long lasting depolarizing potential. A burst of spikes occured often during this potential. This long lasting depolarization occured also when the polarity of the IPSP was reversed. This sequence of synaptic events could also be observed in extracellular recordings: fimbria stimulation induced a sequence of inhibition followed by an excitatory rebound in most SHNs.

Responses to Peripheral Stimulation

A majority of SHNs (68%, n= 155), regardless of the conditions of anaesthesia, were driven by natural peripheral stimulation. In most cases the units were not driven by light cutaneous stimulation but only by strong, noxious mechanical or thermal stimulations (Fig. 2).

Nine neurons only were driven by non-noxious stimulation. The most frequent receptive field (RF) observed comprised the two hindlimbs and the tail (45%). The next frequent type of RF comprised the whole body (38%). RFs located on the ipsi- or contralateral hindlimb were much less frequent (14%). RFs restricted to the tail were rare (1 case). The nature of the stimulus driving the SHNs was difficult to define, i.e. it could not be clearly identified as superficial or deep. The most efficient stimulus was usually a pinch applied on the paws and/or the tail. In most cases the neuronal response to peripheral stimulation was an excitation. In a few cases (8% of the SHNs responsive to peripheral stimulation), an inhibition was observed. In about one-third of the cases (27 out of 81 SHNs under urethane anaesthesia), the response was associated with the accentuation or the appearance of a rhythmic bursting activity. In most cases, the responses to intense mechanical stimulation outlasted the period of stimulation. Increasing the strength of the mechanical stimulation resulted in an increase in the amplitude and duration of the response. These responses could be observed in the absence of any ECoG change.

Forty SHNs were tested for their response to thermal stimulation (hot water bath applied on the tail). They were not responsive to non-noxious thermal stimulation. The threshold for response was between 46°C and 48°C. Responses were excitatory in 29 cases (72%), and inhibitory in 3 cases. Thus the majority (80%) of the SHNs tested were responsive to noxious thermal stimulation.

Microiontophoresis Experiments

Acetylcholine (ACh) excited 70% of the SHNs, whereas 29% were unaffected and only 1% inhibited. This excitation had typically a

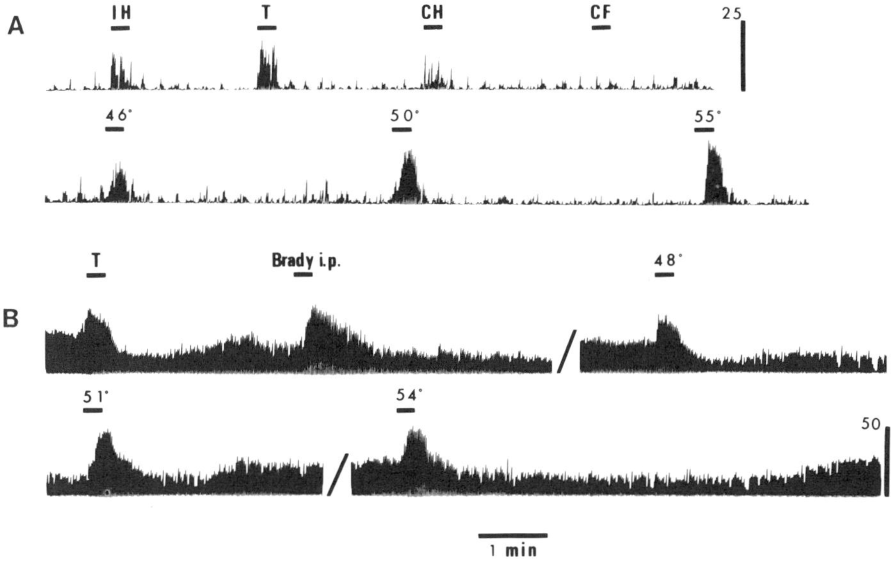

Fig. 2. A. SHN (urethane 2 g/kg i.p.) excited by a pinch applied to ipsilateral hindpaw (IH), tail (T), contralateral hindpaw (CH), but not contralateral forepaw (CF). This SHN was also excited by noxious heat (bottom row). Notice the clear relation between temperature and amplitude of the neuronal response.
B. SHN (urethane 1.5 g/kg i.p.) excited by a pinch applied on the tail (T), by i.p. bradykinin injection (Brady) and by noxious heat. Notice that responses to tail pinch and noxious heat were biphasic.

relatively long latency (several seconds) and long duration. The ACh-induced excitation was prolonged by physostigmine (Fig. 3), readily abolished by atropine but rarely by nicotinic antagonists such as hexamethonium or mecamylamine. Carbachol was, by far, the most potent cholinergic agonist tested. It induced strong, prolonged excitations of SHNs even with low currents. Muscarinic agonists were active on a larger proportion of SHNs than nicotinic agonists. They induced excitatory effects. Inhibitory effects were rarely observed.

Excitatory amino-acids (such as glutamic acid, aspartic acid, homocysteic acid) induced excitations of SHNs. GABA induced strong inhibitions of their spontaneous activity, even when applied with low currents.

Substance P and TRH excited respectively 8 out of 18 and 47 out of 109 SHNs. Responses had a long duration and could be obtained with low currents. Responses to TRH were not abolished by atropine.

DISCUSSION

The present series of experiments is, to our knowledge, the first systematic study of identified septo-hippocampal neurons. Several conclusions can be drawn from our observations. The first conclusion is

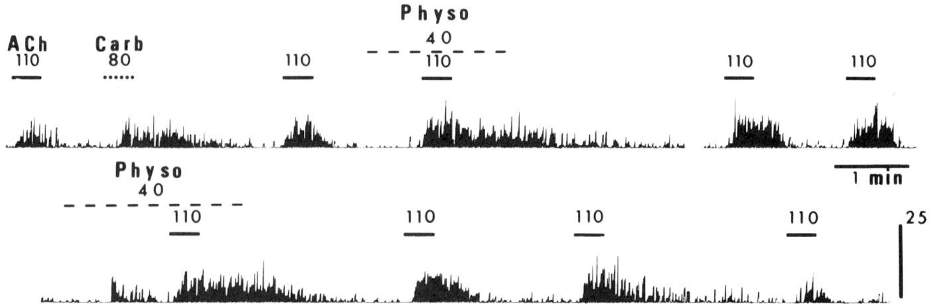

Fig. 3. Effect of acetylcholine (ACh) and carbachol (Carb) on a SHN. This SHN was excited by both substances, applied by microiontophoresis. Horizontal symbols indicate the duration of application ; numbers indicate the current intensity in nA. Vertical calibration bar: 25 impulses. Application of physostigmine (Physo) greatly prolonged the neuronal excitation induced by ACh. This effect was reversible and reproducible.

that SHNs are a non-homogeneous population. Indeed SHNs can be divided in several subgroups on the basis of i) their pattern of spontaneous activity and ii) their conduction velocity (or antidromic latency). About 45% of the SHNs (at least under our experimental conditions) display a rhythmically bursting pattern of discharge. It is known since a long time[6,7,8,9] that a rhythmic electrical activity at 3-7 Hz can be recorded from the hippocampus and from the septum, under specific experimental conditions. This rhythm is urethane resistant and is likely to be under the control of the septo-hippocampal pathway[10,11]. We hypothesize that some rhythmically bursting SHNs are the cholinergic neurons driving the atropine-sensitive hippocampal theta rhythm.

The presence of muscarinic binding sites in the medial septal area[12,13] explains the effect of ACh and muscarinic agonists. Thus, it is likely that cholinergic SHNs can be excited by the iontophoretic application of their own transmitter. Our observations show that SHNs are also sensitive to other neurotransmitters which are supposed to play a physiological role in the septal area: glutamic acid, GABA, substance P, TRH[14,15,16,17,18].

Intracellular recordings provide evidence that SHNs receive strong synaptic influences from the hippocampus. The presence of Cl^-dependent IPSPs is consistent with the view that SHNs receive a dissynaptic GABAergic input from the hippocampus (the GABAergic interneurons being located in the septum itself). The IPSPs trigger in some SHNs a rebound long lasting depolarization which could subserve the bursting activity of SHNs observed under urethane anaesthesia.

Finally we show that SHNs are often sensitive to noxious somatic peripheral stimulation. They could therefore be involved in central mechanisms related to nociception or responses to stressful stimuli.

REFERENCES

1. H.C. Fibiger, The organization and some projections of cholinergic neurons of the mammalian forebrain, Brain Res. Rev., 4, 327 (1982).

2. D.G. Amaral, J. Kurz, and F. Eckenstein, An analysis of the origins of the cholinergic and non-cholinergic septal projections to the hippocampal formation of the rat: a double labeling study using WGA-HRP and an antibody to choline acetyltransferase, Neurosci. Abstr., 10, 612 (1984).
3. R.H. Baisden, M.L. Woodruff, and D.B. Hoover, Cholinergic and non-cholinergic septo-hippocampal projections: a double-label horseradish peroxidase-acetylcholinesterase study in the rabbit, Brain Res., 290, 146 (1984).
4. D.B. Rye, B.H. Wainer, M.M. Mesulam, E.J. Mufson, and C.B. Saper, Cortical projections arising from the basal forebrain: a study of cholinergic and non-cholinergic components employing combined retrograde tracing and immunohistochemical localization of choline acetyltransferase, Neuroscience, 13, 627 (1984).
5. Y. Lamour, P. Dutar, and A. Jobert, Septo-hippocampal and other medial septum-diagonal band neurons: electrophysiological and pharmacological properties, Brain Res., 309, 227 (1984).
6. G. Apostol, and O.D. Creutzfeldt, Crosscorrelation between the activity of septal units and hippocampal EEG during arousal, Brain Res., 67, 65 (1974).
7. O. Macadar, J.A. Roig, J.M. Monti, and R. Budelli, The functional relationship between septal and hippocampal unit activity and hippocampal theta rhythm, Physiol. Behav., 5, 1443 (1970).
8. H. McLennan, and J.J. Miller, The hippocampal control of neuronal discharges in the septum of the rat, J. Physiol. (Lond.), 237, 607 (1974).
9. H. Petsche, C. Stumpf, and G. Gogolak, The significance of the rabbit's septum as a relay station between the midbrain and the hippocampus. I. The control of hippocampus arousal activity by the septum cells, Electroenceph. clin. Neurophysiol., 14, 202 (1962).
10. R. Kramis, C.H. Vanderwolf, and B.H. Bland, Two types of hippocampal rhythmical slow activity in both the rabbit and the rat: relations to behavior and effects of atropine, diethyl ether, urethane and pentobarbital, Expl. Neurol., 49, 58 (1975).
11. J.N.P. Rawlins, J. Feldon, and J.A. Gray, Septo-hippocampal connections and the theta rhythm, Expl. Brain Res., 37, 49 (1979).
12. M.J. Kuhar, and H.I. Yamamura, Localization of cholinergic muscarinic receptors in rat brain by light microscopic radioautography, Brain Res.; 110, 229 (1976).
13. R. Nonaka, and T. Moroji, Quantitative autoradiography of muscarinic cholinergic receptors in the rat brain, Brain Res., 296, 295 (1984).
14. M.J. Brownstein, M. Palkovits, J.M. Saavedra, R.M. Bassiri, and R.D. Utiger, Thyrotropin-releasing hormone in specific nuclei of rat brain, Science, 185, 267 (1974).
15. E. Costa, P. Panula, H.K. Thompson, and D.L. Cheney, The transynaptic regulation of the septo-hippocampal cholinergic neurons, Life Sci., 32, 165 (1983).
16. C. Gall, and R.Y. Moore, Distribution of enkephalin, substance P, tyrosine hydroxylase and 5-hydroxytryptamine immunoreactivity in the septal region of the rat, J. comp. Neurol., 225, 212 (1984).
17. T. Hökfelt, K. Fuxe, O. Johansson, S. Jeffcoates, and N. White, Distribution of thyrotropin-releasing hormone (TRH) in the central nervous system as revealed with immunohistochemistry, Eur. J. Pharmac., 34, 389 (1975).
18. P. Panula, A.V. Revuelta, D.L. Cheney, J.Y. Wu, and E. Costa, An immunohistochemical study on the location of GABAergic neurons in rat septum, J. comp. Neurol., 222, 69 (1984).

MICROMOLAR CONCENTRATIONS OF NEUROTOXIC CATIONS INDUCE PHASE SEPARATION, AGGREGATION AND FUSION IN PHOSPHATIDYLSERINE CONTAINING MEMBRANES

M. Deleers, J.P. Servais and E. Wülfert

Research Center, UCB S.A.
Pharmaceutical Sector
B-1420 Braine-l'Alleud (Belgium)

INTRODUCTION

Neurotoxic effects of aluminum, cadmium and manganese have been documented (1-5), the biochemical basis of these effects is not well established. Aluminum has been considered by several authors to be the toxic causal agent involved in various types of dementia (3-5).

There is also evidence that aluminum, cadmium and manganese strongly inhibit choline transport in erythrocytes and synaptosomes (6-7) by interacting with membranes.

To explore further the mechanism of the neurotoxicity of these cations, we therefore decided to study their effect on phospholipid model membranes.

MATERIALS AND METHODS

Bovine brain phosphatidylserine, egg yolk phosphatidylcholine, egg yolk phosphatidylethanolamine and cholesterol were purchased from Sigma Chemical Co. (St-Louis, Mo.), C_6-NBD-PC was purchased from Avanti Polar Lipids (Birmingham, Al) and 6 carboxyfluorescein (6CF) from Eastman Kodak (Rochester, N.Y.).

Small unilamellar vesicles (SUV) of various lipid compositions were obtained in 0.12 mol/l NaCl/0.02 mol/l tris-HCl, pH 7.4 by ultrasonication.

The NBD or 6CF fluorescence is continuously monitored either with an SLM 4800 Aminco Spectrofluorometer (SLM-Aminco, Urbana, Il.). NBD and 6CF were excited at 475 and 490 nM and monitored at 530 and 550 nM respectively. The aggregation was monitored by the turbidity changes of the unilamellar vesicles suspension at 400 nM using of a Beckman model 24 spectrophotometer (Beckman Fullerton, Ca.).

RESULTS

Quenching of NBD

The effect of increasing concentrations of calcium, manganese, cadmium and aluminum on the quenching of C_6-NBD-PC, 5 mol % incorporated into phosphatidylserine liposomes is demonstrated in figure 1. Approximate values for half maximal effects (ED_{50}) for these ions were respectively 50, 500, 700 and 900 µmol for Al^{3+}, Cd^{2+}, Mn^{2+} and Ca^{2+}.

Quenching of fluorescence depends on the concentration of Al^{3+} and not on the ratio of Al^{3+} to phosphatidylserine.

When liposomes were incubated simultaneously with aluminum and calcium, the sequence of addition of the cations determined the effects observed. As can be seen from table 1, pre-incubation with 1 mmol Ca^{2+} partially inhibited the effect of low Al^{3+} concentration.

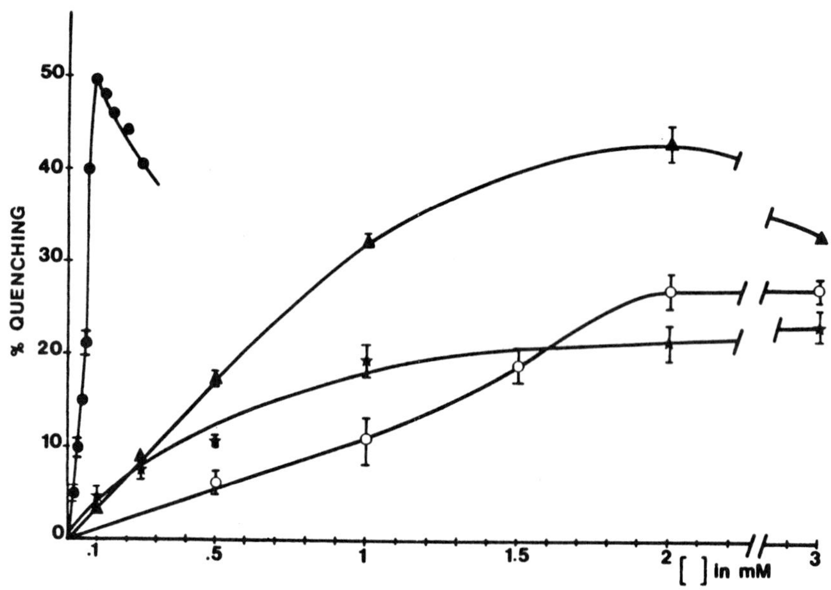

Fig. 1: Al^{3+} , Cd^{2+} , Mn^{2+} and Ca^{2+} -induced fluorescence quenching in phosphatidylserine vesicles as a function of cation concentration. 65 nmol of C_6-NBD-PC: phosphatidylserine (5:95) were suspended in 2 ml of buffer and the cations were added to the final concentration indicated, ● Al^{3+}, ▲ Cd^{2+} , ✶ Mn^{2+} and ○ Ca^{2+} . Each point is the mean of 3 to 4 experiments for the divalent cations and of at least 6 experiments for Al^{3+}.

TABLE 1

	Q_1	Q_2	$Q_{tot.}$
Ca → Al			
1 .025	9.8 ± .3	1.4 ± .8	11.2
1 .050	9.8 ± .3	11.9 ± 1.9	21.8
1 .075	9.8 ± .3	16.0 ± 1.2	25.8
1 1.00	9.8 ± .3	54.0 ± 2.2	63.8
Al → Ca			
.025 1	6.6 ± 1.30	9.9 ± 2.4	16.6
.050 1	17.2 ± 1.10	11.7 ± 1.4	29.0
.075 1	38.9 ± 1.30	10.4 ± 1.6	49.3
1.00 1	50.2 ± .40	9.8 ± 1.8	60

Effect of the sequence of addition of Al^{3+} and Ca^{2+} on quenching. Time between addition of 1st and 2nd cation was 2 min. The concentrations are in mmol and the Q_1, Q_2 and Q_{tot} values represent the quenching due to the first ion added, the quenching due to the second ion added after 2 min and the total quenching respectively. Results are the mean ± S.E.M. of 6-10 experiments.

The quenching effect of Al^{3+} could be partially inhibited by citrate, indicating chelation of Al^{3+} by the tricarboxylic acid. Aluminum-induced quenching of fluorescence was also altered by increasing amounts of phosphatidylcholine in the liposomes. However, the addition of cholesterol did not modify the effect of the cation (see figure 2).

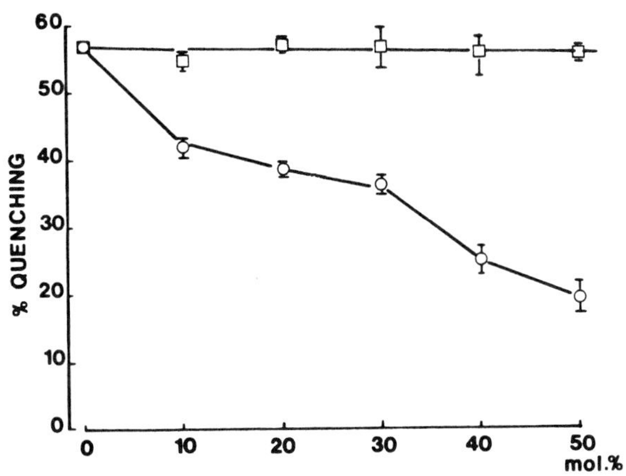

Fig. 2: Aluminum-induced NBD quenching in mixed phosphatidylserine/phosphatidylcholine (○) and in mixed phosphatidylserine/cholesterol vesicles (□). Liposomes consisting of phosphatidylserine and phosphatidylcholine (○) or cholesterol (□) and containing 5 mol % C_6-NBD-PC were incubated in the presence of 100 μmol/l Al^{3+}. The extent of quenching was determined after 4' when quenching reached a plateau value.

Release of 6-Carboxyfluorescein

The release of 6CF from unilamellar phosphatidylserine liposomes by increasing concentrations of Al^{3+} was studied by measuring changes in fluorescence intensity following the addition of the cation.

The effect was concentration dependent and the dequenching of the probe was apparent at concentrations of Al^{3+} less than 75 μmol. When plateau values were plotted against the concentrations of the three cations used, figure 3 was obtained. It is apparent from these data that Al^{3+} has a pronounced effect on the release of the probe from the liposomes, quite distinguishable from the effect seen with Cd^{2+} and Mn^{2+}.

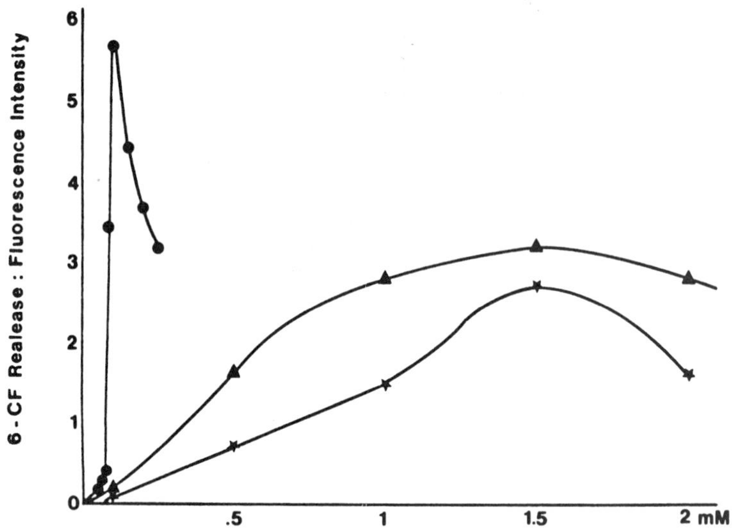

Fig. 3: Al^{3+}, Cd^{2+} and Mn^{2+}-induced 6-carboxyfluorescein release from phosphatidylserine vesicles after 4' as a function of cation concentration ● Al^{3+}, ▲ Cd^{2+} and ✶ Mn^{2+}.

Aggregation of liposomes

Aggregation of pure unilamellar phosphatidylserine liposomes or liposomes containing variable amounts of phosphatidylethanolamine, phosphatidylcholine or cholesterol was studied at increasing concentrations of aluminum. As can be seen from figure 4, phosphatidylethanolamine or phosphatidylcholine did not affect the threshold concentration of Al^{3+} for aggregation but significantly reduced maximum aggregation. A molar ratio of phosphatidylserine: cholesterol of either 8:2 or 6:4 did however slightly shift the concentration threshold for Al^{3+} induced aggregation towards lower concentrations of the cation and also significantly decreased maximum aggregation.

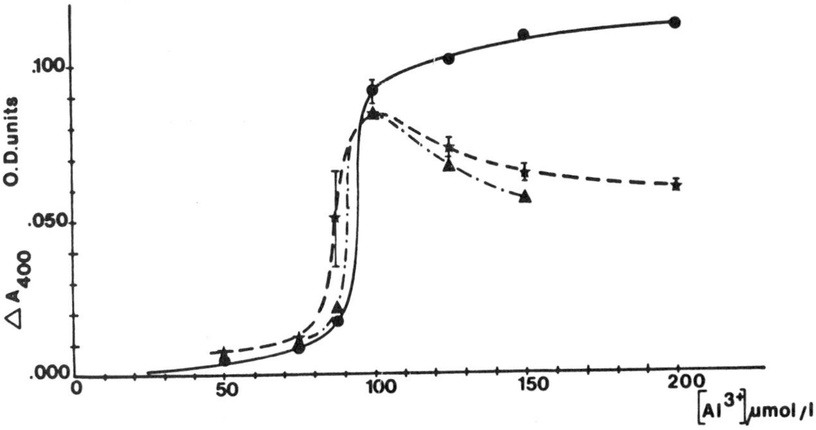

Fig. 4: Turbidity changes after 4' with vesicles (50 µmol/l) of different phospholipid composition versus Al^{3+} concentration. ● phosphatidylserine, ▲ phosphatidylserine - phosphatidylethanolamine (4:1) and ✶ phosphatidylserine - phosphatidylcholine (4:1). (The number of experiments are shown in the figure.

DISCUSSION

The data presented here clearly demonstrate that the three cations used alter the physical state of phosphatidylserine containing membranes. In all the experiments carried out (quenching, aggregation and 6CF release), aluminum always showed the most powerful effect at concentrations at least ten times lower than any of the other cations. ED_{50} ratios were respectively 10, 15 and 18 for Al^{3+}/Cd^{2+}, Al^{3+}/Mn^{2+} and Al^{3+}/Ca^{2+}.

Quenching of C_6-NBD-PC and the release of 6-CF always reached their plateau values after 4 min of incubation with Al^{3+}.

In our experiments with Al^{3+}, an effect of cholesterol on cation-induced quenching was not observed. Our findings with Al^{3+} could be due to particular affinity of this ion for phosphatidylserine lipids.

Several studies have demonstrated that citrate chelates aluminum with a high association constant (10^8 mol^{-1}). Partial inhibition by citrate of the quenching effect of Al^{3+} observed in our experiments suggests high affinity of Al^{3+} for phosphatidylserine lipids. Finally, it is remarkable that quenching, aggregation and release were all observed at the same concentration of aluminum.

The concentrations of Al^{3+}, Cd^{2+} and Mn^{2+} required to obtain half maximum effects (ED_{50}) are close to the ED_{50} values reported for inhibition of choline transport in erythrocytes and brain synaptosomes (6-7). This might suggest that at least some of the toxic effect of Al^{3+} on biological processes could be caused or associated with a direct interaction of aluminum with phospholipid membrane constituents.

This paper presents evidence that Al^{3+} in concentrations only slightly higher than those normally encountered in biological fluids profoundly alters the physical state of phosphatidylserine containing membranes. We believe that these findings constitute a possible rational basis for explaining some of the toxic effects of aluminum at the molecular level.

REFERENCES

1. D.R. Crapper, S.S. Krishnan and S. Quittkat, Aluminum, neurofibrillary degeneration and Alzheimer's disease, Brain 99: 67 (1976)
2. A.C. Alfrey, G.R. Legendre and W.D. Koehny, The dialysis encephalopathy syndrome. Possible aluminum intoxication, N.Engl.J.Med. 294:184 (1976)
3. G.P. Cooper and R.S. Manalis, Cadmium: effect on transmitter release at the frog neuromuscular junction, Eur.J.Pharmacol. 99:251 (1984)
4. W.R. Markesberry, Brain manganese concentration in human aging and Alzheimer's disease, Neurotoxicol. 5:49 (1984)
5. R.M. Garruto, R. Fukatsu, R. Yanagihara, D.C. Gajdusek, G. Hook and C.E. Fiori, Imaging of calcium and aluminum in neurofibrillary tangle bearing neurones in Parkinsonism dementia of Guam, Proc.Natl.Acad.Sci. 81:1875 (1984)
6. J.C.K. Lai, J.F. Guest, T.K.C. Leung, L. Lim and A.N. Davison, The effect of cadmium, manganese and aluminum or sodium-potassium-activated and magnesium-activated adenosine triphosphatase activity and choline uptake in rat brain synaptosomes, Biochem.Pharmacol. 29:141 (1980)
7. R.G. King, J.A. Sharp and A.L.A. Boura, The effect of Al^{3+}, Cd^{2+} and Mn^{2+} of human erythrocytes choline transport, Biochem.Pharmacol. 32:3611 (1983).

MPTP-INDUCED PARKINSONIAN SYNDROMES IN HUMANS AND ANIMALS

I.J. Kopin, S.R. Burns, C.C. Chiueh, and S.P. Markey

National Institutes of Health, National Institute of Neurological and Communicative Disorders and Stroke
Bethesda, Maryland 20205

INTRODUCTION

The illicit synthesis and use of a meperidine analogue containing a side reaction product, 1-methyl-4-phenyl-1,2,3,6-tetrahydropyridine (MPTP), led to the discovery that this contaminant is a neurotoxin which produces in some animals, as well as in humans, a motor disorder which closely resembles Parkinson's Disease (Davis, et al., 1979; Langston, et al., 1983). This discovery has stimulated considerable research in efforts to determine the areas of brain which are involved, the attendant biochemical changes, the mechanisms of toxicity, and the usefulness of the toxin-induced motor disorder as an animal model with which to gain further insight into the pathogenesis and treatment of Parkinson's Disease. It is the purpose of this presentation to recount the history of this discovery, to review our present knowledge of MPTP-induced motor disorders and to examine the implications for understanding spontaneously occurring Parkinson's Disease.

DISCOVERY OF THE PARKINSONISM-PRODUCING TOXICITY OF MPTP

In 1977, a 23 year old college student was referred to the Clinical Center at NIH because of the sudden onset, 3 months earlier, of a parkinsonian syndrome. The severity of the bradykinesia, rigidity and mutism were responsible for the initial diagnosis of catatonic schizophrenia and admission to a psychiatric ward. After failure to respond to electroshock therapy or antipsychotic drugs, he was seen by a neurologist and treatment with L-dopa and benztropine initiated with striking beneficial effects. Due to the unusual nature of the disorder, the patient was referred to the NIH. After admission to NIH, it became apparent that the onset of the illness was related to self-administration of drugs. The patient had used a variety of illicit agents over a period of nine years, but during the summer before admission began to use a mixture of cocaine and a demerol-like compound, 1-methyl-4-phenyl-4 - propionoxy-piperidine (MPPP), synthesized in his home laboratory. He successfully prepared and used several batches of MPPP, but the last batch was sloppily prepared and used without purification. Dr. Sanford Markey obtained from the patient's home the glassware used in the chemical synthesis. Although the patient's mother had washed and stored the equipment, from traces of chemicals remaining on a glass desiccator, Dr. Markey was able to identify a mixture of several compounds which included the precursor chemical, 1-methyl-4-hydroxy-4-phenyl-piperidine (MHPP), the desired product, and a major side product, MPTP.

The patient was treated with L-dopa and bromocryptine, but continued to abuse drugs and died of an overdose of a drug mixture. Autopsy revealed striking nerve cell loss in the substantia nigra, confirming the loss of dopamine neurons which had been suspected from the very low levels of HVA found in the patients cerebrospinal fluid. This first case of a meperidine analogue-induced parkinsonism in human was reported in the literature (Davis, et al., 1979).

Attempts to produce chemical lesions in the brains of rodents were initiated, but failed to produce a parkinsonian syndrome. At about that time, there surfaced in California, several cases in which young drug abusers were admitted to hospitals with a clinical picture similar to that described in our patient. An astute technician in the Drug Abuse Laboratories recalled the published report of induction of parkinsonism from meperidine analogues (Davis, et al., 1979) and when the substances which had been used by these patients were examined, they were found to consist of almost pure MPTP (Langston, et al., 1983).

This stimulated further efforts towards reproducing the disorder in animals and Burns et al. (1983) found that MPTP administered intravenously for several days to monkeys induced a parkinsonian disorder in these animals and produced selective destruction of nigrostriatal dopaminergic neurons (Jacobowitz, et al., 1984). Treatment of these animals with L-dopa reversed the movement disorder and in parallel increased CSF levels of dopamine (Chiueh, et al., 1984a).

SPECIES SPECIFICITY OF MPTP TOXICITY

In all species examined, MPTP administration produces an array of immediate behavioral responses which mimic the effects of compounds which release biogenic amines, particularly serotonin. These effects soon are dissipated and the animals become apparently normal or present relatively minor motor dysfunctions. With time, or after repeated MPTP administration for several days, in monkeys and dogs, as well as in humans, there appears a marked change in motor behavior with features that closely resemble the bradykinesia, rigidity, and tremor of Parkinson's disease. These chronic effects are minimal in guinea pigs, even less obvious in mice, and absent in rats, even after administration of much higher doses of MPTP. The acute pharmacological actions are clearly different from the chronic toxic effects of MPTP.

Acute behavioral effects of MPTP

After it had been determined that a parkinsonian-like disorder might be attributed to the toxic effects of MHPP, MPPP, or MPTP (Davis, et al., 1979) a series of studies were initiated in rats to examine both acute and chronic effects of intravenous administration of these compounds, alone or in combination. The opiate potency of MPPP which had previously been reported (Foster and Carmen, 1947) was confirmed, but MPTP did not appear to have any opiate activity (Johannsen & Markey, 1984). There were, however, striking characteristic behavioral effects which were apparent almost immediately after injection of the MPTP (5-10 mg/kg). Rats become tremulous and adopt a typical hunched posture with hind legs splayed, forelegs placed widely, tail erect, with prominent piloerection, exophthalmos, and profuse salivation. Similar effects are seen in mice. In rats, clonic movements of the forelegs occur and there is a slow retropulsion. These effects which resemble the "serotonin syndrome" (Jacobs 1976), last for 15-30 minutes, after which mobility returns and the animals gradually assume normal posture and locomotor behavior (Chiueh et al. 1984 a,b). The syndrome is almost immediately reversed by intravenous administration of methysergide, a serotonin antagonist; marked hyperactivity replaces the immobility and the animals episodically charge across their cages.

The acute behavioral effects of intravenously administered MPTP in primates, including humans, and dogs, are quite similar to those in the rat. Intense salivation, myoclonic movements and shaking episodes, and signs of enhanced sympathetic discharge dominate the clinical picture. Patients report hallucinations, metallic or medicinal taste, and blurred or dimmed vision (Langston, et al., 1985). The acute signs and symptoms last up to several hours. When administered subcutaneously to rats, higher doses of MPTP are tolerated, the onset of behavioral changes is delayed, and the effects are prolonged (Enz, et al., 1984) but similar to those seen after intravenous administration. MPTP does not produce rotation in animals with unilateral nigrostriatal lesions, suggesting that the drug does not stimulate dopamine receptors. In dogs, the acute effects of intravenously administered MPTP correspond to those observed in other species, but since these animals are even more susceptible to the chronic toxic effects of MPTP than are monkeys, the evolution of the phases of the toxicity can be observed after a single dose (2.5 mg/kg) of MPTP.

Acute pharmacological effects of MPTP on biogenic amines

The acute biochemical effects of MPTP include increases in serotonin (5HT) levels in the median raphe (Chiueh, et al., 1984b) and hypothalamus (Enz, et al., 1984) and decreases in 5-hydroxyindole acetic acid (5HIAA) levels, suggesting a decrease in 5HT metabolism. This could result from either a decrease in 5HT release or metabolism or direct stimulation of 5HT receptors. The effects on dopamine and its metabolite suggest that immediately after MPTP administration, release of this amine is decreased whereas release of norepinephrine is increased, as indicated by declining levels of this amine and increased levels of its metabolite, 3-methoxy-4-hydroxyphenylglycol (MHPG).

The striking increase in signs of peripheral sympathetic activity are attended by elevated plasma norepinephrine levels (Chiueh et al., 1984a) and decreases in catecholamine levels in the heart, mesenteric blood vessels, and adrenal medulla in both rats and mice (Fuller, et al., 1984).

In rhesus monkeys, administration of MPTP is followed by a decline in ventricular cerebrospinal fluid levels (CSF) of HVA, MHPG, and 5HIAA. Levels of dopamine in the putamen and caudate nuclei are increased 24 hours after the fifth daily dose of MPTP (Burns, et al., 1983). These results are consistent with the acute decrease in release of dopamine and 5HT seen in rats, but norepinephrine metabolism also appears to be decreased in monkeys, whereas in rats the rate of norepinephrine metabolites is reported to be increased (Enz, et al., 1984). In guinea pigs, dopamine formation and metabolism is markedly decreased in nucleus accumbens (A10 projection) as well as in the caudate (A9 projection) immediately after treatment with MPTP (Chiueh, et al., 1984a). The low affinity of MPTP for both dopamine and norepinephrine receptors suggests that the drug does not act by directly stimulating these receptors. The biochemical effects on serotonin and its metabolites as well as the reversal of behavioral effects by methysergide are most consistent with the action of MPTP directly on 5HT receptors. This action may produce effects which alter release of dopamine and norepinephrine.

Chronic neurotoxic effects of MPTP

Several days after repeated exposure of primates to MPTP the symptoms of Parkinson's disease gradually appear; there is increasing bradykinesia, rigidity, and episodes of "freezing". The time course of the development may span 3 days to 3 weeks; the degree of final impairment may vary from minimal symptoms to severe parkinsonism. At least 80% of the dopamine must be depleted before symptoms appear. The projections to the dorsolateral striatum of the monkey caudate appear most vulnerable to the toxin (Chiueh, et al., 1985a). The major difference in the clinical picture in monkeys with MPTP-induced parkinsonism and in humans with either MPTP-induced parkinsonism or Parkinson's disease is the characteristics of the tremor. In monkeys, the tremor is related to posture or movement, whereas in humans, the tremor typically occurs at rest. The toxic effects of MPTP in primates appear to be well localized to the nigrostriatal dopamine-containing neurons. In the case reported by Davis, et al. (1979) there was a striking loss of pigmented nerve cells in the substantia nigra with gliosis and extracellular neuromelanin pigment. The locus coreuleus and other amine-containing neuron cell groups appeared to have been spared. This was also observed in other species of primates including rhesus monkeys (Burns, et al. 1983), squirrel monkeys (Langston, et al. 1984a) and the marmoset (Jenner, et al. 1984).

In dogs, a single dose of MPTP (2.5 mg/kg) causes the usual acute sympathomimetic effects, followed by a gradual appearance of a parkinsonian motor disorder. The immediate effects, which include salivation, tachypnea, tachycardia and other indices of autonomic discharge, are attended by motor deficits, with splaying of legs, immobility or slowed gait. During the next few days (1-5) mobility is impaired, eating and drinking cease, eyelid closure and flexed posture becomes more prominent, postural tremors appear and episodes of freezing become superimposed on rigidity and bradykinesia. After this interval there is improvement in mobility, but even after one month, some tremor, bradykinesia, and freezing episodes occur, but the animals are able to eat and drink. During the first week after MPTP administration the animal responds to L-dopa with hyperactivity but tremor is prevented and swallowing improves.

The biochemical alterations in CSF and brain regions are consistent with the observed pathology. In monkeys levels of HVA in CSF remain low for months after MPTP administration, but those of 5-HIAA and MHPG return towards normal (Burns, et al., 1983). The levels of tyrosine hydroxylase and dopa decarboxylase as well as of dopamine are strikingly reduced in the nigrostriatal neuronal regions, but relatively intact in other areas of brain.

In mice, (300-400 mg/kg) MPTP administered in divided doses, up to 50 mg/kg/day, produces striking and persistent decreases in levels of dopamine and its metabolites in the striatum attended by diminished ^{3}H-dopamine uptake (Hallman, et al., 1984; Heikkila, et al., 1984 a,b). The cell number in the zona compacta of the substantia nigra was reported to have been reduced markedly, but subsequent studies by Hallman, et al. (1985), showed that although the dopamine content was reduced in both the striatum and DA cell bodies of the A9 area, there was no reduction in the number of cell bodies which contained immunoreactive tyrosine hydroxylase, suggesting that the nerve terminals but not the cell bodies were destroyed by the toxin. This probably accounts for the complete recovery in mice of the striatal dopamine levels within 6-8 months after administration of even high doses (300 mg/kg) of MPTP (Chiueh, et al., 1985b). Furthermore, in the mouse, the high doses of MPTP used appear to have a similar effect on noradrenergic neuronal projections from the locus coeruleus to the cortex (Hallman, et al., 1985). Thus, in-vitro uptake of tritiated dopamine by striatal tissue and of ^{3}H-norepinephrine by frontal cortex were similarly reduced in MPTP-treated mice. Furthermore, in mice, the norepinephrine contents of the olfactory bulb, frontal cortex, hippocampus, are striatum were reduced to about the same extent as is striatal dopamine. In the dog, although cell death is observed in nigrostriatal neurons, damage to some norepinephrine- and other dopamine-containing neurons appears to be similar to that seen in mice.

Mechanisms of Neurotoxicity of MPTP

Although the mechanisms responsible for the toxic effects of MPTP are unknown, it is evident that a number of factors contribute to the target specificity and species vulnerability. It is also evident that the chronic toxic effects result from factors independent of those accounting for the immediate pharmacologic effects. Factors which contribute to target specificity of a toxin include localization of enzymes which detoxify or activate the chemical substances, mechanisms which concentrate the toxic compound or its metabolite in specific cells, availability of precursors which can form reactive intermediates (e.g., free radicals), capacity of cellular defense mechanisms (which scavenge free radicals or destroy potentially dangerous molecules), and the capacity of cells to repair or replace molecules essential for survival. The apparent relationship of MPTP toxicity to neuromelanin content has been regarded as a clue to both the target vulnerability and species sensitivity to the toxin.

Metabolism of MPTP - MPTP is rapidly oxidized in many tissues to form the pyridinium derivative (Markey, et al., 1984; Langston, et al., 1984b), 1-methyl-4-phenyl pyridinium (MPP^+), which appears to persist in the monkey brain for long periods of time (up to 20 days) but is relatively rapidly removed (within hours) from rodent brain (Johannesen, et al., 1985). The formation of MPP^+ from MPTP (Fig. 1) is prevented by pargyline and deprenyl, but not chlorgyline, suggesting that MAO-B is the enzyme responsible for this conversion (Chiba, Trevor, and Castagnoli, 1984). MAO-B inhibition by administration of either pargy-

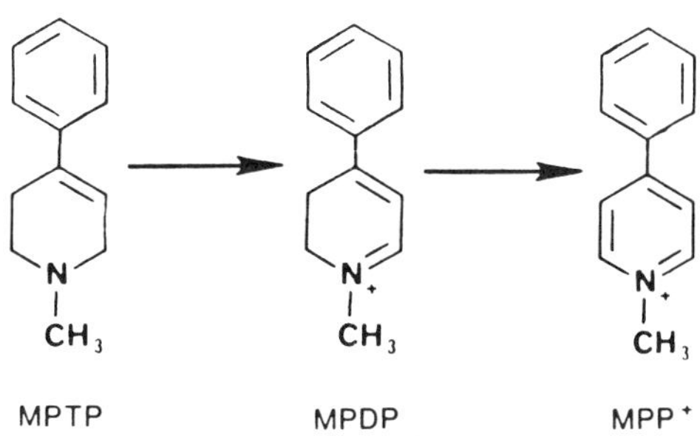

Figure 1. MPTP Metabolism

or deprenyl, prevents the parkinsonian syndrome produced by MPTP in primates (Langston, et al., 1984c) and dogs and protects mice from the dopamine neurotoxic effects of MPTP in this species (Heikkila et al., 1984; Markey, et al., 1984). Using specific antibodies for immunohistochemical localization, MAO-B appears to be well localized in astrocytes and 5-HT containing neurons, whereas dopaminergic neurons contain predominently MAO-A (Richard Denny, personal communication). This suggests that MPP^+ may be formed in MAO-B containing cells and subsequently transferred to dopamine containing cells. If the substantia nigra compacta contains an unusually rich concentration of MAO-B-containing cells relative to other dopamine cell groups, this may be a factor in the selective vulnerability of the nigrostriatal neurons to MPTP effects.

Concentrating Mechanisms - Biogenic amine uptake mechanisms have long been recognized as having a role in the specificity of neurotoxins. Thus 6-hydroxydopamine is selectively accumulated in catecholamine-containing neurons whereas 5,7-dihydroxytryptamine is taken up into serotonergic neurons.

A number of investigators have sought to demonstrate mechanisms for accumulation of MPTP or MPP^+ by dopamine or neuromelanin-containing cells, which might contribute to the selective vulnerability of nigrostriatal neurons to the toxicity of MPTP. Thus MPP^+ has been shown to have a high affinity for the dopamine uptake system (Javitch and Snyder, 1985) and to bind a specific amine neurons in human caudate, substantia nigra, and locus coeruleus (Javitch and Snyder, 1984). Heikkila et al. (1985) demonstrated that while MPTP diminishes serotonin and dopamine binding it has a higher affinity for serotonin uptake sites whereas the reverse is true for its metabolite, MPP^+. ^{3}H-MPTP binding has been related to pargyline binding sites on MAO-B (Del Zompo, et al., 1985; Javitch and Snyder, 1985) while affinity of MPTP for melanin has been demonstrated by Lyden, et al. (1985). None of these observations, however, are completely satisfactory for explaining the species specificity and tissue selectivity of MPTP toxicity since the studies on binding were performed in the rat, which is resistant to the toxic effects of MPTP and even in susceptible species not all cells which form MPP^+ or contain melanin are destroyed by MPTP.

Role of Free Radical Intermediates - Although the toxicity of MPP^+ has not been studied extensively, a related compound, paraquat (Figs. 1 and 2) has received wide attention for its use as a defoliant in controlling marajuana production. Bus, et al. (1976) proposed that the

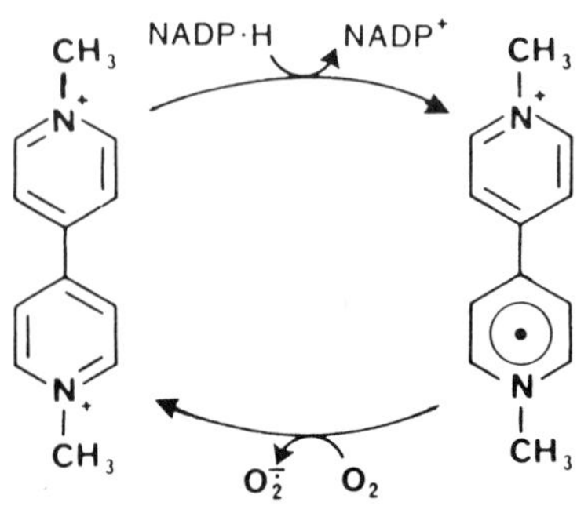

Figure 2. Superoxide generation by paraquat redox cycling

toxicity of paraquat, which involves primarily the lungs, liver, and kidney, is related to the generation of superoxide free radicals (O_2^-). After depletion of protective anti-oxidants (e.g., α-tocopherol, glutathione, etc.), O_2^-, H_2O_2, and ·OH can react with and destroy essential membrane polyunsaturated lipids by initiating chain reactions of lipid peroxidation. Formation of free radicals is a well known and important mechanism by which toxins produce cell damage and tissue injury (Freeman and Crapo, 1982; Trush, Mimnaugh and Gram, 1982). There are several cellular defense mechanisms which effectively remove the highly reactive transient free radicals. Superoxide dismutase, catalase, and glutathione peroxidase-reductase as well as soluble reducing substances e.g. α-tocopherol, ascorbic acid, glutathione and uric acid, contributes to maintenance of low free radical levels. When rates of free radical formation are increased, these mechanisms become ineffective, critical target molecules are attacked and cell injury supervenes. If cell injury proceeds to a point where repair or replacement mechanisms are ineffective, cell death occurs.

Mechanisms involving free radicals have been used to explain the cytotoxic effects of 6-hydroxydopamine (Cohen, 1984) and chronic manganese toxicity (Donaldson and Labella, 1984; Halliwell, 1984). Graham (1984) has suggested that formation of dopamine quinone and semi-quinone products and oxidative free radicals (O_2^-, H_2O_2, and ·OH) are factors in the pathogenesis of Parkinson's disease. Cohen (1984) suggested that dopamine release by MPTP may cause cell damage by a similar mechanism. The obvious similarity of MPP^+ to paraquat (Figs. 1,2) has stimulated speculation that free radical generation is an integral part of the molecular events leading to MPTP neurotoxic effects.

Free radicals can interact with a variety of enzymes, lipids, nucleotides, etc., and thereby disrupt cellular metabolic processes and transport mechanisms. Inability to repair such damage leads to cell death.

Relationship to neuromelanin. Primates have high concentrations of neuromelanin in brain dopaminergic and noradrenergic neurons. Neuromelanin accumulation increases with age; MPTP susceptibility also appears to increase with age. Dogs have high neuromelanin contents in brain catecholaminergic neurons and are susceptible to MPTP toxicity whereas rodents have little or none of the pigment and are resistant to the toxin. The apparent association of neuromelanin with enhanced vulnerability to the cytotoxic effects of MPTP is probably not fortuitous. Neuromelanin accumulations may reflect a low capacity of the cellular defense mechanisms to limit levels of partially reduced oxygen molecules (O_2^-, H_2O_2, ·OH) which promote quinone formation from catechols (Fridovich, 1975). The additional burden of reactive molecules of MPP^+ and the H_2O_2 generated from the action of MAO on MPTP could overwhelm the marginally protective mechanisms of the neuromelanin-containing neurons. Furthermore, neuromelanin may be a participant in the redox cycling of MPP^+ which generates free radicals. Neuromelanin is a redox polymer which has stable free radicals and the semiquinone free radical of melanin can act as an electron acceptor (Van Woert and Ambani, 1974). Since neuromelanin is sequestered in particles, there is little opportunity to react with other organelles (e.g., mitochondria). If soluble MPP^+ can react with the reduced quinone (QH_2 in Fig. 3), the MPP^+-MPP· redox cycle can act as an electron shuttle. The sequestered neuromelanin could then enhance free radical formation at mitochondria (Fig. 3). Similarly MPP^+-MPP· redox cycling might involve dopamine stored in vesicles and formation of toxic quinones (Graham, et al., 1978) might further enhance the toxic effects of MPTP.

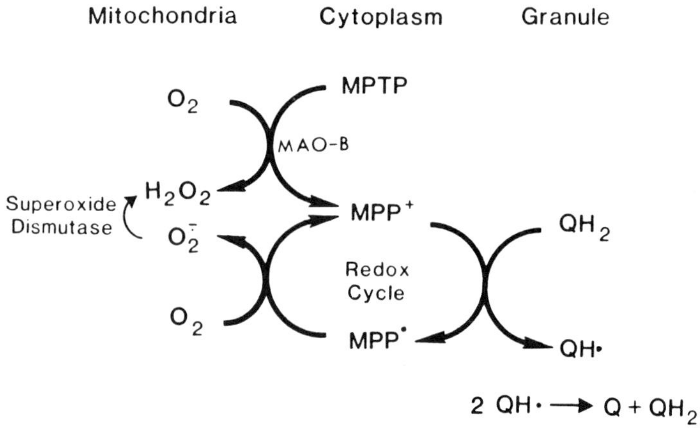

Figure 3. Possible role of melanin in MPTP toxicity

MPTP toxicity as an experimental model for Parkinson's disease

The chemical lesion produced after administration of MPTP, although attended by most of the major clinical features of Parkinson's disease, does, in some aspects differ from the progressive degenerative disease. Biochemical differences reflect sparing of the noradrenergic systems in human MPTP toxicity; the locus coeruleus is frequently involved in Parkinson's disease, but not in MPTP toxicity. Thus in Parkinson's disease there is often a decrease in MHPG levels in cerebrospinal fluid which cannot be attributed to decreased plasma MHPG. In contrast to this, in MPTP toxicity the levels of MHPG in CSF which are derived from brain norepinephrine metabolism are generally elevated (Burns, et al., 1985a), possibly reflecting a compensatory increase in noradrenergic activity. Another difference relates to the course of the disease. MPTP-induced parkinsonism begins acutely, whereas Parkinson's disease has a gradual onset. Although the possible gradual development of a parkinsonian syndrome in subjects exposed to subclinically toxic doses of MPTP cannot yet be excluded, there is some evidence that once MPTP-induced parkinsonism stabilizes, it does not progress rapidly. A young chemist who had developed parkinsonism after massive laboratory exposure to MPTP has been found to have remained at a stable level of motor dysfunction over a period of at least seven years. During this interval he had continous treatment with L-DOPA and a peripheral decarboxylase inhibitor. This course certainly appears to have differed from that of Parkinson's disease and is consistent with a single nonprogressive toxic insult (Burns, et al., 1985b). Furthermore, this case suggests that L-dopa does not contribute to the progress of the degenerative disorder in Parkinson's disease.

Clinical-pathological correlations of neurological deficits in Parkinson's disease which are absent in MPTP-induced parkinsonism may prove useful in relating human brain regions to specific functions. It is clear, however, that involvement of the nigrostriatal pathway alone, as occurs with MPTP, is sufficient to produce the major motor deficits of Parkinson's disease.

The insights which might be provided by MPTP-toxicity into the pathogenesis of Parkinson's disease, however, are perhaps the most exciting aspect of the model motor disorder. Birkmayer, et al (1983) reported that treatment with the MAO-B blocking drug, (-)deprenyl, as a long term adjunct to conventional L-DOPA therapy, appears to have retarded progression of the disease. If there is a relationship between MPTP toxicity, which, as indicated earlier, is blocked by (-)deprenyl, and the mechanisms responsible for the progressive degenerative process in Parkinson's disease, then perhaps agents which interfere with these processes will retard the progression of the disease. Efficacy of agents, such as anti-oxidants or free radical scavengers, might be tested by examining their ability to prevent or delay MPTP-induced parkinsonism in animals. It is clear that future research will provide important answers to questions regarding the mechanisms for selective vulnerability of these neurons to the toxic damage by MPTP and the degenerative processes resulting in Parkinson's disease.

REFERENCES

Birkmayer, W., Knoll,J., Riederer,P., and Youdim, M.B.H., 1983, (-)-Deprenyl leads to prolongation of l-dopa efficacy in parkinson's disease, Mod. Probl. Pharmacopsychiat., 19:170-176.

Burns, R.S., Chiueh, C.C., Markey, S.P., Ebert, M.H., Jacobowitz, D.M., and Kopin, I.J., 1983, A primate model of parkinsonism: selective destruction of dopaminergic neurons in the pars compacta of the substantia nigra by N-methyl-4-phenyl-1,2,3,6-tetrahydropyridine, Proc Natl Acad Sci USA, 80:4546-50.

Burns, R.S., LeWitt, P.A., Ebert, M.H., Pakkenberg, H., Langston, J.W., and Kopin, I.J., 1985a, The clinical syndrome of striatal dopamine deficiency: Parkinsonism induced by MPTP, N Engl J Med, in press.

Burns, R.S., Pakkenberg, H., and Kopin, I.J., 1985b, Lack of progression of MPTP-induced parkinsonism during long term treatment with L-DOPA, Ann Neurol, in press.

Bus, J.S., Cogen, S., Olgaard, M., and Gibson, J.E., 1976, A mechanism of paraquat toxicity in mice and rats. Toxicol. Appl. Pharmacol., 35:501-513.

Chiba, K., Trevor, A., Castagnoli, N.,Jr., 1984, Metabolism of the neurotoxic tertiary amine, MPTP, by brain monoamine oxidase, Biochem. Biophys. Res. Commun, 120:574-578.

Chiueh, C.C., Markey, S.P., Burns, R.S., Johannessen, J.N., Jacobowitz, D.M., and Kopin, I.J., 1984a, Neurochemical and behavioral effects of 1-methyl-4-phenyl-1,2,3,6-tetrahydropyridine (MPTP) in rat, guinea pig, and monkey Psychopharmacol Bull, 20(3):548-553.

Chiueh, C.C., Markey, S.P., Burns, R.S., Johannessen, J.N., Pert, A., and Kopin, I.J., 1984b, Neurochemical and behavioral effects of systemic and intranigral administration of N-methyl-4-phenyl-1,2,3,6-tetrahydropyridine in the rat, Eur. J. Pharmacol., 20:100(2):189-194.

Chiueh, C.C., Burns, R.S., Markey, S.P., Jacobowitz, D.M. and Kopin, I.J., 1985a, Primate Model of parkinsonism: Selective lesion of nigrostriatal neurons by 1-methyl-4-phenyl-1,2,3,6-tetrahydropyridine produces an extrapyramidal syndrome in rhesus monkeys. Life Sci., 36:213-218.

Chiueh, C.C., Johannessen, J.N., Chesselet, M.F., and Markey, S.P., 1985b, Neurotoxic mechanism of 1-methyl-4-phenyl-1,2,3,6-tetrahydropyridine (MPTP) and its oxidative metabolites in the nigrostriatal system of C57BL6 mice., Fed. Proc., 44: 893.

Cohen, G., 1984, Oxy-radical toxicity in catecholamine neurons, Neurotoxicology, 5(1):77-82.

Davis, G.C., Williams, A.C., Markey, S.P., Ebert, M.H., Caine, E.D., Beichert, C.M., and Kopin, I.J., 1979, Chronic parkinsonism secondary to intravenous injection of meperidine analogues, Psychiatry. Res., 1:249-254.

Del Zompo, M., Bocchetta, A., Piccardi, M.P., Pintus, S., Corsini, G.U., 1984, Inhibition of 3H MPTP binding to rat brain by pargyline, Biochem. Pharmacol., 33(24):4105-4107.

Donaldson, J., and LaBella, F.S., 1984, The effects of manganese on the cholinergic receptor in vivo and in vitro may be mediated through modulation of free radicals, Neurotoxicology, 5(1):105-112.

Enz, A., Hefti, F., and Frick, W., 1984, Acute administration of 1-methyl-4-phenyl-1,2,3,6-tetrahydropyridine (MPTP) reduces dopamine and serotonin but accelerates norepinephrine metabolism in the rat brain. Effect of chronic pretreatment with MPTP, Eur. J. Pharmacol., 101(1-2):37-44.

Foster, R.H.K., and Carmen, A.J., 1947, Studies in analgesia: piperidine derivatives with morphine-like activity, J. Pharm. Exp. Ther., 91:195-209.

Freeman, B.A., and Crapo, J.D., 1982, Biology of Disease: Free radicals and tissue injury, Lab. Invest., 47(5):412.

Fridovich, I., 1975, Superoxide Dismutases, Ann. Rev. Biochem., 44:147-159.

Fuller, R.W., Hahn, R.A., Snoddy, H.D., and Wikel, J.H., 1984, Depletion of cardiac norepinephrine in rats and mice by 1-methyl-4-phenyl-1,2,3,6-tetrahydropyridine (MPTP), Biochem. Pharmacol., 33(19):2957-2960.

Graham, D.G., 1978, Oxidative pathways for catecholamines in the genesis of neuromelanin and cytotoxic quinones, Mol. Pharmacol., 14:633-634.

Graham, D.G., 1984, Catecholamine toxicity: A proposal for the molecular pathogenesis of manganese neurotoxicity and parkinson's disease, Neurotoxicology, 5(1):83-96.

Hallman, H., Lange, J., Olson, L., Stromberg, I., and Jonsson, G., 1985, Neurochemical and histochemical characterization of neurotoxic effects of 1-methyl-4-phenyl-1,2,3,6-tetrahydropyridine on brain catecholamine neurons in the mouse, J. Neurochem., 44(1):117-127.

Hallman, H., Olson, L., and Jonsson, G., 1984, Neurotoxicity of the meperidine analogue N-methyl-4-phenyl-1,2,3,6-tetrahydropyridine on brain catecholamine neurons in the mouse, Eur. J. Pharmacol., 97(1-2):133-136.

Halliwell, B., 1984, Manganese ions, oxidation reactions and the superoxide radical, Neurotoxicology, 5(1):113-118.

Heikkila, R.E., Cabbat, F.S., Manzino, L., and Duvoisin, R.C., 1984a, Effects of 1-methyl-4-phenyl-1,2,3,6-tetrahydropyridine on negrostriatal dopamine in mice, Neuropharmacology, 23(6):711-713.

Heikkila, R.E., Hess, A., and Duvoisin, R.C., 1984b, Dopaminergic neurotoxicity of 1-methyl-4-phenyl-1,2,3,6-tetrahydropyridine in mice, Science, 224(4656):1451-1453.

Heikkila, R.E., Manzino, L., Cabbat, F.S., and Duvoisin, R.C., 1984c, Protection against the dopaminergic neurotoxicity of 1-methyl-4-phenyl-1,2,3,6-tetrahydropyridine by monoamine oxidase inhibitors, Nature, 311(5985):467-469.

Jacobs, B.L., 1976, An animal behavior model for studying central serotonin synapses, Life Sci., 19:777.

Javitch, J.A., and Snyder, S.H., 1985, Uptake of MPP^+ by dopamine neurons explains selectivity of parkinsonism-inducing neurotoxin, MPTP, Eur. J. Pharm., 106:455-456.

Javitch, J.A., Uhl, G.R., and Snyder, S.H., 1984, Parkinsonism-inducing neurotoxin,N-methyl-4-phenyl-1,2,3,6-tetrahydropyridine: characterization and localization of receptor binding sites in rat and human brain, Proc Natl Acad Sci USA, 81(14):4591-4595.

Jenner, P., Rupniak, N.M., Rose, S., Kelly, E., Kilpatrick, G., Lees, A., and Marsden, C.D., 1984, 1-methyl-4-phenyl-1,2,3,6-tetrahydropyridine-induced parkinsonism in the common marmoset, Neurosci. Lett., 50(1-3):85-90.

Johannesen, J.N., Chiueh, C.C., Burns, R.S., and Markey, S.P., 1985, Differences in the metabolism of MPTP in the rodent and primate parallel differences in sensitivity to its neurotoxic effects, Life Sci. 36:219-224.

Johannessen, J.N., and Markey, S.P., 1984, Assessment of the opiate properties of two constituents of a toxic illicit drug mixture, Drug Alcohol. Depend., 13(4):367-374.

Langston, J.W., 1985, MPTP neurotoxicity: An overview and characterization of phases of toxicity, Life Sci., 36:201-206.

Langston, J.W., Ballard, P., Tetrud, J.W., and Irwin, I., 1983, Chronic parkinsonism in humans due to a product of meperidine-analog synthesis, Science, 219(4587):979-980.

Langston, J.W., Forno, L.S., Rebert, C.S., and Irwin, I., 1984a, Selective nigral toxicity after systemic administration of 1-methyl-4-phenyl-1,2,3,6-tetrahydropyridine (MPTP) in the squirrel monkey, Brain Res., 292(2):390-394.

Langston, J.W., Irwin, I., Langston, E.B., and Forno, L.S., 1984b, 1-methyl-4-phenylpyridinium ion (MPP^+): identification of a metabolite of MPTP, a toxin selective to the substantia nigra, Neurosci. lett., 49(1):87-92.

Langston, J.W., Irwin, I., Langston, E.B., and Forno, L.S., 1984c, Pargyline prevents MPTP-induced parkinsonism in primates, Science, 225(4669):1480-1482.

Lyden, A., Bondesson, V., Larsson, B.S., and Lindquist, N.G., 1983, Melanin affinity of 1-methyl-4-phenyl,1,2,3,6-tetrahydropyridine an inducer of chronic parkinsonism in humans, Acta Pharmacol. et. toxicol., 53:429-432.

Markey, S.P., Johannsessen, J.N., Chiueh, C.C., Burns, R.S., and Herkenham, M.A., 1984, Intraneuronal generation of a pyridinium metabolite may cause drug-induced parkinsonism, Eur. J. Pharmacol., 102(2):375-377.

Trush, M.A., Mimnaugh, E.G., and Gram, T.E., 1982, Activation of pharmacologic agents to radical intermediates: Implications for the role of free radicals in drug action and toxicity, Biochem. Pharmacol., 31:3335-3346.

Van Woert, M.H., and Ambani, L.M., 1974, Biochemistry of neuromelanin, Adv. Neurology., 5:215-223.

HUMAN AND ANIMAL STUDIES WITH CHOLINERGIC AGENTS: HOW CLINICALLY EXPLOITABLE IS THE CHOLINERGIC DEFICIENCY IN ALZHEIMER'S DISEASE

Michael Davidson, Vahram Haroutunian, Richard C. Mohs,
Bonnie M. Davis, Thomas B. Horvath, and
Kenneth L. Davis

Psychiatry Service (116A)
Bronx VA Medical Center
130 W. Kingsbridge Road, Bronx, NY 10468
and
Departments of Psychiatry and Pharmacology
Mt. Sinai School of Medicine
One Gustave L. Levy Place, New York, NY 10029

INTRODUCTION

Studies of brain neurotransmitter systems in patients with a diagnosis of Alzheimer's Disease (AD) repeatedly demonstrated a deficit in the cholinergic system (Davies and Maloney, 1976) suggesting that a rational treatment approach would be the pharmacologic enhancement of cholinergic activity. Pharmacologic strategies employed in this attempt included: increasing Acetylcholine (ACh) synthesis by precursor loading; limiting ACh breakdown by inhibiting Acetylcholine Esterase (AChE); administration of direct receptor agonists; a combination of two pharmacologic strategies. This paper reviews animal and clinical data that attempt central cholinergic augmentation.

ANIMAL STUDIES

The cholinergic neurons of the nucleus basalis of Meynert (nbM) which project to the cortex degenerate during the course of AD (Price et al, 1982). Lesions of the rat nbM result in the pronounced depletion of cholinergic markers in the cortex (Johnston et al., 1981). Hence, nbM lesioned rats serve as an interesting system to investigate the impact of a cortical cholinergic deficit on cognitive processes (Bartus et al., 1982).

nbM lesion-induced cognitive deficits in rats are demonstrable in a variety of learning and memory paradigms including tests of long term habituation, acquisition and retention of T-maze alternation, spatial matching to sample, and passive avoidance. For example nbM lesioned rats and sham operated controls, were exposed to a novel environment on two consecutive occasions separated by 24 hours. During the initial exposure to the novel experiment, lesioned and control animals engaged in comparable amounts of exploration and locomotor activity. There were also no group differences in the rate of habituation of the exploratory response. Significant differences between the lesioned and sham operated animals emerged however, when the two groups were reintroduced to the test environment 24 hours later. Exploratory behavior was greatly reduced in the sham operated rats on their second exposure to the test chamber. This was probably due to long term habituation and decreased novelty of the test environment. Lesioned rats, on the other hand, showed no long term habituation and behaved in the test chamber in exactly the same manner as they had during their first exposure. Thus exploratory behavior, locomotor capacity, and short term habituation were unaffected by the nbM lesion, while the retention of habituation was severely impaired. Similar results were obtained in a study of the long term habituation of an acoustic startle response. The slope of the within-session habituation curve in this study was comparable in lesioned and sham operated controls, however on retest 24 hours later, the nbM lesioned rats showed no evidence of long term habituation, whereas controls showed significant long term habituation of the acoustic startle response.

Thus, lesions of the nbM area in the rat lead to the impairment of memory for simple tasks. Subsequently experiments examined the effect of nbM lesion on more complex cognitive functions. The ability of nbM lesioned rats to perform in a delayed matching to sample task was investigated. nbM lesioned and sham operated controls were permitted to obtain food reinforcement from one corner of a rectangular test chamber. Thereafter the animals were reinforced only when they returned to the same corner where reinforcement had been previously available. Once the animals mastered this task, short delays (5 min and 10 min) were interposed between phases one and two. Thus reinforcement in phase two was dependent upon the retention of where reinforcement had occurred during phase one. Lesioned and control animals performed comparably during the no-delay portion of the experiment. The introduction of 5 and 10 minute delays between phase one and phase two of each trial resulted in a significant rise in the number of errors made by the lesioned animals relative to the performance of the sham operated controls. As a further test of the effects of cholinergic impairment on the performance of this task, the 5 minute delay condition was repeated under conditions of low dose scopolamine challenge. Control and lesioned animals were injected with scopolamine 15 min prior to the initiation of the 5 min delay condition. Sham operated controls increased their error rated by 18%. Error rate for the lesioned animals on the other hand increased by 84%. A similar impairment of memory for complex tasks in nbM lesioned rats was observed where acquisition of a T-maze alteration task was examined. These experiments demonstrate that nbM lesions produce a deficit in simple and complex learned behavior with no effect on exploratory behavior or locomotor activity,suggesting that cholinergic cells of the nbM have a specific role in cognitive functions. A further step in elucidating the relationship between this experimental cholinergic and cognitive deficit was performed by attempting to reverse the cognitive deficit of nbM lesioned animals by cholinergic enhancement.

Studies focusing on the pharmacological reversal of nbM lesion induced cognitive deficits have used a one trial passive avoidance task. In this passive avoidance task the animals are permitted to enter the dark side of a light/dark shuttle box. Upon entry into the dark chamber the animal receives a foot shock and is injected with either saline, physostigmine 0.03 mg/kg or 0.06 mg/kg. Retention is tested by repeating the above procedures 72 hours later. Latency to cross from the light into the dark compartment of the shuttle box is used as the index of memory. Animals with lesions of the nbM show very poor retention of this passive avoidance task relative to sham operated controls. Typically, nbM lesioned rats enter into the shock chamber during the retention test with crossthrough latencies which are only marginally greater than their initial, pre-shock crossthrough latencies. Physostigmine enhanced the retention of the passive avoidance response in both sham operated and nbM lesioned rats. The dose of physostigmine required to achieve significant enhancement of retention in nbM lesioned rats was twice that which was needed for significant improvement in the sham operated controls. In fact that effective dose of physostigmine in nbM lesioned rats had a detrimental effect on the retention test performance of the sham operated controls. The finding that a larger dose of physostigmine is needed for improved performance in nbM lesioned animals relative to sham operated controls is not surprising in light of the lesion induced decreases in cholinergic projections to the cortex with a concomitant decrease in choline acetyltransferase (CAT) (Haroutunian et al., 1985).

An alternative method of enhancing cholinergic activity is to increase the quantal release of acetylcholine by the cholinergic neuron. The metabolic enhancer 4 - aminopyridine (4 AP) has been shown to increase neurotransmitter release from nerve terminals (Vizi et al., 1977). 4-AP, like physostigmine, can enhance the passive avoidance test performance of non-lesioned adult rats (Haroutunian et al., 1985). When 4-AP was administered to nbM lesioned rats immediately following one trial passive avoidance training significant alleviation of the lesion induced deficit was observed. As was the case with physostigmine, a larger dose of 4-AP was needed to augment the test performance of the nbM lesioned rats compared with the dose effective in sham operated animals.

The principal action of physostigmine and 4-AP are through the modulation of presynaptic cholinergic activity. Since AD involves the progressive degeneration of central cholinergic neurons, direct receptor activation was attempted. The effects of the muscarinic agonist oxotremorine was tested in naive as well as nbM lesioned rats. Low dose oxotremorine (0.1 and 0.2 mg/kg) were potent stimulators of passive avoidance retention in naive rats. When these same doses were administered to nbM-lesioned and sham operated rats a different profile of results was obtained. The 0.1 and 0.2 mg/kg doses effectively enhanced retention test performance in sham operated controls, but neither dose had a significant effect on the performance of nbM lesioned rats. In fact, the 0.2 mg/kg dose appeared to have a deleterious effect on the performance of the lesioned rats. However, smaller doses of oxotremorine, were quite effective in augmenting the test performance of nbM lesioned rats. These data suggest that nbM lesions may lead to increased sensitivity to oxotremorine, necessitating the use of lower doses of oxotremorine in rats with lesion induced cholinergic deficits. This is interesting in light of the marked central cholinergic side effects observed in AD patients treated with oxotremorine.

Taken as a whole, the studies outlined above have shown that the cholinergic cells of the nbM are closely involved in the acquisition and retention of learned behaviors. Furthermore, these studies show that the pharmacological enhancement of cholinergic function can, at least partially, overcome nbM lesion-induced cognitive deficits. Further animal studies should investigate the cognitive effect of other neurotransmitter and neuromodulator deficiencies like norepinephrine and somatostatin which seem to be reduced in the brains of some AD patients. A combined cholinergic and noradrenergic experimental deficiency may be a better model for the study of AD, than an nbM lesion alone.

HUMAN STUDIES

In addition to the animal and postmortem investigations pharmacological studies with the muscarinic receptor blocker scopolamine suggest cholinergic enhancement as a treatment modality in patients with AD. Scopolamine administration produces a transient cognitive impairment in normal subjects in a pattern that shares some characteristics with AD (Drachman, Levitt, 1974).

ACh precursor loading has been an often used strategy in clinical trials attempting to enhance cholinergic transmission in AD patients, mainly due to safety and ease of administration. Despite preclinical evidence that precursors can increase ACh brain levels (Cohen et al., 1976), clinical trials with choline and lecithin showed minimal or no improvements in symptoms of AD patients (Thal et al., 1981; Etienne, 1983), probably because under normal conditions precursors availability does not increase choline neuronal uptake or ACh release (Bierkamper and Goldberg, 1979). However, under conditions of increased neuronal firing precursor availability may augment ACh release (Goldberg 1982). This hypothesis was tested in clinical trials combining lecithin with the metabolic enhancer piracetam, a drug thought to enhance release of ACh and therefore the uptake of choline. A study of 10 patients given piracetam combined with 3 doses of lecithin, each dose for one week, produce mainly negative results. This is in agreement with a similar piracetam/choline study which reported minimal improvement in AD symptom (Friedman et al., 1981). Another presynaptic strategy, presently in clinical trial, is based on the ability of 4-AP to augment the amount of neurotransmitter released per nerve impulse. This in conjunction with precursor loading, may prove a useful approach in some AD patients. Indeed, a presynaptic approach may have the advantage of mimicking the phasic action of the cholinergic cells. Unfortunately this strategy also has serious limitations. Many AD patients have an extensive cholinergic cell loss. This is in addition to the limited overlapping cholinergic projections (Coyle et al., 1983) which may preclude the surviving cells from compensating functionally for the lost neurons, makes a presynaptic strategy ultimately, a flawed one.

Administration of physostigmine, an AChE inhibitor augments the amount of ACh available in the synaptic cleft. In order to establish the effect of this drug on cognitive symptoms of AD patients physostigmine was initially administered IV (Davis et al,1982). Thirteen out of 16 patients infused with 3 different doses of physostigmine showed a statistically significant but moderate transient improvement on the visual recognition memory test. In spite of the theoretical importance of this finding, confirmed by others (Christie et al, 1981), its clinical applicability is limited by the short action of intravenous physostigmine. A meaningful evaluation of the drug therapeutic potential in AD required a better and safer delivery route which would enable a comprehensive evaluation of this drug over an extended period of time. Such a comprehensive evaluation needs to assess cognitive and non cognitive symptoms and possess the flexibility to include AD patients in different stages of this progressive disease. Alzheimer Disease Rating Scale (ADRS) (Rosen et al., 1984) is such an instrument. It is specifically designed to evaluate severity of symptoms in pharmacological studies. Cognition and language are assessed by task such as object naming, following commands, orientation, constructional and ideational praxis. Non cognitive behaviors are assessed by item such as depression, cooperation, psychotic symptoms, motor activity and vegetative signs. The scale includes a broad range of tasks so that both very severe and mildly symptomatic patients can be evaluated. A higher score on the scale represents a more severe form of illness. Using this scale in conjunction with repeated oral administration of physostigmine provides a framework to study the more chronic effects of this treatment. The ability of oral physostigmine to improve AD symptoms depends on the drug absorption, central penetrance, and the number of functioning cholinergic neurons still intact. It should be anticipated that in patients with extensive cholinergic cell loss or major abnormalities in other neurotransmitter systems physostigmine would be either unlikely to increase neurotransmission or improve symptoms. Consequently, it is necessary to obtain a measure of physostigmine biological effect in the central nervous system along with measures of symptom severity. Cortisol secretion may be a potential indicator of physostigmine effect on cholinergic activity, as suggested by human and animal studies demonstrating that cholinergic drugs increase and anticholinergic suppress cortisol nocturnal secretion (Davis et al., 1982; Davis et al., 1983). Hence, plasma cortisol levels were measured in a study examining the effect of physostigmine on symptoms of AD patients.

Twelve patients with a diagnosis of probable AD by the recent NINCDS-ADRDA criteria (McKhann et al., 1984) were given 4 doses of oral physostigmine. The drug was given Q 2 h each dose for 3 to 4 days. The dose associated with the best response and placebo were repeated for 5 additional days. This dose-finding/replication design was chosen based on previous finding showing that cholinergic drugs enhance memory in a narrow low dose range (Davis and Mohs, 1978), and that different optimal doses may be required for each patient. Plasma cortisol was measured on the last night of each treatment condition in the replication phase. Eleven of 12 patients studied had lower (better) ADRS scores on a dose of physostigmine which was maintained in 7 patients during the replication phase. Only about a 1/3 of patients showed a consistent and clinically evident improvement on physostigmine. However, it is encouraging to note that patients who improved during the replication phase also tended to show the greatest improvement during the dose finding phase. Examination of percent increase in mean nocturnal cortisol revealed a strong linear relationship between percent increase in cortisol and symptoms improvement suggesting that patient's symptoms improved only to the extent that physostigmine enhanced central cholinergic activity. Physostigmine induced improvement in some AD patients reported here is in agreement with most (Sullivan et al., 1982; Muramoto et al., 1984; Thal et al., 1983), but not all reported studies (Ashford et al., 1981), with consistently more robust effect being noted. Undoubtedly the heterogeneity of the condition of cholinergic neurones and the variable involvement of other neurotransmitters and neuromodulators contributes to the differences among studies. However, it is likely that the use of biological measures (e.g. nocturnal cortisol, CSF AChE) will help further studies identify patients who should benefit from cholinergic manipulations.

Several additional questions raised by the recent attempts to enhance cholinergic neurotransmission in AD patients need to be addressed in order to meaningfully evaluate this therapeutic approach. Clinician's diagnostic impressions are incorrect in almost a third of patients as indicated by long term follow-up (Marsden and Harrison, 1972). Such patients have other neurologic disorders or lack the characteristic histopathologic findings required for postmortem validation of AD (Liston and Rue, 1983). Even rigorous diagnostic criteria have a 10% error rate. Hence typical pharmacological trials, with relatively small sample size are less likely to find statistically significant group means if they include the inevitable misdiagnosed patients. The existence of a subgroup of demented patients deficient in a neurotransmitter in addition to ACh is another problem that may limit the utility of cholinomimetic therapies. Noradrenergic cells of the locus coeruleus are reported to be lost in some AD patients with presenile onset (Bondareff et al., 1982). The neuropeptide somatostatin is a neuromodulator reported to be decreased in the neocortex of AD patients (Rossor et al., 1980). Even if a subgroup of patients with an isolated cholinergic deficiency is identified, an extensive destruction of cholinergic neurons would make the efficacy of a cholinesterase inhibitor improbable. Under these circumstances an alternate strategy for treating the cholinergic deficit might be a direct cholinergic agonist. Studies with the cholinergic agonists oxotremorine and RS86 have begun but in our experience are seriously hampered by cholinergic side effects like depression, anxiety, chills, tremors, bradycardia and hypotension, particularly with oxotremorine. Further, an unanswered question is the extent to which the more tonic effects of a receptor agonist will mimic the more phasic effects of endogenous acetylcholine. Despite these concerns arecoline has been reported to improve the symptoms of AD (Christie et al., 1981), encouraging further trials with direct receptor agonists. Indeed the use of more specific m_1 and m_2 agonists might improve the efficacy of these agents, while diminishing their adverse effects.

In addition to developing safer cholinergic agonists, future studies should investigate specific neurotransmitter abnormalities which would identify pharmacological manipulations required for individual AD patients. For example, combined neurotransmitter enhancement may be the answer to a generalized transmitter deficiency.

REFERENCES

Ashford, J.W., Soldinger, S., Schaeffer, J., Cochran, L., Jarvik, L.F., Physostigmine its effect in six patients with dementia, 1981, Am J Psychiat., 138: 829.

Bartus, R.T., Dean, R.L., Beer, B. and Lippa, A.S. The cholinergic hypothesis of genetic memory dysfunction, 1982, Science, 217: 408.
Bierkamper, G.G., and Goldberg, A.M., 1979, The effect of choline in the release of acetylcholine from the neuromuscular junction in: Nutrition and Brain Vol. 5, Barbeau, A., Growden, J.H., Wurtman, R.J., eds., Raven Press, New York.
Bondareff, W., Mountjoy, C.Q., Roth, M: Loss of neurons of origin of the adrenergic projection to cerebral cortex (nucleus locus coeruleus) in senile dementia, 1982, Neurology 32: 164.
Christie, J.E., Shering, A., Ferguson, J., Glen, A.M., 1981, Physostigmine and arecoline: Effects of intravenous infusion in Alzheimer presenile Brit J Psychiat., 138: 46.
Cohen, E.G., Wurtman, R.J: Brain acetylcholine: control by dietary choline, 1976, Science, 191: 561.
Coyle, J.T., McKinney, M., Johnston, M.V., Hedreen, J.C. , 1983, Synaptic neurochemistry of the basal forebrain cholinergic projection, Psychopharmacol Bull., 19: 441.
Davies, P., and Maloney, A.J.F., 1976, Selective loss of central cholinergic neurons in Alzheimer's disease, Lancet, 2: 1403.
Davis, K.L., and Mohs, R.C., 1982, Enhancement of memory processes in Alzheimer's disease with multiple dose intravenous physostigmine, Am J Psychiat., 139: 1421.
Davis, K.L., Mohs, R.C., Tinklenberg, J.R., Pfefferbaum, A., Hollister, L.E. Kopell, B.S., 1978, Physostigmine improvement of long term memory processes in normal humans, Science, 201: 272.
Davis, B.M., Brown, G.M., Miller, M., Friesen, H.G., Kastin, A.J., Davis, K.L., 1982, Effect of cholinergic stimulation of pituitary hormone release. Psychoneuroendocrinol., 7: 3671.
Davis, B.M., Mathé, A.A., Mohs, R.C., Levy, M.I., 1983, Effects of propantheline bromide on basal growth hormone cortisol and prolactin levels, Psychoneuroendocrinol., 18: 103.
Drachman, D.A., and Levitt, J., 1974, Human memory and the cholinergic system. Arch Neurol. 30: 112.
Etienne, P., 1983, Treatment of Alzheimer's disease with lecithin in: Alzheimer's Disease, B. Reisberg ed., The Free Press, New York.
Friedman, E., Sherman, K.A., Ferris, S.H., 1981, Clinical response to choline plus piracetam in senile dementia: relation to red cell choline levels. N Engl J Med., 304: 1490.
Goldberg, A.M., 1982, The interaction of neuronal activity and choline transport on the regulation of acetylcholine synthesis in: Alzheimer's Disease: A Report of Progress in Research, Vol. 19, Corkin, S., Davis, K.L., Growden, J.H. eds., Raven Press, New York.
Haroutunian, V., Barnes, E., and Davis, K.L., Cholinergic modulation of memory in rats. Psychopharmacology (in press).
Haroutunian, V., Kanof, P. and Davis, K.L. Pharmacological alleviation of the cholinergic lesion induced meory deficit in rats, Life Science (in press).
Johnston, M.V., McKinney, M. and Coyle, J.T., 1981, Neocortical cholinergic innervation: A description of extrinsic and intrinsic components in the rat. Exp. Brain Research, 43: 159.
Liston, E.H., Rue, A.L., 1983, Clinical differentiation of primary degeneration and multi-infarct dementia: A critical review of the evidence. Biol. Psychiat., 12: 1451.
Marsden, C.D., Harrison, M.J.G., 1972, Outcome investigation of patients with presenile dementia. Br J Psychiat., 1: 240.
McKhann, G., Drachman, D., Folstein, M. Katzman, R., Price, D., Stadlan, E.M., 1984, Clinical diagnosis of Alzheimer's disease: Report of NINCDS-ADRDA Work Group under the auspices of the Department of Health and Human Services. Task force of Alzheimer's disease, Neurology, 34: 939.
Muramoto, O., Sugishita, A., Anolo, K., 1984, Cholinergic system and constructional praxis: A further study of physostigmine in Alzheimer's disease. J Neurol Neurosurg Psychiat., 47: 485.
Price, D.L., Whitehouse, P.J., Struble, R.G., Clark, A.W., Coyle, J.T., DeLong, M.R. and Hedreen, J.C., 1982, Basal forebrain cholinergic systems in Alzheimer's

disease and related dementias, Neurosci. Commentaries, 1:84.
Rosen, W.G., Mohs, R.C., Davis, K.L., 1984, A new rating scale for Alzheimer's disease, Am J Psychiat., 141: 11, 1356.
Rossor, M.N., Emerson, P.C., Mountjoy, C.Q., 1980, Reduced amounts of immunoreactive somatostatin in the temporal cortex in senile dementia of Alzheimer type. Neuroscience Letter 20: 373.
Sullivan, E.V., Shedlack, K.J., Corkin, S., 1982, Physostigmine and lecithin in Alzheimer Disease in: Alzheimer Disease: A Report of Progress, S. Corkin, K.L. Davis, J.H. Growdon, E. Usdin, R.J. Wurtman, eds., Raven Press, New York.
Thal, L.J., Fuld, P.A., Masur, D.M., 1983, Oral physostigmine and lecithin improve memory in Alzheimer's disease. Ann Neurol 13: 491.
Thal, L.J., Rosen, W., Sharpless, N.S., 1981, Choline chloride fails to improve cognition in Alzheimer's disease. Neurobiology of Aging 2: 205.
Vizi, E.S., van Dijk, J., Folders, F.F., 1977, The effect of 4-aminopyridine on acetylcholine release. J. Neurol. Trans., 41: 265.

PHARMACOLOGICAL ACTIVITY OF NOVEL ANTICHOLINESTERASE AGENTS OF POTENTIAL USE IN THE TREATMENT OF ALZHEIMER'S DISEASE

Marta Weinstock[1], Michal Razin[1], Michael Chorev[2] & Zeev Tashma[2]
Departments of Pharmacology[1] and Medicinal Chemistry[2]
School of Pharmacy, Hebrew University, Ein Kerem, Jerusalem
Israel

INTRODUCTION

In dementia of the Alzheimer type there is a selective loss in the cerebral cortex of choline acetyltransferase (CAT), the enzyme that synthesizes acetylcholine (ACh)[1,2]. The degree of dementia and memory impairment that occurs in this condition is well correlated with the decrement in cortical cholinergic transmission[3]. Moreover, scopolamine, a cholinergic antagonist, can cause memory impairment in normal individuals similar to that in aging[4]. These findings suggest that impaired cortical cholinergic transmission may be at least in part responsible for the symptomatology of Alzheimer disease. In support of this suggestion it was found that physostigmine, which prevents the destruction of ACh, can cause memory improvement in Alzheimer patients[5]. The extent of improvement of the symptomatology was closely related to the degree of inhibition of acetylcholinesterase (AChE) in the spinal fluid, and thus to the amount of physostigmine reaching the central nervous system[6].

As potential therapy for dementia, physostigmine has a number of disadvantages, the most serious of which is its low therapeutic ratio. In most studies in which any improvement in symptomatology was reported, the dose range in which this occurred was very narrow (1-2.5mg orally[6] or 0.25-0.5mg, i.v.[7]), with higher doses causing a decrement in performance or distressing side effects due to peripheral cholinergic overactivity. Another disadvantage is its low chemical stability[8] and short duration of action, which necessitate frequent dosing. Its oral bioavailability is also unpredictable, and it only appears to produce improvement in Alzheimer symptomatology by this route if it is given with lecithin[9].

The purpose of the present study was to synthesize anticholinesterase agents which readily reach the CNS after parenteral and oral administration; which have a higher therapeutic ratio than that of physostigmine, greater chemical stability, and a longer duration of action. These advantages should make them more suitable than physostigmine for the long term treatment of conditions associated with a deficit in cholinergic transmission in the central nervous system.

Apart from physostigmine, all of the carbamate anticholinesterases which are used medicinally, have a quaternary N-function and thus do not penetrate the CNS to any significant extent[10]. Almost all the synthetic carbamates with a tertiary N were designed as insecticides, and have a monomethyl substituent on the N of the carbamate. They are thus relatively unstable at physiological pH and of short duration[10]. One such carbamate, miotine, has only been used clinically as a miotic[11]. The dimethyl analogue, has only been used as an insecticide[12]. The effect of other mono or dialkyl substitution on the N of the carbamate of this structure on AChE activity _in vitro_ or _in vivo_ does not appear to have been studied. Accordingly we prepared and tested a series of mono and alkyl derivatives of miotine, the activities of some of which are described. (A patent has been applied for the novel structures). Particular emphasis is placed on their abilities to inhibit brain AChE and on their relative toxicities.

METHODS

Preparation of mono- and di-substituted phenyl carbamates

The N-monoalkyl and N,N-dialkyl substituted phenyl carbamates were synthesized from α-m-hydroxyphenylethyl-dimethylamine (I), which was itself prepared according to the procedure described by Stedman and Stedman[11] with minor modifications, as shown in the scheme below:

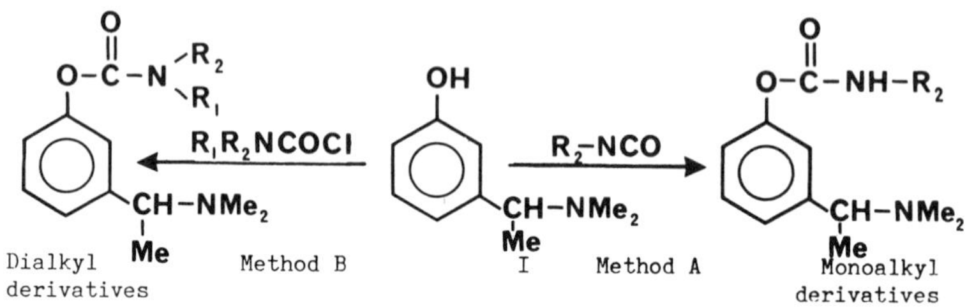

For the synthesis of the monoalkylphenyl carbamates, a 2-3 fold molar excess of the alkyl isocyanate was reacted with phenol I in dry benzene at room temperature overnight (see Scheme 1 method A). For the synthesis of the N,N-dialkyl-substituted phenyl carbamates, 1.5-2 fold molar excess of the corresponding carbamoyl chloride was allowed to react with phenol I in dry acetonitrile in the presence of a similar excess of sodium hydride (see Scheme 1 method B). The weak acidity of phenol I required the use of a strong base such as sodium hydride to produce the phenolate which acts as the nucleophile.

All carbamates were obtained as hydrochloride salts by saturating their etheral solutions with HCl(g). These salts were purified by re-crystallization from ethanol-ether. Purity was assessed by t.l.c. on precoated silica gel plates, reversed-phase HPLC, elemental microchemical analysis and ^{1}H-n.m.r.

Measurement of antiAChE activity in vitro

Male mice (Sabra strain) weighing 30-40g were sacrificed by cervical dislocation and the whole brain minus cerebellum rapidly removed and weighed. The brains from 10 mice were homogenized in 1ml/100g wet weight phosphate buffer 0.1M pH 8.0, centrifuged at 12,000 rpm and the supernatant, discarded. The pellet was mixed with a similar volume as above of buffer 0.1M pH 8.0 containing 1% Triton using a Vortex Genie at maximum speed for 1 min. The mixture was centrifuged and the supernatant which contained most of the solubilized AChE was used for subsequent determinations of anticholinesterase activity.

The effect of at least three different concentrations of each inhibitor was measured on the rate of hydrolysis of 20 µl of 0.075M acetylthiocholine iodide by 25 µl of solubilized AChE. The enzyme was incubated with the inhibitor for periods ranging from 2-180 mins at 37°C before the addition of the substrate. The rate of hydrolysis was measured by the spectrophotometric method of Ellman et al.[13]. From these data the molar concentration of each agent that inhibited the activity of the enzyme by 50% (IC50) at the time of peak activity (30-120 min) was calculated.

Measurement of antiAChE activity in vivo

At least three doses of each drug were administered subcutaneously (s.c.) or orally to mice. Animals were sacrificed at different times ranging from 0.25 to 7 hours after drug administration. The presence or absence of side effects reminiscent of cholinergic hyperactivity (tremors, salivation, defecation, fasciculations, difficulty in breathing) were noted for each drug. The brain was rapidly removed at the given times stated above and the enzyme AChE extracted and solubilized as described in the previous section. The activity of the enzyme removed from drug treated mice was measured as described above and compared with that of mice given saline (control).

Assessment of acute toxicity

Male mice were given one of at least three different doses of each drug orally or s.c., a minimum of 10 mice being alotted to each dose. The number of animals that died in each group within 3 hours was determined, and from these data the LD50 (dose in µmoles/kg which was lethal to 50% of the mice) was computed.

Table 1. Relationship between chemical structure, relative hydrophobicity and molar refractivity of phenyl carbamates

Drug	R^1	R^2	Capacity factor (k')*	Mol. Refractivity
RA2 (miotine)	H	Me	0.5	5.65
RA6	H	Et	0.83	10.30
RA15	H	n-Pr	1.48	14.96
RA13	H	i-Pr	1.37	14.96
RA14	H	Allyl	1.33	14.49
RA12	H	c-Hexyl	6.17	26.69
RA10	Me	Me	1.33	11.30
RA7	Me	Et	2.33	15.95
RA8	Et	Et	4.33	20.60

* Capacity factor defined as ratio of difference between retention time of the compound and that of the unretained solute to that of the unretained solute on a reversed phase (C18) HPLC column (solvent; 70% of 0.1% aqueous TFA soln. + 30% methanol). This factor is a measure of the relative hydrophobicity of the compound.

This experiment was repeated in animals which had been pretreated 15 mins previously with either atropine methylnitrate (ATMN 5mg/kg) which block only peripheral muscarinic receptors[14] or atropine sulphate, (5mg/kg) which blocks both central and peripheral muscarinic receptors, and the anticholinesterase agents were injected s.c.

Measurement of antiAChE activity in different areas of rat brain

Male and female Sabra rats weighing 150-350g were injected s.c. with either saline, physostigmine 0.15mg/kg, RA6 1.0mg/kg. RA7 0.5mg/kg or RA15 0.5mg/kg (six animals were used for each treatment group). The cerebral cortex, hippocampus, corpus striatum and medulla oblongata were rapidly dissected on ice, weighed individually, homogenized in phosphate buffer and extracted and solubilized as described above for mouse brain. The activity of the enzyme from treated and control rats was also measured as described above.

The percent inhibition of AChE by each drug was computed for the different brain areas by comparison with the pooled mean of the control values (n=12) for each area.

Statistical analyses. Data from the experiment on the effects of drugs on AChE in different areas of rat brain were analysed by 2-way analysis of variance, followed by Neuman Keul's post hoc comparisons.

RESULTS

The relationship between the N alkyl substituents, relative hydrophobicity and molar refractivity is shown in Table 1. In general both the latter parameters increased as the size of the mono or disubstituted alkyl groups became larger.

Table 2. The effect of the novel compounds on AChE activity in mouse brain *in vitro* and *in vivo*

Drug	IC50 µM	Relative Potency to Physostigmine	ED50 µMoles/kg	Relative Potency to Physostigmine
Physostigmine	0.011	100	0.92	100
RA2	0.013	85	0.92	100
RA6	0.40	3	8.47	11
RA15	0.11	10	2.80	33
RA13	12.10	0.1	40.0	2
RA14	0.43	3	6.01	15
RA12	0.093	12	7.24	13
RA10	0.027	41	1.14	81
RA7	3.00	0.4	4.20	22
RA8	35.0	0.03	56.0	2

AntiAChE activity in mouse brain

The inhibitory activities of the novel carbamates and physostigmine on a solubilized preparation of AChE of mouse whole brain *in vitro* are summarized in Table 2. The monomethyl substituted derivative, RA2, (miotine), was found to be the most potent inhibitor of brain AChE, both *in vitro* and *in vivo*. It has a rapid onset of action which is of a relatively short duration (90-120 min *in vivo*) like that of physostigmine (Table 3). Increase in the size of the alkyl radical to ethyl (RA6), resulted in a large reduction (>30 fold) in *in vitro* activity, but only a 6-fold decrease, *in vivo*. Larger substituents, n-propyl, and c-hexyl proved to be more potent inhibitors than N-ethyl, or N-allyl, but less so, than N-methyl, while introduction of an i-propyl group resulted in a 1000-fold decrease in AChE activity. In general, all the novel monosubstituted carbamates were more active *in vivo* by factors of 2-20 times, than one would have expected from the activities on the isolated enzyme when compared to physostigmine or miotine. [Table 2].

Comparison of the data in Tables 1 and 2, reveals that there is no correlation between *in vitro* anticholinesterase activity (IC50) of the monosubstituted carbamates and any of the physical parameters examined, e.g. chain length in extended conformation, methyl (RA2), <ethyl (RA6), <n-propyl (RA15); molar refractivity, cf. c-hexyl (RA12), ethyl and i-propyl (RA13); hydrophobicity, cf n-propyl and i-propyl.

The disubstituted carbamates were generally less active *in vitro* than the corresponding monosubstituted derivatives. Among the three analogues there appeared to be a negative correlation between inhibitory potency, and both hydrophobicity and molar refractivity volume.

Introduction of a second methyl group on the N of the carbamate caused only a small reduction in inhibitory activity. However, when one group was substituted by ethyl, (RA7) *in vitro* activity fell by 2 orders of magnitude. Surprisingly, this compound was considerably more potent than one would have expected from the *in vitro* data when it was injected into the whole animal Under these conditions its activity was only reduced to 1/3rd of that of the dimethyl derivative.

Table 3. Duration of action of carbamates on brain AChE in mice

Drug	Time of peak inhibition (min.)	% inhibition ± s.e. by ED50 at 3 hrs	ED50 oral / ED50 s.c.
Physostigmine	15	0	4.3
RA2	15	0	1.3
RA6	30-120	47±1	2.6
RA15	15-30	26±5	4.0
RA14	30	41±3	3.8
RA12	30-60	36±3	3.0
RA10	15	0	3.4
RA7	60-120	33±3	1.5
RA8	30-120	31±6	1.4

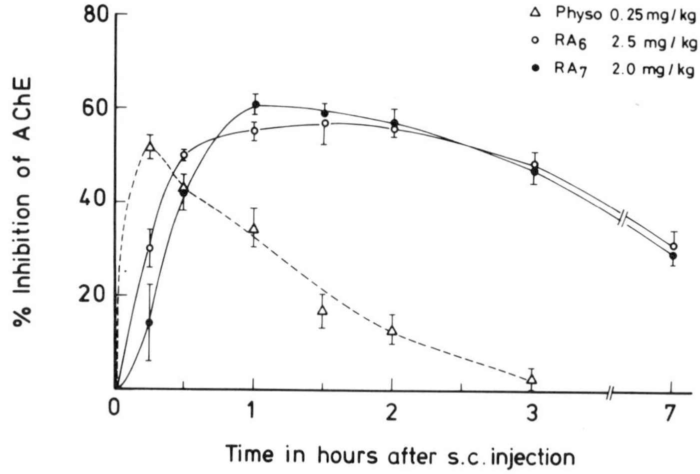

Fig. 1: Duration of inhibition of brain AChE after s.c. injection of physostigmine, RA6 and RA7 in mice

The diethyl substituted compound, RA8, proved to be a weak inhibitor, with an IC50 of only 35 µM. All the compounds having a substitutent larger than methyl, had a slower onset of action, both on the isolated solubilized enzyme and in the whole animal, and a longer duration of action *in vivo*, than methyl derivatives and physostigmine (Table 3). The latter drugs ceased to inhibit brain AChE 2-3 hours after injection, while all the novel compounds with alkyl substituents larger than methyl caused significant inhibition for 3-7 hours [Fig. 1].

The maximum inhibition of the brain AChE after oral administration of any dose of physostigmine, did not exceed 50%. This was achieved at about a 4 times larger dose than the ED50 after s.c. injection [Table 3]. Higher doses, caused marked respiratory distress, fasciculations and tremors. With the possible exception of RA10, a greater than 70% inhibition of brain AChE was obtained after oral administration of all the other compounds. The incidence of untoward symptoms due to cholinergic overactivity was also much lower with these compounds.

Acute toxicity

The acute toxicity of the anticholinesterase agents is shown in Table 4, when these were given alone or after pretreatment with ATMN or atropine. The therapeutic ratios, defined as the LD50/ED50, of all the compounds except RA2 were about 3 times greater than that of physostigmine, which was only 3.3. Blockade of peripheral muscarinic receptors by ATMN, caused a similar increase in LD50 (1.5-2.2 fold) in all the compounds. When muscarinic receptors in the CNS were also blocked by atropine, the LD50 of physostigmine and the majority of the compounds rose by 2.2-3.5 fold. The disubstitued compounds, RA10 and RA7, however, showed a 6-11 fold increase in LD50.

AntiAChE activity in different areas of rat brain

The AChE activity of different areas of rat brain is shown in Table 5. While the cerebral cortex, hippocampus and medulla showed approximately similar amounts of enzyme activity, that in the striatum was about 10-fold higher.

Fig. 2 shows the effect of physostigmine and three novel carbamates on AChE activity in 4 areas of rat brain. The doses of the 4 drugs were chosen which gave the same degree of inhibition of AChE in the cerebral cortex. At these doses, RA6, RA7 and RA15 caused significantly less inhibition in the medulla ($P<0.05$) and RA7 caused a lower effect in the striatum, than in the cortex. RA6 and RA7 also produced significantly less inhibition in the medulla than did physostigmine. The effect of RA15 in the hippocampus was significantly greater than that of all the other drugs when given at a dose that inhibited the enzyme in the cortex to a similar extent.

DISCUSSION

In the present series of carbamate derivatives *in vitro* inhibition (IC50) of brain AChE varied 3000-fold from the most to least potent drug. In the mono-alkylated derivatives, no correlation was found between the IC50 values and hydrophobicity, molar refractivity, or length of the most extended conformation of the carbamate moiety. Thus, the largest substituent, c-hexyl, showed a much smaller decrease in inhibitory potency compared to miotine, than did the monoethyl derivative. On the other hand, introduction of an i-propyl resulted in a 1000-fold decrease in activity, while n-propyl, which has the same molar refractivity and hydrophobicity, was only 10 times less potent than miotine.

Table 4. Acute toxicity of carbamates in mice

Drug	LD50 µmoles/kg s.c.	Therapeutic ratio (LD50/ED50)	Degree of protection** afforded by pretreatment with ATMN*	Atropine*
Physo.	3.0	3.3	1.8	3.0
RA2	4.50	4.9	1.8	2.4
RA6	95.7	11.3	1.5	2.7
RA15	30.5	10.9	1.5	3.0
RA14	64.8	10.8	1.8	2.2
RA12	41.5	9.8	1.2	3.5
RA10	12.4	10.9	1.6	5.8
RA7	46.0	11.0	2.2	10.9
RA8	>568	>10.0	-	

* Drug injected 15 min. after atropine methyl nitrate 5 mg/kg or atropine sulphate 5 mg/kg

** $\frac{\text{LD50 after ATMN or atropine pretreatment}}{\text{LD50 of drug alone}}$

Table 5. AChE activity in different areas of rat brain

Brain Area	μM of substrate hydrolysed per min per mg. tissue ± s.e.
Cerebral cortex (11)	2.73±0.09
Hippocampus (12)	3.43±0.09
Medulla (12)	5.55±0.27
Corpus striatum (11)	27.10±1.10

Furthermore, no clear correlation could be demonstrated between anti AChE activity of the carbamates on the isolated enzyme taken from mouse brain and that obtained *ex vivo* after injection of the drug into mice. All the novel carbamates were relatively much more active *in vivo* in relation to physostigmine or miotine, than *in vitro*. This discrepancy was especially evident in the disubstituted analogues, RA7 and RA8. These compounds were 50-60 times more effective *in vivo* than one would have predicted from the data on the isolated enzyme.

The relatively greater activity of the larger monoalkyl and dialkyl substituted drugs in the whole animal may be due to a greater chemical stability. It has previously been shown that monomethyl carbamates are much less stable that dimethyl derivatives at physiolgical pH[10]. The relatively long duration of enzyme inhibition (>7 hours) of all the larger alkyl derivatives *in vivo*, (compared with about 2 hours for physostigmine) suggests that they are chemically more stable at body pH and are more slowly metabolized.

Another reason for the greater *in vivo* activity of the RA compounds may be their higher lipid solubility, which should enable a greater proportion of the drug to reach the central nervous system. This property could also explain the more efficient absorption from the gastro-intestinal tract of several of these carbamates, particularly RA7 and RA8.

Comparison of the acute toxicity of the RA compounds with that of physostigmine in mice, showed the former to have considerably higher therapeutic ratios, 10-12, compared with 3.3 for physostigmine and 4.5 for miotine. Furthermore, signs of cholinergic overactivity, fasciculations, tremors, salivation and defecation were seen at the ED50 dose (which caused 50% inhibition of the whole brain enzyme) of physostigmine but not of the other carbamates. The greater therapeutic ratios of the RA compounds appears at first sight to be surprising since the mortality is a direct result of AChE inhibition, and is due to the presence of excess AChE in the medulla, which causes respiratory arrest[15]. This was demonstrated in the present study by pretreating the animals with atropine which prevents the centrally induced respiratory depression[14], and which raises the LD50 of all the monosubstituted carbamates by a factor of about 3. In the presence of such muscarinic blockade, death from overdose then results from respiratory muscle paralysis due to excess ACh at the neuromuscular junction. At this stage, no antidotes are effective and only artificial ventilation can prevent loss of life. The fact that the LD50 of RA7 can be increased 11-fold by muscarinic receptor blockade, demonstrates a relative lack of effect of this drug on somatic muscle. This is a distinct advantage in terms of its therapeutic potential.

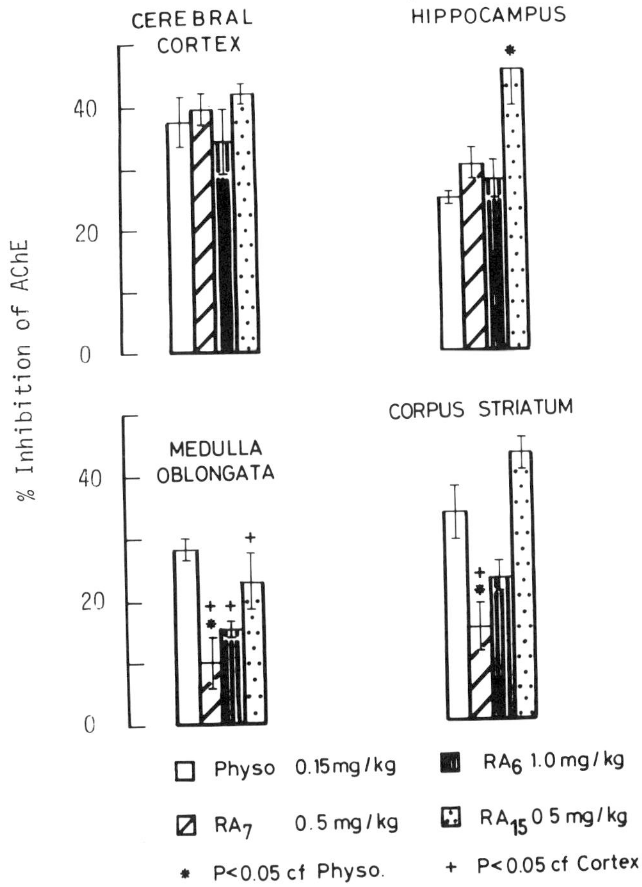

Fig. 2. Inhibition of AChE in different areas of rat brain by physostigmine and 3 novel carbamates
* Significantly different from physostigmine in same brain area $P<0.05$
\+ Significantly different from value in cortex for same drug $P<0.05$

In order to explain the lower toxicity of the RA compounds an attempt was made to determine whether they have a selective effect in different brain areas. It was found that physostigmine inhibited AChE to the same extent in four areas in the rat brain in spite of the fact that these areas contain different amounts of enzyme. In contrast, RA6, RA7 and RA15 given in doses which blocked AChE in the cerebral cortex by 35-40%, caused significantly less inhibition in the medulla. The most striking difference was seen with RA7 which only reduced AChE in the medulla by 10%. Since the ED50 was determined in whole brain, of which the cerebral cortex contributes a major portion compared to the medulla, this differential effect of the drugs serves to explain their higher therapeutic ratio.

The selective effect may result from a difference in the distribution of the drugs to these brain areas. Alternatively, it may be due to the presence of AChE isoenzymes, which could have different affinities for the inhibitors. Such a differential sensitivity of multiple forms of AChE has been demonstrated for organophosphates[10]. It remains to be determined whether multiple forms of AChE are present in rat brain, and whether they are selectively inhibited by RA compounds.

The data from this study show that larger monoalkyl or dialkyl derivatives of miotine, possess several advantages over physostigmine for potential therapeutic application in conditions involving reduced cholinergic transmission in the cerebral cortex. If the therapeutic effect of these agents results from inhibition of AChE in this brain area, compounds RA6, RA15, RA14, RA12, RA10, RA7 and RA8 all have considerably higher therapeutic ratios than physostigmine and show fewer side effects at ED50 doses. This may be due to a selective inhibition in cortical areas sparing the medulla. RA7 and RA10 have an additional advantage in the fact that the lethal effects of drug overdose can be prevented by atropine. While the duration of significant enzyme inhibition after physostigmine is less than 2 hours, all the above drugs (except RA10) act for periods of 7 hours or more after a single injection. The longer duration is a distinct advantage in the treatment of chronic conditions such as Alzheimer's disease. Furthermore, RA6, RA7 and RA8 show a significantly more efficient oral absorption since their potencies when given by this route closely resemble those after parenteral administration.

Acknowledgement. This research was supported by a grant from the Israeli National Council for Research and Development No. 2248.

REFERENCES

1. P. Davies, and A.J.F. Maloney, Selective loss of central cholinergic neurons in Alzheimer's disease, Lancet 2:1403 (1976).
2. J.A. Richter, E.K. Perry, and E.B. Tomlinson, Acetylcholine and choline levels in post-mortem human brain tissue: preliminary observations in Alzheimer's disease, Life Sci., 26:1683 (1980).
3. E.K. Perry, B.E. Tomlinson, G. Blessed, K. Bergmann, P.H. Gibson, and R.H. Perry, Correlation of cholinergic abnormalities with senile plaques and mental test scores in senile dementia, Br. Med. J., 2:1457 (1979).
4. D.A. Drachman, and J.B. Leavitt, Human memory and the cholinergic system, Arch. Neurol., 30:113 (1974).
5. K.L. Davis, R.C. Mohs, and J.R. Tinklenberg, Enhancement of memory by physostigmine, N. Engl. J. Med., 301:946 (1979).
6. L.J. Thal, P.A. Fuld, M.S. Masur, and N.S. Sharpless, Oral physostigmine and lecithin improve memory in Alzheimer's disease, Ann. Neurol., 13:491 (1983).
7. K.L. Davis, and R.C. Mohs, Enhancement of memory processes in Alzheimer's disease with multiple-dose intravenous physostigmine, Am. J. Psychiat., 139:1421 (1982).
8. E. Stedman, Studies on the relationship between chemical constitution and physiolgical action. I. Position isomerism in relation to miotic activity of synthetic methanes. Biochem. J. 20: 719 (1926).
9. B.H. Peters, and H.S. Levin, Effects of physostigmine and lecithin on memory in Alzheimer's disease. Ann. Neurol. 6: 219 (1979).
10. A.R. Main, Mode of action of anticholinesterases. Pharmacol. Therap. 6: 579 (1979).
11. E. Stedman, and E. Stedman, Methyl urethans of the isomeric α hydroxyphenylethyldimethylamines and their miotic activity. J. Chem. Soc. 609 (1929).

12. J. Meltzer, and H.B.A. Welle, Insecticidal activity of substituted phenyl N-methyl carbamates. Entomol. Exp. Appl. 12:169 (1969).
13. G.L. Ellman, K.D. Courtney, V. Andres Jr., and R.M. Featherstone, A new and rapid colorimetric determination of acetylcholinesterase activity. Biochem. Pharmacol. 7: 88 (1961).
14. A. Herz, H. Teschamacher, A. Hofstetter, and K. Kurg, Importance of lipid solubility for the central action of cholinolytic drugs. Int. J. Neuropharmacol. 4, 207 (1965).
15. X. Machne, and K.W.R. Unna, Actions at the central nervous system, in: "Cholinesterases and Anticholinesterase Agents", G.B. Koelle, ed., Springer-Verlag, Berlin (1963).

SULFONYL FLUORIDES AS POSSIBLE THERAPEUTIC AGENTS IN ALZHEIMER'S DISEASE: STRUCTURE/ACTIVITY RELATIONSHIPS AS CNS SELECTIVE CHOLINESTERASE INHIBITORS[1]

D. E. Moss, L. A. Rodriguez, W. C. Herndon,
S. P. Vincenti, and M. L. Camarena

Departments of Psychology and Chemistry
University of Texas at El Paso
El Paso, Texas 79968

INTRODUCTION

Senile dementia of the Alzheimer's type (SDAT) is a disease that produces gross pathological changes in the brain. However, it has also been recently associated with specific changes in neurotransmitters such as somatostatin (Davies, Katzman and Terry, 1980; Rossor et al., 1980; Rogers and Morrison, 1984), amino acids (Arai, Kobayashi, Ichimiya, Kosaka and Iizuka, 1984) and acetylcholine (Davies and Maloney, 1976; Whitehouse et al., 1982). Although SDAT is not a disorder of a single neurotransmitter, deterioration of cholinergic function in the CNS appears to be correlated with dementia. For example, loss of the cholinergic system related to the nucleus basalis of Meynert (nbM) is associated with dementia in other disorders including Parkinson's disease (Nakano and Hirano, 1984), parkinsonism-dementia complex of Guam, and boxer's dementia (Nakano and Hirano, 1983). It is the apparent association between deterioration of the cholinergic system and dementia that is the basis for the cholinergic strategies for treating SDAT (e.g., Davies, 1981; Bartus, Dean, Beer and Lippa, 1982). In fact, physostigmine, a cholinesterase[2] inhibitor that acts within the CNS as well as peripherally, has been reported to produce clinical improvement in tests with SDAT patients (e.g., Davis and Mohs, 1982; Brinkman and Gershon, 1983). This limited success has led to interest in developing a system for delivering cholinergic drugs directly into the CNS (Harbaugh, Roberts, Coombs, Saunders and Reeder, 1984) as well as the development of new long-lasting carbamate cholinesterase inhibitors that may have improved efficacy (Weinstock, Razin and Chorev, this volume).

Because of the apparent involvement of the CNS cholinergic system and the initial limited success with physostigmine, the development of CNS selective cholinesterase inhibitors was specifically suggested by Davies (1981) as an alternative possible treatment strategy for SDAT. Recently, we discovered that a few selected sulfonyl fluorides are interesting

----

[1]Supported in part by NIMH, the MBRS Program, the Robert A. Welch Foundation of Houston, Texas, and the Moss Family.

[2]The term "cholinesterase" is used as a generic label for all forms of the enzyme including acetylcholinesterase (E.C. 3.1.1.7) and butyrylcholinesterase (E.C. 3.1.1.8) (see Massoulie and Bon, 1982).

cholinesterase inhibitors with a high inherent selectivity for the CNS and, therefore, potential therapeutic agents in the treatment of SDAT (Moss, Rodriguez, Selim, Ellett, Devine and Steger, 1985).

The sulfonyl fluorides are long-lasting irreversible cholinesterase inhibitors which form a covalent sulfonyl-enzyme complex similar to the phosphonyl-enzyme complex formed by the organic phosphate inhibitors (Fahrney and Gold, 1963; Kitz and Wilson, 1962; Myers and Kemp, 1954). Phenylmethanesulfonyl fluoride (PMSF, also known as phenylmethylsulfonyl fluoride and alpha-toluenesulfonyl fluoride) was found to produce up to 80% inhibition of rat CNS cholinesterase after a single large dose with less than 50% inhibition in the peripheral cholinergic systems (skeletal muscle, smooth muscle and heart). In addition, because CNS synthesis of new enzyme is slow relative to peripheral tissues, it was demonstrated that repeated administrations of small doses of either PMSF or methanesulfonyl fluoride (MSF) could produce up to 90% inhibition within the CNS with less than 30% inhibition in the peripheral tissues with no appearance of gross cholinesterase toxicity (Moss et al., 1985b). Other research has shown that PMSF and MSF do not suppress extrapyramidal motor behaviors like other CNS active inhibitors (Moss, Rodriguez and McMaster, 1985). In view of the potential therapeutic applications in SDAT and related disorders, the purpose of the present experiments was to attempt to determine which of several sulfonyl fluorides are CNS selective cholinesterase inhibitors.

METHOD

In the original experiments (Moss et al., 1985b), only four closely related compounds (PMSF, MSF, benzenesulfonyl fluoride, and para-toluenesulfonyl fluoride) were studied. In the present experiments, an additional 33 sulfonyl fluorides of widely varying structure were screened for reactivity against CNS and peripheral cholinesterase. As in the earlier experiments (Moss et al., 1985b), the compounds were dissolved in Emulphor EL-620, a polyoxyethylated vegetable oil (GAF Corp., Los Angeles) immediately before use and tested _in vivo_ by an initial i.p. injection of 0.575 mmole/kg (a dose equal to 100 mg/kg PMSF). The animals were observed for two to four hours after injection for gross toxic effects. If the animals did not survive, a lower dose was tested. If the animals survived, the experimental animals and placebo injected controls were sacrificed by decapitation 18 hours after injection and tissues were taken for cholinesterase assays. The tissues taken were: forebrain (as a sample of CNS), last one cm of the ileum next to the ileocecal junction, a sample of pectoralis major, and the heart (as samples of peripheral cholinesterase containing tissues). The tissue samples were removed quickly and cooled to 0° in ice cold 0.1 M (Na) PO_4 buffer, pH 7.0. The assays were completed as quickly as the tissues could be prepared, typically within 3 hours of death. There was no significant change in enzyme activity during this period of time.

The enzyme assays were conducted in triplicate according to the spectrophotometric method of Ellman et al. (1961), $25^{o}C$ except that the assays were conducted at pH 7.0 in a spectrophotometer specially equipped with continuous stirring in the sample compartment in order to maintain an even suspension of the tissues. The homogenates were diluted 1:30 (0.1 ml homogenate into a total of 3.0 ml) into the assay media containing substrate and Ellman's reagent (5',5'-dithio-bis-(2-nitrobenzoic acid), Sigma Chemical Co., St. Louis) for determination of enzyme activity. Therefore, the muscle tissues were assayed at a final dilution of 1:900 and brain at 1:1500. For the simple determination of cholinesterase activity remaining after treatment with the various compounds tested, the assays were conducted at 500 μM acetylthiocholine substrate (Sigma Chemical). At this level of substrate (five to ten times K_m, depending upon tissue), activity is a function of the amount of enzyme remaining in the tissue and the reaction is linear for several minutes. The details of this modified method are reported by Moss et al. (1985b). The data are expressed as the percent of the enzyme activity in the control animals.

Rats reared in the animal colony at the University of Texas at El Paso from Sprague-Dawley albino stock served as subjects. The precaution of rearing insured no exposure to popular cholinesterase-inhibiting pesticides. All of the test compounds were obtained from Aldrich Chemical Company or the subsidiary Alfred Bader Library of rare chemicals (Milwaukee) as sulfonyl fluorides or sulfonyl chlorides. The chlorides were converted to fluorides according to the general methods of Millington, Brown and Pattison (1956). Briefly, ethanesulfonyl chloride, isopropylsulfonyl chloride, 4-fluorobenzenesulfonyl chloride and pentafluorobenzenesulfonyl chloride were converted to the corresponding fluoride by adding an excess of potassium fluoride in a concentrated aqueous mixture, stirring overnight at room temperature with additional stirring for 2 hours at 70°C. The mixture was diluted with additional water and extracted several times with ether. The ether was removed by evaporation and the remaining material was dried overnight with anhydrous sodium sulfate. The final product was distilled at about 1 mm Hg vacuum and the purity was determined by IR spectra. The remaining compounds were available as fluorides. All test materials were stored desiccated at 0°C under nitrogen and protected from light until used.

RESULTS

All of the larger molecular weight compounds (e.g., m-(hexadecylsulfamoyl)-benzenesulfonyl fluoride, ethyl-4-chloro-2(p-fluorosulfonylphenyl)-6-quinoline carboxylate, and 4-(hexadecylsulfonyl)-metanilyl fluoride) and compounds with two or more rings (e.g., 5-nitro-1-naphthalenesulfonyl fluoride, 1,3-bis(m-fluorosulfonylphenyl) urea, bis-[para-(fluorosulfonyl)-phenyl]-succinate, and 4-fluorosulfonyl-1-hydroxy-2-napthoic acid) were virtually without effect at the standard test dose (0.575 mmole/kg).

Other, smaller compounds which produced no significant effect in the CNS and no significant effects in peripheral tissues included:

4-Fluorobenzenesulfonyl fluoride
Pentafluorobenzenesulfonyl fluoride
p-Fluorosulfonylbenzenesulfonyl chloride
4-Chloro-3,5-dinitrobenzenesulfonyl fluoride
3-Bromosulfanilyl fluoride
2,4-Dimethyl-5-nitrobenzenesulfonyl fluoride
o-Aminobenzenesulfonyl fluoride
4-Methyl-3-nitrobenzenesulfonyl fluoride
m-Acetylbenzenesulfonyl fluoride
4-(Methylsulfonyl)-metanilyl fluoride
o-Nitrobenzenesulfonyl fluoride
m-Aminobenzenesulfonyl fluoride
4-(tert-butyl)-3-nitrobenzenesulfonyl fluoride
Sulfanilyl fluoride
m-Nitrobenzenesulfonyl fluoride
2-Mesitylenesulfonyl fluoride
4-(Fluorosulfonyl)-benzoic acid
4-(Fluorosulfonyl)-phthalic acid
4-Chloro-3-nitrobenzenesulfonyl fluoride

Table 1 presents a detailed summary of the compounds which produced significant inhibition in the CNS as well as a comparison to additional examples of inactive but structurally related compounds.

Table 1. Effects of Selected Sulfonyl Fluorides on CNS and Peripheral Cholinesterases

Compound Name	Structure	B	I	H	P[a]
<u>Examples</u> <u>of</u> <u>CNS</u> <u>active</u>:					
Phenylmethanesulfonyl fluoride	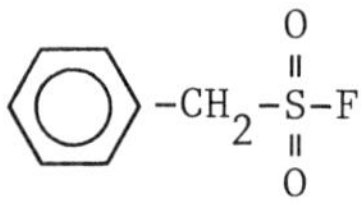	++++	+	++	++[b]
3-Amino-4-methylbenzene sulfonyl fluoride	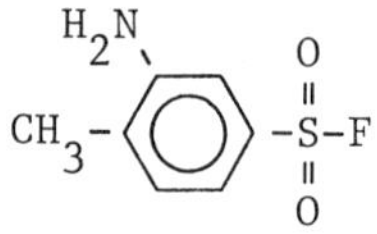	++++	++	++	++
4-Methoxymetanilyl fluoride	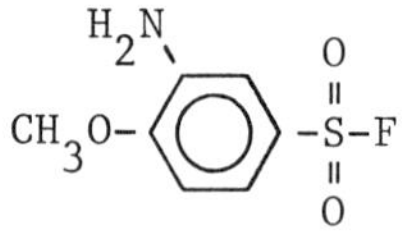	++++	0	++	++
Ethanesulfonyl fluoride	$CH_3CH_2-SO_2-F$	+++++ ++++ ++	++ ++ +	+++ +++ ++	++[c] ++[d] 0[e]
<u>Examples</u> <u>of</u> <u>inactive</u>:					
Benzenesulfonyl fluoride	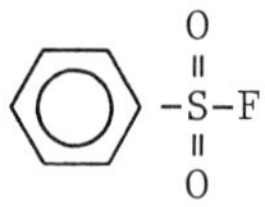	0	+	0	+
p-Toluenesulfonyl fluoride	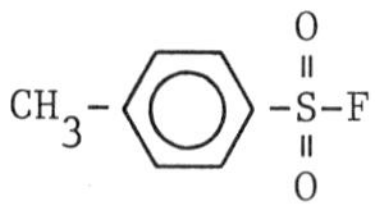	0	0	0	0
3-Amino-4-ethoxybenzene sulfonyl fluoride	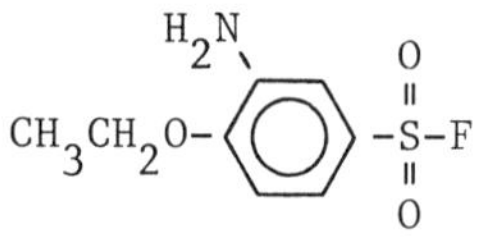	+	++	0	0
3-Amino-4-chlorobenzene sulfonyl fluoride	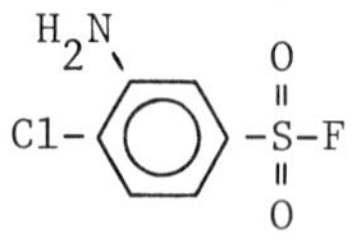	0	++	0	0
Isopropylsulfonyl fluoride	$(CH_3)_2CH-SO_2-F$	0	0	0	0[f]

[a] B=Brain, I=Ileum, H=Heart, P=Pectoral Muscle.
[b] Each "+" represents approximately 20% inhibition, 0 shows no effect.
[c] Ethanesulfonyl fluoride at 16 mg/kg.
[d] Ethanesulfonyl fluoride at 8 mg/kg.
[e] Ethanesulfonyl fluoride at 3 mg/kg.
[f] Isopropylsulfonyl fluoride tested only at 15 mg/kg and 30 mg/kg.

DISCUSSION

The results presented in Table 1 and those of earlier experiments (Moss et al., 1985b) demonstrate that a few sulfonyl fluorides have inherent selectivities to inhibit CNS cholinesterase. The mechanism responsible for inducing selectivity is currently obscure. These results, when combined with earlier research (Moss et al., 1985b), suggest that PMSF, MSF, 3-amino-4-methylbenzenesulfonyl fluoride, and 4-methoxymetanilyl fluoride are all sufficiently selective for the CNS to justify additional evaluation.

It must be noted that the initial level of selectivity represented by the data presented above does not represent the potential practical therapeutic value of the compounds. As was reported earlier (Moss et al., 1985b), cholinesterase within the CNS appears to be synthesized at a slower rate (half-time of 11 days) than peripheral enzymes (half-times of 1 day, 3 days, and 6 days for ileum, heart, and skeletal muscle, respectively). Therefore, a very high level of CNS cholinesterase inhibition (e.g., 90%) can be produced with minimum peripheral inhibition (e.g., 30% or less) by small doses of inhibitor given every other day or even less often (Moss et al., 1985b).

One of the problems with the sulfonyl fluorides is their relatively low biological activity (i.e., large amounts of material are required to produce significant inhibition). With the exception of MSF, a therapeutic dose equivalent in rats would be in the range of 50 to 100 mg/kg. With MSF, the dose would be approximately 0.5 mg/kg (Moss et al., 1985b). Corresponding to the low level of biological activity, the gross toxicity is also relatively low for this type of agent. The LD_{50} was determined to be 200 mg/kg, 20 mg/kg and 2 mg/kg for PMSF, ethanesulfonyl fluoride and MSF, respectively. With the notable exception of 4-(methylsulfonyl)-metanilyl fluoride, these compounds were remarkably low in toxicity. 4-(Methylsulfonyl)-metanilyl fluoride was quite toxic at one tenth the standard test dose and the toxicity was not related to the very minimum effects this compound produced on cholinesterase. However, because the sulfonyl fluorides are generally low in reactivity, it may be that these compounds will produce less non-specific toxicity than other, more reactive compounds such as the organic phosphates. An example of toxicity which must be avoided in any agent for chronic use is "Ginger Jake" paralysis, a delayed demyelinating neurotoxic effect produced by exposure to sublethal doses of certain organophosphorus compounds (Brimblecombe,1974). Finding compounds with increased potency and selectivity as CNS cholinesterase inhibitors without increased toxicity would be desirable.

REFERENCES

Arai, H., Kobayashi, K., Ichimiya, Y., Kosaka, K. and Iizuka, R., 1984, A preliminary study of free amino acids in the postmortem temporal cortex from Alzheimer-type dementia patients. Neurobiol. Aging, 5:319-321.

Bartus, R. T., Dean, R. L., III, Beer, B. and Lippa, A., 1982, The cholinergic hypothesis of geriatric memory dysfunction. Science, 217:408-417.

Brimblecombe, R. W., 1974, "Drug Actions on Cholinergic Systems", University Park Press, Baltimore.

Brinkman, S. D. and Gershon, S., 1983, Measurement of cholinergic drugs effects on memory in Alzheimer's disease. Neurobiol. Aging 4:139-145.

Davies, P., 1981, Theoretical treatment possibilities for dementia of the Alzheimer's type: The cholinergic hypothesis, in: "Strategies for the Development of an Effective Treatment for Senile Dementia", T. Crook and S. Gershon, eds., Mark Powley, New Canaan (Conn.). pp 19-34.

Davies, P., Katzman, R. and Terry, R.D., 1980, Reduced somatostatin-like immunoreactivity in cerebral cortex from cases of Alzheimer disease and Alzheimer senile dementia. Nature, 288:279-280.
Davies, P. and Maloney, A. J. R., 1976, Selective loss of central cholinergic neurons in Alzheimer's disease. Lancet, 2:1403.
Davis, K.L. and Mohs, R. C., 1982, Enhancement of memory processes in Alzheimer's disease with multiple-dose intravenous physostigmine. Amer. J. Psychia., 139:1421-1424.
Delfs, J. R., 1984, Possible role of somatostatin in Alzheimer's disease, in: "Proceedings of the Fifth Tarbox Parkinson's Disease Symposium: "The Norman Rockwell Conference on Alzheimer's Disease", J. T. Hutton and A. D. Kenny, eds., Alan R. Liss, Publishers; New York. In press.
Delfs, J. R., Zhu, C.-H. and Dichter, M. A., 1984, Coexistence of acetylcholinesterase and somatostatin-immunoreactivity in neurons cultured from rat cerebrum. Science, 223:61-63.
Ellman, G. L., Courtney, K. D., Andres, V. and Featherstone, R. M., 1961, A new and rapid colorimetric determination of acetylcholinesterase. Biochem. Pharmacol., 7:88-95.
Fahrney, D. E. and Gold, A. M., 1963, Sulfonyl fluorides as inhibitors of esterases. I. Rates of reaction with acetylcholinesterase, chymotrypsin, and trypsin. J. Amer. Chem. Soc., 85:997-1000.
Harbaugh, R. E., Roberts, D. W., Coombs, D. W., Saunders, R. L. and Reeder, T. M., 1984, Preliminary Report: Intracranial cholinergic drug infusion in patients with Alzheimer's disease. Neurosurgery, 15:514-518.
Kitz, R. and Wilson, I. B., 1962, Esters of methanesulfonic acid as irreversible inhibitors of acetylcholinesterase. J. Biol. Chem., 237:3245-3249.
Massoulie, J. and Bon, S., 1982, The molecular forms of cholinesterase and acetylcholinesterase in vertebrates. Ann. Rev. Neurosci., 5:57-106.
Millington, J. E., Brown, G. M. and Pattison, F. L. M., 1956, Toxic flurine compounds. VIII. Fluoroalkanesulfonyl chlorides and fluorides. J. Amer. Chem. Soc., 78:3846-3847.
Moss, D. E., Rodriguez, L. A. and McMaster, S. B., 1985a, Comparative behavioral effects of CNS cholinesterase inhibitors. Pharmacol. Biochem. Behav., 22(3), in press.
Moss, D. E., Rodriguez, L. A., Selim, S., Ellett, S. O., Devine, J. V. and Steger, R. W., 1985b, The sulfonyl fluorides: CNS selective cholinesterase inhibitors with potential value in Alzheimer's disease, in, "Proceedings of the Fifth Tarbox Parkinson's Disease Symposium: The Norman Rockwell Conference on Alzheimer's Disease", J. T. Hutton and A. D. Kenny, eds., Alan R. Liss, Publishers; New York. In press.
Myers, D. K. and Kemp, A., 1954, Inhibition of esterases by the fluorides of organic acids. Nature, 173:33-34.
Nakano, I. and Hirano, A., 1983, Neuron loss in the nucleus basalis of Meynert in parkinsonism-dementia complex of Guam. Ann. Neurol., 13:87-91.
Nakano, I. and Hirano, A., 1984, Parkinson's disease: Neuron loss in the nucleus basalis without concurrent Alzheimer's disease. Ann. Neurol., 15:415-418.
Rogers, J. and Marrison, J. H., 1984, CO-localization of somatostatin immunoreactivity with neuritic plaques in Alzheimer's disease. Amer. Aging Assoc. Abstr., Abstr. #48, p. 14.
Rossor, M. N., Emson, P. C., Mountjoy, C. Q., Roth, M. and Iverson, L. L., 1980, Reduced amounts of immunoreactive somatostatin in the temporal cortex in senile dementia of the Alzheimer's type. Neurosci. Lett., 20:373-377.
Whitehouse, P. J., Price, D. L., Struble, R. G., Clarke, A. W., Coyle, J. T. and DeLong, M. R., 1982, Alzheimer's disease and senile dementia: Loss of neurons in the basal forebrain. Science, 15:1237-1239.

A NOVEL TRANSDERMAL THERAPEUTIC SYSTEM AS A POTENTIAL TREATMENT FOR ALZHEIMER'S DISEASE

Drora Levy, Peretz Glikfeld, Yona Grunfeld, Jacob Grunwald, Moshe Kushnir, Aharon Levy, Yacov Meshulam, Michael Spiegelstein, Dov Zehavi and Abraham Fisher

Israel Institute for Biological Research
Ness-Ziona, 70450, ISRAEL

INTRODUCTION

Alzheimer's disease (AD) is mainly characterized by cognitive impairments as well as by a selective cholinergic hypofunction in certain brain areas (1,2). Therefore, clinical improvement in AD might be expected from drugs which elevate cholinergic activity in the brain. These drugs include centrally active acetylcholinesterase inhibitors such as physostigmine (3,4) and direct acting agonists such as arecoline and oxotremorine administered parenterally (4) or bethanechol infused intracerebroventricularly (5). Unfortunately, some of these drugs as exemplified by physostigmine, have a short biological half-life and a narrow therapeutic index, which limit their clinical application.

One way to overcome these difficulties is to administer systemically active drugs through the skin, using a transdermal delivery system. The few transdermal delivery systems presently available employ only drugs which penetrate the skin at rates high enough to yield therapeutic levels in the plasma (6). However, the majority of drugs do not penetrate the skin at rates sufficiently high to achieve therapeutic efficacy.

The purpose of the present work was to develop and evaluate a transdermal drug delivery system for the treatment of central cholinergic disorders (7). The permeation promoting delivery system, comprising a vehicle and ratelimiting laminate, was particulary designed for physostigmine and other related drugs.

MATERIALS AND METHODS

System Design

The Cholinergic Percutaneous Device (CPD) is composed of three layers (Figure 1):

1. A backing layer that provides a physical barrier to loss of physostigmine.

2. A drug reservoir, containing physostigmine and a permeation promoting vehicle (formula P) providing a continuous supply of the drug for several days.

3. A laminate based on ethylene-vinylacetate (EVA) copolymer for rate controlled delivery of physostigmine. The laminate also contains an adhesive formulation that permits passage of the drug and provides effective attachment to the skin.

In-Vivo Studies

Albino guinea pigs of either sex of a local strain (Dunkin-Hartley origin, 300-400 g), and female pigs of the Large White and Landrace strain (8-12 weeks of age, 8-14 kg) were used. A solution of physostigmine base (Sigma) in Formula P (50% w/v) incorporated into the CPD, was applied to dorsal test-sites of the experimental animal. At 30 minutes prior to CPD application, the hair at the test sites was closely clipped. Blood samples were obtained at specified times by cardiac puncture in guinea-pigs and venipuncture from the superior vena-cava in pigs. The biological effect of physostigmine was determined by measuring the decrease of whole blood cholinesterase (ChE) (8,9). Physostigmine concentration in plasma was measured by high performance liquid chromatography (HPLC) on a Varian 5020 HPLC unit, using Whelpton's method (10), with modification of the extraction procedure. For comparison, the effect of intramuscular injection and a constant rate intravenous infusion of physostigmine was determined in guinea-pigs and pigs, respectively.

In-Vitro Studies

Measurements of penetration rates through excised pig skin were carried out; as a screening method to compare various physostigmine-vehicle mixtures; to investigate permeation characteristics of different laminates; and to determine the rate limiting effect of the laminates on physostigmine diffusion. Full intact skin placed in diffusion cells (1 cm2 of bare area, 37oC) was used and an excess of drug mixture was applied. Fractions were collected at 2 hours intervals, from a continuously flowing perfusate (2.4 mM phosphate buffer, NaCl, pH=7.3, flow rate, 10 ml/hr). Physostigmine concentration in the perfusate samples, was determined by an enzymatic method (11) modified by us.

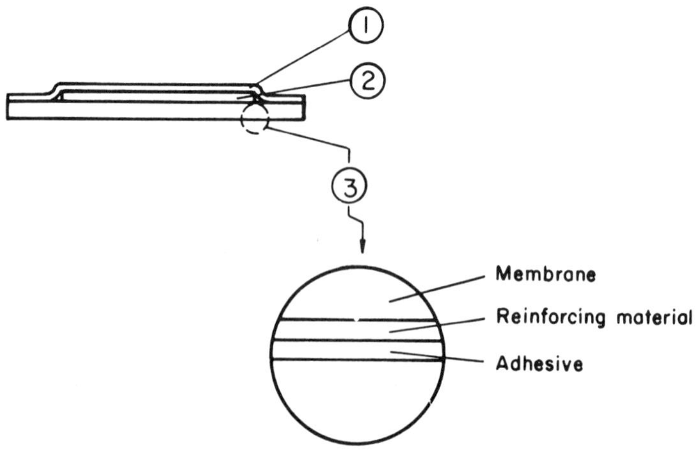

Figure 1: System design of CPD

RESULTS

Figure 2 demonstrates the limitations of physostigmine administered by a conventional pulsed method (injection) as compared to administration by CPD.

1. The short half-life of the drug (2 hr) requires a dosage regimen of multiple doses over a 24-hour period, which is inconvenient and often results in non-compliance.

2. Fluctuations, lowering the level of blood ChE inhibition, may cause side effects.

The main advantages of CPD are illustrated in Figure 3. Physostigmine administered by CPD, showed a zero order kinetics, thus maintaining a constant ChE inhibition level within the desired range (20-40% inhibition), for several days. The ChE inhibition pattern correlated with plasma concentrations of physostigmine measured by HPLC (Figure 4). The rate of permeation of Formula P dissolved physostigmine through pig skin was estimated by comparing ChE inhibition profiles of transdermally administered and infused physostigmine (Figure 5), and was found to be $7{+}2$ ug/cm^2 hr.

Typical in vitro penetration curves of physostigmine are presented in Figure 6a. The EVA laminate confined physostigmine flux to the desired concentration range and kept it constant for about 80 hours (Figure 6-b). The permeation rate of the drug could be altered by using a different thickness of the laminate. In vitro physostigmine penetration through pig skin in conjunction with a laminate showed a lower permeation rate and a longer lag-time (Figure 6-c).

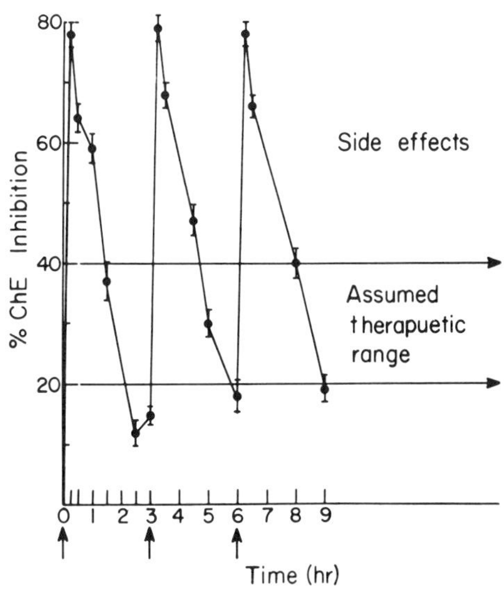

Figure 2: Blood ChE inhibition profile, following repeated injection (arrows) of physostigmine (125 ug/kg), in guinea-pigs.

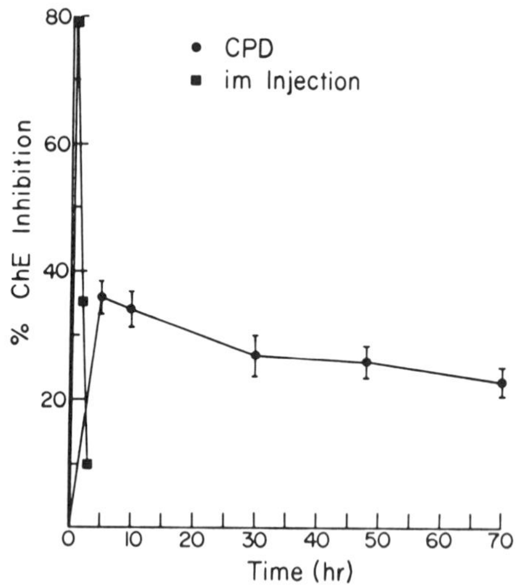

Figure 3: Blood ChE inhibition profile, following a single application of physostigmine CPD (1.5 cm^2/kg), compared to a single intramuscular(im) injection (125 ug/kg) in guinea-pigs.

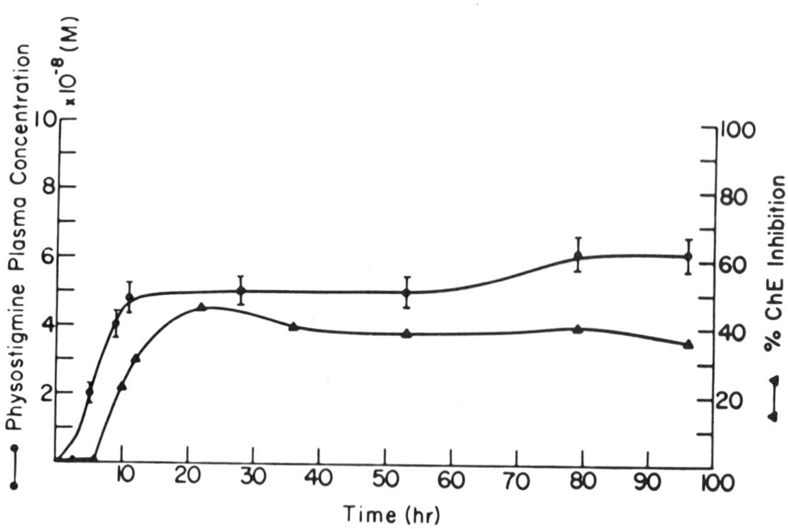

Figure 4: Correlation between physostigmine plasma levels (HPLC) and blood ChE inhibition in pigs treated with physostigmine CPD.

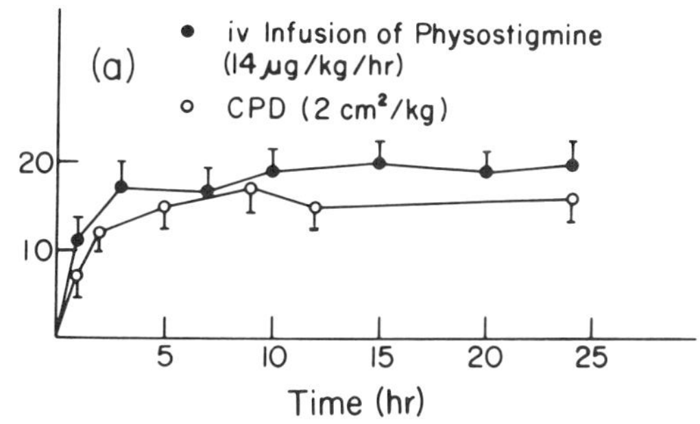

Figure 5: Blood ChE inhibition profile, following transdermal application of physostigmine versus infusion in pigs.

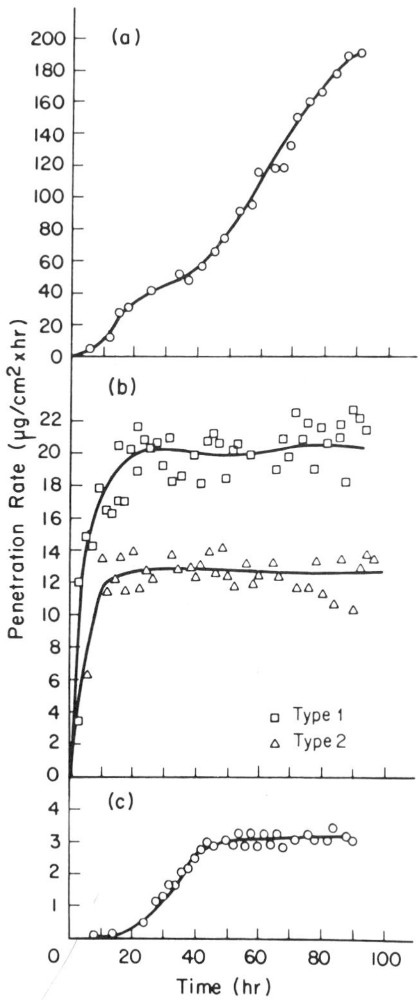

Figure 6: *In vitro* physostigmine (in Formula P) penetration rate profile through pig skin (a), through different laminates (b) and through skin protected by a laminate (c).

DISCUSSION

The results presented in this paper demonstrate that our transdermal delivery system has attributes which are superior to other modes of systemic drug administration:

1. It allows a continuous administration of the drug to the circulation over a prolonged period of time.

2. It provides an essentially stable drug level in the blood, thus limiting side effects due to overdosing and lack of effect as a result of underdosing.

3. It permits use of pharmacologically active drugs with short half lifes.
4. It simplifies the medication regimen.

In this study we selected physostigmine for our transdermal delivery system, but other related drugs may as well be utilized. These include tetrahydroaminoacridine and/or arecoline already used in AD or oxotremorine that has been suggested for treatment (4 and references cited therein).

The above mentioned drugs have the same drawbacks as physostigmine: e.g. a short biological half-life and relatively narrow therapeutic index. They are however active at doses of a few mg/day and therefore constitute excellent candidates for the described transdermal delivery system. Presently, these drugs and their applicability for incorporation into the transdermal system are under investigation in our laboratory.

In case of physostigmine delivered into the circulation via the transdermal route, inhibition of AChE in the blood was 40% or less. It must be noted, however, that this level of inhibition does not necessarily reflect that considered suitable for therapeutic efficacy in AD. It has been indicated that in AD patients, AChE is already reduced in selected brain areas, such as the cortex and the hippocampus, in particular. Therefore, physostigmine administered by the transdermal route should mainly affect these brain areas, while rendering other regions relatively unaffected due to the fact that only small amounts of the drug are delivered at each time point during treatment. The outcome of such an apparent selectivity could diminish the adverse side effects caused by parenterally administered physostigmine, in both healthy age-matched controls and AD patients.

Obviously, it will be imperative to conduct clinical trials to demonstrate the validity of these assumptions. Such studies with healthy volunteers and AD patients are planned for the near future.

REFERENCES

1. R.T. Bartus, R.L. Dean III, B. Beer, A.S. Lippa. The cholinergic hypothesis of geriatric memory dysfunction. Science, 217, 408-417 (1982).
2. J.T. Coyle, D.L. Price, M.R. Delong. Alzheimer's disease: A disorder of cortical cholinergic innervation. Science, 219, 1184-1190 (1983).
3. L.J. Thal, P.A. Fuld, M.S. Masur and N.S. Sharpless. Oral physostigmine and lecithin improve memory in Alzheimer's disease, Ann Neurol, 13, 491-496 (1983).

4. M. Davidson, V. Haroutunian, R.C. Mohs, B.M. Davis, T.M. Horvath, K.L. Davis. Human and animal studies with cholinergic agents: How clinically exploitable is the cholinergic deficiency in Alzheimer's disease? This volume.
5. R.E. Harbaugh, D.W. Roberts, D.W. Combs, R.L. Saunders and T.M. Reeder. Preliminary report: Intracranial cholinergic drug infusion in patients with Alzheimer's disease. Neurosurgery, 15, 514-518 (1984).
6. Y.M. Chein. Logic of transdermal contolled drug administration, Drug Develop Indust. Pharm. 9, 497-520 (1983).
7. A. Fisher, D. Levy, Y. Grunwald, M. Kushnir, A. Levy and M.Y. Spiegelstein. Drug delivery system. Israeli Patent No. 72684 (1984).
8. G.L. Ellman, K.D. Curtney, V.A.Jr. and R.M. Featherstone. A new and rapid colorimetric determination of acetylcholinesterase activity. Biochemical Pharmacology, 7, 88-95 (1961).
9. C.D. Johnson and R.L. Russell. A rapid simple radiometric assay for cholinesterase, suitable for multiple determinations. Anal. Biochem. 64, 229-238,(1975).
10. R. Whelpton. Analysis of plasma physostigmine concentration by liquid chromatography. J. Chromatog., 272, 216-220 (1983).
11. H.O. Michel. An electrometric method for the determination of red blood cell and plasma cholinesterase activity. J. lab. clin. Med., 34, 1564-1568 (1949).

DIFFERENCES IN THE AGONIST BINDING PROPERTIES OF MUSCARINIC RECEPTOR SUBPOPULATIONS IN THE RAT CEREBRAL CORTEX AND MYOCARDIUM

Nigel J.M. Birdsall and Edward C. Hulme

Physical Biochemistry Division
National Institute for Medical Research, Mill Hill, London
NW7 1AA, U.K.

INTRODUCTION

Low levels of presynaptic cholinergic markers such as choline acetyltransferase seem to be a characteristic feature of certain brain regions of people with senile dementia of the Alzheimer type (see eg. Bartus et al., 1982; Coyle et al., 1983 for reviews). In contrast, there seems to be little if any change in the density of muscarinic receptors located on the target cells of the cholinergic neurones (10 references cited in Bartus et al., 1982). As the muscarinic cholinergic system is thought to be involved in the storage and retrieval of newly acquired information it has been considered that a muscarinic agonist might be used therapeutically to compensate for the "cholinergic deficit" in senile dementia of the Alzheimer's type and alleviate some of the memory problems associated with the disease. Very recently, the muscarinic agonist RS 86 has been shown to improve general cognitive functions in a minority of Alzheimer's patients (Wettstein and Spiegel, 1984). In general however, the doses of muscarinic agonists which can be used for this purpose are limited by additional effects produced by their actions on muscarinic receptors in other tissues. What is required is an agonist which will selectively stimulate specific muscarinic functions in the cerebral cortex.

The results of whole tissue pharamacological studies on muscarinic receptor responses show that there are receptor subclasses which may be discriminated by selective antagonists. (For recent reviews see Birdsall and Hulme, 1983; Hammer and Gaichetti, 1984). The selectivity demonstrated by drugs such as pirenzepine, gallamine and 4-diphenylacetoxy-N-methyl piperidine methiodide has been confirmed in binding studies (Hammer et al., 1980; Stockton et al., 1983; Birdsall et al., 1980).

There is less evidence from functional studies for the existence of selective agonists (Caulfield and Straughan, 1983; Lambrecht and Mutschler, 1984). Some of the difficulties in elucidating the molecular basis of such selectivity using a functional approach arise because it is not easy to estimate agonist <u>affinity</u> constants for whole tissue responses to full agonists. Hence it may not be possible to say whether the selectivity of a given agonist arises from an increased affinity or increased efficiency of receptor-response coupling.

An alternative approach is to determine from binding studies whether the muscarinic receptor subclasses have different agonist binding properties and to relate these results to those of functional studies. We have in fact been able to show that McN-A-343 (Roszkowski, 1961) binds to myocardial muscarinic receptors in a different manner to that of other agonists (Birdsall et al., 1983). In general, the agonist binding properties of muscarinic receptors are complex (Hulme et al., 1975; Birdsall and Hulme, 1976; Birdsall et al., 1978) and there appear to be subpopulations of binding sites (or binding states), termed SH, H and L which have very similar or identical affinities for conventional antagonists such as atropine. In contrast the affinities for a potent agonist for the SH state can be up to 3000 times greater than its affinity for the L site (Birdsall et al., 1978). The agonist binding properties of muscarinic receptors also vary from region to region of the brain (Birdsall et al., 1980). However it is difficult to determine unambiguously whether the differences in the binding are due to (1) differences in the proportions of SH, H and L subpopulations, (2) variations in the agonist affinities for the SH, H and L states, or (3) changes in both parameters. Our previous studies suggested that the major regional variations were due to differences in the proportions of SH, H and L sites.

In this chapter we describe experiments to characterize the binding properties of the highest affinity state (SH) of two postulated muscarinic receptor subpopulations in the rat cerebral cortex and the predominant receptor subpopulation found in the myocardium and demonstrate differences in both the agonist and antagonist binding properties of these states. This was accomplished using low concentrations of the potent tritiated agonist [^{3}H]-oxotremorine-M ([^{3}H]-oxoM) (Birdsall et al., 1978; Waelbroeck et al., 1982; Harden et al., 1983; Hulme et al., 1983) to monitor the SH states of the receptors.

MATERIALS AND METHODS

EDTA-washed membranes from rat cerebral cortex and myocardium were prepared as described by Hulme et al. (1983). The KCl/pyrophosphate/EDTA extracted membranes were prepared by the method of Berrie et al. (1984). This preparation gave the same binding properties as the EDTA-washed myocardial membranes but a lower non-specific binding of [^{3}H]-oxoM. The membrane preparations were frozen and stored at -20° or -70° for no more than two weeks before use. The frozen membranes were homogenized at 0° in 20 mM NaHepes pH 7.5 which was then supplemented with 1 mM $MgSO_4$. Binding assays were carried out at 30° for 15 minutes in the 20 mM NaHepes/1 mM Mg^{2+} pH 7.5 buffer using the microcentrifugation technique described previously (Hulme et al., 1983). 3-quinuclidinylbenzilate (10^{-6} M) was used to define non-specific binding. Assays were generally carried out in duplicate and were repeated 4-6 times. (-)-[^{3}H]-N-methylscopolamine (NMS) (83.4 Ci/mmole) and [^{3}H]-oxotremorine-M (82 Ci/mmole) were obtained from New England Nuclear. Oxotremorine-M, methylfurmethide, 4-diphenylacetoxy-N-methyl piperidine methiodide and 3-quinuclidinylbenzilate were synthesised in our laboratory.

Pirenzepine and McN-A-343 were kind gifts from Dr. R. Hammer, Istituto de Angeli, Milan.

RESULTS

The composition of the incubation buffer for the binding assays was chosen such that the agonist binding was maximized (Hulme et al., 1983). Pretreatment of the membranes with EDTA followed by the addition of 1 mM Mg^{2+} was also found to enhance agonist binding and promote, where possible,

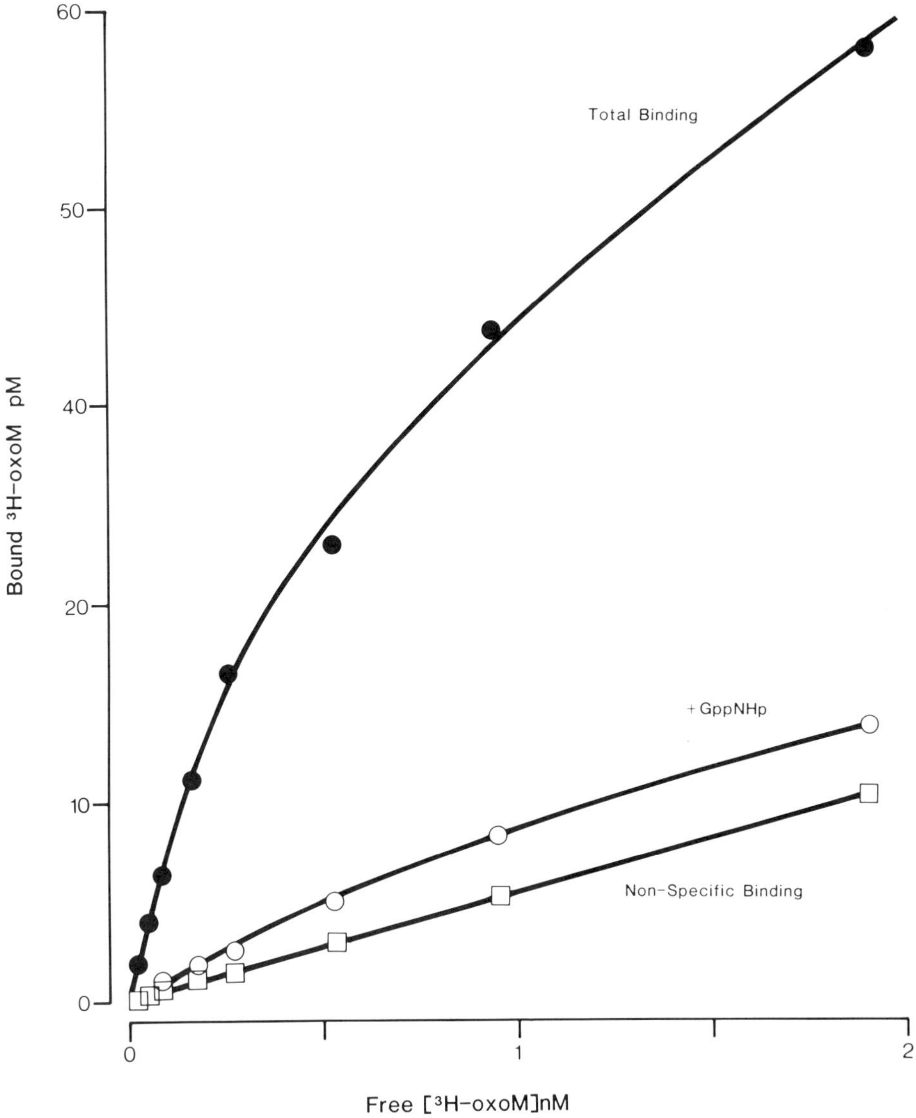

Figure 1

The binding of [^{3}H]-oxotremorine-M to muscarinic receptors in membrane preparations from rat myocardium in the presence (o) and absence (o) of 5′-guanylylimidodiphosphate (10^{-4} M).

the agonist mediated coupling of the receptor to a guanine nucleotide protein or proteins.

Binding of [^{3}H]-oxoM in the Myocardium and Cerebral Cortex

The binding of the radiolabelled agonist to muscarinic receptors in the two tissues was measured in the absence and presence of the GTP analogue, 5-guanylylimidodiphosphate (GppNHp, 10^{-4} M). GppNHp promotes the dissociation of muscarinic receptor - guanine nucleotide binding protein complexes (Berrie et al., 1984) and decreases the binding potency of muscarinic agonists by up to 100 fold (Berrie, et al., 1979; Ehlert et al., 1981; Wei and Sulakhe, 1979).

The [^{3}H]-oxoM binding curves in the myocardium (Figure 1) show that a high percentage of receptor-specific binding is inhibited by GppNHp. Subtraction of the [^{3}H]-oxoM bound in the presence of GppNHp from the total bound [^{3}H]-oxoM gives the guanine nucleotide sensitive component (G-sensitive component). Non-linear least squares analysis demonstrated that the data could be fit adequately to a one-site model with a [^{3}H]-oxoM affinity of 1.9 x 10^9 M^{-1}, the estimate of the concentration of binding sites being 40 pM. A similar analysis of the guanine nucleotide insensitive (G-insenstive) [^{3}H]-oxoM binding curve, obtained by subtraction of the non-specific binding from [^{3}H]-oxoM binding in the presence of GppNHp, gave 5.5 pM binding sites with an affinity of 1.0 x 10^9 M^{-1}. The total concentration of binding sites (estimated with [^{3}H]-NMS) was 104 pM. Therefore the G-sensitive and G-insensitive high affinity [^{3}H]-oxoM binding components represent respectively ca 40% and 5% of the total muscarinic binding sites in the myocardium under these conditions.

In analogous experiments on the binding of [^{3}H]-oxoM to muscarinic receptors in a membrane preparation from rat cerebral cortex the estimates of oxoM affinity were 1.8 x 10^9 M^{-1} and 1.1 x 10^9 M^{-1} for the G-sensitive and G-insensitive components. The percentage of total receptor binding sites which had the very high affinity for [^{3}H]-oxoM but were G-insensitive is about the same (6%) as found in the myocardium but the GppNHp sensitive SH sites in the cortex had a lower relative abundance (12%) in agreement with previous findings (Hulme et al., 1983; Nukada et al., 1983).

Binding Properties of the High Affinity [^{3}H]-oxoM binding sites

In both the myocardium and cortex we have been able to delineate populations of high affinity [^{3}H]-oxoM binding sites which are either sensitive or insensitive to GppNHp. As the G-insensitive [^{3}H]-oxoM binding component in the myocardium is of such low abundance and concentration (5-10 pM in a typical assay), it was decided to investigate only the G-sensitive [^{3}H]-oxoM binding sites in the myocardium but both the G-sensitive and G-insensitive sites could be assayed in the cerebral cortex. We used three protocols for the binding assays. Firstly, the ability of muscarinic drugs to inhibit the binding of low concentrations of [^{3}H]-oxoM (0.3 nM) to myocardial membranes was examined. As 85-95% of the receptor specific [^{3}H]-oxoM is inhibited by GppNHp, this binding assay monitors predominantly the G-sensitive high affinity sites in the myocardium. Secondly, drug inhibition of the binding of [^{3}H]-oxoM (0.3 nM) to muscarinic receptors on cortical membranes was measured as a monitor of <u>both</u> the G-sensitive and G-insensitive high affinity [^{3}H]-oxoM binding sites as, under these conditions, only 60-80% of [^{3}H]-oxoM binding is inhibited by GppNHp.

TABLE 1

Antagonist potencies (-log IC_{50}*) for inhibition of [^{3}H]-oxoM binding

	Heart	Cortex	
	-GppNHp	-GppNHp	+GppNHp
N-Methylscopolamine	9.26 ± 0.20	9.30 ± 0.10	9.12 ± 0.15
Atropine	8.59 ± 0.06	8.61 ± 0.02	8.48 ± 0.07
4-Diphenylacetoxy-N-methylpiperidine methiodide	8.67 ± 0.12	8.36 ± 0.08	8.42 ± 0.20
Pirenzepine	6.22 ± 0.15	6.62 ± 0.04#	6.26 ± 0.06
Gallamine	7.25 ± 0.09°	6.38 ± 0.08°	6.17 ± 0.05°

* Values are means ± range (n=2) or ± s.e. (n=3-5) and (with the exception of gallamine) can be increased by 0.2 log unit to correct for [^{3}H]-oxoM occupancy and give an estimate of the affinity constant in the absence of GppNHp. In the presence of GppNHp the factor is 0.1.

\# Binding curves had a Hill slope of ca. 0.8

° Inhibition was not competitive and reached a maximum of 92-96% at high concentrations of gallamine.

Thirdly, drug inhibition of [^{3}H]-oxoM binding in the cortex <u>in the presence of GppNHp</u> provides a description of the G-insensitive sites. Comparison of the binding data for the second and third assays gives an estimate of the affinity for the G-sensitive sites in the cerebral cortex.

The log IC_{50} values for the ability of 5 antagonists to inhibit [^{3}H]-oxoM binding to muscarinic receptors in the cerebral cortex and heart are shown in Table I. The conventional antagonists N-methylscopolamine (NMS) and atropine have almost identical affinities in the three assays, the values for NMS after correction for receptor occupancy by [^{3}H]-oxoM agreeing with the values estimated directly by [^{3}H]-NMS binding. Somewhat surprisingly the selective antagonist, 4-diphenylacetoxy-N-methylpiperidine methiodide, (Barlow et al., 1976) had a slightly higher affinity in the myocardium than in the cortex. This is in contrast to results found at higher ionic strengths (100 mM NaCl + 10 mM Mg^{2+}) where this drug had an 8-fold lower affinity for myocardial than for cortical receptors (Birdsall et al., 1980). Pirenzepine however still exhibits some selectivity, binding with low affinity to the G-sensitive sites in the myocardium and the G-insensitive sites in the cerebral cortex. The inhibition curve in the cerebral cortex in the absence of GppNHp is not mass action (Hill coefficient 0.8) and the IC_{50} value is decreased. These results point qualitatively to the G-sensitive [^{3}H]-oxoM binding sites in the cerebral cortex having a high affinity for pirenzepine, a finding which has been confirmed using [^{3}H]-pirenzepine as a monitor of the high affinity pirenzepine subpopulation of binding sites (Birdsall et al., 1984). Analysis of the binding data indicates the pirenzepine affinity for the G-sensitive [^{3}H]-oxoM sites in the cerebral cortex is 2×10^7 M^{-1}.

Gallamine, which binds to a second binding site on muscarinic receptors and allosterically modifies the binding of drugs such as NMS to the conventional acetylcholine binding site (Stockton et al., 1983), exhibits the same non-competitive behaviour in modulating [^{3}H]-oxoM binding. The inhibition reaches a plateau of 92-96% inhibition at high concentrations of gallamine indicating that gallamine and [^{3}H]-oxoM are binding simultaneously to the muscarinic receptor but the [^{3}H]-oxoM affinity is decreased by a factor of 20-40 in this ternary complex. The cardioselectivity of gallamine shown by binding studies and functional studies is maintained under these conditions with gallamine having a 10 times higher affinity for the myocardial receptors than for the cortical receptors. In addition, gallamine is 10-20 times more potent than is found in buffers of higher ionic strength.

It is clear therefore that the major qualitative differences in the antagonist binding properties of the subpopulations of muscarinic receptors are retained under these conditions but for some drugs the differences are attenuated.

The potencies of ten agonists for inhibiting [^{3}H]-oxoM in the three binding assays are given in Table 2. With one exception, the inhibition curves approximated closely to mass action curves. In general the log IC_{50} values in the three assays agreed closely, the values for the G-insensitive sites being slightly lower than the G sensitive sites in the myocardium (difference after correction for [^{3}H]-oxoM occupancy, 0.29 ± 0.07 log unit, mean $\pm$ s.e.m. n = 10) and the G-sensitive sites in the cortex (difference 0.17 ± 0.05 log unit). These differences in affinity were also found in the [^{3}H]-oxoM saturation curves described earlier. However not all agonists exhibited an identical pattern of behaviour. Certain agonists such as furmethide had almost identical affinities for the three [^{3}H]-oxoM binding sites whereas oxotremorine exhibited the greatest dispersity in affinity of the agonists examined. Under these conditions oxotremorine binds with an affinity of 2×10^9 M^{-1} to the myocardial [^{3}H]-oxoM binding sites but with only 5×10^8 M^{-1} to the G-insensitive cortical sites. There were further small differences in the relative potencies of the agonists for the three receptor subpopulations. Pilocarpine appears to have a slightly higher affinity for the G-insensitive sites than the G-sensitive sites in the cortex, whereas methylfurmethide shows a selectivity for the cortical G-sensitive sites. Although these differences in affinities are small, the results clearly show that the structure-binding relationships for the three [^{3}H]-oxoM binding sites (SH states) are different. The binding curve for McN-A-343 in the heart did not reach 100% inhibition at high concentrations but levelled off at 96% confirming our previous finding that McN-A-343 binds to the allosteric site on myocardial receptors (Birdsall et al., 1983).

TABLE 2

Agonist potencies for inhibition of [^{3}H]-oxoM binding (-log IC_{50})*

	Heart	Cortex	
		-GppNHp	-GppNHp
oxotremorine	9.13 ± 0.09	8.73 ± 0.11	8.60 ± 0.23
oxotremorine-M	9.08 ± 0.11	8.96 ± 0.04	8.68 ± 0.12
carbachol	8.06 + 0.14	7.91 + 0.14	7.87 + 0.13
methylfurmethide	8.06 ± 0.16	8.15 ± 0.16	7.90 ± 0.04
muscarine	7.60 ± 0.23	7.49 ± 0.12	7.38 ± 0.12
furmethide	7.27 ± 0.28	7.30 ± 0.09	7.29 ± 0.04
pilocarpine	7.15 ± 0.21	6.88 ± 0.18	7.15 ± 0.21
bethanechol	6.98 ± 0.16	6.72 ± 0.03	6.71 ± 0.02
McN-A-343	6.65 ± 0.19#	6.72 ± 0.10	6.70 ± 0.20
propyltrimethylammonium	5.64 ± 0.10	5.62 ± 0.16	5.48 ± 0.02

* Values are means ± range (n=2) or ± s.e. (n=3-6). The [^{3}H]-oxoM occupancy correction is 0.1 (cortex, + GppNHp) and 0.2 (heart, cortex, -GppNHp).

\# The inhibition curves levelled off at 96%.

DISCUSSION

Previous studies of the binding of selective ligands to muscarinic receptors have used [^{3}H]-antagonists as markers for the receptor. We have proposed that [^{3}H]-antagonists are likely to monitor receptors in both the ground state and excited state, but have not been able to exclude the possibility that certain antagonists may bind predominantly to the ground state of the receptor (Birdsall, et al., 1980). In this chapter, the interaction of agonists and antagonists with the SH state of the muscarinic receptors in different tissues is compared. This is the state of the receptor to which potent agonists such as [^{3}H]-oxoM bind with the highest affinity.

The affinity of agonists for the SH sites appears to be highly predictive of the pharmacological potency (Birdsall et al., 1978) and there is evidence that, at least in the myocardium, the SH sites represent a complex between the receptor and nucleotide binding protein (Hulme et al., 1984). Thus one can justifiably regard the SH state as an activated state of the receptor and it is clearly important to determine whether there are subtypes of the activated state. This is most important for agonists, for which it might reasonably be expected to be the state of the receptor in which the binding selectivity and pharmacological selectivity would be manifest.

The binding assay conditions were chosen so that the generated data provided information on the binding properties of receptor subtypes which are distinguished by antagonists (pirenzepine and gallamine) and by effector coupling mechanisms (G-sensitive or G-insensitive).

The major finding is that at least one agonist, oxotremorine, distinguishes to a marked extent (4-fold) between SH sites in the myocardium and the cortex. Differences are also seen for oxotremorine-M and, to a smaller extent, for some other agonists. A component of this selectivity appears to arise from an ability to distinguish between guanine nucleotide-sensitive and -insensitive sites. This is particularly true for oxotremorine-M but does not appear to account fully for the selectivity of oxotremorine.

Recently Bevan (1984) and Vickroy et al. (1984) have reported pharmacological differences in the high affinity agonist binding states of muscarinic receptors in the cerebral cortex and heart. The conditions used for the binding assays were somewhat different from those described in this paper and complex binding isotherms were found for certain agonists and antagonists. As a consequence, it is difficult to make comparisons between these data sets.

The binding selectivity of oxotremorine may be related to the suggestion from pharmacological studies that presynaptic receptors are selectively activated by oxotremorine (Kilbinger and Wessler, 1980) and that N-methyl-N-(1-methyl-4-pyrrolidino-2-butynyl) acetamide behaves as a presynaptic antagonist and a postsynaptic agonist (Nordstrom et al., 1983). The fact that oxotremorine-M also exhibits a similar binding selectivity to oxotremorine argues that a feature of the oxotremorine structure might be important.

The binding selectivity of oxotremorine for the myocardial muscarinic receptor suggests that it may be possible to develop more selective potent agonists. It will be interesting to determine whether putative selective agonists such as 3-acetoxy-N-methylpiperidine methiodide, acetyl tropine methiodide (Barlow et al., 1980), 2-methyl-spiro-(1,3-dioxolane-4,3′)-quinuclidine (Fisher et al., 1976) or some of the agonists recently described by Lambrecht and Mutschler (1984) behave in a similar or opposite manner to that of oxotremorine.

In view of the fact that the SH states have differing affinities for agonists and antagonists, it is no longer possible to assume that all muscarinic receptors can exist in just three agonist binding states, SH, H and L. It appears that each receptor subclass can probably exist in closely related but different SH, H and L states. The binding approach described here provides a further dissection of the complex binding properties of muscarinic receptors and may be useful in the development of selective muscarinic agonists.

REFERENCES

Barlow, R.B., Berrv, K.J., Glenton, P.A.M., Nikolau, N.M. and Soh, K.S. (1976) Br. J. Pharmacol. 58, 613-620.

Barlow, R.B., Burston, K.M. and Vis, A. (1980) Br. J. Pharmacol. 68, 141P.

Bartus, R.T., Dean, R.L., Beer, B. and Lippa, A.S. (1982) Science 217,408-417.

Berrie, C.P., Birdsall, N.J.M., Burgen, A.S.V. and Hulme, E.C. (1979) Biochem. Biophys. Res. Commun 87, 1000-1004.

Berrie, C.P., Birdsall, N.J.M, Hulme, E.C., Keen, M. and Stockton, J.M. (1984) Br. J. Pharmacol. 82, 853-861.

Bevan, P. (1984) Eur. J. Pharmacol., 101, 101-110.

Birdsall, N.J.M., Burgen, A.S.V. and Hulme, E.C. (1978) Mol. Pharmacol. 14, 723-736.

Birdsall, N.J.M., Burgen, A.S.V., Hulme, E.C., Stockton, J.M. and Zigmond, M.J. (1983) Br. J. Pharmacol. 78, 257-259.

Birdsall, N.J.M. and Hulme, E.C. (1976) J. Neurochem. 27, 7-14.

Birdsall, N.J.M. and Hulme, E.C. (1983) Trends Pharmacol. Sci., 4, 459-463.

Birdsall, N.J.M., Hulme, E.C. and Burgen, A.S.V. (1980). Proc. R. Soc. Lond. B. 207, 1-12.

Birdsall, N.J.M., Hulme, E.C., Hammer, R. and Stockton, J. (1980) In: Psychoparmacology and Biochemistry of Neurotransmitter Receptors. Eds. H.I. Yamamura, R.W. Olsen and E. Usdin. Elsevier, N.Y. 97-101.

Birdsall, N.J.M., Hulme, E.C. and Stockton, J.M. (1984) Trends Pharmacol. Sci. Suppl., 4-8.

Caulifeld, M. and Straughan, D. (1983) Trends Neurosci. 6, 73-75.

Coyle, J.T., Price, D.L. and DeLond, M.R. (1983) Science 219, 1184-1189.

Ehlert, F.J., Roeske, W.R. and Yamamura, H.I. (1981) Fed. Proc. 40, 153-159.

Fisher, A., Weinstock, M., Gitter, S. and Cohen, S. (1976) Eur. J. Pharmacol. 37, 329-338.

Hammer, R., Berrie, C.P., Birdsall, N.J.M., Burgen, A.S.V. and Hulme, E.C. (1980) Nature (Lond.) 283, 90-92.

Hammer, R. and Giachetti, A. (1982) Life Sci. 31, 2991-2998.

Hammer, R. and Giachetti, A. (1984) Trends Pharmacol. Sci. 5, 18-20.

Harden, T.K., Meeker, R.B. and Martin, M.W. (1983) J. Pharm. Exp. Ther. 227, 570-577.

Hulme, E.C., Berrie, C.P., Birdsall, N.J.M. and Burgen, A.S.V. (1981) Eur. J. Pharmacol. 73, 137-142.

Hulme, E.C., Berrie, C.P., Birdsall, N.J.M., Jameson, M. and Stockton, J.M. (1983) Eur. J. Pharmacol. 94, 59-72.

Hulme, E.C., Burgen, A.S.V. and Birdsall, N.J.M. (1975) INSERM 50, 49-70.

Kilbinger, H. and Wessler, I. (1980) Arch. Pharmakol. 314, 259-266.

Luber-Narod, J. and Potter, L.T. (1982) Soc. Neurosci. Abstr. 8, 238.

Mutschler, E. and Lambrecht, G. (1984) Trends Pharmacol. Sci. Suppl. 39-44.

Nukada, T., Haga, T. and Ichiyama, A. (1983) Mol. Pharmacol. 24, 366-373.

Nordstrom, O., Alberts, P., Westlind, A., Unden, A. and Bartfai, T. (1983) Mol. Pharmacol. 24, 1-5.

Roszkowski, A.P. (1961) J. Pharmacol. Exp. Ther. 132, 156-170.

Stockton, J., Birdsall, N.J.M., Burgen, A.S.V. and Hulme, E.C. (1983) Mol. Pharmacol. 23, 551-557.

Vickroy, T.W., Roeske, W.R. and Yamamura, H.I. (1984) J. Pharmacol. Exp. Therap. 229, 747-755.

Waelbroeck, M., Robberecht, P., Chatelain, P. and Christophe, J. (1982) Mol. Pharmacol. 21, 581-588.

Watson, M., Yamamura, H.I. and Roeske, W.R. (1983) Life Sci. 32, 3001-3011.

Wei, J.-W. and Sulakhe, P.V. (1979) Eur. J. Pharmacol. 58, 91-92.

Wettstein, A. and Spiegel, R. (1984) Psychopharmacology 84, 572-573.

CHOLINOCEPTOR CHARACTERIZATION

RECONSIDERED IN THE LIGHT OF DIVERSITY OF RESPONSE

Rachel Rubinstein, Nathan Dascal and Sasson Cohen

Department of Physiology & Pharmacology
Tel Aviv University Sackler Faculty of Medicine
Tel Aviv, Israel 69978

INTRODUCTION

The current concern with central cholinergic hypofunction as a unique pathophysiological correlate of Alzheimer disease and related disabilities is perhaps behind the recent revival of interest in the pharmacology of the cholinoceptive site (1). Conceivably, and given the assumption that such sites are sufficiently dissimilar among different tissues, say brain and muscle, to allow a differential response to a cholinomimetic molecule, then the prospects of drug-based management of such disabilities could be set on a rational basis. Historically, the issue of possible heterogeneity among cholinoceptive sites of the so-called muscarinic type had a relatively early head-start when it was realized that such drugs as acetylcholine (ACh) and carbachol (CCh) were not proportionately active in the heart on one hand and the intestine or bladder on the other (2), thus suggesting some organ or tissue specificity in the respective molecule. The pharmacological history of the cholinoceptor does not lack other examples of tissue or rather effect specific agents (3-8). These, however, failed to evoke sufficient interest as potential probes for cholinoceptor characterization. The prevailing approach regarded antagonists as unequivocal probes, and their relative affinity to the cholinoceptor, expressed as the equilibrium dissociation or association constant, as an index of its identity. Thus, and for long, atropine or a related molecule served as a universal touchstone for the unfailing identification of the cholinoceptor. The popularity of these probes is due to a rare combination of high potency and high specificity. Yet, they could not discriminate among receptor subtypes; so much so, that leading investigators found no reason to assume the existence of cholinoceptor subtypes. The emergence of even more potent antagonists such as QNB which heralded the advent of the popular radioligand binding assay (9), opened additional avenues for cholinoceptor characterization, but then an almost dogmatic adherence to "affinity" remained the major criterion for defining cholinoceptor identity which remained uniform with only a few suggestions to the contrary (10, 11).

Paradoxically, relatively weak antagonists proved to be better probes for the detection of heterogeneity among cholinoceptor subclasses. The underlying hypothesis was presented earlier (12) and recently rationalized on thermodynamic grounds (13). Among these, one could cite a quinuclidine derivative AF-14 (12) and the tricyclic molecules pirenzepine (14, 15) and nortriptyline (16). Yet, all these probes are antagonists, hence any evidence of heterogeneity they provide must reflect a difference in topology rather than one in function or response. For the same reason, reliance on an "affinity" term in the interaction between a cholinoceptor and a given agonist is not likely to provide more information than in the use of antagonists, because affinity constants do not relate to response (17). The alternative course is to seek a system of classification based on some characteristic of the evoked response. The various approaches to response quantification as a basis for receptor classification have been reviewed recently by Kenakin (18). The present article is not meant to discuss the relative merit or limitation of a given approach. Its objective is the presentation of experimental evidence showing that taxonomy of the cholinoceptor might be physiologically meaningless, unless referred to the type and magnitude of the response evoked.

EVIDENCE FROM CONTRACTILE RESPONSE IN ISOLATED PREPARATIONS

Under proper conditions, the diversity of response to cholinomimetics could be observed in this classical bioassay. Following an earlier observation that the response to histamine in guinea pig ileum or bladder reveals more information when carried out in Krebs solution rather than the customary Tyrode solution (19), a re-investigation of the contractile response of these preparations to cholinomimetics in Krebs solution seemed timely.

In the guinea pig bladder, maximum contractile response evoked by ACh was on the average 40% of that of CCh maximum and never exceeded 60% (Fig. 1). Conceivably, the reduced efficacy of ACh with respect to CCh in this preparation could be ascribed to its spontaneous hydrolysis by acetylcholinesterase (AChE). Indeed, when this enzyme had been inhibited by prior incubation with neostigmine, maximum contractile response to ACh increased to the level of that evoked by CCh. Yet, this contention, alone, is not sufficient to explain the profile of response to ACh which, in the presence of intact enzyme, maintained a steady level throughout the relatively wide range of 5 µM to 100 µM and often beyond it to about 1000 µM. The almost constant level of response to ACh throughout this wide range could be rationalized by assuming either of two alternative mechanisms, not necessarily exclusive of each other. First, one may assume an increase in turnover number of membrane-bound AChE with an increase in substrate concentration, in analogy with the finding with solubilized AChE (20). If this is indeed the case, then any increase in ACh concentration beyond 5 µM must be almost fully balanced by a proportional increase in enzyme activity. However, Michaelis-Menten kinetics also require that the enzyme have a finite maximum rate which, in the case of the solubilized enzyme, is close to 3 mM (20). In view of this, the concentration-response curve ought to have assumed a course of slow and continuous rise to reach a steady state at the maximum response of the preparation upon full saturation of the membrane-bound enzyme. Obviously, the experimental results are different. The alternative approach is to assume non-competitive antagonism of ACh-induced response through an agent which must arise in the presence of the intact enzyme. The most likely candidate is choline. In fact, 10 to 100 µM choline depressed almost equipotentially the maximum response, whether evoked by CCh or ACh in the presence of neostigmine, but had only a slight effect on the maximum of ACh in presence of the intact enzyme (Fig. 1). Since antagonism by choline is non-competitive, one expects ACh to act as a non-competitive antagonist of CCh in the presence of the intact enzyme. This is indeed the case, as the joint effect of CCh and ACh applied together proved to elicit a lower response than the calculated sum of the responses of each of these agents when applied separately (Fig. 2).

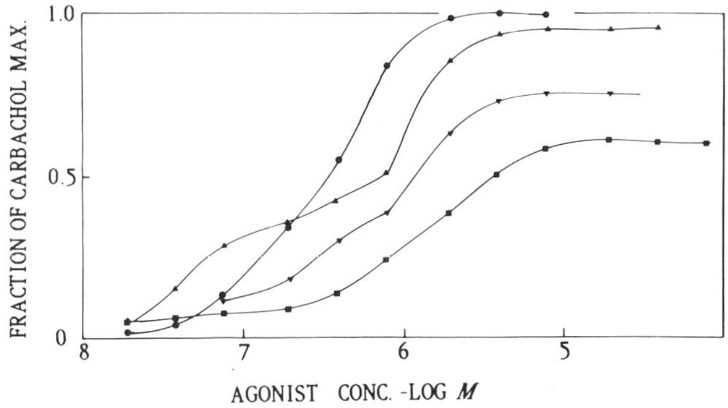

Fig. 1. Relative contractile response evoked in a single isolated guinea pig bladder in Krebs solution by: ● CCh; ■ ACh; ▲ ACh after incubation with neostigmine 100 nM; ▼ ACh after incubation with neostigmine 100 nM and choline chloride 100 μM.

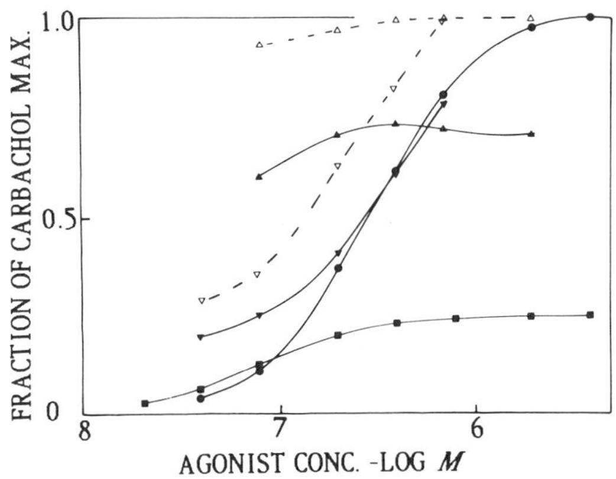

Fig. 2. Relative contractile response evoked in a single isolated guinea pig bladder in Krebs solution by: ● CCh; ■ ACh; ACh in presence of 800 nM CCh, found ▲ , versus calculated △ ; CCh in presence of 800 nM ACh, found ▼ , versus calculated ▽ .

The response of the guinea pig ileum differed from that of the bladder on two counts: First, in a few preparations, both CCh and ACh produced the same amplitude in maximum response, which was never observed in the bladder; but in most cases, maximum ACh response was about 60% of carbachol maximum, an observation first documented by Bolton and Clark (21) (Fig. 3). This last effect of apparent partial agonism by ACh cannot be detected in Tyrode solution where both CCh and ACh produce the same amplitude (Fig. 4). Again, neostigmine raised ACh maximum to the level of CCh maximum (Fig. 3), and in both cases maximal response of the preparation was reduced in the presence of 10 to 100 μM choline to a level of 60-70% of the maximum. In the presence of the intact enzyme, choline produced a similar depression of response in those preparations where response to ACh reached CCh maximum, but was much less effective when response to ACh was about 50% of that of CCh maximum.

The other point of distinction between bladder and ileum is the substantial response of the ileum to concentrations of ACh or CCh in the range of 1 to 100 nM. This early phase of response was less evident in the bladder and proved more convenient to study in the ileum. Neostigmine potentiated it, often considerably (Fig. 3), but this effect was also followed by tachyphylaxis manifested as lack or reduced response to further ACh application, if the preparation had not been allowed sufficient time to recover after washout. Pirenzepine, 50 nM reduced or eliminated the early contractile phase without affecting the late phase of response (Fig. 5). Since pirenzepine is not known to block ganglia, at least at this concentration, then one might conclude that the early phase of response is mediated through a muscarinic cholinergic receptor that is distinct from the one mediating the late phase of contraction. The usual ganglion blocker, hexamethonium 10 μM, had no effect on the early phase, thus reducing even further the likelihood of involvement of nicotinic receptors in parasympathetic ganglia. Remarkably, the selective muscarinic antagonist AF-14 produced a dual effect in the contractile response of the ileum. At concentrations in the range of 1 to 30 μM, it antagonized competitively the ACh-induced contractile response. At much lower concentrations, however, 10 to 300 nM, it potentiated the early phase of response (Fig. 6). Since this drug has negligible nicotinic activity and is a poor AChE inhibitor (12), its observed effect on the early phase could be ascribed to either of two possibilities: direct activation of the muscarinic receptor mediating the early phase, AF-14 presumably being a partial agonist in this respect; or more probably, selective inhibition of a presynaptic inhibitory receptor modulating ACh release, in analogy with the model offered by Kilbinger (22).

To summarize, the effect of ACh in the guinea pig bladder and often in the ileum is self-limiting presumably through the release of choline which reduces the amplitude of the contractile response. In these preparations, ACh seems to act as a partial agonist and could antagonize the effect of carbachol. Also, there is evidence that either drug is capable to cause release of endogenous ACh when applied at concentrations that are not sufficient to evoke a direct contractile effect in the muscle. This early effect of ACh or CCh could be inhibited with pirenzepine or potentiated with AF-14 when either of these drugs is applied at concentrations that do not interfere with the late phase of response evoked by ACh or CCh.

EVIDENCE FROM TRANSMEMBRANE CURRENTS EVOKED IN XENOPUS LAEVIS OOCYTE

The diversity of response to ACh is not restricted to multicellular tissue. It could be shown to occur also in a single cell. Single mammalian cells do not lend themselves easily to such an undertaking, but the

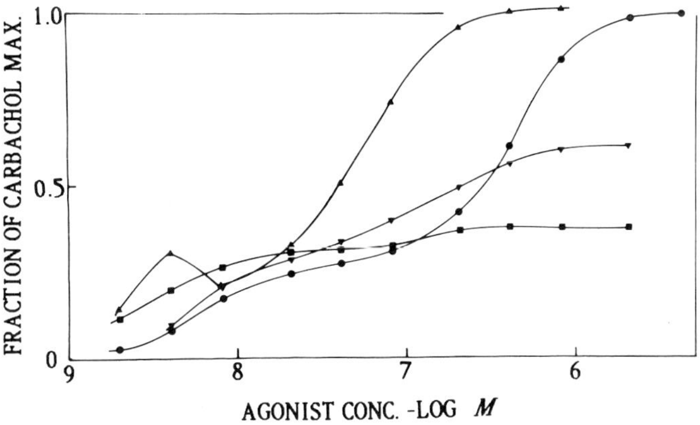

Fig. 3. Relative contractile response evoked in a single guinea pig ileum preparation by: ● CCh; ■ ACh; ▲ ACh after incubation with neostigmine 100 nM; ▼ ACh after incubation with neostigmine 100 nM and choline chloride 100 μM.

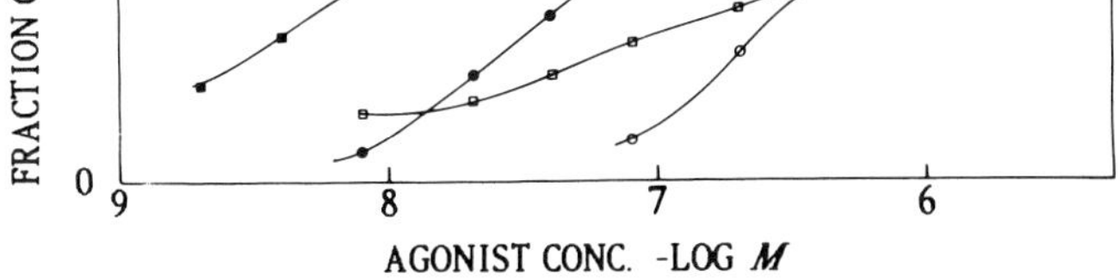

Fig. 4. Relative contractile response evoked in a single guinea pig ileum preparation by: ● CCh and ■ ACh in Krebs solution; ○ CCh and □ ACh in Tyrode solution. Krebs solution composition (mM): NaCl 118; KCl 4.75; $CaCl_2$ 3.36; $MgCl_2$ 1.19; $NaHCO_3$ 25; KH_2PO_4 1.18; glucose 11, pH 7.2. Tyrode solution (mM): NaCl 136.9; KCl 2.68; $CaCl_2$ 1.80; $MgCl_2$ 1.05; $NaHCO_3$ 11.90; NaH_2PO_4 0.42; glucose 5.55; pH 7.0.

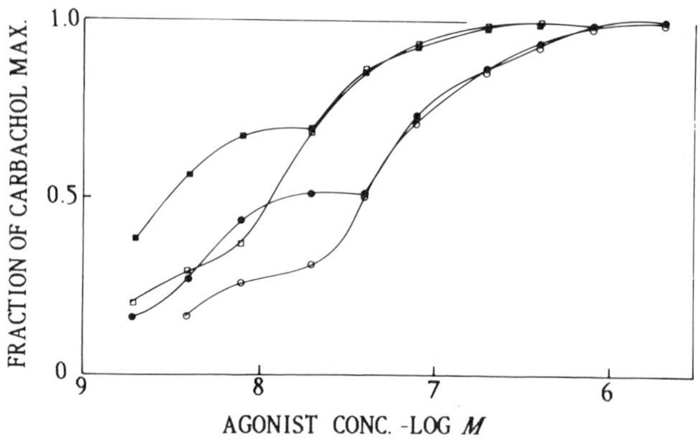

Fig. 5. Relative contractile response evoked in a single guinea pig ileum preparation in Krebs solution by: ● CCh; ○ CCh in presence of 50 nM pirenzepine; ■ ACh; □ ACh in presence of 50 nM pirenzepine. In this particular preparation, ACh and CCh maxima had the same amplitude.

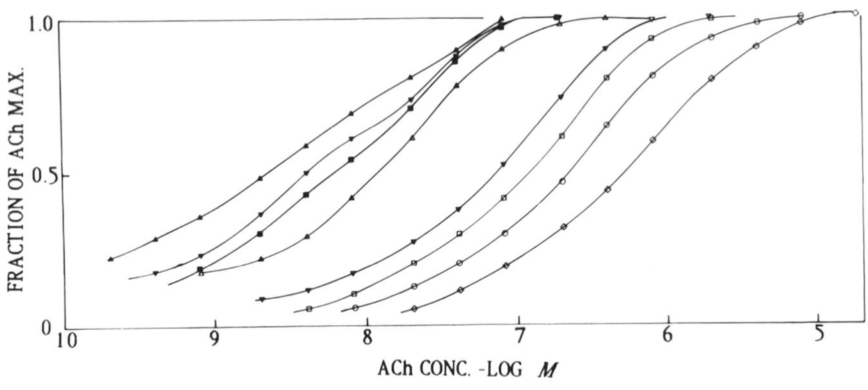

Fig. 6. Relative contractile response evoked in a single guinea pig ileum preparation in Krebs solution by: ■ ACh; and ACh in presence of the following concentrations of AF-14 (μM): ▲ 0.01; ▼ 0.3; △ 1; ▽ 6; □ 10; ○ 20; ◇ 30.

Xenopus laevis denuded oocyte has proved recently to offer a convenient medium for the study of the multiplicity of responses evoked by ACh (23-25). Cholinergic innervation of the oocyte has never been demonstrated, so that the presence of any cholinergic surface receptors on this cell must be inferred from the response elicited by ACh, as a transmembrane current. By use of voltage-clamp technique and intracellular microelectrode recording, it has been shown that ACh could elicit four distinct and independent electrophysiological events (25): A fast transient inward (depolarizatory) current, D_1; followed by a longer lasting inward current, D_2; then an almost overlapping but usually much smaller outward current (hyperpolarizatory), H; as a rule, both D_2 and H are accompanied by large inward current fluctuations, F. Selective isolation of each of the four components of the response to ACh could be performed by applying an appropriate technique: voltage clamping at the Cl^- or K^+ equilibrium potential; blockade of the H response with tetraethylammonium; or of the F response at low molarity. Also, D_1 and D_2 display differential sensitivity to extracellular calcium (25). Thus, the oocyte as a model seemed admirably well suited to investigate the diversity of response to ACh or related cholinomimetics in one single cell. Whether these different responses arise in correspondingly different cholinoceptors must remain for the time a matter of conjecture. The current evidence however, could be interpreted either way, in accordance with one's premise of similarity or dissimilarity among receptors.

Analysis of fractional response, in this case the observed current amplitude, with respect to ACh concentration dwelt on the assumption that a single ACh molecule binds to a single receptor site, that such binding follows mass action kinetics, and that the intensity of the evoked current, whether carried by Cl^- or K^+, is a linear function of $(\text{occupancy})^n$, n being an integer $\geqslant 1$. "Occupancy" is defined as $[ACh] / [ACh]+K$, where $[ACh]$ is the applied concentration and K is the equilibrium dissociation constant of the ACh-receptor entity. This assumption enabled the derivation of an estimate of the affinity of ACh to the putative cholinoceptor presumably mediating the particular response being considered.

For most cells studied, the D_1 response relative to $[ACh]$ was sigmoidal and steep with a Hill coefficient $\geqslant 2.5$. The data proved consistent with a model in which ACh effect is mediated jointly by two distinct sets of receptor sites, response being a linear function of the sum total of $(\text{occupancy})^3$ at either site as follows:

$$\text{observed } D_1 = D^*_{1(\max)} \left\{ \frac{[ACh]}{[ACh] + K^*_{D_1}} \right\}^3 + D_{1(\max)} \left\{ \frac{[ACh]}{[ACh] + K_{D_1}} \right\}^3 \qquad (1)$$

where (*) denotes parameters that characterize the site with the higher affinity to ACh.

The data for the D_2 response proved to be consistent with the same model; but in this case the response appeared to arise from the stimulation of a single site, as follows:

$$\text{observed } D_2 = D_{2(\max)} \left\{ \frac{[ACh]}{[ACh] + K_{D_2}} \right\}^3 \qquad (2)$$

hence,

$$(1/D_2)^{1/3} = (1/D_{2(\max)})^{1/3} + (K_{D_2}/D_{2(\max)})^{1/3} \cdot 1/[ACh] \qquad (3)$$

Such being the case, D_1 and D_2 share a common dependence on occupancy, are both carried by Cl^-, yet differ in time-sequence and, partly, in the affinity of ACh to the putative cholinoceptive sites. In making this conclusion, it is conceded that the model offered in accordance with eq. (1) and (2) is unusual. In the more current model of positive cooperativity (26), amplitude of evoked D_2 response ought to have been expressed as follows:

$$\text{observed } D_2 = D_{2(max)} \cdot \frac{[ACh]^3}{[ACh]^3 + K_{D_2}} \tag{4}$$

hence,

$$1/D_2 = 1/D_{2(max)} + K_{D_2}/D_{2(max)} \cdot 1/[ACh]^3 \tag{5}$$

However, a plot of $1/D_2$ against $1/[ACh]^3$ failed to comply with linearity, while a plot of $(1/D_2)^{1/3}$ against $1/[ACh]$ did. $D_{2(max)}$ and K_{D2} could then be calculated from the double reciprocal plot in the usual way. The phenomenological interpretation of this modification of positive cooperativity implies that three cholinoceptive sites must be occupied concomitantly for any response to arise. A similar model was proposed to account for the effect of calcium in transmitter release (27).

For a proper recording of the H response, interference from D_2 had to be eliminated by voltage clamping of the membrane very close to the Cl^- equilibrium potential. The dose-response relationship was consistent with a simple Langmuir isotherm with a Hill coefficient close to 1. In this case, analysis by the double reciprocal plot gave an estimate of the affinity of ACh to the putative cholinoceptor involved. The various parameters derived from the concentration-response relationship of ACh in the oocyte are summarized in Table 1.

Table 1. Parameters derived from the concentration-response relationship of three ACh-induced currents in denuded Xenopus oocytes.

Response	Current	Hill coefficient	Calcd K, uM	N
D_1	Cl^-	1.39±0.16	0.032±0.028	5
		2.53±0.14	0.31 ±0.26	4
D_2	Cl^-	2.61±0.08	0.29 ±0.09	3
H	K^+	1.02±0.12	0.39 ±0.28	4

It is remarkable that the K estimates correspond to the data of Birdsall (28) for the "superhigh" and "high" affinity sites found in mammalian brain. In the present case, the two sets of sites could be declared dissimilar on account of the wide difference in their relative affinity to ACh. By the same token, the sites mediating the D_2 and H responses could be declared similar in view of the very close values of the estimates of their respective affinities to ACh. However, and if one were to rely on the criterion of function or response as an index of receptor characterization, then obviously the H response must be ascribed to sites having different characteristics than those mediating the D_1 or D_2 response.

Further characterization of the sites mediating these three responses was attempted by use of the selective muscarinic agonist McN-A343 which is a ganglion-specific agent, and pirenzepine which is a CNS-specific antagonist. The first elicited, at most, a small inward current or had no observable effect in cells which otherwise exhibited pronounced responses to ACh. Pirenzepine inhibited almost equipotentially all three responses at a median inhibitory concentration of about 0.5 μM, without discriminating between D_1 and D_2 or these and H. These findings imply that cholinoceptive sites on the oocyte may share some properties with post-synaptic muscarinic receptors in mammalian peripheral tissues, but not in ganglia or the CNS (29).

CONCLUSION

It is not known whether the present findings are of physiological significance and whether they have a parallel in the intact organism. But they do illustrate the diversity of response mediated by cholinoceptive sites that would otherwise seem to belong into a single class. Any strategy based on a premise of cholinoceptor heterogeneity should perhaps give more weight to the diversity of response than done so far.

ACKNOWLEDGMENT

These investigations were supported by the Mauerberger Chair of Neuropharmacology provided to S.C.

REFERENCES

1. M. Caulfield and D. Straughan, Muscarinic receptors revisited, Trends in Neurosci. 6: 73 (1983).
2. G. B. Koelle, Parasympathomimetic agents, in "The Pharmacological Basis of Therapeutics". L.S. Goodman and A. Gilman ed., 5th ed., McMillan, London (1975).
3. A.P. Roszkowski, An unusual type of ganglion stimulant, J. Pharmacol. exp. Ther. 132: 156 (1961).
4. D. V. Franko, J. W. Ward and R. S. Alphin, Pharmacological studies of N-benzy-3-pyrrolidyl acetate methobromide (AHR-602), a ganglion stimulating agent, J. Pharmacol. exp. Ther. 139: 25 (1963).
5. J. C. Smith, Observations on the selectivity of stimulant action of 4-(m-chlorophenyl)carbamyloxy-2-butynyltrimethylammonium chloride on sympathetic ganglia, J. Pharmacol. exp. Ther. 153: 266 (1966).
6. R. J. Marshall, A new muscarinic agent: 1,4,5,6-tetrahydro-5-phenoxypyrimidine (AH-6405), Br. J. Pharmacol. 39: 191 (1970).
7. S. I. Ankier, R. T. Brittain and D. Jack, Investigation of central cholinergic mechanisms in the conscious mouse, Br. J. Pharmacol. 42: 127 (1971).
8. A. Fisher, M. Weinstock, S. Gitter and S. Cohen, A new probe for heterogeneity in muscarinic receptors: 2-methyl-spiro-(1,3-dioxolane-4,3')quinuclidine, Europ. J. Pharmacol. 37: 329 (1976).
9. H. I. Yamamura and S. H. Snyder, Muscarinic cholinergic binding in rat brain, Proc. Nat. Acad. Sci. USA 71: 1725 (1974).
10. R. B. Barlow, F. M. Franks, J. D. M. Pearson and A. A. Butt, A comparison of the affinities of antagonists for acetylcholine receptors in the ileum, bronchial muscle and iris of the guinea pig, Br. J. Pharmacol. 46: 300 (1972).
11. Y. Kloog, Y. Egozi and M. Sokolovsky, Characterization of muscarinic acetylcholine receptors from mouse brain: evidence for regional heterogeneity and isomerization, Mol. Pharmacol. 15: 545 (1979).
12. A. Fisher, Y. Grunfeld, M. Weinstock, S. Gitter and S. Cohen, A study of muscarinic receptor heterogeneity with weak antagonists, Europ. J. Pharmacol. 38: 131 (1976).
13. S. Cohen and F. Haberman, Enthalpy-entropy relationship in drug-cholinoceptor interaction: a new approach (in manuscript).
14. R. Hammer, C. P. Berrie, N. J. M. Birdsall, A. S. V. Burgen and E. C. Hulme, Pirenzepine distinguishes between different subclasses of muscarinic receptors, Nature 283: 90 (1980).

15. R. Hammer and A. Giachetti, Muscarinic receptor subtypes: M1 and M2 biochemical and functional characterization, Life Sci. 31: 2991 (1982).
16. R. Rubinstein, I. Nissenkorn and S. Cohen, Affinity of nortriptyline to muscarinic receptors in the bladder and ileum of man and guinea pig, Europ. J. Pharmacol. 100: 21 (1984).
17. R. F. Furchgott and P. Bursztyn, Comparison of dissociation constants and relative efficacies of selected agonists acting on parasympathetic receptors, Ann. N. Y. Acad. Sci. 144: 882 (1967).
18. T. P. Kenakin, The classification of drugs and drug receptors in isolated tissues, Pharmacol. Rev. 36: 165 (1984).
19. R. Rubinstein and S. Cohen, Histamine-mediated acetylcholine release in the guinea pig ileum, Europ. J. Pharmacol. (in press).
20. S. Ehrenpreis, Molecular aspects of cholinergic mechanisms, in "Drugs affecting the Peripheral Nervous System", A. Burger ed., M. Dekker, New York (1967).
21. T. B. Bolton and J. P. Clark, Actions of various muscarinic agonists on membrane potential, potassium efflux, and contraction of longitudinal muscle of guinea pig intestine, Br. J. Pharmacol. 72: 319 (1981).
22. H. Kilbinger, Facilitation and inhibition of muscarinic agonists of acetylcholine release from guinea pig myenteric neurones: mediation through different types of neuronal muscarinic receptors, Trends in Pharmacol. Sci. 5 (suppl.): 49 (1984).
23. K. Kusano, K. Miledi and J. Stinnakre, Cholinergic and catecholaminergic receptors in the Xenopus oocyte membrane, J. Physiol. 328: 143 (1982).
24. N. Dascal and E. M. Landau, Cyclic GMP mimics the muscarinic response in Xenopus oocyte: identity of ionic mechanisms, Proc. Nat. Acad. Sci. USA 79: 3052 (1982).
25. N. Dascal, E. M. Landau and Y. Lass, Xenopus oocyte resting potential, muscarinic responses and the role of calcium and cyclic GMP, J. Physiol. 352: 551 (1984).
26. D. Colquhoun, The relation between classical and cooperative models for drug action, in "Drug Receptors", H. P. Rang ed., McMillan, New York (1973).
27. F. Dodge and R. Rahamimoff, cooperative action of Ca ions in transmitter release at the neuromuscular junction, J. Physiol. 193: 419 (1967).
28. N. J. M. Birdsall, E. C. Hulme and J. M. Stockton, Muscarinic receptor heterogeneity, Trends in Pharmacol. Sci. (suppl) 5: 4 (1984).
29. N. J. M. Birdsall and E. C. Hulme, Muscarinic receptor subclasses, Trends in Pharmacol. Sci. 4: 459 (1983).

STRUCTURE-ACTIVITY RELATIONSHIPS OF RS 86 ANALOGUES

G. Bolliger, J.M. Palacios, A. Closse, G. Gmelin,
J. Malanowski

Preclinical Research, Sandoz Ltd.
CH-4002 Basle, Switzerland

INTRODUCTION

The recent discovery (Rossor, 1982; Coyle et al., 1983, for reviews) of a marked decrease in presynaptic cholinergic markers in the brains of patients dying of Alzheimer's disease has stimulated the interest for the search of orally active, safe and long-acting centrally active muscarinic cholinergic agonists which could be of therapeutic value in the treatment of this disease.

Different approaches have been proposed for obtaining tissue or organ selective cholinergic agonists. This may include targeting specific muscarinic receptor subtypes or use of partial agonists or allosteric regulators (see Jenden and Ehlert, 1984, for a review).

Classical cholinomimetics such as physostigmine, arecoline or oxotremorine are short-acting and have many unwanted side effects. The spiro-succinimide **RS 86** (compound **1**) appears to be an orally active well tolerated, long-lasting central muscarinic cholinergic agonist (Spiegel, 1984; Spiegel et al., 1984; Wettstein and Spiegel, 1984).

In an effort to expand our knowledge of the muscarinic receptor we have investigated some structure-activity relationships in a series of RS 86 analogues.

CHEMISTRY

RS 86 and the analogues **2** to **10** were prepared according to methods previously described (Jucker and Süess, 1961). Compound **11** was obtained by regiospecific reduction of RS 86 (Süess, 1977) whereas the partially reduced compound **12** had to be prepared by a different multi-step synthesis not depicted here.

The sulphur analogues **13** to **15** were obtained as a mixture by refluxing RS 86 with Lawesson's reagent (Lawesson et al., 1978) in dry benzene. Chromatographic separation of the crude reaction product yielded the pure compounds. Figure 1 outlines the different chemical approaches used to prepare RS 86 and its congeners. For structural details see Table I.

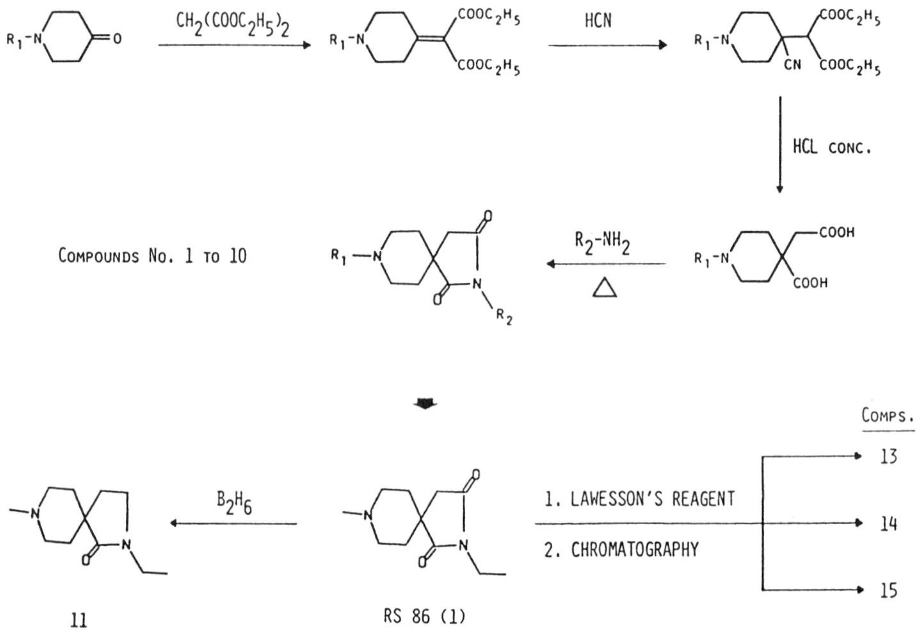

Figure 1

PHARMACOLOGY

The pharmacological activity of these analogues was assessed by using a battery of _in vitro_ and _in vivo_ tests for cholinergic activity.

The affinity of these compounds for muscarinic cholinergic receptors was measured in muscarinic agonist and antagonist binding assays using ^{3}H-cis-methyldioxolane (Bittiger and Heid, 1981) and ^{3}H-pirenzepine (Watson et al., 1983) as ligands and rat cortex membranes as receptor preparations. _In vitro_ functional assays such as the guinea-pig ileum and the rat superior cervical ganglion were used to measure affinity and efficacy.

Central _in vivo_ muscarinic cholinergic activity was evaluated by measurement of hypothermia and tremor in mice. In addition, a number of characteristic peripheral parasympathomimetic effects such as salivation, lacrimation and diarrhoea were observed in mice and scored. The signs were scored as absent (0), present (1) or intense (2). A detailed description of the methodology has been presented elsewhere (Palacios et al., 1985).

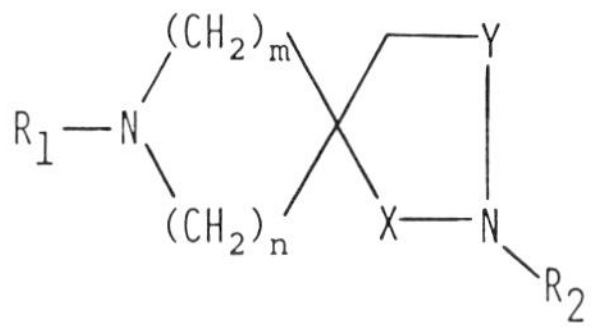

Table I. Chemical Structure of RS 86 and Analogues

COMPOUND	R_1	R_2	X	Y	m	n
RS 86 (1)	CH_3	C_2H_5	C=O	C=O	2	2
2	H	C_2H_5	C=O	C=O	2	2
3	C_2H_5	C_2H_5	C=O	C=O	2	2
4	CH_3	CH_3	C=O	C=O	2	2
5	H	CH_3	C=O	C=O	2	2
6	CH_3	H	C=O	C=O	2	2
7	H	H	C=O	C=O	2	2
8	H	C_2H_5	C=O	C=O	3	1
9	CH_3	C_2H_5	C=O	C=O	3	1
10	CH_3	CH_3	C=O	C=O	3	2
11	CH_3	C_2H_5	C=O	CH_2	2	2
12	CH_3	CH_3	CH_2	C=O	2	2
13	CH_3	C_2H_5	C=O	C=S	2	2
14	CH_3	C_2H_5	C=S	C=O	2	2
15	CH_3	C_2H_5	C=S	C=S	2	2

RESULTS AND DISCUSSION

Table II summarizes the results obtained with the different spirosuccinimide derivatives in the *in vitro* tests for muscarinic activities. In analyzing the binding data two factors have to be taken into account. First, in one case the ligand is an agonist (^{3}H-cis-methyldioxolane) and in the other an antagonist (^{3}H-pirenzepine). Muscarinic agonists present higher affinities for agonist binding sites than for antagonist sites (Birdsall et al., 1984). Second both ligands probably label the proposed muscarinic receptor subtypes in a differential way. Thus, while ^{3}H-pirenzepine labels the M_1 subtype (Hammer et al., 1980) the exact nature of the sites labeled by ^{3}H-cis-methyldioxolane is still a matter of discussion (Vickroy et al., 1984). Regarding the functional models the guinea pig ileum (longitudinal muscle) is enriched in "M_2" sites while the superior cervical ganglion is a "M_1" preparation.

Variations in the substituents of the piperidine and/or succinimide nitrogens (compound **1** to **7**) lead to modifications of the affinities for both binding sites as well as in the activity of these compounds in the functional assays. A relatively good parallelism was found between the variation of affinity for the ^{3}H-agonist binding site and the activity in the functional assays. Thus, loss of affinity by methyl (compounds **4** and **5**) or hydrogen (compounds **6** and **7**) substitution at the succinimide nitrogen was reflected in similar loss of activity. Substitution at the piperidine nitrogen beyond the methyl group (compound **3**) led to a dramatic loss of affinity and activity. The ^{3}H-antagonist binding reflected with less accuracy changes in activity. Examples of that are compounds **3**, **4** and **5** which were equipotent in displacing ^{3}H-pirenzepine although compound **3** was inactive but **4** and **5** were active in the functional models.

Alteration of the position of the nitrogen in the piperidine ring (compounds **8** and **9**) or of the size of this ring (compound **10**) resulted in changes in both affinity and activity which did not however, always run in parallel. Thus, while compound **8** presented lower affinities than compound **10** in both binding assays, the first but not the latter was active in the functional assays.

Reduction of one of the two oxygens in the succinimide ring (compounds **11** and **12**) led to a marked decrease in affinity (around 20-fold) and activity (about 10-fold). Apparently these effects were more pronounced when the oxygen in position α to the spirocarbon, (compound **12**) rather than that in position β, (compound **11**) was reduced.

Table II. Affinities and Activities of RS 86 Analogues in Different Receptor Binding and Functional Assays of Muscarinic Receptors

COMPOUND	IC_{50} (nM) FOR THE BINDING IN RAT CORTEX		GUINEA-PIG ILEUM		RAT SUPERIOR CERVICAL GANGLION	
No.	^{3}H-CIS-METHYLDIOXOLANE	^{3}H-PIRENZEPINE	pD_2	pA_2	pD_2	pA_2
1	87	765	6.1		6.7	
2	75	475	5.9		6.3	
3	6250	3600	INACTIVE		INACTIVE	
4	175	4050	5.3		6.0	
5	350	3000	5.1		5.8	
6	6100	13200	INACTIVE		INACTIVE	
7	5400	6795	INACTIVE		INACTIVE	
8	2250	6250	4.2		4.6	
9	10000	10000	INACTIVE		INACTIVE	
10	1455	555	INACTIVE		INACTIVE	
11	1600	11300	5.0		5.7	
12	2050	9200	4.4		5.1	
13	200	110	5.2		6.0	
14	2950	490		5.4		5.5
15	665	145		6.3		6.6

CNS

HYPOTHERMIA

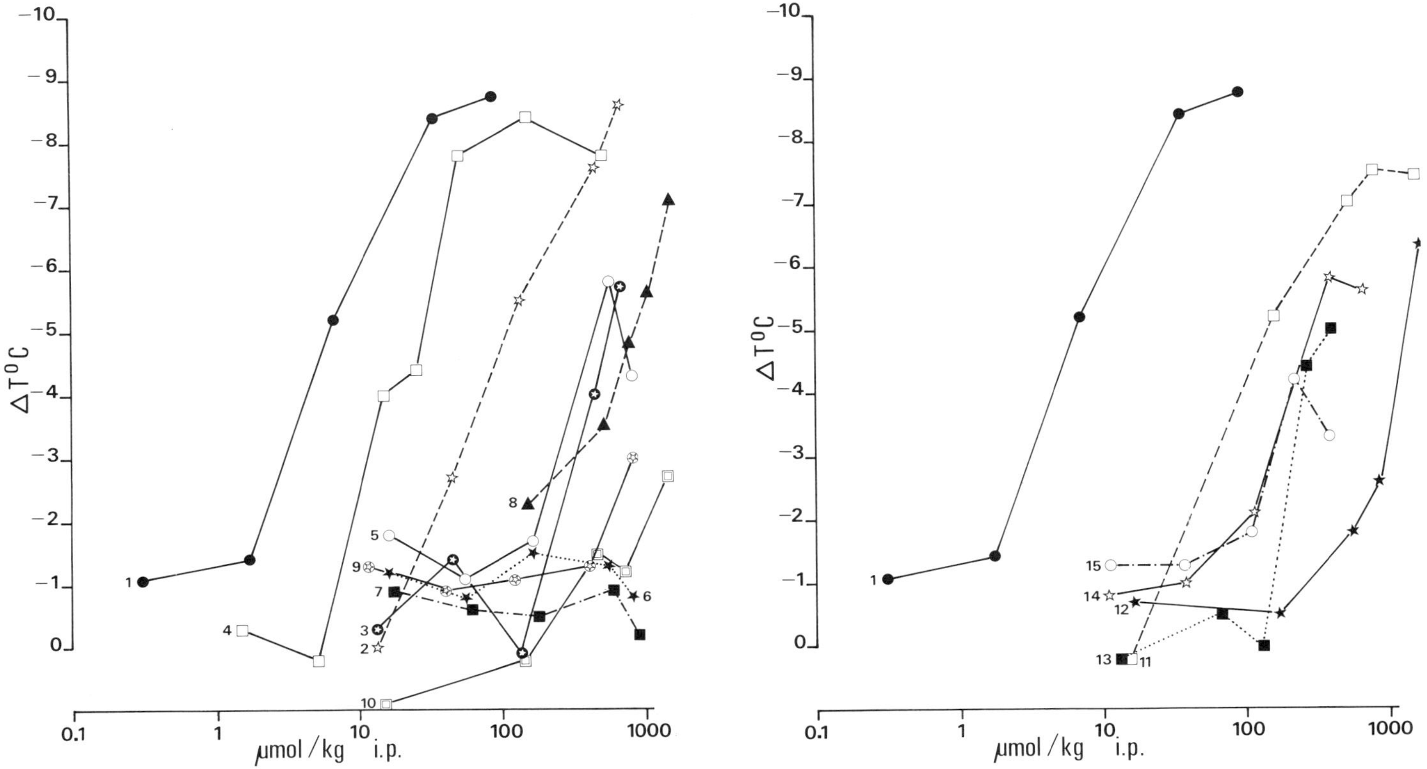

Figure 2

Dose-response curves of **RS 86 (1)** and the analogues **2** to **15** for a typical central muscarinic effect (hypothermia).

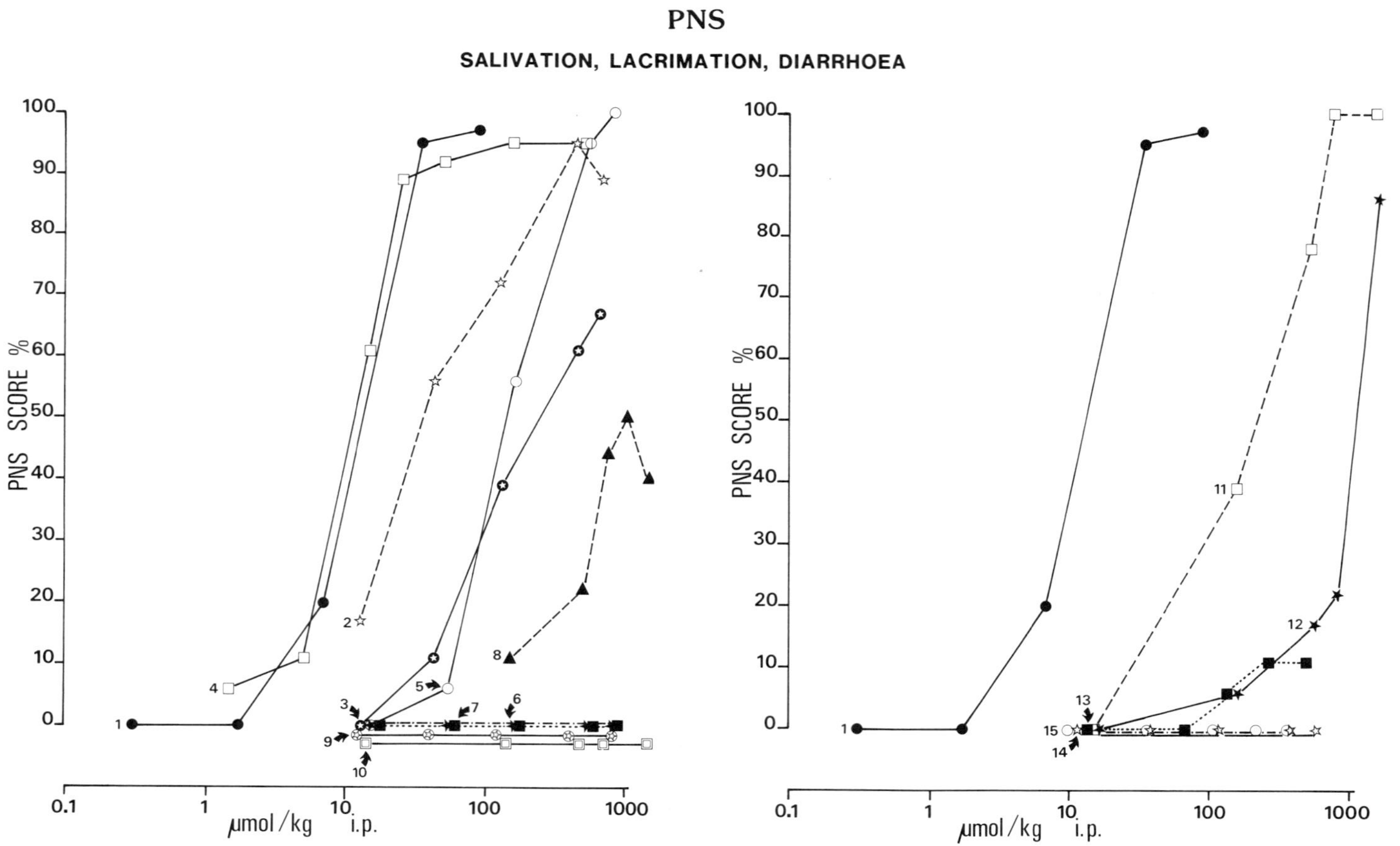

Figure 3

Dose-response curves of **RS 86 (1)** and the analogues 2 to 15 for various peripheral muscarinic effects.

Finally, the effects of the substitution of one or both oxygen atoms by sulphur (compounds **13**, **14** and **15**) was followed by changes not only in the affinity but also in the activity and the character of this muscarinic activity. Again substitution of the α oxygen (compound **14**) resulted in a more pronounced loss of affinity for ^{3}H-agonist binding sites than substitution of the β oxygen (compound **13**). In both cases an increase in the affinity for the ^{3}H-antagonist sites was observed. In addition, while compound **13** was an agonist, compound **14** was a weak antagonist in both functional tests. Substitution of both oxygen atoms by sulphur (compound **15**) again led to marked decrease in affinity for ^{3}H-agonist sites and to a higher affinity for the ^{3}H-antagonist sites. This was paralleled by an increased antagonistic activity in the functional in vitro tests.

The dose dependency of both central (hypothermia) and peripheral (sum scored of salivation, lacrimation and diarrhoea) effects for compounds **1** to **15** is depicted on Figures 2 and 3. While there was some correlation between in vivo effects and in vitro affinity and activity this correlation was far from being perfect. Compound **1** (RS 86) was the most active in vivo compound of the series, both centrally and peripherally. Compound **4** was the second most active compound followed by compound **2** although in vitro the opposite was true. Compounds **11** and **12** were one and two orders of magnitude less active than **RS 86** (compound **1**), respectively. This is in good agreement with the in vitro data. Also in good agreement with in vitro results, compounds **6**,**7**,**9** and **10** were inactive in vivo and compound **8** presented only a low activity. This was not the case for compound **3** which although inactive in vitro presented an in vivo activity which was about one to two orders of magnitude lower than that of **RS 86**. Finally, compound **13**, as well as the in vitro antagonists **14** and **15**, although they did not elicit peripheral muscarinic activity did show hypothermic effects, an activity considered to be an expression of central agonistic activity. Biotransformation to agonistic metabolites is a very likely explanation for these findings.

In summary all these results demonstrate that very strict structural requirements for muscarinic activity exist in the series of analogues of the spiro-succinimide **RS 86**. This compound represented the optimal structure for both in vitro and in vivo agonistic activity. The lack of complete parallelism between in vitro and in vivo activities suggests that metabolic factors could play an important role in determining the in vivo activity of these compounds. These studies add further to our knowledge of the exquisite molecular requirements for the activation of the muscarinic cholinergic receptor.

REFERENCES

Birdsall, N.J.M., Hulme, E.C. and Stockton, J.M., 1984, Muscarinic receptor heterogeneity, Trends Pharmacol. Sci. (Supp. Jan.), 4.

Bittiger, H. and Heid, J., 1981, Radioreceptor assay for muscarinic agonists using ^{3}H-cis-methyldioxolane, Experientia, 37:638.

Coyle, J.T., Price, D.L. and DeLong, M.R., 1983, Alzheimer's disease: A disorder of cortical cholinergic innervation, Science, 219:1184.

Hammer, R., Berrie, C.P., Birdsall, N.J.M., Burgen, A.S.V. and Hulme, E.C., 1980, Pirenzepine distinguishes between different subclasses of muscarinic receptors, Nature, 283:90.

Jenden, D.J. and Ehlert, F.J., 1984, Heterogeneity of cholinergic receptors, in: "Alzheimer's Disease: Advances in Basic Research and Therapies", R.J. Wurtmann, S.H. Corkin and J.H. Growdon, eds., Center for Brain Sciences and Metabolism Charitable Trust, Cambridge, USA, pp. 123.

Jucker, E. and Süess, R., 1961, Ueber neuartige Spiro-Succinimide, Arch. Pharmaz., 294/66:210.

Lawesson, S.-O., Pederson, B.S. and Scheibye, S., 1978, Studies on organophosphorus compounds XXI. The dimer of p-methoxyphenylthionophosphine sulfide as thiation reagent. A new route to thiocarboxamides, Bull. Soc. Chim. Belg., 87:229.

Palacios, J.M., Bolliger, G., Closse, A., Enz, A., Gmelin, G. and Malanowski J., The pharmacological assessment of RS 86 (2-ethyl-8-methyl-2,8-diazospiro-[4,5]-decan-1,3-dion hydrobromide). A potent, specific muscarinic cholinergic agonist, Europ. J. Pharmacol., submitted.

Rossor, M.N., 1982, Dementia (Neurotransmitters and CNS Disease), The Lancet, ii:1200.

Spiegel, R., 1984, Effects of RS 86, an orally active cholinergic agonist, on sleep in man, Psychiatry Research, 11:1.

Spiegel, R., Azcona, A. and Wettstein, A., 1984, Frist results with RS 86, an orally active muscarinic agonist, in healthy subjects and in patients with dementia, in: "Alzheimer's Disease: Advances in Basic Research and Therapies", R.J. Wurtman, S.H. Corkin, and J.H. Growdon, eds., Proc. of the 3rd Meeting of the International Study Group on the Treatment of Memory Disorders Associated with Aging, Zürich, Switzerland, pp. 391.

Süess, R., 1977, Regiospezifische Reduktionen von 1,3,3-trisubstituierten Succinimiden mit Diboran, Helv. Chim. Acta, 60:1650.

Vickroy, T.W., Roeske, W.R. and Yamamura, H.I., 1984, Pharmacological differences between the high-affinity muscarinic agonist binding states of the rat heart and cerebral cortex labeled with (+)-^{3}H-cis-methyldioxolane, J. Pharmacol. Exp. Ther., 229:747.

Watson, M., Yamamura, H.I. and Roeske, W.R., 1983, A unique regulatory profile and regional distribution of [^{3}H]pirenzepine binding in the rat provide evidence for distinct M_1 and M_2 muscarinic receptor subtypes, Life Sci., 32:3001.

Wettstein, A. and Spiegel, R., 1984, Clinical trials with the cholinergic drug RS 86 in Alzheimer's Disease (AD) and Senile Dementia of the Alzheimer Type (SDAT), Psychopharmacology, 84:572.

THE LIPID REGIMEN

Meir Shinitzky

Department of Membrane Research
The Weizmann Institute of Science
Rehovot 76100, ISRAEL

INTRODUCTION - GENERAL PATTERNS IN MEMBRANE AGING

In the early phase of tissue aging, the turnover rate of metabolic processes is slowed down to a level that cannot cope effectively with external stress, as can the young tissue. At this phase, the continuous accumulation of serum lipids (e.g., cholesterol and sphingomyelin) in cell membranes is not fully compensated for by fluidity homeostasis (Sinensky, 1974) and a progressive decrease in membrane fluidity takes place. This phase is therefore characterized by changes in lipid composition, mostly increase in cholesterol and sphingomyelin, while the population of proteins and other functional entities remains to a large extent unaffected. Table 1 summarizes changes in membrane lipid composition of various tissues with age, all of which correlate with decrease in fluidity. It seems that these changes precede the decline in the overt physiological functions and in some way induce it. The lipid regimen is based on the supposition that restoration of normal membrane fluidity in aging cells, notably neurites, can rectify deteriorated physiological, as well as behavioural patterns which are characteristic of aging.

STRATEGIES FOR MEMBRANE FLUIDIZATION

Inasmuch as the composition of membrane lipids can be altered by passive exchange with external pools, it is in principle possible to design special lipid mixtures that can fluidize rigidified cell membranes at a relatively fast rate which can override the rate of metabolic clearance. The agent used must be non-toxic, preferably natural lipid, should freely cross the blood-brain barrier and exert its effect before being metabolized, namely, within several blood cycles (i.e.,minutes). For lipid fluidization of aged tissues the best candidate is lecithin (Phosphatidyl choline, PC) which is the most common membrane fluidizer in nature. However, when PC is introduced into the blood it forms stable bilayers or integrates into serum lipoproteins, both of which are slow in affecting the cell membrane fluidity (i.e., hours). The introduced PC is therefore mostly degraded before it can significantly fluidize "hyperviscous" cell membranes. However, the rate of membrane fluidization by PC can be markedly increased when PC is loosly integrated in structures which facilitate processes of lipid exchange between the membrane and the serum.

Table 1. Increased Content of Membrane Lipids with Age

Tissue	Species	Cholesterol	Sphingomyelin	Glycosphingolipids	Saturated lipids	Reference
Synapse	Rat	+			+	Shinitzky et al.(1983) Hitzemann et al.(1984)
Brain	Man	+	+	+		Rouser et al. (1972) Rouser and Yamamato (1968)
Brain	Rat	+	+	+		Rouser et al. (1972) Shinitzky et al. (1983)
Myelin	Rat	+	+	+		Curzner and Davison (1968) Dalal and Einstein (1969)
Adipocyte	Rat				+	Hubbard and Garratt (1980)
Lymphocyte	Man	+				Rivnay et al. (1980)
Lymphocyte	Mouse	+				Rivnay et al. (1979)
Erythrocyte	Man	+				Araki and Rifkind (1980)

A mixture of lipids which provides such structures, termed as Active Lipid (AL), has been recently designed for effective membrane fluidization *in vivo* and *in vitro* (Lyte and Shinitzky, 1985). The constituents of this mixture are neutral lipids (NL), mostly triglycerides, phosphatidyl choline (PC) and phosphatidyl ethanolamine (PE) all from hen egg yolk. The optimal composition of AL, for membrane fluidization, as determined by *in vitro* experiments with normal and cholesterol enriched leukocytes, was found to be NL/PC/PE=7/2/1. A typical fluidization experiment, which verifies the potency of this particular composition, is shown in Figure 1. The same composition (AL 721) was found to be the most effective in the rate of extraction of excess ^{3}H-cholesterol from cell membranes (see Figure 2). Unexpectedly, however, introduction of PC from AL 721 into the cell membranes of leukocytes was found to be ineffective. Only brain membranes (P_2m from rat cortex) were found to accumulate PC from AL in a relatively short incubation time (less than 1 hr). It seems, therefore, that the fluidization effect of AL 721 on rigid cell membranes operates predominantly via cholesterol extraction and to a lesser extent by insertion of PC.

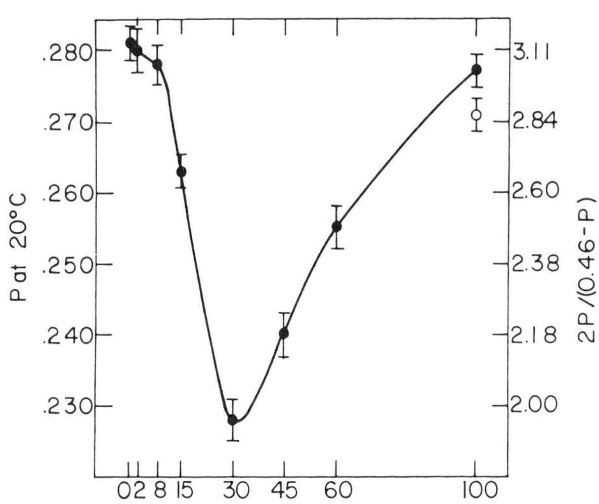

Fig. 1. Membrane fluidization of human lymphocytes by AL of PC/PE=2/1 and increasing amounts of NL. Peripheral blood lymphocytes from 19 humans were treated *in vitro* for 2 hrs with 0.5 mg/ml AL. The degree of DPH fluorescence polarization, P, and the corresponding scale of membrane microviscosity, 2P/(0.46-P), were determined (Shinitzky and Barenholz, 1978). The results shown represent the mean ± S.D. AL 721 reduced the membrane microviscosity by about 35% whereas PC at the same concentration (Φ) had a much smaller effect (from Lyte and Shinitzky, 1985).

THE EFFECT OF ACTIVE LIPID ON THE SYNAPTIC MEMBRANE

Like most other body tissues, nerve tissues also acquire more rigid membranes upon aging (see Table 1). Of particular relevance to Alzheimer's disease is the finding that the membrane of synapses in old animals is similarly impaired (Shinitzky et al. 1983; Hitzemann et al. 1984). It was also observed that emerging neurites are of a particularly fluid membrane (De Laat et al. 1979) and that artificial manipulation of the membrane lipid fluidity of regenerating neurites can markedly affect their extent of outgrowth (Pollak et al. 1985). Results of recent experiments carried out in Prof.M.Schwartz's laboratory, which clearly demonstrate the suppressive effect of cholesterol and the stimulating effect of AL on neurite extention, are shown in Figure 3.

The information presented above, though scarce, lends a conceptual support to the lipid regimen approach for treatment of dementia. Along this line, it is likely that part of the positive effects previously reported for treatments with phosphatidyl choline (Wurtman, 1979) or phosphatidyl serine (Drago et al. 1983) actually emerged from their action as membrane fluidizers.

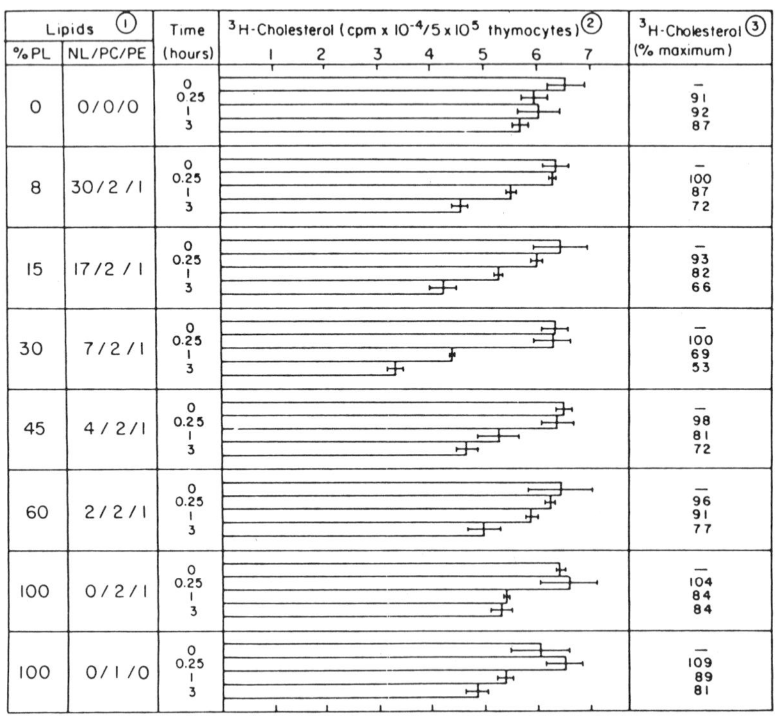

Fig. 2. Effect of various AL compositions and PC on the rate of extraction of cholesterol from the plasma membrane of mouse thymocytes. ^{3}H-cholesterol was incorporated into the cell plasma membranes by exchange with the external medium. The rate of reduction in radioactive counts upon incubation with lipid containing medium was determined. In the control experiment (upper panel) the rate of reduction in ^{3}H-cholesterol represents the rate of exchange with the control medium which should be taken as the baseline. The results are shown as mean $\pm$ S.D. of triplicate.

THE ACTIVE LIPID DIET

The most convenient route of AL administration is *per os* together with lipid free food. It is assumed that the processes of the lipid absorption in the small intestine, which entail hydrolysis and reacylation, do not change significantly the physical nature of AL which reassembles in the serum. The fatty acid compositions of the NL, PC and PE from hen egg yolk are very similar to each other and also to that of their blood serum analogues. It is therefore expected that when AL is given in a diet which contains no other lipids and after overnight fasting the absorbed lipids will appear in the serum in chylomycron assemblies of a membrane fluidization capacity similar to that of an *in vitro* dispersion of AL (Lyte and Shinitzky, 1985). Disintegration and digestion of AL is expected to be rather fast with an estimated clearing time of less than an hour. If the given dose of AL exceeds the amount of the residual serum lipids after overnight fasting (approximately 10 gr in humans) it may be expected that within the clearing time AL will impart some fluidization effect on the rigidified cell membranes (see Figure 1). In such a lipid regimen it is reasonable to assume that brain tissues are susceptible to changes induced by the lipid diet similarly to other tissues, since serum lipids can passively pass the blood-brain barrier and can thus participate in the lipid exchange processes with the aged brain cell membranes. The cumulative effect of the AL diet is expected to be noticeable within several days.

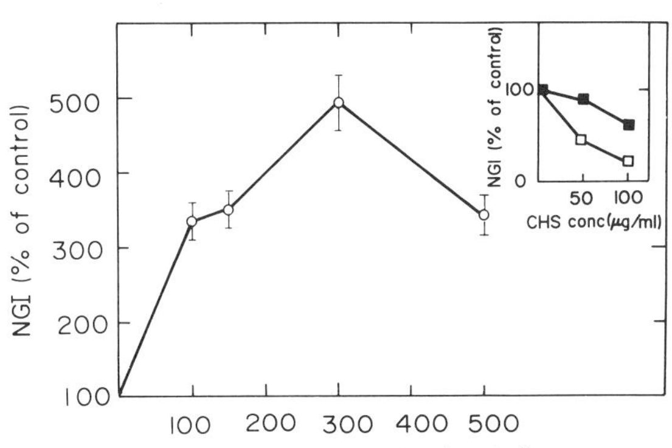

Fig. 3. The effect of AL concentration on neurite outgrowth from goldfish retina in culture. The retina were excised at 8-14 days after the optic nerve crush. Each point represents the results obtained by screening 40-60 retinal pieces which were taken from a pool of 20-30 different retina . The nerve index (NGI) is represented relatively to the control values (% of control) ± SEM. The inset shows the inhibitory effect of cholesteryl hemisuccinate (CHS) added on day 7 (■) and 9 (□) in culture (Pollak, N., Mizrachi, Y., Samuel, D. and Schwartz, M. unpublished results).

Our current mice diet consists of purina chow (which is relatively low in lipids) supplemented with 4-6% AL. The recommended human diet consists of 7-15 gr AL given with lipid free food. Since up to now our results were positive (see below) and no adverse effect was noticed we have used a more acute treatment (e.g. iv or intraperitoneal injections) only in studies where a rapid recovery of lipid fluidity was essential (Heron et al. 1982).

BLOOD LEUKOCYTES AS MONITORS FOR CHANGES IN THE CNS

The major obstacle in the development of therapeutic approaches to aging is the lack of quantitative physiological scale for monitoring brain function *in vivo*. Blood leukocytes, notably platelets, were found to reflect biochemical and pharmacological changes related to nerve endings in various psychological disorders (Rotman, 1983; Kafka et al. 1980), as well as in Alzheimer's disease (Zubenko, 1984). The systemic change in lipid composition of cell membranes in aging (Table 1) occurs more or less at a similar rate on all metabolically active non-dividing cells. This implies that the increased rate of net incorporation of serum lipids, notably cholesterol and sphingomyelin, into cell membranes in aging is probably similar in the CNS and in blood leukocytes. If this presumption is indeed valid, it opens a way for indirect monitoring the effect of treatment (e.g. AL diet) on changes of lipid composition and fluidity, as well as physiological activity, in the CNS. Stimulation of peripheral blood leukocytes by plant mitogens is one of the most reproducible quantitative tests known for biological activity of intact cells. This test is simple and can be performed daily and may reflect the efficacy of the lipid regimen in restoration of brain function. Yet, the full evaluation of the correlation between the mitogenic response of blood leukocytes and brain function in the aged is awaiting verification in large scale studies which are currently under planning.

The effect of AL 721 on immune functions of leukocytes from old animals and men is summarized in the following.

RECTIFICATION OF IMMUNE COMPETENCE IN THE AGED

The overt immune response can be monitored by the responsiveness of lymphocytes to mitogens like Con A or PHA. As expected, there is a good correlation between the lymphocyte membrane fluidity, or level of cholesterol, and their response to mitogens (Rivnay et al. 1979, 1980). *In vitro* experiments demonstrated that treatment of lymphocytes from aged mice or men with AL 721 increased markedly their membrane fluidity and their response to mitogenic stimulation. Similarly, lymphocytes which were artificially enriched with cholesterol, and thus acquired a rigid plasma membrane and resistance to mitogenic stimulation, could be reactivated by *in vitro* treatment with AL 721. It should be noted that in all the *in vitro* experiments with lymphocytes, lecithin by itself was found to be much less active as a membrane fluidizer or as a rectifier of mitogenic responsiveness (Rivnay et al. 1983), again indicating that its membrane fluidizing capacity becomes effective only when integrated in special lipid assemblies.

Restoration of immune competence in aged mice and rats by AL diet was examined in a large scale study. Mitogenic stimulations of splenocytes and lymph node leukocytes were determined for each individual animal with Con A and PHA at various stimulation doses. Results of a typical experiment are shown in Figure 4. As indicated, splenocytes from old rats on a standard diet are considerably less responsive to mitogenic

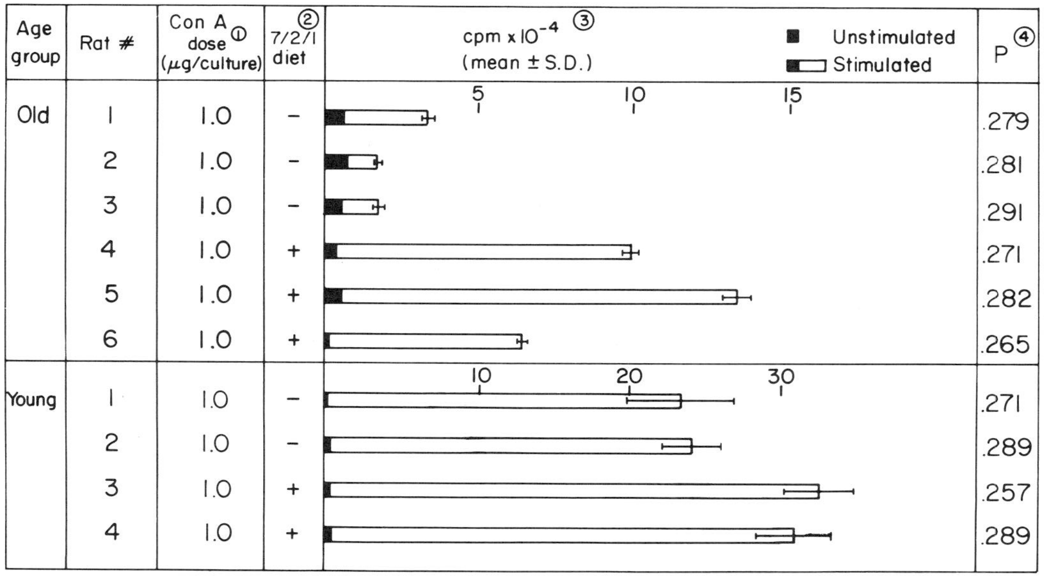

Fig. 4. The effect of AL 721 diet compared to standard diet on ConA stimulation of rat splenocytes. Young (3-5 months) and old (22-24 months) rats were given AL diet for 1 month and their splenocytes were tested *in vitro* for mitogenic response by Con A stimulation and ^{3}H-thymidine incorporation. The results are presented for each individual rat as mean $\pm$ S.D. of triplicates.

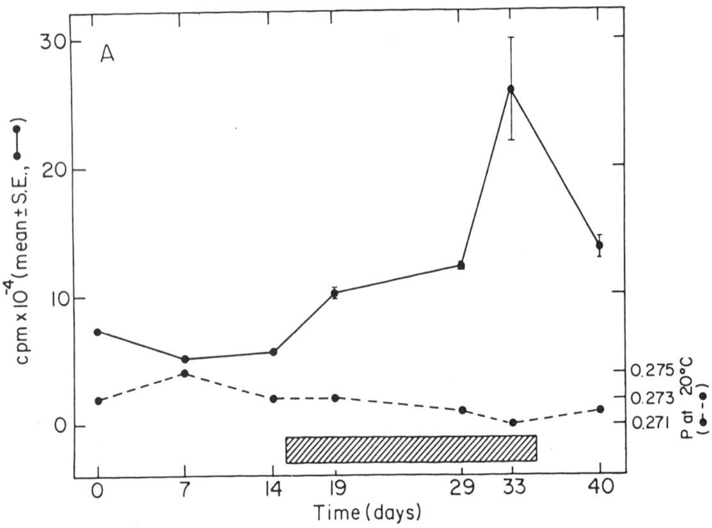

Figure 5A. (See legend on next page)

stimulation than splenocytes from young rats (Rivnay et al. 1979). AL diet in the old increased the splenocyte responsiveness by about 5-fold to a level similar to that found in the young (Figure 4). Splenocytes from young were only slightly activated by the AL diet. Similar results were also obtained with lymph node cells from mice and rats.

The overall restoration of immune competence by AL diet was examined by increase in survival of old animals infected with pathogenic bacteria. Again, the average ability of the old animals to cope with the infectious disease has increased markedly by AL diet and reached a level similar to that of the young animals (to be published).

Human Studies

Inasmuch as AL is a par excellence nutrient, no adverse reactions could be expected when given to men. This was verified by acute and chronic toxicology studies in animals, which opened the way for studies with human subjects under well defined AL diet. In our immunological study we have selected participants over 75 years of age who were immune suppressed but did not display any organic disease and were not taking immunosuppressive drugs. The study and the experimental protocol were carried at the Meir Hospital, Kfar Saba, Israel and was conducted under the supervision of Prof. A. Klajman and Dr. H. Rabinowich. The mitogenic responsiveness of peripheral blood lymphocytes was tested in each of the 10 participants at least 3 times within 3 weeks before entering the study in order to well define their basal immune competence. The AL diet of 10 gr was given each morning during a period of several weeks and the responsiveness of peripheral blood lymphocytes to mitogens was tested every several days. The AL diet was then stopped and the effect on mitogenic stimulation was measured 7 days later. The trend that was observed is the following: Already after several days of AL diet a significant increase in response to mitogens was observed. After about 3 weeks it reached a level typical to that found in the young. Upon cessation of the diet the lymphocyte responsiveness slowly declined towards the initial basal level. Typical results obtained in 3 subjects are shown in Figure 5.

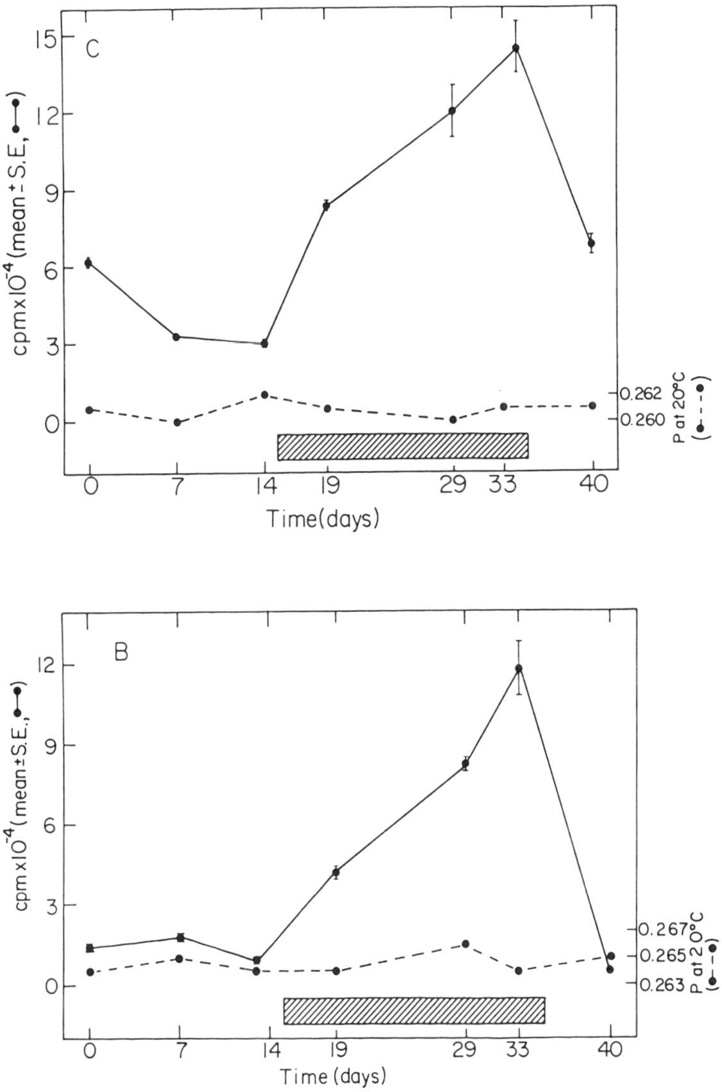

Figure 5B and C.

Responsiveness of peripheral blood lymphocytes to PHS stimulation before, during (▨) and after AL diet in 3 human subjects over 75 years of age (Rabinowich et al. submitted for publication).

REFERENCES

Araki, K., and Rifkind, J.M., 1980, Erythrocyte membrane cholesterol : An explanation of the aging effect on the rate of hemolysis. Life Sci., 26:2223.

Barbeau, A., Growdon J.A., and Wurtman, R.J., eds., 1979,"Choline and Lecithin in Brain Disorders," Raven Press, New-York.

Curzner, M.C., and Davison, A.N., 1968, The lipid composition of rat brain myelin and subcellular fractions during development, Biochem. J., 106:29.

Dalal, K.B., and Einstein, E.R., 1969, Biochemical maturation of the central nervous system: I. Lipid changes, Brain Res., 16:441.

De Laat, S.W., Van Der Saag, P.T., Elson, E.L., and Schlessinger, J., 1979, Lateral diffusion of membrane lipids and proteins is increased specifically in neurites of differentiating neuroblastoma cells, Biochim. Biophys. Acta, 558:247.

Drago, F., Toffano, G., Catalano, L., Danielli, R., Continella, G., and Scapagnini, 1983, Phosphatidyl serine facilitates learning and memory processes in aged rats, in: "Aging of the Brain", D. Samuel, S. Algeri, S. Gershon, V.E. Grimm, and G. Toffano, eds. Raven Press, New-York.

Heron, D., Shinitzky, M., and Samuel, D., 1982, Alleviation of drug withdrawal symptoms by treatment with a potent mixture of natural lipids, Eur. J. Pharmacol., 83:253.

Hubbard, R.E., and Garratt, , 1980, The composition and fluidity of adipocyte membranes prepared from young and adult rats, Biochim. Biophys. Acta, 600:701.

Kafka, M.S., Van Kammen, D.P., Kleinman, J.E., Nurnberger, J.I., Siever, L.J., Uhde, T.W., and Polinsky, R.J., 1980, Alfa-adrenergic receptor function in schizophrenia, affective disorders and some neurological diseases, Comm. in Psychopharmacol., 4:477.

Lyte, M., and Shinitzky, M., 1985, A special lipid mixture for membrane fluidization, Biochim. Biophys. Acta, 812:133.

Pollak, N., Mizrachi, Y., Samuel, D., and Schwartz, M., 1985, Membrane fluidity and neuronal regeneration in lower vertebrates. J. Neurochem. in press.

Rivnay, B., Globerson, A., and Shinitzky, M., 1979, Viscosity of lymphocyte plasma membranes in aging mice and its possible relation to serum cholesterol, Mech. Age. Dev., 40:71.

Rivnay, B., Bergman, B., Shinitzky, M., and Globerson, A., 1980, Correlation between membrane viscosity, serum cholesterol, lymphocyte activation and aging in man, Mech. Age. Dev.,12:119.

Rivnay, B., Orbital-Harel, T., Shinitzky, M., and Globerson, A., 1983, Enhancement of the response of ageing mouse lymphocytes by *in vitro* treatment with lecithin, Mech. Aging Dev., 23:329.

Rotman, A., 1983, Blood platelets in psychopharmacological research, Prog. Neuro-Psychopharmacol. Biol. Psychiat., 7:135.

Rouser, G., Kritchevsky, G., Yamamoko, A., and Baxter, C.F., 1972, Lipids in the nervous system of different species as a function of age: Brain, spinal cord, peripheral nerves, purified whole cell preparations and subcellular particulates: Regulatory mechanisms and membrane structure, Adv. Lipid Res., 10:261.

Rouser, G., and Yamamoko, A., 1968, Curvilinear regression course of human brain lipid composition changes with age, Lipids, 3:284.

Shinitzky, M., and Barenholz, Y., 1978, Fluidity parameters of lipid regions determined by fluorescence polarization, Biochim. Biophys. Acta, 525:367.

Shinitzky, M., Heron, D.S., and Samuel, D., 1983, Restoration of membrane fluidity and serotonin receptors in the aged mouse brain, in: "Aging of the Brain", D. Samuel, S. Algeri, S. Gershon, V.E. Grimm, and G. Toffano, eds. Raven Press, New-York.

Sinensky, M., 1974, Homeoviscous adaptation : A homeostasis process that regulates the viscosity of membrane lipids in E. coli, Proc. Natl. Acad. Sci. USA, 71:522.

Zubenko, G.S., Cohen, B.M., Growdon, J., and Corkin, S., 1984, Cell membrane abnormality in Alzheimer's disease, Lancet, 2:235.

SPATIAL DISCRIMINATION AND PASSIVE AVOIDANCE BEHAVIOR IN THE RAT: AGE-RELATED CHANGES AND MODULATION BY CHRONIC DIETARY CHOLINE ENRICHMENT

F.J. van der Staay, W.G.M. Raaijmakers, and T.H. Collijn

Comparative & Physiological Psychology, University of Nijmegen, P.O.Box 9104, 6500 HE Nijmegen, The Netherlands

INTRODUCTION

Because the number of elderly suffering from Alzheimer's disease is increasing (Coyle et al., 1983), the problem of an age-associated decrease of memory has gained growing attention. Although different causes have been postulated for the memory impairments, the 'cholinergic hypothesis of geriatric memory' (Bartus et al., 1982) has received the most convincing support. This hypothesis states that central cholinergic dysfunction is the major cause of memory impairment. Consequently, there have been attempts to modulate cholinergic activity pharmacologically. One approach, characterized as precursor therapy (Bartus et al., 1984), tries to improve memory by enhancing the availability of the acetylcholine precursor choline (or lecithin). The rationale of this approach is twofold. Firstly, cholinergic activity can be increased by enhanced precursor availability (e.g. Haubrich et al., 1975). Hence, increased precursor availability is able to compensate for cholinergic dysfunctioning. Secondly, enhancement of cholinergic activity should be accompanied by a reduction of cognitive impairment (Bartus et al., 1984).

Age-related memory impairment is not restricted to humans. It has been documented for a great variety of species -including rats and mice-, and for a wide variety of testing paradigms including spatial discrimination learning and avoidance learning. Among the spatial discrimination tasks sensitive to memory impairment accompanying aging are the Stone 14-unit maze (Goodrick, 1968, 1975; Michel& Klein, 1978), the Morris water maze (Gage et al., 1984), the circular platform and the radial maze (Barnes, 1979; Barnes et al., 1980; Wallace et al., 1980; Davis et al., 1983; de Toledo-Morrell et al., 1984). We used a holeboard task for which we recently found age-related memory deficits in 2.5-year-old rats when compared with 6-month-old rats (in prep.).

Age-related impairment in passive avoidance retention has been well documented for rats (e.g. McNamara et al., 1977; Gold et al., 1981). For mice, studies are available in which successful attempts have been made to ameliorate age-associated retention deficits by chronic dietary choline enrichment (Bartus et al., 1980; Davis et al., 1984; Mervis et al., 1984).

The aim of our study was to evaluate effects of chronic dietary choline enrichment on performance in the holeboard and the passive avoidance task in two age groups of rats.

METHODS

Subjects: Fourteen 12-month-old former female breeder rats and twelve female weanling rats of the inbred CPBB strain were used in our study. Subjects were housed individually in standard Makrolon cages under a reversed light-dark cycle, light being on from 2000 to 0800. After pairwise matching based on ad lib body weight, one rat of each pair was randomly assigned to a choline enriched group. All rats received standard chow (Hope Farms, containing approximately 1.6 mg choline/gram) and tap water ad libidum Choline enrichment consisted of 2.5 mg choline chloride/ml tap water (Bartus et al., 1980). After four months, the choline concentration was doubled (5 mg choline chloride/ ml water).

Apparatus: The holeboard (70*70*40 cm) was constructed according to the description given by Oades (1981). There were 16 holes in the floor with a diameter of 3.5 cm; distance between holes was 10 cm. All walls were made of transparent PVC. Under each hole, a cup filled with twenty 45 mg food pellets was placed in order to supply equivalent food-associated sensory cues in all holes. A perforated aluminium disk covered each cup, thus making up the bottom of a hole and preventing the rats from reaching the pellets in the cup.

The passive avoidance apparatus consisted of a light compartment and a dark compartment, each measuring 40 * 25 * 40 cm. The light compartment was made of transparent perspex. A bulb mounted above provided an illumination of 1500 lux at the floor of the compartment. The dark compartment was made of opaque, black perspex. It was covered by a black lid. The floor consisted of a metal grid (diameter of stainless steel bars: 3.3 mm, free space between bars: 9.9 mm) connected to a shock scrambler. A guillotine door separating both compartments could be raised 10 cm.

Procedure: Holeboard training started when rats were seven and eighteen months old, respectively, after gradual deprivation to 90% of their free feeding weights. Rats were habituated to the holeboard for five consecutive days (Oades, 1981). Habituation and formal training were carried out between 0900 and 1200.

During 54 acquisition trials and 12 retention trials (five weeks after acquisition was terminated) a fixed set of four holes was baited with one 45 mg food pellet. A trial was initiated by raising the guillotine door between start box and holeboard; it was terminated when the rat had found the fourth food pellet. On the first day of acquisition, two trials were given, all subsequent daily sessions consisted of four trials. Hole visits were registered manually using a keyboard with 16 keys, which was connected to an Apple//e micro computer. A "holevisit" was scored when the nose of the rat turned to the edge of a hole, moved over it or was placed in it (Oades, 1981).

Three measures will be discussed:

1) Working memory: (number of food-rewarded visits) / (number of visits and revisits to the baited set of holes). The working memory holds information which is only useful for a specific trial in a specific task.

2) Reference memory: (number of visits and revisits to the baited set of holes) / (number of visits and revisits to all holes). The reference memory holds information which is valuable across trials in a specific task.

3) Choice correspondence from trial to trial. Choice correspondence was calculated as follows: The sequence of the first four holevisits of two subsequent trials was compared and the length of the longest common sequence of choices was determined. This measure could range from zero to four. Zero was scored if none of the holevisits within the first four choices of a specific trial returned in the first four visits of the following trial. A score of four was assigned if the same holes were visited, and order of holevisits was completely identical on both trials. The higher the score on choice accuracy, the less variable is the pattern

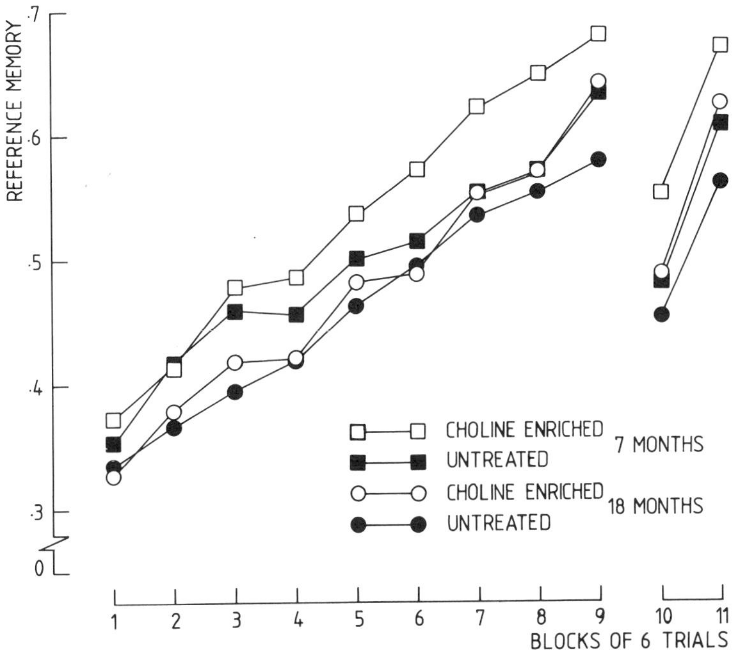

Figure 1. Reference memory of choline treated and untreated female CPBB rats of two different ages in a holeboard task. Means of blocks of six trials are presented. Acquisition (blocks 1-9) and retesting (blocks 10,11) were separated by a five weeks retention interval.

of visiting holes from trial to trial.

Block means of six trials were analyzed by a one-way, two-factorial (age * treatment) ANOVA. Effects of the retention interval were analyzed by a two-way, three-factorial ANOVA (age * treatment * retention interval) with repeated measures on the last factor (last trial block of acquisition vs. first trial block of retention).

Between holeboard training and passive avoidance testing, all rats were subjected to operant conditioning in the Skinnerbox (reported elsewhere). Passive avoidance was tested when the age groups were 12 and 23 months old (e.g. after 11 months of dietary treatment). Two 10 min habituation sessions were given on consecutive days. On the third day, the guillotine door was lowered as soon as the rat had entered the dark compartment with its four paws and a footshock (1 mA, 0.5 s) was administered. Each rat was returned to its homecage immediately after footshock. In two retention sessions (24 hours and 4.5 months after shock administration) step-through latencies (latencies of entering the dark) were measured. Rats which did not enter the dark within 10 minutes were assigned a latency of 600 s.

RESULTS AND DISCUSSION

In the holeboard, neither age nor treatment effects were found for working memory. With respect to reference memory, older rats performed worse than the younger rats throughout the whole experiment (table 1 and figure 1). Choline treated rats performed better than untreated controls from trial block eight on. Retention interval decreased performance [$F(1,22)=70.08$, $p<.01$] but the differences which existed between the age groups [$F(1,22)=5.70$, $p<.05$] and between choline enriched and untreated

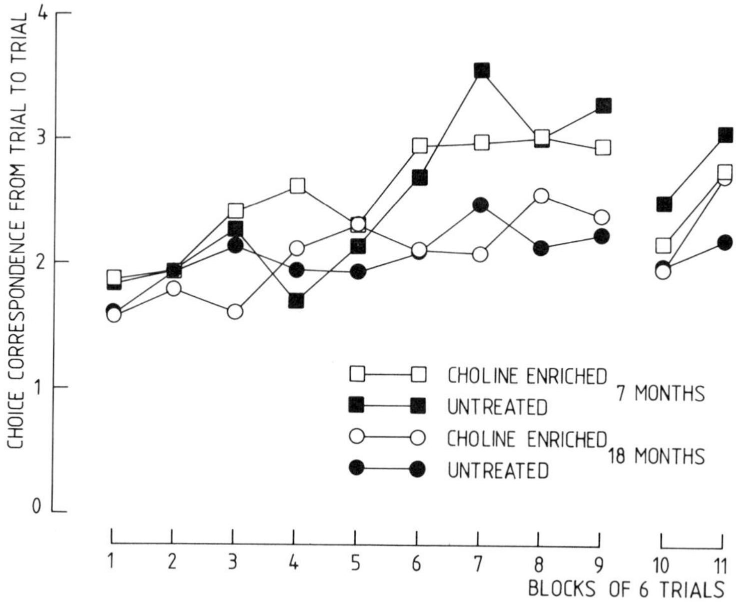

Figure 2. Choice correspondence from trial to trial in a holeboard task by choline treated and untreated female CPBB rats of two different ages. Means of blocks of six trials are presented.

rats [$F(1,22)=7.68$, $p<.05$] remained unaffected.

On choice correspondence (table 1 and figure 2) age differences were found in trial blocks 3,6,7,8, and 11. Young subjects apparently learned to visit holes in a less variable way than the older subjects. Retention interval reduced choice correspondence [$F(1,22)=14.01$, $p<.01$], but differences between age groups remained unchanged [$F(1,22)=7.07$, $p<.05$]. No treatment effects were found, except in trial block eight. Most

Table 1. F-ratios (df 1,22) for age differences and treatment effects in reference memory and choice correspondence (trial blocks represent means of 6 trials; blocks 10 and 11 reflect the retention phase). None of the age * treatment interactions reached significance (F-ratios not reported).
+ : p<.10, * : p<.05, ** : p<.01.

Trial block	Reference memory Age		Reference memory Treatment		Choice correspondence Age		Choice correspondence Treatment	
1	3.21	+	0.12		2.50		0.01	
2	5.87	*	0.09		0.29		0.24	
3	12.47	**	1.55		6.08	*	1.32	
4	5.20	*	0.43		0.29		7.66	*
5	4.00	+	1.43		0.15		1.13	
6	5.13	*	1.08		7.51	*	0.19	
7	3.21	+	2.87		10.78	**	2.55	
8	5.16	*	4.65	*	5.67	*	0.79	
9	2.47		3.55	+	8.53	**	0.08	
10	4.53	*	5.73	*	2.09		0.53	
11	5.03	*	9.00	**	4.45	*	0.07	

likely, this isolated treatment effect was caused by an accidental reduction of choice correspondence in the younger, untreated group. As the effect did not return in other phases of the experiment, it was judged to be of minor importance.

Our results corroborate the findings of other studies (e.g. Barnes 1979; Barnes et al., 1980; de Toledo-Morrell et al., 1984; Davis et al., 1983; Gage et al., 1984; Ingram et al., 1981; Wallace et al., 1980) where complex spatial discrimination tasks like the Morris water maze, the circular platform, or the radial maze were used. In the radial maze test usually all arms are baited; hence, all errors made by a subject are errors of the working memory. The holeboard task used in our study makes it possible to distinguish between a working and a reference memory component. We found, that differences in memory performance could be ascribed to the reference memory component alone. Working memory was completely unaffected by age or treatment.

Goodrick (1968,1973) reported that aged rats make more repetitive errors in a complex maze. On the basis of this finding, he characterized aged rats as behaviorally rigid. We did not find evidence for behavioral rigidity in our older groups. On the contrary, the younger groups of rats seemed to use a more rigid search pattern, taking into consideration their increasingly higher choice correspondence. The difference in reference memory found between treated and untreated groups, however, cannot be accounted for by differences in choice correspondence.

Passive avoidance retention was tested when the younger groups had reached the age of one year, and the older groups were nearly two years old. In other studies, age differences between comparable age groups have been reported (e.g. McNamara et al., 1979; Gold et al., 1981) and female rats have consistently been reported to show poorer avoidance retention (Van Oyen et al., 1979) than male rats. Conversely, in our study retention was excellent in both age groups. Only five of the 26 subjects used in this experiment failed to avoid the dark compartment (i.e. entered the dark within 600 s). Three non-avoiders belonged to the untreated older group, two of them were untreated younger rats. Because of irremovable inhomogeneity of variance, results were analyzed by Fisher exact probability test. Choline enrichment enhanced passive avoidance retention ($p<.02$). Treatment effects were not age-dependent.

Before the second retention test could be performed, two animals had died (one untreated younger and one untreated older animal). One older untreated animal was excluded because of illness. Even after a 4.5 months retention interval, 2 rats did not enter the dark within 600 s. After transformation to the natural logarithm, step-through latenties were analyzed by a two factorial analysis of variance (age * treatment). Choline enriched animals tended to avoid the dark more than the untreated controls [$F(1,19)=3.49$, $p<.10$]. Age differences were not found.

Amelioration of passive avoidance retention by chronic dietary choline enrichment corroborates results of earlier studies with mice (Bartus et al., 1982; Davis et al., 1984; Mervis et al., 1984). However, an interpretation of our results in terms of a compensation for an age-related memory impairment can be questioned, because the chronic dietary choline enrichment enhanced performance in both tasks irrespective of age. Moreover, the CPBB strain is not characterized by an early onset of an age-related memory impairment especially in view of the nearly perfect retention in the passive avoidance task. The effect of a chronic dietary choline enrichment appears to be strain dependent; in comparable experiments with rats of two other inbred strains the choline treatment had no effects on memory (reported elsewhere). Thus the present results may not be generalized without some caution.

REFERENCES

Barnes, C.A. (1979). Memory deficits associated with senescence: A neurophysiological and behavioral study in the rat. Journal of Comparative and Physiological Psychology, 93(1), 74-104.

Barnes, C.A., Nadel, L., & Honig, W.K. (1980). Spatial memory deficit in senescent rats. Canadian Journal of Psychology/Review of Canadian Psychology, 34(1), 29-39.

Bartus, R.T., Dean, R.L., Goas, J.A., & Lippa, A.S. (1980). Age-related changes in passive avoidance retention: Modulation with dietary choline. Science, 209, 301-303.

Bartus, R.T., Dean III, R.L., Beer, B., & Lippa, A.S. (1982). The cholinergic hypothesis of geriatric memory dysfunction. Science, 217, 408-417.

Bartus, R.T., Dean III, R.L., & Beer, B. (1984). Cholinergic precursor therapy for geriatric cognition: Its past, its present, and a question of its future. In J.M. Ordy, D. Harman, & R. Alfin-Slater (Eds.). Nutrition in Gerontology, New York: Raven Press, pp. 191-225.

Coyle, J.T., Price, D.L., & DeLong, M.R. (1983). Alzheimer's disease: A disorder of cortical cholinergic innervation. Science, 219, 1184-1190.

Davis, H.P., Idowu, A., & Gibson, G.E. (1983). Improvement of 8-arm maze performance in aged Fischer 344 rats with 3,4-diaminopyridine. Experimental Aging Research, 9(3), 211-214.

de Toledo-Morrell, L., Morrell, F., & Fleming, S. (1984). Age-dependent deficits in spatial memory are related to impaired hippocampal kindling. Behavioral Neuroscience, 98(5), 902-907.

Gage, F.H., Dunnett, S.B., & Bjorklund, A. (1984). Spatial learning and motor deficits in aged rats. Neurobiology of Aging, 5, 43-48.

Gold, P.E., McGaugh, J.L., Hankins, L.L., Rose, R.P., & Vasquez, B.J. (1981). Age dependent changes in retention in rats. Experimental Aging Research, 8, 53-58.

Goodrick, C.L. (1968). Learning, retention, and extinction of a complex maze habit for mature-young and senescent Wistar albino rats. Journal of Gerontology, 23(3), 298-304.

Goodrick, C.L. (1975). Behavioral rigidity as a mechanism for facilitation of problem solving for aged rats. Journal of Gerontology, 30(2), 181-184.

Haubrich, D.R., Wang, P.F.L., Clody, D.E., & Wedeking, P.W. (1975). Increase in rat brain acetylcholine induced by choline and deanol. Life Sciences, 17, 975-980.

Ingram, D.K., London, E.D., & Goodrick, C.L. (1981). Age and neurochemical correlates of radial maze performance in rats. Neurobiology of Aging, 2, 41-47.

McNamara, M.C., Benignus, V.A., Benignus, G., & Tiller, Jr. A.T. (1977). Active and passive avoidance in rats as a function of age. Experimental Aging Research, 3, 3-16.

Mervis, R.F., Horrocks, L.A., Wallace, L.J., & Naber, E. (1984). Influence of chronic choline containing diets on neurobehavioral parameters in the C57Bl mouse. Society of Neuroscience Abstracts, 10, 976.

Michel, M.E., & Klein, A.W. (1978). Performance differences in a complex maze between young and aged rats. Age, 1, 13-16.

Oades, R.D. (1981). Types of memory or attention? Impairments after lesions in the hippocamus and the limbic ventral tegmentum. Brain Research Bulletin, 7, 221-226.

van Oyen, H.G., van de Poll, N.E., & de Bruin, J.P.C. (1979). Sex, age and shock-intensity as factors in passive avoidance conditioning. Physiology and Behavior, 23, 915-918.

Wallace, J.E., Krauter, E.E., & Campbell, B.A. (1980). Animal models of declining memory in the aged: Short-term and spatial memory in the aged rat. Journal of Gerontology, 35(3), 355-363.

HIPPOCAMPAL MORPHOMETRY IN THE RAT: AGE-RELATED CHANGES AND MODULATION BY CHRONIC DIETARY CHOLINE ENRICHMENT

W.G.M. Raaijmakers, F.J. van der Staay, T.H. Collijn, and J.G. Veening *

Comparative & Physiological Psychology, and * Anatomy & Embryology, University of Nijmegen, P.O.Box 9104, 6500 HE Nijmegen, The Netherlands

INTRODUCTION

In an accompanying paper in this volume (Van der Staay et al., 1985) we reported on positive behavioral effects of chronic dietary choline enrichment in a spatial discrimination task and in a passive avoidance task. An age-related decline of performance was found in the spatial discrimination task, but not in the passive avoidance task. The absence of age differences in passive avoidance behavior appears to be a strain-related phenomenon since an age-related decline in performance has been shown to exist in other strains of rats and in mice.

The hippocampus has been related extensively to memory, especially spatial memory (e.g. O'Keefe & Nadel, 1978; Olton et al., 1979). Age-related changes in anatomical and physiological parameters of this structure have been studied (see Barnes, 1983, for a review of this literature). The granule cells of the fascia dentata are the target cells for the perforant pathway, the main hippocampal input, arising in the entorhinal cortex. In the fascia dentata the number of granule cells appears to increase substantially even during the second half of the first year of life in the rat (Bayer et al., 1982), but it is unknown how this late neurogenesis relates to the behavioral function of the hippocampus.

In adult mice genetically-associated variations have been found in dentate granule cell numbers (Wimer & Wimer, 1982) and in distribution and volume of the mossy fiber system, which consists of the axons and terminals of the dentate granule cells (Schwegler & Lipp, 1983). A striking correlation between active avoidance performance in a shuttlebox and part of the mossy fiber projection system in the regio inferior of the hippocampus in mice was found by Schwegler & Lipp (1983). Using Timm's silver sulfide stain, the different layers of the rat hippocampus are clearly distinguishable and their boundaries can be accurately defined (West et al., 1978).

In view of the apparent plasticity of the fascia dentata (Cotman & Scheff, 1979), the behavioral correlates of the relative volume of the mossy fiber system (Schwegler & Lipp) and our own behavioral findings (Van der Staay et al., 1985), we decided to perform a morphometric analysis of the hippocampus regio inferior. It was hypothesized that aging and chronic dietary choline enrichment affect the relative volumes of the different layers in this region.

METHODS

Animals and treatment: Female rats of two ages (18 and 29 months old) of a hooded inbred strain (CPBB) were used. Half of the animals had been given a choline enriched diet by adding choline chloride (5mg/ml) to their drinking water. The animals were tested behaviorally (see Van der Staay et al., 1985) before being used in this study. Of these animals, two rats died, so that 24 rats were left: five control 18-month-old, six treated 18-month-old, six controls 29-month-old and seven treated 29-month-old rats. In all groups the treated animals had been on the choline enriched diet for 17 months.

Histochemical technique: We used essentially the same staining procedure as West et al. (1978). Under deep barbiturate anesthesia the animals were perfused through the left ventricle with solutions of saline followed by buffered sodium sulfide (pH 7.35) for 20 min. Brains were removed and postfixed for 60 min in the same solution after which they were put in a 20% sucrose solution for about 24 hours. Using a cryostat microtome the brains were horizontally sectioned at 25 µm. The sections were thawed on slides and developed in Timm's solution at 28° C in the dark for 1-2 hour. After fixation and dehydration the sections were coated with Entellan and coverslipped.

Morphometry: Boundaries between regio inferior and regio superior and between the different layers of regio inferior were defined according to West et al. (1978) and are schematically shown in figure 1. Starting at a midseptotemporal level immediately below the most ventral extension of the septal hippocampal pole and using every fourth section, per rat a total of five sections of the left hippocampus was analyzed. Colorslides of the sections were projected on a screen of 30x30 cm (Vanguard Instrument Corporation, U.S.A.) fitted with a transparent square lattice which had a line distance of 15 mm. Measurements were performed at a final magnification of 65x. The volume densities (i.e. relative volumes) of the different layers were determined by computerized point counting according to standard procedures described by Weibel (1979). The regio inferior was divided into stratum oriens, stratum pyramidale, mossy fiber layer, stratum radiatum, stratum lacunosum-moleculare and hilus fasciae dentatae, according to the criteria given by West et al. (1978). No differentiation was made between supra-, infra-, and intra-pyramidal mossy fibers (cf. Schwegler & Lipp, 1983).

RESULTS AND DISCUSSION

The results are summarized in table 1. For each layer the mean volume density and standard error of the ratio (SER) is given. The volume densities or proportions of the different layers are comparable to the values given by Schwegler & Lipp (1983) for rats. Analysis of variance revealed that age decreases the volume density of the mossy fiber system (14 percent)[$F(1,20) = 5.21$; $p<.03$] while an increase (11 percent) was found for stratum oriens [$F(1,20) = 7.26$; $p<.02$]. The stratum oriens is that layer of the hippocampus which contains the basilar dendritic tree of pyramidal neurons. Afferents to this layer are primarily from the contralateral hippocampus and ipsilateral septal region. The choline treatment tended to increase the volume density of stratum oriens (8 percent)[$F(1,20) = 3.86$; $p<.07$]. The other layers of the hippocampal regio inferior were unaffected by age or choline treatment. No differences were found with respect to total volume of regio inferior.

A potential source of error in morphometric studies of this kind

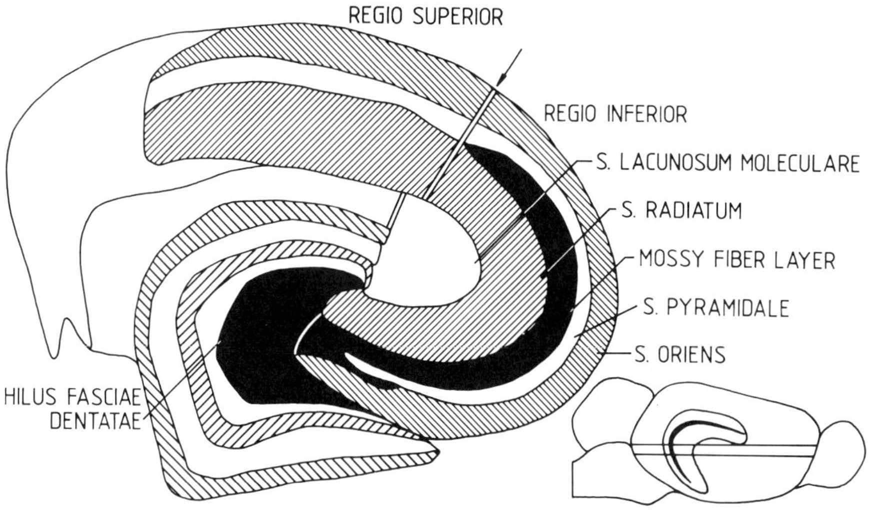

Figure 1. Schematic illustration of the hippocampal layers in a Timm's stained horizontal section (modified from West et al., 1978). The arrow in the figure indicates the boundaries within the layers between regio superior and regio inferior. In the lower right corner the position of the hippocampus within the rat brain is shown schematically. The upper and lower sampling planes for morphometry are indicated (modified from Schwegler & Lipp, 1983).

consists of variability in cutting plane. The influence of this source of error was minimized. Firstly, we used sections through a part of the hippocampus which is relatively homogeneous, irrespective of small differences in inclination of sectioning (West et al., 1978). Secondly, relative volumes (volume densities) rather than absolute volumes were analyzed (cf. Schwegler & Lipp, 1983).

The Timm's stain indicates the presence of heavy metals; the intense staining of the mossy fiber system is caused by a high concentration of zinc in the nerve endings or giant boutons (Haug, 1967). Zinc ions are not only associated with metalloenzymes in presynaptic endings, but they may also participate more directly in synaptic transmission, since they are released upon stimulation (Assaf & Chung, 1984) and are preferentially taken up by mossy fibers and dentate granule cells (Howell et al., 1984). Zinc deficiency produces an abnormal response decrement upon repetitive stimulation, specifically in mossy fibers (Hesse, 1979).

The observed age-dependent decrease in volume density of the mossy fiber system might well be related to an age-dependent decrease in mossy fiber function resulting from a decrease in the extent of mossy fiber projections.

The presumed age-dependent decrease in extent of mossy fiber terminal field does not support the assumption that the mossy fiber system is unaffected by aging (Barnes, 1983). This assumption followed from the observation of a constant number of dentate granule cells during aging on the basis of estimations made from ultrastructural studies on 3-month-old vs 25-month-old rats (Geinisman et al., 1978). These results, however, are at variance with the data of Bayer et al. (1982) who showed that the number of dentate granule cells increases substantially in the rat during the first year of life. These different results might be reconciled by assuming that the number of granule cells decreases after the age of one year so that no difference is observable between the ages of 3 and 25

Table 1. Volume densities of the different layers of hippocampus regio inferior. Mean values and SER (between brackets) are shown.

	18-month-old control n=5	18-month-old chol-enr n=6	29-month-old control n=6	29-month-old chol-enr n=7
s.oriens	24.7(.02)	26.8(.04)	27.5(.02)	29.3(.01)
s.pyramidale	9.8(.01)	8.2(.03)	10.9(.03)	9.5(.04)
mossy fibers	16.8(.02)	16.8(.02)	14.2(.02)	14.8(.03)
s.radiatum	27.4(.03)	27.6(.02)	26.5(.01)	25.9(.02)
s.lac/mol	8.2(.01)	8.1(.01)	8.4(.01)	8.9(.02)
hilus	13.0(.04)	12.9(.02)	12.4(.02)	11.6(.02)

months. Such a decrease could also explain our finding of an age-related decrease in volume density of the mossy fiber system.

The effects of aging and choline treatment on the stratum oriens are difficult to explain. The stratum oriens contains the basal dendrites of the CA3 pyramidal neurons. Changes in volume density of the stratum oriens might be caused by changes in the proportion of synaptic endings in this layer. Chronic dietary choline enrichment has been found to increase the number of spines at the terminal tips of dendritic trees of neocortical pyramidal cells in the C57Bl/6j mouse (Mervis, 1981; Mervis & Bartus, 1981). In view of the generally accepted notion of an overall reduction of synaptic contacts during aging, however, it is difficult to interpret the age-related increase in volume density of the stratum oriens found in our study as an increase in synaptic contacts.

An alternative explanation might be hypertrophy of astrocytes. Lindsey et al. (1979) reported that with increasing age extensive hypertrophy of astrocytes occurs in the hippocampal synaptic fields radiatum and stratum oriens. Apart from the interpretion of the changes in volume density of the stratum oriens, however, there remains a basic difficulty; how can we explain the fact that aging and choline treatment induce similar changes? It is possible that both neuronal and glial changes are involved differentially, but our results do not allow for any conclusion in this respect. In our behavioral study we found opposite effects of aging and choline treatment (Van der Staay et al., 1985).

The choline treatment effect was manifest in both age groups. However, since the younger group was relatively old and since we have no data of a young control group we cannot draw any conclusions on possible interactions between age and treatment. Comparing 18-month-old and 29-month-old rats, there is no differential effect of the diet on hippocampal morphology, but it is still possible that an interaction between age and diet might be found, if relatively young rats were analyzed too.

In summary, the Timm's staining technique seems to be useful to study changes in hippocampal morphometry associated with aging and chronic dietary treatments. The results of the present study indicate that both aging and chronic dietary choline enrichment modulate the volume density of the stratum oriens in the regio inferior of rats. Aging also appears to be associated with a decrease in volume density of the mossy fiber terminal field.

REFERENCES

Assaf, S.Y., & Chung, S.-H. (1984). Release of endogenous Zn2+ from brain tissue during activity. Nature, 308, 734-736.

Barnes, C.A. (1983). The physiology of the senescent hippocampus. In: W. Seifert (ed.) Neurobiology of the hippocampus. London: Academic Press, pp. 87-108.

Bayer, S.A., Yackel, J.W., & Puri, P.S. (1982). Neurons in the rat dentate gyrus granular layer substantially increase during juvenile and adult life. Science, 216, 890-892.

Cotman, C.W., & Scheff, S.W. (1979). Synaptic growth in aged animals. In A. Cherkin et al. (Eds.). Physiology and Cell Biology of Aging (Aging Volume 8). New York: Raven Press.

Geinisman, Y., Bondareff, W., & Dodge, J.T. (1978). Dendritic atrophy in the dentate gyrus of the senescent rat. American Journal of Anatomy, 152, 321-330.

Haug, F. M.-S. (1967). Electron microscopical localization of the zinc in hippocampal mossy fiber synapses by a modified sulfide silver procedure. Histochemie, 8, 355-368.

Hesse, G.W. (1979). Chronic zinc deficiency alters neuronal function of hippocampal mossy fibers. Science, 205, 1005-1007.

Howell, G.A., Welch, M.G., & Frederickson, C.J. (1984). Stimulation-induced uptake and release of zinc in hippocampal slices. Nature, 308, 736-738.

Lindsey, J.D., Landfield, P.W., & Lynch, G. (1979). Early onset and topographical distribution of hypertrophied astrocytes in hippocampus of aging rats: A quantitative study. Journal of Gerontology, 34, 661-671.

Mervis, R.F. (1981). Cytomorphological alterations in the aging animal brain with emphasis on Golgi studies. In: J.E. Johnson Jr. (ed.). Aging and cell structure, vol.1. New York: Plenum Press, pp. 143-186.

Mervis, R.F., & Bartus, R.F. (1981). Modulation of pyramidal cell dendritic spine population in aging mouse neocortex: Role of dietary choline. Journal of Neuropathology and Experimental Neurology, 40, 313.

O'Keefe, J., & Nadel, L. (1978). The hippocampus as a cognitive map. Oxford: Oxford University Press.

Olton, D.S., Becker, J.T., & Handelmann, G.E. (1979). Hippocampus, space and memory. The Behavioral and Brain Sciences, 2, 313-365.

Schwegler, H., & Lipp, H.P. (1983). Hereditary covariations of neuronal circuitry and behavior: Correlations between the proportions of hippocampal synaptic fields in the regio inferior and two-way avoidance in mice and rats. Behavioural Brain Research, 7, 1-38.

Van der Staay, F.J., Raaijmakers, W.G.M., & Collijn, T.H. (1985). Spatial discrimination and passive avoidance behavior: Age-related changes and modulation by chronic dietary choline enrichment. This volume.

Weibel, E.R. (1979). Stereological methods. Vol.1. Practical methods for biological morphometry.London: Academic Press.

West, M.J., Danscher, G., & Gydesen, H. (1978). A determination of the volumes of the layers of the rat hippocampal region. Cell and Tissue Research, 188, 345-359.

Wimer, R.E., & Wimer, C.C. (1982). A biometrical-genetic analysis of granule cell number in the area dentata of house mice. Developmental Brain Research, 2, 129-140.

NERVE GROWTH FACTOR PROMOTES SURVIVAL OF SEPTAL CHOLINERGIC NEURONS AFTER INJURY

F. Hefti

Department of Neurology
University of Miami
Miami, FL 33010, U.S.A.

INTRODUCTION

Alzheimer's disease is associated with a selective loss of cholinergic neurons located in the basal forebrain. Even though some other neuronal systems are also affected, the loss of cholinergic neurons seems to be a principal factor responsible for the memory loss that is characteristic for Alzheimer's disease (for review see Bartus et al, 1982). A treatment preventing the degeneration of these neurons therefore would be of great value in the therapy of this disease. Such a therapeutic tool might promote the survival of remaining cholinergic neurons in mildly affected patients and might therefore prevent the normally progressive behavioral deterioration.

Findings obtained in recent years suggest the possibility that the survival of the cholinergic neurons affected in Alzheimer's disease is influenced by a neurotrophic factor. It has been found that the ascending cholinergic neurons of the basal rat forebrain, i.e. neurons homologous to the cholinergic neurons degenerating in human Alzheimer's disease, respond to nerve growth factor (NGF). These findings are surprising, since NGF normally is believed to be a selective neurotrophic factor for sympathetic and sensory neurons of the peripheral nervous system. Survival and maintenance of function of these cells is dependent on NGF (for review see Greene and Shooter, 1980; Thoenen and Barde, 1980). The following findings suggst that NGF might have a similar role in the function of cholinergic neurons from the basal forebrain: First, NGF as well as the mRNA coding for NGF are present in the rat brain and their levels seem to be highest in the hippocampus, i.e. in a target area of forebrain cholinergic neurons (Crutcher and Collins, 1982; Korsching and Thoenen, 1984; Shelton and Reichhardt, 1984). Second, NGF injected into target areas of forebrain cholinergic neurons (i.e. hippocampus and cortex) is taken up by nerve terminals and is transported retogradly to the cholinergic cell bodies located in the basal forebrain (Schwab et al., 1979; Seiler and Schwab, 1984). Since NGF uptake is mediated by specific receptors, these findings suggest the existence of NGF receptors on cholinergic neurons. Third, stimulation of NGF receptors on cholinergic neurons results in an elevation of the activity of choline acetyltransferase (CAT), the key enzyme in the synthesis of acetylcholine, in cholinergic neurons. NGF increases CAT activity in cultures containing cholinergic neurons of the fetal rat forebrain (Hefti et al., 1985; Honegger and Lenoir, 1980), in brains of neonatal rats (Gnahn et al., 1983), and in the brain of adult rats with partial lesions of a cholinergic pathway (Hefti et al., 1984). Fourth, the notion that NGF acts as a neurotrophic factor for forebrain cholinergic neurons is supported by results from lesion studies. Destruction of the cholinergic input to the hippocampus results in an ingrowth of peripheral sympathetic fibers which matches the previous distribution of cholinergic terminals in the hippocampus (Crutcher et al., 1979; Loy and Moore, 1977; Stenevi and Bjorklund, 1978). Since peripheral sympathetic neurons react to NGF, it has been postulated that the hippocampal signal attracting sympathetic fibers is identical to NGF and that, in intact brains, NGF acts upon and is taken up by the cholinergic terminals in this area (Crutcher and Davies, 1981).

I now report that NGF is able to promote survival of forebrain cholinergic neurons _in vitro_ and _in vivo_. First, NGF was given intraventricularly to rats with lesions of the cholinergic septo-hippocampal pathway. Such lesions reduce the number of cholinergic cell bodies in the septum. NGF was found to strongly attenuate this lesion-induced degeneration of cholinergic cell bodies. Second, the effect of NGF was studied on cholinergic neurons in cultures prepared from the septal region of neonatal rats. NGF was found to increase the number of cholinergic neurons surviving under these culture conditions.

EFFECT OF NGF ON SURVIVAL OF SEPTAL CHOLINERGIC NEURONS AFTER TRANSSECTION OF THE FIMBRIA

The group of ascending cholinergic neurons of the basal forebrain is composed of cells located in septum, diagonal band of Broca, substantia innominata and nucleus basalis. These neurons form a topographically organized projection to hippocampus, olfactory bulb and cortex (for review see Mesulam et al., 1983; Wainer et al., 1984). The cholinergic septo-hippocampal projection represents the best characterized part of this projection system. It is formed by cells located in the medial septal nucleus and the vertical limb of the diagonal band, and which innervate the hippocampus (McKinney et al., 1983; Mesulam et al., 1983). The vast majority of their fibers course through the fimbria (Meibach and Siegel, 1977; Segal and Landis, 1974). Since its anatomy is well described and since the fimbria are easily accessible for lesioning, the septo-hippocampal pathway was chosen for studying the effects of NGF on the survival of cholinergic neurons after injury.

The cholinergic septo-hippocampal fibers were transsected in adult rats by cutting the fimbria. A specially designed knife was lowered into the brain at the antero-posterior level A6000 (according to the atlas of Koenig and Klippel, 1963) and at a position 1.0mm lateral to the midline. The knife was moved vertically into the brain until its tip reached the dorso-ventral level +0.5mm. The knife was then moved laterally to 4.0mm lateral to the midline and was

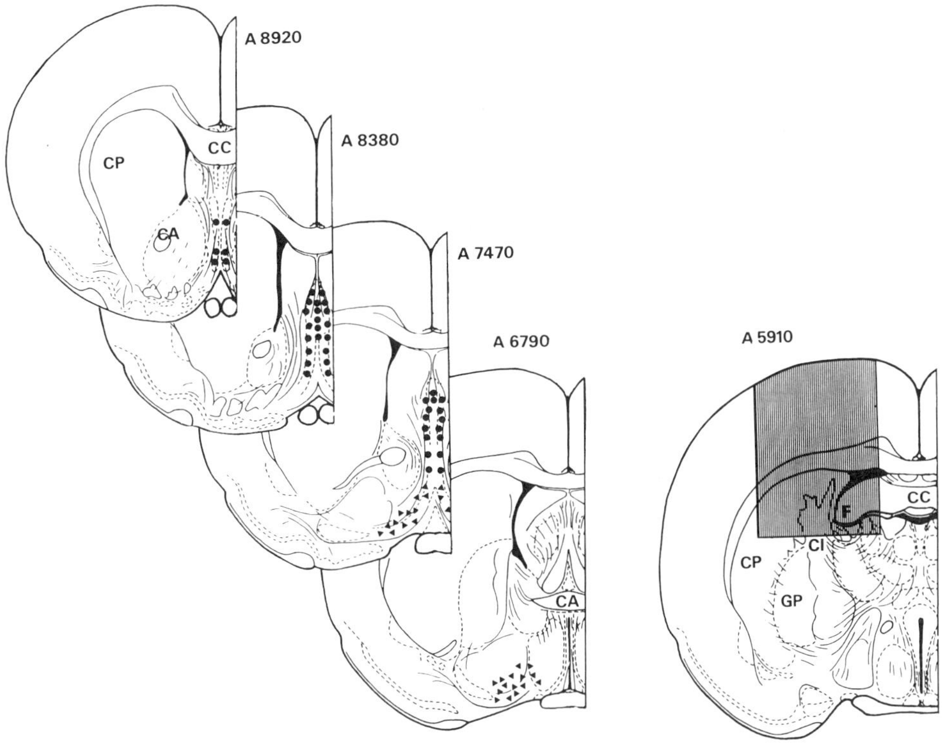

Figure 1: Fimbrial transsections and counting of cholinergic neurons in the septal area. The fimbria was unilaterally transsected in adult rats by making a cut through the brain as indicated by the shaded area. Because of the elasticity of the fimbria and to ascertain its transsection, the knife had to be moved to a distant lateral position. To quantify the effect of the lesions on the number of cholinergic neurons, brains were sectioned in a standardized manner. Twentyfour sections of 30μm thickness were taken between antero-posterior levels A9000 and A6700 (Koenig and Klippel, 1963). Cholinergic neurons were visualized using AChE-histochemistry (after DFP-pretreatment) and were ascribed to one of the following two groups: first, to medial septal nucleus and vertical limb of the diagonal band of Broca (i.e. areas containing cholinergic neurons projecting to the hippocampus, indicated in the figure by dots), or, second, to horizontal limb of the diagonal band and substantia innominata (i.e. areas containing cholinergic neurons not projecting to the hippocampus, indicated by triangles). The total number of cholinergic cells was calculated by multiplying the number of counted cells in 24 sections by 3, thereby accounting for the fact that every third section only was taken for analysis. CA = anterior commissure; CC = corpus callosum; CI = internal capsule; CP = caudate putamen; F = fimbria; GP = globus pallidus.

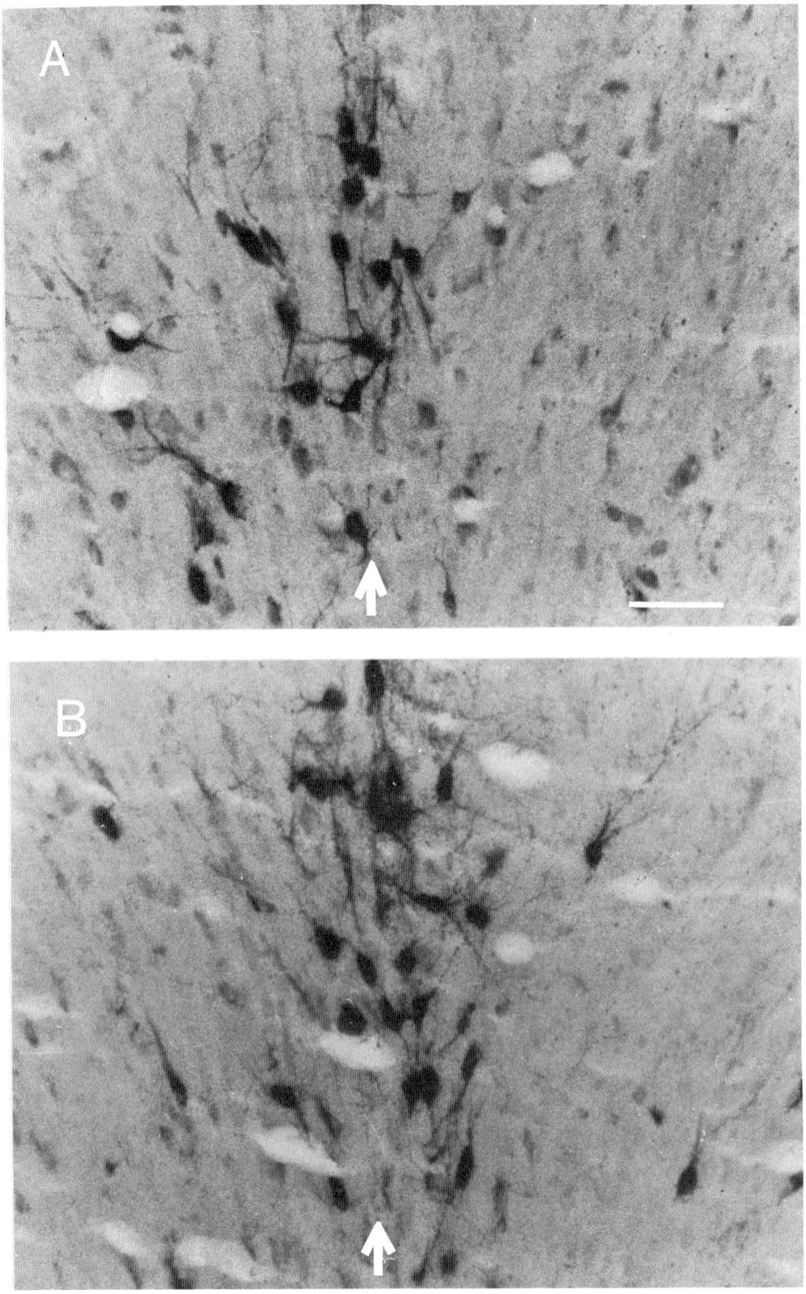

Figure 2: Effect of intraventricular administration of NGF on survival of cholinergic neurons in the medial septal nucleus after injury of their axons. Rats received unilateral fimbrial transsections, and were then injected intraventricularly during 4 weeks with NGF (10µg twice weekly) or with equal amounts of a control protein. Panel A shows the medial septal nucleus of a lesioned control animal, panel B shows the same area of a lesioned animal treated with NGF. Cholinergic neurons were visualized with AChE-histochemistry. The arrows indicate the median of the brain, the bar represents 100µm.

retrieved at this position (fig. 1). After performing the lesion, a cannula was inserted into the lateral ventricle of the lesioned side and was permanently fixed with dental cement. Twice weekly, the lesioned animals received intraventricular injections of mouse salivary gland 2.5S NGF (10µg in 5µl) or of an equal amount of control protein (cytochrome c, which has similar biochemical properties to NGF but no activity on NGF receptors). Four weeks after lesioning, the animals were taken for the histochemical visualization of cholinergic cell bodies. They were pretreated with diisopropylfluorophosphate (DFP, 2mg/kg) and were then perfused intracordially. Brains were frozen and frontal sections of 30µm thickness were cut and stained for acetylcholinesterase (AChE) according to Geneser-Jensen and Blackstad (1971). AChE is a reliable marker for cholinergic neurons in the septal area, since 80-90% of all AChE-positive neurons were found to be co-stained for CAT (Levy et al., 1983 ; Eckenstein and Sofroniew, 1983). To facilitate counting of cholinergic cells in the septal area, brains of lesioned animals were cut in a standardized manner. The first frontal section was taken at level A9000. Further sections were taken every 90µm until the level of the anterior commissure (A6800, cf. fig. 1). The sectioned part of the brain contained the entire medial septal nucleus and the diagonal band of Broca, i.e. the areas containing cell bodies projecting to the hippocampus (McKinney et al., 1983).

Table 1: Effect of intraventricular injections of NGF on the number of cholinergic neurons surviving in basal forebrain nuclei after fimbrial transsections. Animals were lesioned as shown in figure 1 and injected intraventricularly during 4 weeks with NGF (10µg twice weekly) or with equal amounts of a control protein (controls). Cholinergic neurons were visualized by AChE-histochemistry and counted and grouped as indicated in fig. 1.

	medial septum and ventrical limb of diagonal band	horizontal limb of diagonal band and sub. innominata
CONTROLS (9)		
control side	1428 ± 114	1407 ± 120
lesioned side	696 ± 69*	1260 ± 111
(% of control side)	(49.9±3.9%)	(89.8±2.3%)
NGF-TREATED (10)		
control side	1377 ± 93	1263 ± 99
lesioned side	1209 ± 99**	1242 ± 93
(% of control side)	(87.8±6.2%)**	(98.8±2.1%)

means ± S.E;M., numbers in brackets indicate number of animals analyzed.
*different from corresponding control side, **different from lesioned side of control animals, p<0.01 (analysis of variance).

In lesioned control animals, treated during 4 weeks with a control protein, the fimbrial transsections resulted in a pronounced reduction of the number of AChE-positive cell bodies in the medial septal nucleus and in the vertical limb of the diagonal band on the brain side ipsilateral to the lesion (fig. 2A). Cholinergic neurons located in the horizontal limb of the diagonal band and the substantia innominata were not affected. These findings confirm that cholinergic neurons projecting to the hippocampus are located in medial septal neucleus and the vertical limb of the diagonal band (McKinney et al., 1983; Mesulam et al., 1983). In lesioned animals chronically treated with NGF, there was no obvious difference in the number of AChE-positive cells between the lesioned and the control side in all areas containing cholinergic cell bodies (fig. 2B). These findings indicate that the fimbrial transsections resulted in a degeneration of part of the cholinergic neurons in the septal area and that chronic intraventricular injections of NGF were able to attenuate this lesion-induced degeneration of cholinergic neurons.

For quantitative comparisons, cholinergic neurons projecting to the hippocampus (i.e. those located in the medial septal nucleus and the vertical limb of the diagonal band) were grouped together and were compared with neurons not projecting to the hippocampus (i.e. those located in the horizontal limb of the diagonal band and the substantia innominata). In lesioned control animals, the fimbrial transsections reduced the number of AChE-positive cell bodies in medial septal nucleus and vertical limb of the diagonal band to 50% of the number counted on the unlesioned side. In lesioned animals chronically treated with NGF, the number of AChE-positive cell bodies in these areas was only marginally reduced on the lesioned side, i.e. to 88% of control values (table 1). There was no difference in the number of AChE-positive cells between NGF-treated and control animals on the unlesioned sides of the brain. Furthermore, the number of AChE-positive cell bodies in the horizontal limb of the diagonal band and the substantia innominata, which was not significantly reduced by fimbrial transsections, was equal in control and NGF-treated animals. Staining intensity of AChE-positive cell bodies was not enhanced in NGF- treated animals, in confirmation of earlier findings showing that NGF does not stimulate the expression of AChE activity by cholinergic neurons (Gnahn et al., 1983; Hefti et al., 1984; 1985).

EFFECTS OF NGF ON SURVIVAL OF SEPTAL CHOLINERGIC NEURONS IN CULTURE

Cholinergic neurons are not easily accessible in living animals and many questions arising from the findings presented in the previous section cannot be addressed by studies in vivo. To establish the dose-response relationship and the specificity of NGF's effect on survival of forebrain cholinergic neurons, further experiments were therefore carried out in vitro. To come most close to the situation of injury studied in adult rats, cholinergic neurons were dissociated from the septal area of postnatal animals, i.e. from a developmental stage, when the septal cholinergic neurons had already started to invade hippocampal tissue (Crutcher, 1982; Milner et al., 1983, Nadler et al., 1974). Neurons taken for culture from such animals lost their processes during the dissociation procedure and they therefore were comparable to neurons submitted to axonal transsection in vivo.

The septal area was dissected from brains of rats of postnatal day P2. The area dissected contained cholinergic cell bodies belonging to the medial septal nucleus, the diagonal band of Broca and the substantia innominata. Cells were dissociated using enzymatic and mechanical procedures. Aliquots of the cell suspension were plated in culture dishes coated with polylysine. Cultures were grown in a modified L15 medium containing 10% horse serum and 1% fetal calf serum (for experimental details cf. Hefti et al., 1985). After 10

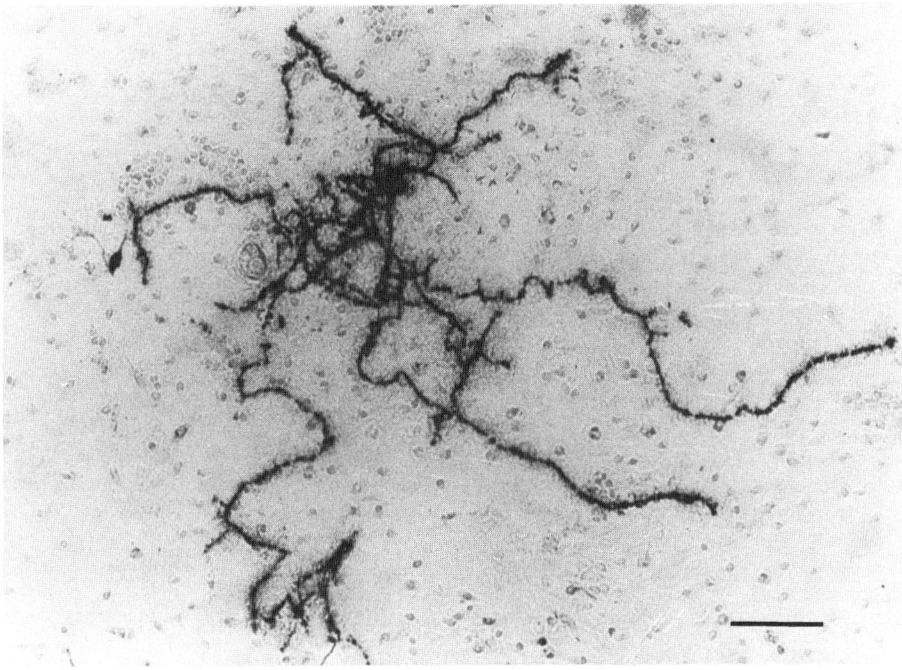

Figure 3: Typical cholinergic neuron in culture of septal cells dissociated from postnatal rat brains. Cholinergic neurons were visualized using AChE-cytochemistry. The bar represents 100μm.

Table 2: Effect of NGF and anti-NGF on survival of cholinergic neurons in cultures of septal cells dissociated from postnatal rats. Cultures were grown for 10 days and cholinergic neurons were then visualized using AChE-cytochemistry.

	AChE-positive cells per culture dish
controls	21.0 ± 0.9
NGF 3ng/ml medium	26.7 ± 4.4
10	33.3 ± 4.2*
30	32.5 ± 3.2*
100	37.1 ± 2.8*
1000	38.5 ± 3.4*
NGF 100ng/ml + anti-NGF[1)]	8.6 ± 4.2*
anti-NGF[1)]	9.2 ± 1.3*

means ± S.E.M. n= 5-12
*different from controls, $p<0.05$ (analysis of variance)
1) 2µl/ml of sheep anti-mouse NGF serum (Suda et al., 1978).

days incubation, cultures were fixed and cholinergic neurons were visualized using AChE-cytochemistry. Earlier studies with co-staining of AChE and CAT have shown that AChE is a reliable marker for cholinergic neurons in these cultures (Hefti et al., 1985). The number of cholinergic neurons was counted in cultures grown in presence of 2.5S NGF, of an antiserum to NGF (Suda et al., 1978), or without any further additions (controls).

NGF significantly elevated the number of AChE-positive cells surviving in the cultures. Addition of 100ng/ml of 2.5S NGF increased the number of AChE-positive cells by 92% as compared to control cultures. The stimulatory effect of NGF was prevented by the addition of an antiserum to NGF, indicating that the effect was specific for NGF. Cultures grown in presence of both NGF and anti-NGF or in presence of anti-NGF alone contained significantly fewer AChE-positive cells than control cultures. These findings suggest that NGF is formed be neurons or glial cells growing in the cultures, in sufficient quantities to support the survival of an intermediate number of cholinergic cells. The ED_{50} of NGF's effect on survival of cholinergic neurons was found to be approximately 10ng/ml (corresponding to 4×10^{-10}M). This concentration is in the range of concentrations necessary to stimulate NGF receptors on sympathetic and sensory neurons (Greene and Shooter, 1980; Thoenen and Barde, 1980). The findings obtained on cell cultures indicate that NGF promotes survival of injured cholinergic neurons by acting at specific receptors.

CONCLUSIONS

Results of the present study indicate that NGF promotes the survival of forebrain cholinergic neurons after injury. A beneficial effect of NGF on survival was observed after transsection of axons of septo-hippocampal cholinergic neurons in vivo. In vitro, NGF promoted the survival of septal cholinergic neurons which had lost their processes during the dissociation procedure. Earlier findings had demonstrated that NGF was able to elevate CAT levels in forebrain cholinergic neurons studied in vivo and in vitro (Gnahn et al., 1983; Hefti et al., 1984; 1985; Honegger and Lenoir, 1980). Based on these findings it had been concluded that the role of NGF in the function of forebrain cholinergic neurons is rather limited (Hefti et al., 1985). The findings of the present study significantly broaden the role of NGF in the function of forebrain cholinergic neurons by indicating that NGF is able to rescue these neurons after transsection of their processes.

I have earlier hypothesized that the selective loss of cholinergic neurons in Alzheimer's disease might be caused by lack of NGF available to these neurons (Hefti, 1983). The idea was based on the general hypothesis of Appel (1981), who suggested that diseases associated with selective neuronal degenerations might be due to absence of the corresponding neurotrophic factor. I furthermore drew attention to the possibility that NGF or drugs mimicking NGF's actions might be useful in the treatment of Alzheimer's disease. The new findings indicating that, in experimental animal models, NGF promotes the survival of cholinergic neurons after injury, strongly support this notion.

REFERENCES

Appel, S.H., 1981, A unifying hypothesis for the cause of amyotrophic lateral sclerosis, parkinsonism, and Alzheimer's disease. Ann. Neurol., 10:499-505.

Bartus, R.T., Dean, R.L., Beer, B. and Lippa, A.S., 1982, The cholinergic hypothesis of geriatric memory dysfunction. Science, 217:408-417.

Crutcher, K. A., 1982, Development of the rat septo-hippocampal projection: a retrograde fluorescent tracer study. Develop. Brain Res., 3:145-150

Crutcher, K.A. and Collins, F., 1982, In vitro evidence for two distinct hippocampal growth factors: basis of neuronal plasticity? Science, 217:67-70.

Crutcher, K.A. and Davis, J.N., 1981, Sympathetic noradrenergic sprouting in response to central cholinergic denervations. Trends Neurosci., 4:70-72.

Crutcher, K.A., Brother, L. and Davis, J.N., 1979, Sprouting of sympathetic nerves in the absence of afferent input. Exp. Neurol., 66:778-783.

Eckenstein, F., and Sofroniew, M.V., 1983, Identification of central cholinergic neurons containing both choline acetyltransferase and acetylcholinesterase and of central neurons containing only acetylcholinesterase, J. Neurosci., 3:2286-2291.

Geneser-Jensen, F.A., and Blackstad, T.E., 1971, Distribution of acetylcholinesterase in the hippocampal region of the guinea pig. I. Entorhinal area, parasubiculum, and pre-subiculum. Z. Zellforsch., 114:460-481.

Gnahn, H., Hefti, F., Heumann, R., Schwab, M., and Thoenen, H., 1983, NGF-mediated increase of choline acetyltransferase (ChAT) in the neonatal forebrain; evidence for a physiological role of NGF in the brain? Dev. Brain Res., 9:45-52.

Greene, L.A., and Shooter, E.M., 1980, The nerve growth factor: biochemistry, synthesis, and mechanism of action. Ann Rev. Neurosci., 3:353-402.

Hefti, F., 1983, Alzheimer's disease caused by a lack of nerve growth factor? Ann. Neurol., 13:109.

Hefti, F., Dravid, A., and Hartikka, J., 1984, Chronic intraventricular injections of nerve growth factor elevate hippocampal choline acetyltransferase activity in adult rats with partial septo-hippocampal lesions, Brain Res., 293:305-309.

Hefti, F., Hartikka, J., Eckenstein, F., Gnahn, H., Heumann, R., and Schwab, M., 1985, Nerve growth factor (NGF) increases choline acetyltransferase but not survival or fiber growth of cultured fetal septal cholinergic neurons. Neuroscience, 14:55-68.

Honegger, P., and Lenoir D., 1983, Nerve growth factor (NGF) stimulation of cholinergic telencephalic neurons in aggregating cell cultures. Dev. Brain Res., 3:229-238.

Koenig, J.F.R., and Klippel, R.A., 1963, The rat brain. A stereotaxic atlas of the forebrain and lower parts of the brain stem. Williams and Wilkins, Baltimore, MD.

Korsching, S., and Thoenen, H., 1984, Regulation of nerve growth factor synthesis in target tissues of the peripheral and central nervous system. Proc. Soc. Neurosci., 10:1056.

Levey, A.I., Wainer, B.H., Mufson, E.J., and Mesulam, M.M., 1983, Co-localization of acetylcholinesterase and choline acetyltransferase in the rat cerebrum. Neuroscience, 9:9-22.

Loy, R., and Moore, R.Y., 1977, Anomalous innervation of the hippocampal formation by peripheral sympathetic axons following mechanical injury. Exp. Neurol., 57:645-650.

McKinney, M., Coyle, J.T., and Hedreen, J.C., 1983, Topographic analysis of the innervation of the rat neocortex and hippocampus by the basal forebrain cholinergic system. J. Comp. Neurol., 217:103-121.

Meibach, R.C., and Siegel, A., 1977, Efferent connections of the septal area in the rat: an analysis utilizing retrograde and anterograde transport methods. Brain Res., 119:1-20.

Mesulam, M.M., Mufson, E.J., Wainer, B.H., and Levey, A.I., 1983, Central cholinergic pathways in the rat: an overview based on an alternative nomenclature (Ch1-Ch6). Neuroscience, 10:1185-1201.

Milner, T.A., Loy. R., and Ameral, D.G., 1983, An anatomical study of the development for the septo-hippocampal projection in the rat. Dev. Brain Res., 8:343-371.

Nadler, J.V., Matthews, D.A., Cotman, C.W., and Lynch, G.S., 1974, Development of cholinergic innervation in the hippocampal formation of the rat. Develop. Biol., 36:142-154.

Schwab, M., Otten, U., Agid, Y., and Thoenen, H., 1979, Nerve growth factor (NGF) in the rat CNS: absence of specific retrograde axonal transport and tyrosine hydoxylase induction in locus coeruleus and substantia nigra. Brain Res., 168:473-483.

Segal, M., and Landis, S., 1974, Afferents to the hippocampus of the rat studied with the method of retrograde transport of horseradish peroxidase. Brain Res., 78:1-15.

Seiler, M., and Schwab, M.E., 1984, Specific retrograde transport of nerve growth factor (NGF) from neocortex to nucleus basalis in the rat. Brain Res., 300:33-36.

Shelton, D.L., and Reichardt, L.F., 1984, Expression of the nerve growth factor gene correlates with the density of sympathetic innervation in effector organs. Proc. Natl. Acad. Sci. USA, 81:7951-7955.

Stenevi, U., and Bjorklund, A., 1978, Growth of vascular sympathetic axons into the hippocampus after lesions of the septo-hippocampal pathway; a pitfall in brain lesion studies. Neurosci. Lett., 7:219-224.

Suda, K., Barde, Y.A., and Thoenen, H., 1978, Nerve growth factor in mouse and rat serum: correlation between bioassay and radioimmunoassay determinations. Proc. Natl. Acad. Sci. USA, 75:4042-4046.

Thoenen, H., and Barde, Y.A., 1980, Physiology of nerve growth factor, Physiol. Revs., 60:1284-1335.

Wainer, B.H., Levey, A.I., Mufson, E.J., and Mesulam, M.M., 1984, Cholinergic systems in mammalian brain identified with antibodies against choline acetyltransferase, Neurochem. Int., 6:163-182.

CAN SEPTAL GRAFTING FACILITATE RECOVERY FROM PHYSIOLOGICAL AND BEHAVIORAL DEFICITS PRODUCED BY FORNIX TRANSECTIONS?

Menahem Segal and Norton W. Milgram

Center for Neurosciences and Behavioral Research
Weizmann Institute of Science
76100 Rehovot, Israel

INTRODUCTION

There is now considerable evidence which links the severe memory deficit of dementia of the Alzheimer type (AD) to degeneration of cholinergic basal forebrain neurons and a corresponding reduction in forebrain acetylcholine (ACh) (1-5). The significance of such correlations are strengthened by observations of memory deficits in animals produced by either pharmacological blocking of ACh or by specific brain lesions (6). In spite of this evidence, attempts to alleviate memory deficits in AD patients by pharmacological manipulation of acetylcholine has had only limited success (7). It is consequently of considerable importance to evaluate the feasibility of treating cognitive dysfunctions by other means such as the recently developed procedure of grafting fetal neural tissue into adult hosts (8,9,10). The present studies were undertaken with this purpose in mind. We have been studying the effects of grafted cholinergic neurons on an animal model of AD produced by denervation of the cholinergic input of the hippocampus.

Functions of the cholinergic-hippocampal system

The hippocampal cholinergic innervation originates from a discrete region in the basal forebrain including the medial septal and the diagonal band nuclei (6). The hippocampus in turn projects back to the septal region forming a feedback loop. The fornix-fimbria (FF) is the major fiber pathway connecting the hippocampus to the basal forebrain. Transection of the FF eliminates nearly 90% of the cholinergic hippocampal innervation and also deprives the basal forebrain regions, the septal nuclei and the hypothalamus of their hippocampal input. The behavioral deficits produced are markedly similar to those resulting from direct hippocampal lesions.

Physiologically, the muscarinic cholinergic receptor in the hippocampus produces a long lasting depolarization, with an associated increase in excitability and input resistance (11). The mechanisms underlying these effects involve closure of several types of K channels (11-14). At a more molar level, the cholinergic system has been implicated in the production of hippocampal theta rhythm, a unique rhythmic slow activity consisting of 6-12 Hz waves which is associated with locomotion (15-16). It is generally assumed that theta rhythm is triggered by rhythmically firing medial septal neurons, as both cholinergic antagonists and medial septal lesions can block theta (17-19). There is also evidence for theta having two components; a cholinergic one, which is modulated by muscarinic drugs and a noncholinergic one, associated with locomotion which is abolished by lesions of the entorhinal cortex (15). The importance of the cholinergic contribution is not thoroughly understood. Nearly half of the septo-hippocampal neurons are not cholinergic; in fact, there is no evidence that the bursting septal neurons are cholinergic. Furthermore, ACh has a slow action in the hippocampus and is unlikely to be involved in the rapid changes of hippocampal EEG in the behaving rat. The position of the septal nuclei, among ascending and descending fiber pathways makes it difficult to study their involvement in theta rhythm in relative isolation. The graft technique therefore provides a means of studying the role of ACh in the generation of hippocampal theta, and allows the examination of the septo hippocampal connection under controlled conditions. Behaviorally, this cholinergic system seems important in memory processes. There is now a voluminous literature dealing with numerous behavioral deficits produced by hippocampal damage (6), including retardation in acquisition of spatial tasks. Similar deficits also occur following either fornix transections, medial septal lesions, or cholinergic blockade (6).

Brain grafting techniques

It has only recently been recognized that the CNS of the adult mammal can exhibit considerable plasticity. There is now evidence that injured neurons can regenerate and intact neurons can grow new processes in response to remote damage. In addition, it has been convincingly documented that immature brain tissue can be grafted into host brain with which it will develop an extensive network of fibers (8,9,20-24). These findings raise the possibility that grafting can be used to treat degenerative neurological disorders. Support for this suggestion is provided by evidence of correction of neuroendocrine deficits by grafting (20,22); there have also been reports of improvement in motor abilities following grafting of embryonic nigral tissue into rat suffering from damage to the substantia nigra (21,25). Finally, and most relevant to AD, are reports of improved learning following intra-hippocampal grafts of cholinergic septal cells both in aged rats which exhibited learning deficits and in fornix transected rats which are deficient in acquisition of spatial maze (10,21,25). In view of the obvious relevance of these findings in the treatment of age related degenerative CNS diseases, it is clearly necessary to substantiate and extend such observations. The research which is reported here was done with this goal in mind. Specifically, we have attempted to correlate behavioral, physiological and anatomical indices of recovery of function following grafting of septal nuclei into FF transected rats.

METHODOLOGY

Surgical procedures using adult male Wistar rats were accomplished in either two or three phases. First, the cholinergic input to the hippocampus was removed by either transection of the FF with a microknife, or by electrolytic lesions of the medial septal area. The second phase, transplantation of embryonic septal tissue, followed a one week recovery interval. Brains of 16 day rat embryos were removed under sterile conditions and maintained in cold modified Krebs solution. Each piece of brain tissue was individually minced, sucked into a 10ul Hamilton syringe and slowly injected into the host hippocampus in a total volume of 1ul over a 5-10 minute interval (10). The needle was withdrawn slowly during the injection. The third phase involved the implantation of recording electrodes constructed from twisted lengths of nichrome insulated wire which were placed in areas of the hippocampus selected to produce robust theta activity (16).

Behavioral testing commenced from one to three months following the grafting, depending on the specific experiment. In some cases behavioral tests were repeated at later intervals in an attempt to trace the time course of behavioral recovery. Other animals were only used for electrophysiological studies and were sacrificied without undergoing behavioral testing. In all of these experiments, AChE staining (26) was used to determine to what extent the graft had innervated the host. The histology supported previous experiments which revealed a progressive spread of cholinergic fibers. Initially, a cluster of AChE neurons was found in the injection site which was usually in or below the dentate gyrus. Fibers began to grow out of the graft in about a week, and by three months the hippocampus was densely innervated (Fig. 1), and AChE staining extends some 4-5 mm away from the graft into nearly the entire length of the hippocampus. The pattern of innervation was similar to the normal case in all major divisions of the host hippocampus.

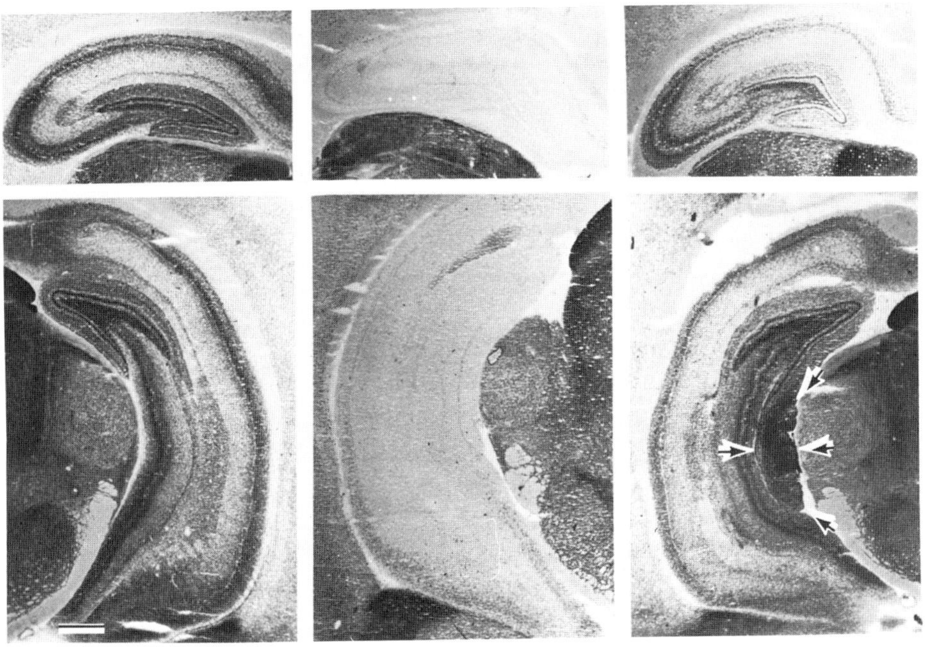

Fig. 1. Acetylcholine-esterase (AChE) staining of normal control hippocampus (left) fornix fimbria (FF) transected (middle) and FF transected with septal grafts rats. The animals were sacrificied three months after the transplantation. The top row is of the dorsal hippocampus and the bottom raw of the main body of the hippocampus. The transplant is marked with arrowheads in the ledlevel of the hipposampus. Calibration 0.5mm. Note that the AChE staining did not reach the entire extent of the dorsal hippocampus in the transplanted rat.

RESULTS

Experiments with hippocampal slices

In order to study the physiological interrelation between the host and the grafted tissue, the hippocampus was sectioned into 350um transverse slices which were immediately placed into an interface chamber. Studies were done on slices in which the transplants was clearly visible. For control, slices were cut from animals where the graft was clearly not viable. In most cases, the initial penetration was directed into the graft in an attempt to record intracellularly from the grafted cells. Extracellular unit activity from the graft was recorded on several occasions, but we have not yet recorded good intracellular signals from grafted septal neurons.

Slices were used successfully in several experiments which examined how electrical stimulation of the graft affects the host hippocampus. Stimulating microelectrodes were placed in the transplant and intracellular activity was recorded from either dentate granule cells or CA1 pyramidal cells, depending on the locus of the graft. Several neurons were found to be responsive to stimulation of the graft, and the results were consistent with the hypothesis that stimulation produced release of acetylcholine into the host tissue (Fig. 2). Graft stimulation produced a slow, voltage dependent depolarization which was enhanced by physostigmine and blocked by atropine (24). In addition, graft stimulation inhibited the pronounced hyperpolarization which typically follows burst discharges from CA1 pyramidal neurons (12). This slow afterhyperpolarization is probably caused by activation of a Ca^{++} dependent K^{+} current in the host cells. The effects exerted by the graft stimulation can also be produced by topical application of ACh (14,24).

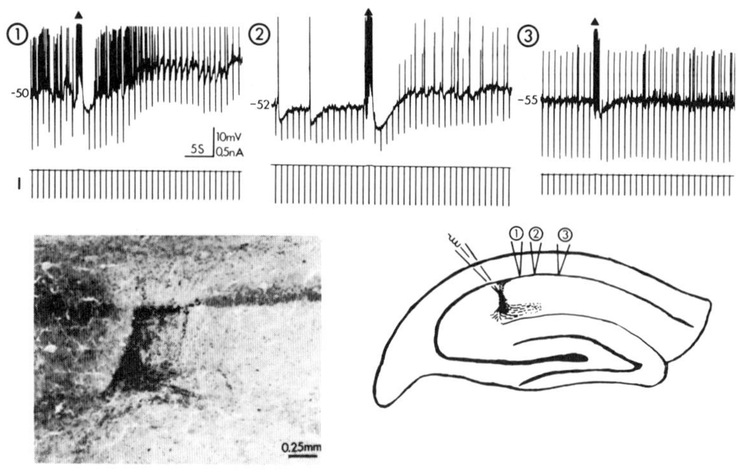

Fig. 2. Stimulation of a 4-week old graft depolarizes nearby but not remote neurons. Three cells were recorded in one hippocampal slice at different distances from the explant as depicted schematically in the diagram at the bottom right. Hyperpolarizing current pulses, downward deflection, bottom traces, are applied at a rate of 1 Hz to measure input resistance of the cell. Stimulation of the graft (10 Hz for 1 sec, triangle) is followed by a brief hyperpolarization which is replaced by a slow 1-5 mV depolarization. Lower left, the graft stained for AChE histochemistry illustrates the extent of the spread of AChE associated fibers (From Segal et al. 1985).

Extracellular recording of evoked field potentials was also used to study the effects of graft stimulation. In two experiments, the stratum oriens was stimulated to evoke field potentials in CA1. Stimulation of the graft produced a marked atropine sensitive enhancement of the evoked Ca1 population spike. This effect was time and stimulation intensity-dependent. Thus, activation of the graft can facilitate reactivity of the host hippocampus to afferent stimulation.

Recording of EEG activity

As anticipated from previous work, there was a robust relationship between hippocampal EEG and behavioral state in normal rats. As illustrated in figure 3, during quiescence, the dominant EEG pattern is a low voltage signal which has both high and low frequency components, while, during locomotion, the dominant pattern is a high voltage slow rhythmic activity in the 9-11 Hz frequency range (theta activity). To quantitate this data, spectral density histograms were calculated under computer control using averages of segments taken during different behavioral states (Fig. 3). Following either medial septal lesions or transection

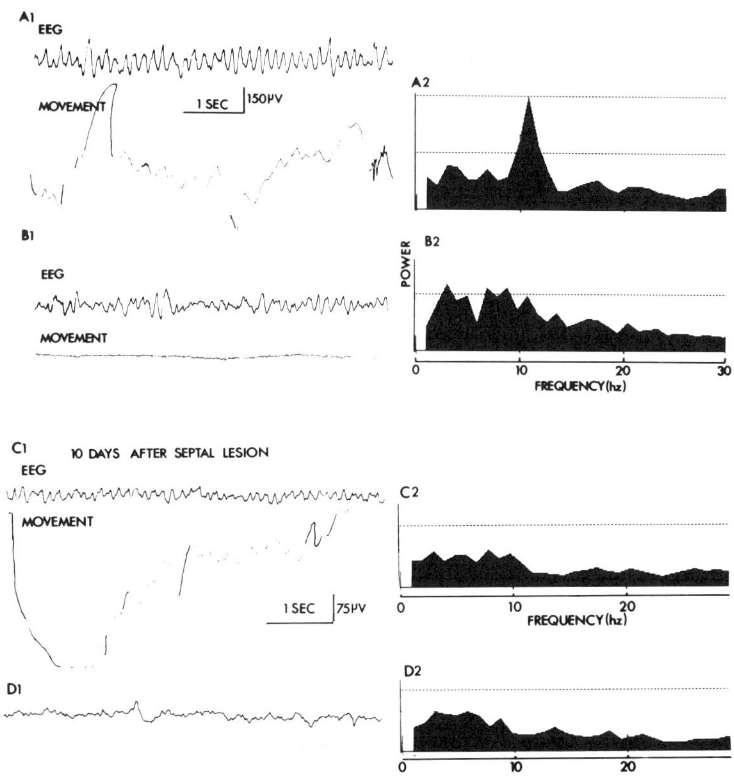

Fig. 3. EEG recording from awake rat hippocampus. A&B in normal conditions a theta rhythm top trace is associated with locomotion see bottom trace in each pair of traces. When the rat is motionless, the pattern of rhythmic activity disappears. A2 & B2 power spectrum analysis of the activity illustrated at left. Note the peak at 11 Hz that is missing when the rat stands still. C & D Same conditions as in A & B, 10 days after an electrolytic lesion of the medial septal nucleus.

of the FF, the movement related theta activity was almost entirely eliminated. We could not confirm the suggestion that the effect was specific to nonmovement related theta activity (15,16). The cholinergic dependence of these connections was examined using atropine (25 mg/Kg i.p.) to block postsynaptic muscarinic receptors and physostigmine (0.025-0.1 mg/Kg i.p.) to enhance cholinergic activity in normal rats. 25 mg/kg of atropine blocked the appearance of hippocampal theta, although this effect was largely due to atropine potentiating 2-3Hz activity. In several instances spectral analyses revealed that the absolute magnitude of the movement related activity was undiminished when compared to the preatropine baseline levels. The results with physostigmine, were more variable: in some cases physostigmine produced the expected decrease in frequency of theta activity; in other cases physostigmine produced a marked attenuation of all activity.

Transplantation of septal tissue did not restore the normal relationship between theta rhythm and behavior. However, there were several instances of the development of an anomalous theta activity which was virtually indistinguishable from the normal movement related theta, except that it was not correlated with movement. The most dramatic case is presented in Fig. 4 which shows an example of 9Hz theta which occurred only during inactivity. These experiments raise the intriguing possibility that grafting of septal tissue restores the mechanisms underlying the driving of theta, but does not affect the lesion-induced dissociation between theta and movement. These experiments have only been carried out up to 4 months after grafting and it remains to be determined whether more normal theta will develop over a longer survival time.

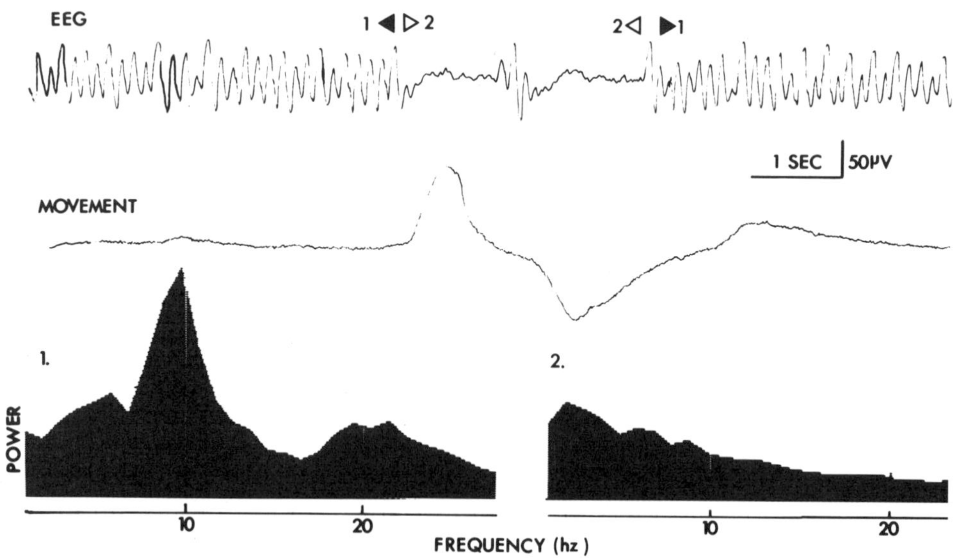

Fig. 4. EEG activity in aFF transected rat implanted with a septum in the hippocampus. Note the regular activity, depicted in the power spectrum during inactivity but disappears when the rat begins to walk.

Behavioral experiments

In three different experiments, FF transected rats, septal lesioned rats and their respective controls were tested in open field, passive avoidance and water maze tasks tested at various times after the lesion and after intrahippocampal grafting of septal tissue. The water maze (27) proved to be the most sensitive task to be affected to the lesions. Normal rats learned to locate a hidden platform in a water bath using spatial, extramaze cues within 3-5 two-minute trials (Fig. 5). FF lesioned animals, on the other hand, showed severe deficits, and only in

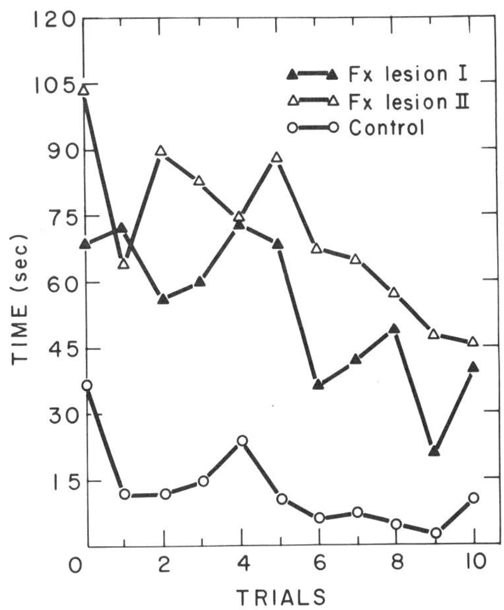

Fig. 5. Learning in a water maze in normal controls and in two groups of FF transected rats. Each group consists of 7-8 rats. See text for details.

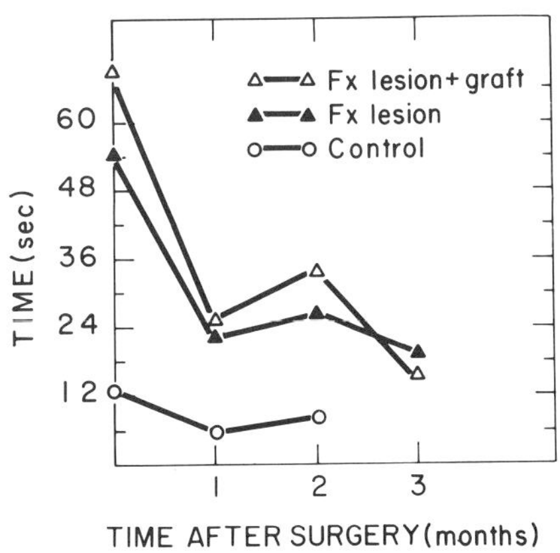

Fig. 6. Progressive improvement of performance in a water maze by both FF transected control and transplanted rats. Each test consists of 10 trials and the values are the mean time to reach the platform in 10 trials. Note the better trend of improvement seen in the grafted rats.

exceptional instances did any learn within a 10 trial daily session. The septal lesioned animals appeared intermediate between the controls and FF group. Both lesioned and grafted groups improved performance in the water maze after repeated training. When tested within three months after grafting, the grafted rats were still not significantly better than lesioned controls (Fig. 6).

DISCUSSION

These experiments confirm previous reports that embryonic neurons can grow and establish viable connections with host tissue, while also maintaining their original neurochemical specificity (8,9,10). Thus, AChE staining revealed an extensive reinervation of the hippocampus by cholinergic fibers within three months after grafting of septal neurons. Moreover, stimulation of the graft produced similar effects to those observed following the direct administration of ACh and proved effective in modulating hippocampal activity yet the graft did not reinstate normal septo-hippocampal functions.

The septo-hippocampal cholinergic neurons belong to a unique class of central nervous system neurons which includes noradrenergic neurons of the nucleus locus coreleus, serotonergic neurons of the raphe nucleus, and dopaminergic neurons of the substantia nigra. In each instance, the cell bodies originate in a small nucleus and project in a widespread but diffuse manner to large parts of the brain. In addition, they all can be grafted into a host brain where they produce an extensive innervation of the host tissue. The functional analysis of these cell groups is hindered by their complex innervation patterns, lack of specific connections and lack of conventional synaptic mechanisms. The physiological evidence reported here suggests that grafting provides a relatively simple short axon system which can be used as a tool for studying these diffuse forebrain systems.

The results dealing with the functional significance of the grafts have been more disappointing thus far. We have no evidence of any recovery of lost behavioral functions, although there is reason to expect that behavioral recovery may require a longer survival interval (25). We also did not find recovery of normal hippocampal EEG. However, we have observed rhythmic theta activity which was unrelated to movement. The presence of theta in grafted animals raises the intriguing possibility that the graft is able to support rhythmic electrical activity which is of new behavioral significances, even though the innervation of the graft is different from that of the intact septal area. This indicates that the septum can function in support of rhythmic activity irrespective of its inputs. Direct support for this possibility is suggested by observations of rhythmicity in medial septal cells which have been deprived of their normal input in a slice preparation (unpublished observations). We have also observed pronounced theta activity a few hours following medial septal lesions, when the septal generators are presumably dead. This result appears to reflect the spontaneous release of ACh from the intact terminals, and provides further evidence that theta does not require the presence of septal afferents which control bursting.

In evaluating these results, it is important to consider that the lesions have effects other than those intended. In the case of FF lesions, the damage is not limited to afferent septal cholinergic fibers. In this respect the behavioral difference between septal lesioned animals and the FF group may reflect an additional deficit due to the damage to noncholinergic inputs to the hippocampus. It is also clear that some of the transplanted neurons were noncholinergic.

In view of these considerations, it is not surprising that the establishment by grafting of viable cholinergic synapses leads to only a partial recovery of theta activity, a gross physiological function, while the grafting does not facilitate the recovery of behavioral functions - at least within the time limits monitored in the present experiments. On the other hand, grafting has proven to be the method of choice in promoting recovery from neuroendocrine disorders (20,23). The difference may reflect behavior, but not neuroendocrine function being under direct environmental control.

In conclusion, the present results are encouraging for those attempting to use brain grafting to study specific neurochemical pathways. On the other hand, we have not found evidence supporting the use of grafting to restore complex cognitive processes produced by neurological insult with short survival times. Future research in this area should also consider possible ways of establishing connections between grafted tissue and appropriate sources of input. Similar studies should explore the role of growth factors in facilitation of recovery of lost functions following brain grafting.

SUMMARY

The present experiments examined the efficacy of using neural grafting to restore physiological and behavioral functions following damage to the cholinergic sept-hippocampal system. Embryonic septal regions were injected into the hippocampi of fimbria-fornix transected rats. The grafts developed an extensive innervation with the host hippocampus and, when stimulated, produced a slow depolarizing response that was blocked by atropine and facilitated by physostigmine. There was also evidence that the graft restored hippocampal theta rhythm which had been eliminated by FF transactions: however, unlike unlesioned controls, theta in grafted animals was not correlated with movement. Performance in a water-maze which was markedly impaired by fornix transection, showed no improvement three months after transplantation. The results indicate that grafting may provide a useful tool for studying some neurotransmitter systems: but they do not support using this technique for treating cognitive disorders of neurological origin, at short survival times.

ACKNOWLEDGEMENTS

We would like to thank Ms. V. Greenberger for the histological assistance, Dr. M. Routtenberg for participating in the behavioral experiments and to Ms. G. Yagur for typing the manuscript. Supported by a grant from the Israeli Ministry of Health.

REFERENCES

1. E.K. Perry, R.H. Perry, P.H. Gibson, G. Blessed and B.E. Tomlinson, A cholinergic connection between normal aging and senile dementia in the human hippocampus, Neurosc. Lett. 3:88 (1977).
2. E.K. Perry, B.E. Tomlinson, G. Blessed, K. Bergmann, P.H. Gibson and R.H. Perry, Correlation of cholinergic abnormalities with senile plaques and mental test scores in senila dementia, Br. Med. J. 2:1457 (1978).
3. D.A. Drachman and J.R. Hughes, Memory and the hippocampal complex III aging and temporal EEG abnormalities, Neurology 21:1 (1971).
4. B.T. Hyman, G.W. Van Hoesen, A.R. Damasio and C.L. Barnes, Alzheimer's disease: cell specific pathology isolates the hippocampal formation, Science 225:1168 (1984).

5. A.S. Lippa, D.J. Critchett, F. Ehlert, H.L. Yamamura, S.J. Enna and R.T. Bartus, Age related alterations in neurotransmitter receptors: an electrophysiological and biochemical analysis. Neurobiol. of Aging 2:3 (1981).
6. J. O'Keefe and L. Nadel, The hippocampus as a cognitive map, Clarendon Press, Oxford, 1978.
7. S. Corkin, K.L. Davis, J.H. Growdon, E. Usdin and R.J. Wurtman, Alzheimer's disease : a report of progress in research, Raven Press, N.Y. (1982).
8. A. Björklund, F.H. Gage, U. Stenevi and S.B. Dunnett, Survival and growth of intrahippocampal implants of septal cell suspensions, Acta Physiol. Scand. Suppl. 522:49 (1983).
9. A. Björklund, U. Stenevi, R.H. Schmidt, S.B. Dunnett and F.H. Gage, Introduction and general methods of preparation, Acta Physiol. Scand. Suppl. 522:1 (1983).
10. S.B. Dunnett, W.C. Low, S.D. Iversen, U. Stenevi and A. Björklund, Septal transplants restore maze learning in rats with fornix fimbria lesions, Brain Res. 251:335 (1982).
11. K. Krnjevic, R. Pumain and L. Renaud, The mechanism of excitation by acetylcholine in the cerebral cortex, J. Physiol. (Lond.) 215:247 (1971).
12. A.E. Cole and R.A. Nicoll, Acetylcholine mediates a slow synaptic potential in hippocampal pyramidal cells, Science 221:1299 (1983).
13. J.V. Halliwell and P.R. Adams, Voltage clamp analysis of muscarinic excitation in hippocampal neurons, Brain Res. 250:71 (1982).
14. M. Segal, Multiple actions of acetylcholine at a muscarinic receptor in rat hippocampal slices, Brain Res. 246:77 (1982).
15. G. G. Buzsaki, L.W.S. Leung and C.H. Vanderwolf, Cellular bases of hippocampal EEG in the behaving rat, Brain Res. Reviews 6:139 (1983).
16. C.H. Vanderwolf, R. Kramis, L.A. Gillespie and B.H. Bland, Hippocampal slow activity and neocortical low voltage fast activity: relations to behavior, in: "The Hippocampus", Vol. 2, R.L. Issacson and K. Pribram, eds., Plenum Press, N.Y. (1975).
17. H. Petsche, C.H. Stumpf and G. Gogolak, The significance of the rabbit's septum as a relay station between the midbrain and the hippocampus. I. Control of hippocampal arousal activity by the septum cells. Electroencephalog. Clin. Neurophysiol. 14:202 (1962).
18. O. Macadar, J.A. Roig, J.M. Monti and R. Budelli, The functional relationship between septal and hippocampal unit activity and hippocampal theta rhythm, Physiol. Behav. 5:1443 (1970).
19. G. Gogolak, C.H. Stumpt, H. Petsche and F. Sterc, The firing patterns of septal neurons and the form of hippocampal theta wave. Brain Res. 7:201 (1968).
20. R. Drucker-Colin, R. Aguilar-Roblero, F. Garcia Hernandez, F. Fernandez-Cancino and F. Bermudez Rattoni, Fetal suprachiasmatic nucleus transplants: diurnal rhythm recovery of lesioned rats, Brain Res. 311:353 (1984).
21. S.B. Dunnett, S.T. Bunch, F.H. Gage and A. Björklund, Dopamine-rich transplants in rats with 6-OHDA lesions of the ventral tegmental area: 1. Effects on spontaneous and drug-induced locomotor activity. Behavioral Brain Res. 13:71 (1984).
22. D. Gash, J.R. Sladek and S.D. Sladek, Functional developmental of grafted vasopressin neurons, Science 210:1367 (1980).
23. W.C. Low, P.R. Lewis, T.S. Bunch, S.B. Dunnett, S.R. Thomas, S.D. Iversen, A. Björklund and U. Stenevi, Functional recovery following neural transplantation of embryonic septal nuclei in adult rats with septohippocampal lesions, Nature 300:260 (1982).
24. M. Segal, A. Björklund and F.H. Gage, Transplanted septal neurons

make viable cholinergic synapses with a host hippocampus, Brain Res. (1985) in press.

25. F.H. Gage, S.B. Dunnett, U. Stenevi and A. Björklund, Aged rats: recovery of motor impairments by intrastriatal nigral grafts, Science 221:966 (1983).

26. B. Srebro and S.I. Mellgren, S.I., Changes in postnatal development fo acetylcholinesterase in the hippocampal region after early septal lesion in the rat, Brain Res. 79:119 (1974).

27. R. Morris, Developments of a water-maze procedure for studying spatial learning in the rat, J. Neurosci. Methods 11:47-60 (1984).

STRUCTURAL ANALOGS OF AF64A: SYNTHESIS AND THEIR EFFECTS ON HIGH AFFINITY CHOLINE TRANSPORT AND QNB BINDING

J.S. Mistry and D.J. Abraham
Depts. of Medicinal Chemistry
University of Pittsburgh, Pittsburgh, PA 15261

I. Hanin
Dept. of Pharmacology and Experimental Therapeutics
Loyola University Stritch School of Medicine
Chicago, Illinois

INTRODUCTION

A chronic deficiency in central cholinergic function has been demonstrated in a number of neuropsychiatric diseases, including Alzheimer's disease.[1-6] Until recently, animal models that simulate the neurochemical conditions which appear to cause these diseases in humans, as a result of a direct manipulation of the central cholinergic system, were not available. Over the past few years, however, we have been successful in developing a compound, ethylcholine mustard aziridinium ion (AF64A), which has the potential to serve as a novel toxin in developing animal models of human brain disorders in which a cholinergic hypofunction has been implicated.

We originally designed AF64A by keeping the reactive toxin structure as close as possible to the natural substrate, choline. For example, a look at the structures of choline and the aziridinium ion of AF64A reveals a similar molecular volume, polar and charge distribution.

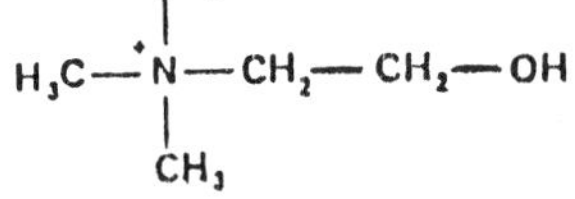

CHOLINE

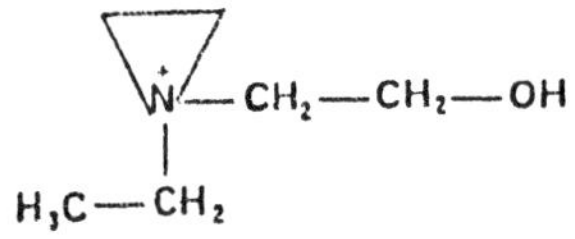

AF64A

AF64A induces, *in vivo*, a persistent central cholinergic hypofunction of presynaptic origin, to the apparent exclusion of other neurotransmitter systems.[7-10]

Although AF64A is a strikingly promising cholinotoxin, we decided to design, synthesize and screen other potential cholinotoxic agents which might possess more selective activity or other effects not exhibited by AF64A. We also anticipated that synthesis of close structural analogs of AF64A would help us identify the optimal structure-activity relationships required for the future development of other selective *in vivo* cholinergic neurotoxins.

In this chapter we describe the synthesis of several structural analogs of AF64A (Scheme I) and report preliminary neurochemical findings vis-a-vis their potential as specific inhibitors of the cholinergic system, by evaluating them for their ability to inhibit high affinity choline transport (HAChT) and their affinity towards brain muscarinic receptors by displacing quinuclidinyl benzilate (QNB).

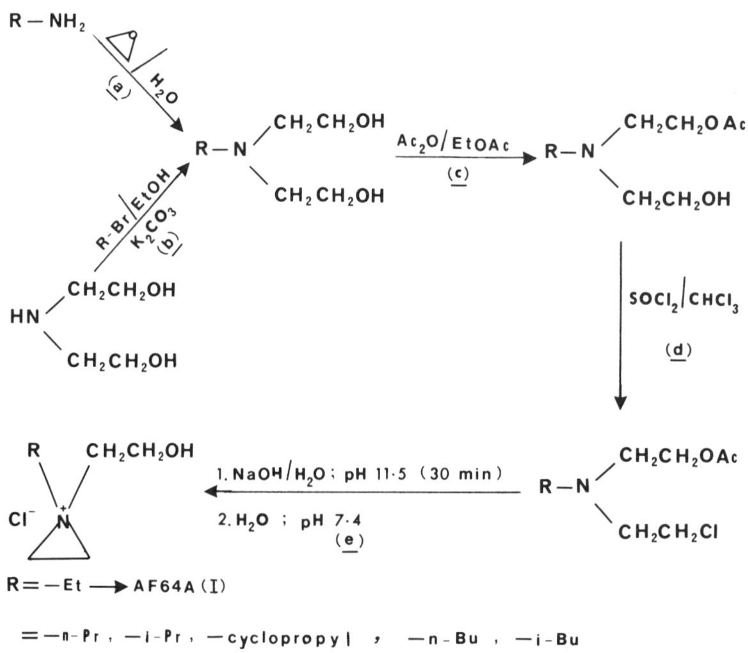

SCHEME I.

BIOLOGICAL RESULTS AND DISCUSSION

1. HaChT:

The procedure used to measure the transport of a toxin into synaptosomes, was an adaptation of the method described by Yamamura and Snyder[11] and later modified by Bader.[12] The inhibitory potency of a toxin on the HAChT system *in vitro* was determined in terms of concentration of the toxin required to inhibit 50% of the transport of $[^3H]$-choline (IC_{50}) into synaptosomes. The IC_{50} values for the various cholinotoxins were determined by plotting the concentration of toxin vs. percent inhibition on semi-log paper. The results for the inhibition of HAChT are presented in Table I. It is clear that increasing the chain length reduces the activity (increased IC_{50}) whereas branching or cyclization of propyl analogs (R = i-Pr, cyclopropyl) produced compounds with activity (IC_{50}) similar to choline and AF64A. This suggests that the HAChT system does possess structural requirements for the inhibitors.

Table I: IC_{50} Values for HAChT System

R-	IC_{50} (μM)*
Et	1.5
n-Pr	7.5
i-Pr	2.6
cyclopropyl	3.9
i-Bu	31
n-Bu	> 1000

*IC_{50} Value for choline = 16 μM

2. QNB Binding:

The assay procedure used to measure the affinity of the above-mentioned potential cholinotoxins towards brain muscarinic cholinergic receptors, was an adaptation of the procedure developed by Yamamura and Synder.[13] The affinity of a toxin to bind to brain muscarinic receptors *in vitro* was determined in terms of percent QNB displaced from the receptors at 50 μM concentration of a toxin. A graph of concentration of toxin vs. percent QNB displacement was plotted on semi-log paper and percent QNB displaced at 50 μM concentration of the toxin was determined from the graph.

Table II compares the toxins under investigation, for their ability to displace QNB *in vitro* from brain muscarinic receptors.

Table II: Data for QNB Binding Studies

R-	% QNB displaced*
Et	18
n-Pr	16
i-Pr	9
cyclopropyl	90
i-Bu	6
n-Bu	9

*at 50 μM concentration of the corresponding toxin

The cyclopropyl analog was found to have a dramatically high affinity for the postsynaptic muscarinic brain receptors, while the other analogs have very low affinity. The cyclopropyl analog displaces 50% of the QNB from the receptors, at concentrations as low as 6.25 μM (= IC_{50}), which is equivalent to the inhibitory activity of the highly potent muscarinic agonist, oxotremorine. This dual effect of the cyclopropyl analog, both on HAChT and on cholinergic receptors, could be advantageous, since the net result should produce a more extensive cholinergic hypofunction within the CNS.

CONCLUSIONS

Our findings show that an increase in aklyl chain length on our toxins, reduces HAChT inhibition, but that branching or cyclization of the alkyl moiety produces similar results as those found for AF64A. This difference in inhibitory activity between long chain and branched alkyl group is probably due to the steric requirements involved at the receptor binding site.

The high affinity of the cyclopropyl aziridinium analog for the postsynaptic muscarinic brain receptors is noteworthy. This result has given us impetus for further designing and synthesizing structural analogs of the cyclopropyl derivative. Without such derivatives we cannot speculate about structure-activity relationships. There may, however, be some correlations between our recent findings and the ideas published by Chothia[14] on the differentiation between muscarinic and nicotinic binding by different conformations of ACh.

Finally, it should be noted that AF64A has been reported as non-specific by some workers.[15-18] This phenomenon, in our hands, appears to be one of dose related response with specificities occurring at very low concentrations of AF64A. It is hoped that this analog study and future work will produce compounds with a greater selectivity, at all dose ranges.

ACKNOWLEDGEMENTS

We gratefully acknowledge the technical assistance of Matthew Clancy. We also wish to thank Dr. Steven Leventer for his advice and consultation. The work described in this chapter has been supported by NIMH Grant #MH34893.

REFERENCES

1. P. Davies and A.J.F. Maloney, Selective loss of central cholinergic neurons in Alzheimer's Disease. Lancet 2:1403 (1976).
2. K.L. Davis and J.A. Yesavage, Brain Acetylcholine and Disorders of Memory, in "Brain Acetylcholine and Neuropsychiatric Disease", Plenum Press, New York and London (1978).
3. S. Corkin, Acetylcholine, aging and Alzheimer's disease. Implication for treatment. Trends in Neurosci., 287 (1981).
4. P.J. Whitehouse, D. Price, A. Clark, J.T. Coyle, and M. Delong, Alzheimer's disease: evidence for a selective loss of cholinergic neurons in the nucleus basalis. Ann. Neurol. 10:122 (1981).
5. M. McKinney, J. Hedreen and J.T. Coyle, Alzheimer's Disease: Report of Progress in Research, in "Aging Vol. 19", Eds. S. Corkin, K. Davis, J. Growdon, G. Usdin and R.J. Wurtman, Raven Press, New York (1982).
6. R.T. Bartus, R.L. Dean, B. Beer, and A.S. Lippa, The cholinergic hypothesis of geriatric memory dysfunction. Science 217:408 (1982).
7. C.R. Mantione, A. Fisher, and I. Hanin, Possible mechanisms involved in the presynaptic cholinotoxicity due to ethylcholine aziridinium (AF64A) in vivo. Life Sci. 35:33 (1984).
8. A. Fisher, C.R. Mantione, D.J. Abraham, and I. Hanin, Long-term central cholinergic hypofunction induced in mice by ethylcholine aziridinium ion (AF64A) in vivo. J. Pharmacol. Exp. Therap., 222:140 (1982).
9. C.R. Mantione, A. Fisher, and I. Hanin, AF64A-treated mouse: Possible model for central cholinergic hypofunction. Science 213:579 (1981).
10. I. Hanin, W.C. DeGroat, C.R. Mantione, J.T. Coyle, and A. Fisher, Chemically-Induced Cholinotoxicity in vivo: Studies Utilizing Ethylcholine Aziridinium Ion (AF64A), in "Banbury Report 15: Biological Aspects of Alzeheimer's Disease", Ed. R. Katzman, Cold Spring Harbor Laboratory (1983).
11. H.I. Yamamura and S.H. Snyder, High affinity transport of choline into synaptosomes of rat brain. J. Neurochem. 21:1355 (1973).
12. C.R. Bader, R.W. Baughman and J.L. Moore, Different time course of development for high affinity choline uptake and choline acetyl transferase in the chicken ratina. Proc. Natl. Acad. Sci. (U.S.A.) 75:2525 (1978).
13. H.I. Yamamura and S.H. Snyder, Muscarinic cholinergic binding in rat brain. Proc. Natl. Acad. Sci. (U.S.A.) 71:1725 (1974).
14. C. Chothia, Interaction of acetylcholine with different cholinergic nerve receptors. Nature 225:36 (1970).

15. J.W. Asante, A.J. Cross, J.F.W. Deakin, J.A. Johnson and H.R. Slater, Evaluation of etylcholine mustard aziridinium ion (EMA) as a specific neurotoxin of brain cholinergic neurons. Brit. J. Pharmacol. 80:573 (1983).
16. A. Levy, G.J. Kant, J.L. Meyerhoff, and L.E. Jarrard, Non-cholinergic neurotoxic effects of AF64A in substantia nigra. Brain Res. 305:169 (1984).
17. L.E. Jarrard, G.J. Kant, J.L. Meyerhoff, and A. Levy, Behavioral and neurochemical effects of intraventricular AF64A administration in rats. Pharmacol. Biochem. and Behavior 22:273 (1984).
18. L. Villani, A. Contestabile, A. Poli, P. Migani, and F. Fonnum, Neurotoxic effects of the presumed cholinergic toxin, AF64A. Neurosci. Lett., Supplement 18, S228 (1984).

IN VIVO EVALUATION OF ^{125}I-LABELED IODOCLEBOPRIDE AND IODOAZIDOCLEBOPRIDE BINDING TO THE DOPAMINE D_2 RECEPTOR

D.R. Elmaleh*, S. Padmanabhan*, H.B. Niznik[+++], P. Seeman[+++], J-H Guan[+] and J.L. Neumeyer[++]

*Massachusetts General Hospital, Boston, MA
[+]Research Biochemicals Inc., Wayland, MA
[++]Northeastern University, Boston, MA and the
[+++]Department of Pharmacology, University of Toronto
Ontario, Canada

INTRODUCTON

The observation that dopamine (DA) in basal ganglia is markedly decreased in Parkinson's disease led to the development of its precursor, L-DOPA as substitution therapy (1,2,3). Following a favourable initial therapeutic response lasting for several years, long-term L-DOPA treatment often loses its effectiveness or is increasingly accompanied by various side effects due possibly to a progressive degeneration of dopaminergic neurons, a loss of DA receptors, or supersensitivity of DA receptors and post-receptor mechanisms (4,5). Symptoms observed in Parkinson's Disease are most likely related to reduced tonic stimulation of dopaminergic D_2 receptors (6,7). Indeed, stimulation of D_2 receptors by dopamine agonists relieves parkinsonism, whereas blockade of D_2 receptors by dopamine antagonists, exacerbates parkinsonian symptoms (8).

Although the dopamine D_2 receptor has been solubilized by several laboratories (9), attempts to isolate and purify the protein by affinity chromatography (10) or photoaffinity labeling (11,12) have been relatively unsuccessful (13,14). Similarly, commercially available irreversible ligands have been too low in receptor affinity and/or selectivity to be of value in dopamine D_2 receptor isolation (10,15-17).

Selective photoaffinity compounds have been extremely useful for the molecular characterization of adrenoceptors (18-20). Clebopride <u>Ia</u> has been reported as a selective D_2 receptor antagonist (21-23). Its derivative, azidoclebopride <u>Ib</u> on photoactivation with light is capable of forming a covalent bond at or near the binding site (24,26). We speculated that the incorporation of radioactive moieties such as ^{125}I into clebopride and azidoclebopride might yield a ligand of sufficiently high specific activity and affinity to be used for in vitro and in vivo evaluation of the D_2 receptors.

We report here the preparation of ^{125}I-iodoaminoclebopride and ^{125}I-iodoazidoclebopride and their in vivo evaluation in rats.

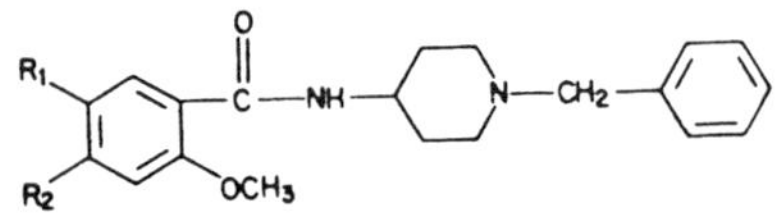

Ia	R_1 = Cl	R_2 = NH_2	Clebopride
Ib	R_1 = Cl	R_2 = N_3	Azidoclebopride
Ic	R_1 = H	R_2 = NH_2	
Id	R_1 = I	R_2 = NH_2	Iodoclebopride
Ie	R_1 = I	R_2 = N_3	Iodoazidoclebopride (IAC)
If	R_1 = ^{125}I	R_2 = NH_2	^{125}I-Iodoclebopride
Ig	R_1 = ^{125}I	R_2 = N_3	^{125}I-Iodoazidoclebopride (^{125}IAC)

MATERIALS OF METHODS

The iodine-125 used in this study was a carrier-free solution of $Na^{125}I$ (ca 100 mCi/ml) in reductant-free 0.1 N NaOH obtained from New England Nuclear Corporation. The commercial solution was diluted immediately prior to use with deionized distilled water to a radioiodide concentration of 5 mCi/0.1 ml. Radioactivity was quantified with a CRC-4R radioisotope callibrator. Synthesis of Ia–Ie is reported elsewhere (27).

TLC analyses were performed on 25 x 20 cm silica gel coated plastic sheets (Kodak 60F-25). The plates were analyzed by autoradiography immediately after development and drying. The solvent systems and the respective R_f values for each system are as follows:

(If), $CHCl_3/CH_3OH/NH_4OH$ (9:1:0.1), R_f = 0.75
(Ig), $CHCl_3/CH_3OH/NH_4OH$ (9:1:0.1), R_f = 0.85

Synthesis of {^{125}I}-Iodoaminoclebopride (If): Exchange Radioiodination): Twenty-five mg of an aqueous solution of iodoclebopride was placed in a 10 ml rubber stoppered test tube to which 5 mg of ammonium sulfate and 5 mCi of $Na^{125}I$ were added. One ml of dry acetone was added and the solvent removed under a flow of nitrogen at 70° C. The mixture was heated to dryness in an oil bath and the dry reaction mixture was maintained at 140-145° for 90 minutes. The mixture was cooled, 2 ml of 5% sodium metabisulphite solution added, and the mixture extracted with ether (3 x 2 ml). The ether extract was washed with water pH 7 (1 x 2 ml) and dried over anhydrous magnesium sulfate. After filtration the solvent was removed yielding pure (If), activity 800 Ci (14 Ci/mmole).

Synthesis of {^{125}I}-iodoazidoclebopride (Ig): Treatment of 100 Ci of (Ig) with acidic sodium nitrite and sodium azide yielded pure ^{125}IAC (Ig) in quantitive yield (100μCi).

Tissue distribution studies: CD Fischer rats (175-225 g) were used to determine the tissue distribution of ^{125}I-iodoclebopride (If) and ^{125}IAC (Ig). Under ether anesthesia the rats were injected intravenously via a tail vein with a normal saline-ethanol (9:1) solution containing the radiochemical (2 μCi/0.1 ml). Groups of rats (6 per group) were sacrificed by ether asphyxiation at 5, 60, 120 and 240 minutes after injection. The various sections of the brain-viz, striatum, cerebellum, thalamus, rest of brain-heart and thyroid were excised, blotted dry, weighed and counted in a gamma well scintillation counter. Blood was obtained from a tail vein in the thoracic cavity and the radioactivity assayed. The concentrations of radioactivity as percent of injected dose per gram of tissue and per organ were calculated.

RESULTS AND DISCUSSION

In vivo evaluation of ^{125}I-labeled iodoclebopride and iodoazidoclebopride for the dopamine D_2 receptors: Iodoclebopride and iodoazidoclebopride were radiolabeled with ^{125}I with a specific activity of 14 Ci per mmol by a simple radiodiodination exchange reaction (28). Both agents were evaluated in rats for their blood, brain and thyroid distribution. Tables 1-4 present the biodistributions performed with the labeled agents. The uptake in the different tissues is expressed as percent dose per gram or percent dose per organ.

In Table I the activity distribution of ^{125}I-iodoclebopride initially shows a relatively high brain uptake. The total percent dose per organ was .85% at 5 minutes which decreased quickly to .29 at 1 hour and to .18 at 2 hours. Striatum to cerebellum concentration decreased from 1.81 at 5 minutes to 1.1 at 2 hours. These data show that iodoclebopride was taken up by the brain and then rapidly eliminated. The fast washout could be associated with the in vivo deiodination of iodoclebopride as indicated by the thyroid uptake which increased from 1.04% dose per gram at 5 minutes to 14.2% at 2 hours. In the case of ^{125}I-iodoazidoclebopride, the total brain uptake in % dose per organ was 1.25 at 5 minutes and 1.03 at two hours. The ratio of striatum to cerebellum was 2.23 at 1 hour and did not change appreciably after two hours, (2.37). The high standard deviation for striatum at 1 hour could be due to its small size. It is worth noting that although the total brain uptake showed significant washout, the striatum concentration remained the same during two hour period at a level over 2.5% dose per gram.

The specificity of the in vivo binding of ^{125}IAC was assessed by co-injecting a potent dopaminergic agonist, (-) apomorphine (8 mg/kg) with ^{125}IAC. The brain distribution in the different sections was studied at the time of sacrifice. This study showed that the total brain uptake at 5 minutes with and without the agonist was 1.25%; it decreased to 1% at 1 and 2 hours. The striatum uptake on the other hand decreased three folds as compared to the measured uptake without (-) apomorphine. The striatum to cerebellum ratio became .68 at two hours as compared to a ratio of 2.37 without the (-) apomorphine.

In this study we selected the substituted benzamide as a ligand that has an inherent affinity for the binding site of D_2 receptors and introduced the azido group as a photosensitive functional group replacing the amino group in Ia. On photoactivation of either lb or le with light these ligands showed the capability of forming the covalent bond at or near the binding site of the D_2 receptors (24,25,26).

The association with a recognition site will ordinarily be reversible until photolysis is initiated. The covalent bond thus formed between the photoprobe and the binding site will facilitate the characterization and isolation of a dopamine D_2 receptor. The irradiation of the striatum membrane in the presence of azidoclebopride or iodoazidoclebopride reduced the specific binding of ^{3}H-spiperone in a concentration dependent fashion. Maximal photoinactivation was attained with 1 micromolar azidoclebopride lb or 300 nanomolar iodoazidoclebopride le and typically represented a loss of 60-80% of the total number of sites labeled by ^{3}H-spiperone. These and other data demonstrated that dopamine D_2 receptors can be selectively photoinactivated by azidoclebopride and protection against photolysis was provided by dopaminergic agonists and antagonists with an appropriate pharmacologic profile (25,26). In this study, the in vivo distribution

Table 1 ^{125}I-Radioactivity following intravenous injection in rats of ^{125}I-iodoclebopride

Organ	% injected dose/organ tissue		
	5 min	1 hr	2 hr
Blood	.29±.05*	.14±.02	.09±.01
Heart	.67±.11	.26±.03	.22±.06
Cerebellum	.43±.09	.21±.02	.17±.01
Thalamus	.51±.15	.22±.03	.17±.02
Striatum	.78±.36	.26±.11	.19±.08
R.O.B.	.42±.09	.18±.02	.11±.04
Thyroid	1.04±.29	2.8±2.4	14.2±9.3
Striatum/ Cerebellum	1.81	1.24	1.11

Organ	% dose/organ		
	5 min	1 hr	2 hr
Blood	3.91±.50	1.82±.26	1.35±.14
Heart	.48±.08	.19±.02	.15±.04
Cerebellum	.11±.03	.05±.01	.04±.00
Thalamus	.05±.01	.02±.01	.02±.00
Striatum	.06±.03	.04±.04	.02±.00
R.O.B.	.63±.12	.18±.03	.10±.05
Thyroid	.05±.01	.12±.12	.58±.29
Total Brain	0.85	0.29	0.18

*Mean ± S.D. for 6 animals

Table 2 Comparative tissue distribution (% dose/gram ± S.D.) in rats after intravenous administration of ^{125}IAC and ^{125}IAC plus (-) apomorphine*.

^{125}IAC

Organ	5 min	1 hr	2 hr
Blood	.53±.11	.34±.03	.32±.05
Heart	2.76±.46	1.61±.18	1.34±.10
Cerebellum	1.16±.14	1.13±.16	1.06±.07
Thalamus	1.28±.25	1.25±.32	1.12±.15
Striatum	2.09±1.16	2.52±1.51	2.52±.64
Rest of Brain	0.91±.21	.78±.10	.73±.06
Striatum/ Cerebellum	1.83	2.23	2.37

^{125}IAC plus (-) apomorphine*

Organ	5 min	1 hr	2 hr
Blood	.10±.01	.08±.03	.08±.03
Heart	.58±.08	.45±.08	.41±.08
Cerebellum	.88±.08	.70±.07	.69±.10
Thalamus	.85±.15	.72±.09	.70±.06
Striatum	.63±.10	.43±.05	.47±.01
Rest of Brain	.80±.11	.61±.07	.60±.06
Striatum/ Cerebellum	.72	.69	.68

*8mg/kg

Table 3 Comparative tissue distribution (% dose/organ $\pm$ S.D.) in rats after intravenous administration of ^{125}IAC and ^{125}IAC plus (-) apomorphine*.

^{125}IAC

Organ	5 min	1 hr	2 hr
Blood	4.33$\pm$.73	2.74$\pm$.17	2.62$\pm$.30
Heart	1.22$\pm$.09	.70$\pm$.06	.59$\pm$.06
Cerebellum	.21$\pm$.05	.19$\pm$.06	.18$\pm$.02
Thalamus	.16$\pm$.05	.11$\pm$.03	.11$\pm$.02
Striatum	.10$\pm$.03	.09$\pm$.07	.05$\pm$.01
Rest of Brain	.80$\pm$.20	.70$\pm$.11	.69$\pm$.07
Total Brain	1.25$\pm$	1.09	1.03
Thyroid	.12$\pm$.04	.29$\pm$.16	.66$\pm$.32

^{125}IAC plus (-) apomorphine*

Organ	5 min	1 hr	2 hr
Blood	1.23$\pm$.16	.90$\pm$.19	.82$\pm$.16
Heart	.30$\pm$.04	.23$\pm$.06	.27$\pm$.03
Cerebellum	.26$\pm$.03	.20$\pm$.03	.19$\pm$.03
Thalamus	.15$\pm$.03	.16$\pm$.02	.16$\pm$.03
Striatum	.05$\pm$.01	.03$\pm$.00	.06$\pm$.00
Rest of Brain	.79$\pm$.08	.58$\pm$.07	.58$\pm$.07
Total Brain	1.25	.97	.99
Thyroid	.11$\pm$.05	.21$\pm$.09	.17$\pm$.01

*8mg/Kg

Table 4 Brain to blood concentration ratios of various radiolabeled neuroleptics

Radioligand	Species	Hours After Injection	Brain-to-Blood Concentration Ratios	Ref
{^{11}C}spiroperidol	mouse	0.5	67	31
{^{18}F}haloperidol	rat	1.0	12	32
{^{82}Br}bromperidol	rat	1.0	2.2	32,33
1-(4,4)-bis-(p-fluorophenyl)butyl -{3,4-^{3}H}-pimozide	rat	0.5	21	34
^{125}IAC	rat	1.0	16.7	present study

of iodoazidoclebopride 1g showed selective and high affinity binding to the striatum in an irreversible manner without light irradiation. The mechanism for this covalent binding is not fully understood. However, we speculate, that the concentration of free radicals and other environmental conditions in the brain are such that covalent bonding of the iodoazidoclebopride to the striatal and tissue can take place.

Table 4 contains brain to blood concentration ratios of several neuroleptics labeled with different isotopes including pimozide, bromoperidol and spiroperidol. Iodoazidoclebopride compared to haloperidol and bromoperidol showed a much higher ratios which will serve to increase further the statistical accuracy of regional receptor concentration measurements by reducing the correction for the vascular component of radioactivity within the brain tissue. In contrast to the striatum to cerebellum concentration ratios, the high brain concentrations (Table 4) and brain to blood concentration ratios are probably not related to receptor binding. Bioavailability to brain tissue, localization in and redistribution from from other tissue (29,30), and metabolism and excretion are most likely responsible for the observed differences in brain concentrations among neuroleptics.

The use of a site specific tracer for the central D_2 receptor such as ^{125}IAC should further our understanding of dopamine receptor populations in healthy and in Parkinson's disease patients before and after therapy, and would benefit the development of new direct-acting DA agonists with long-lasting and selective pharmacological actions, restricted to the D_2 receptors.

Acknowledgement

These studies were supported in part by Research Biochemicals Inc., Wayland, Ma, NIH Grant NS15439, The Ontario Mental Health Foundation, The Medical Research Council of Canada and National Cancer Institute T32CA09362-5.

REFERENCES

1. A. Barbeau, G.F. Murphy and T.L. Sourkes: Science 133:1706 (1961).

2. W. Birkmayer and O. Hornykiewicz, Wien. Klin. Wschr. 73:787 (1961).

3. G.C. Cotzias, van M.H. van Voert, and L.M. Schiffer, N. Engl. J. Med. 276:374 (1967).

4. G. Cohen, J. Neural Transm. Suppl. 19:89-103 (1983).

5. M. Da Prada, H,H, Keller, L. Pieri, R. Keltler and W.E. Haefely, Experientia. 40:1165-1172 (1984).

6. V.H. Sethy, Eur. J. Pharmacol. 60:397-398 (1979).

7. B. Scalton, J. Pharmac. Exp. Ther. 220:197-220 (1982).

8. M.D. Thorner, E. Fluckiger and D.B. Calne in: Bromocriptine-A Clinical and Pharmacological Review. Raven Press, New York, 1980.

9. B.K. Madras, A. Davis and P. Seeman, Eur. J. Pharmacol. 78:431 (1982).

10. J. Ramwani and R.K. Mishra, Fed. Proc. Am. Soc. Exp. Biol., 41:1325 (1982).

11. K. Nishikori, O. Noshiro, K. Sano and H. Maeno, J. Biol. Chem., 255:10909-10915 (1980).

12. K. Thermos, R.B. Murphy and D.I. Schuster, Biochem. Biophy. Res. Commun. Commun. 106:1469-1477 (1982).

13. B. Davis, L. Abood and A.M. Tometsko, Life Sci. 26: 85-88 (1980).

14. G. Testylier, D. Daveloose, F. Letterrier, O. Buchman and M. Shimoni, Photochem. Photobiol., 39:273-276 (1984).

15. J-H. Guan, J.L. Neumeyer, C.N. Filer, D.G. Ahern, L. Lilly, M. Watanabe, D. Grigoriadis and P. Seeman, J. Med. Chem. 27:806-810 (1984).

16. M.W. Hamblin and I. Creese, Life Sci. 32:2247-2255 (1983).

17. D.I. Schuster, W.L. Holden, A.P.S. Nunila and R.B. Murphy, Eur. J. Pharmacol. 77:313-316 (1982).

18. G.L. Stiles, M.G. Caron and R.J. Lefkowitz, Physiol. Rev. 64:661-743 (1984).

19. L.M.F. Leeb-Lundberg, K.E.J. Dickinson, S.L. Heall, J.E.S. Wikberg, P.O. Hagen, J.F. DeBernardis, M. Winn, D.L. Arendsen, R.J. Lefkowitz and M.G. Caron, J. Biol. Chem. 259:2579-2587 (1984).

20. C.E. Seidman, H.J. Hess, C.J. Homey and Graham R.M., Hypertension 6:7-11 (1984).

21. P.N.C. Elliott, P. Jenner, G. Huizing, G.D. Marsden and R. Miller, Neuropharmacology 16:333-342 (1977).

22. S. Fleminger, H. Vand de Waterbeemed, N.M.J. Rupniak and C. Reavill, B. Testa, P. Jenner and C.D. Marsden, J. Pharm. Pharmacol. 35:363-368 (1983).

23. J.W. Kebabian and D.B. Calne, Nature (London) 277:93-96 (1979).

24. H.B. Niznik, J-H. Guan, J.L. Neumeyer and P. Seeman, Eur. J. Pharmacol. 104:387-390 (1984).

25. H.B. Niznik, J-H. Guan, J.L. Neumeyer and P. Seeman, Molecular Pharmacol. 27:293-299 (1985).

26. H.B. Niznik, A. Dumbrille-Ross, J-H Guan, J.L. Neumeyer and P. Seeman, Neurosci. Lett. 55:267-272 (1985).

27. J.L. Neumeyer, J-H. Guan, H.B. Niznik, A. Dumbrille-Ross, P. Seeman, S. Padmanabhan and D.R. Elmaleh, J. Med. Chem. 28:405-407 (1985).

28. T.J. Magner, J.L. Wu and D.M. Wieland, J. Org. Chem. 47:1484-1488 (1982).

29. Y.S. Bakhle and J.R. Vane, Physiol. Rev., 54:1007-1045 (1974).

30. E.A. Brown, Drug Metab. Rev., 3:33-87 (1974).

31. J.S. Fowler, C.D. Arnett and A.P. Wolf, J. Nucl. Med., 23:437-445, (1982).

32. G.A. Digenis, S.H. Vincent and C.S. Kook, J. Pharm. Sci., 70:985-989 (1981).

33. S.H. Vincent, M.V. Shambhu and G.A. Digenis, J. Med. Chem., 23:75-79 (1980).

34. Y. Givant, M.J. Shani and G. Goldhaber, Arch. Int. Pharmacodyn. Ther. 205:317-327 (1973).

MONOAMINE OXIDASE TYPE B INHIBITORS IN HUMAN AND ANIMAL PARKINSONISM

M.B.H. Youdim,
J.P.M. Finberg,
P. Riederer* and
R.E. Heikkila**

Rappaport Family Institute
and Department of Pharmacology
Faculty of Medicine
Technion
Haifa, Israel
*Ludwig Boltzmann Institute
Vienna, Austria
**Department of Neurology
Rutger Medical School
New Jersey, U.S.A.

INTRODUCTION

The introduction of levodopa for the treatment of Parkinson's disease opened up a new era in the treatment of this ailment. The clinical pharmacological action of levodopa as it is known today is dopamine replacement therapy (1). The benefit gained from levodopa surpasses its side effects. Thus the quality of life for Parkinson's patients has been raised almost to the normal level, at least for a few years. However, long-term therapy with levodopa has shown (a) response to the drug falls after the first two to three years, (b) increased incidents of "on-off" phenomenon, and (c) levodopa treatment does not modify the progression of the underlying pathology and the natural course of Parkinson's disease. Therefore, many problems still remain and the search for new strategies in the treatment continues. These directions include development of drugs which directly stimulate the brain dopamine receptor (2,3), or inhibit dopamine uptake (4) or inhibit the brain enzymes responsible for degradation of dopamine (5). Both monoamine oxidase (MAO) and catechol-O-methyltransferase are known to be involved in the inactivation of dopamine.

In this paper the readers' attention will be directed to the exciting development in pharmacology of MAO and its selective inhibitors on the one hand and the recent discovery of the compound N-methyl-4-phenyl-1,2,5,6-tetrahydropyridine (MPTP), which causes Parkinsonism in human subjects and animals (6,7,8). The fact that MAO type B inhibitor, l-deprenyl (l-selegiline), has been proven to have anti-Parkinson activity (9,10,11) as well as preventing the selective nigra striatal lesion induced by MPTP (12,13) may very well shed a new light on our assumption about aetiology of Parkinson's disease and the role of MAO in the brain.

MONOAMINE OXIDASES AND THEIR SELECTIVE INHIBITORS

Numerous investigations have shown that interneuronal monoamine oxidase (MAO) has a direct role in keeping the cytoplasmic level of amine neurotransmitter, dopamine, serotonin and noradrenaline low within the neuron (14,15,16). Thus the resultant of in vivo MAO inhibition in control and reserpinized animals is a significant increase in brain levels of the above neurotransmitters. It is interesting to note that in the absence of vesicular storage sites, as is the case in reserpinized animals, substantial accumulation of brain amines can still occur when MAO is fully inhibited (16,17). This may indicate the the neurons have some other "amine-storage" system besides the vesicles. MAO inhibitor pretreated rats given levodopa develop a behavioural syndrome of hyperactivity and stereotypy reminiscent of that observed with the dopamine agonist, apomorphine (15). This behavioural syndrome can be blocked by dopamine antagonists, e.g. haloperidol (18), suggesting the increased release of dopamine formed from levodopa acts postsynaptically. Evidence is available to support the concept that it is the newly formed dopamine which is preferentially released into the "functional pool" and MAO regulates the size of this pool (19,20).

The physiological role of MAO in the regulation of dopamine deamination is further substantiated by the observation that during postnatal development dopamine MAO activity in rat striatum increases, reaching its maximum by the 4-5th week. Subsequent parallel increases of dopamine deaminated metabolites, dihydroxyphenylacetic acid (DOPAC) and homovanilic acid (HVA) also occurs (Fig. 1.) (21). The rate at which MAO activity increases with age differs in various regions of the rat brain (22). While highest MAO activities are found in the hypothalamus and basal ganglia, low activity is present in cerebral cortex. This is true for both animal and human brains using a variety of substrates of MAO.

The presence of multiple forms of MAO having different substrate specificity and inhibitor sensitivity in animal and human brain was predicted by us when purified MAO was separated electrophoretically into a number of active bands (23). These data were confirmed by the discovery of MAO inhibitors having selectivity for the different enzyme forms using a variety of substrates (24,25). The current hypothesis regarding multiple forms of MAO holds that there are two forms of MAO, type A and type B. However, subgroups of MAO A and B types may also exist (25). Type A enzyme deaminates hydroxylated amines such as serotonin, adrenaline, noradrenaline and octopamine and is sensitive to inhibition by clorgyline. Type B enzyme is thought to be responsible for the deamination of non-hydroregulated amines, benzylamine and phenylethylamine. This enzyme form is selectively inhibited by l-deprenyl and AGN 1135 (Fig. 2.) (14). The specificity of these inhibitors and related compounds has also been established in vivo. Selective inhibition of brain MAO A results in increase of serotonin and noradrenaline while inhibition of MAO B induces an elevation of phenylethylamine (27,28). Evidence is available to indicate that interneuronal MAO activity is, to a large extent, mainly type A (29). However, recent data also speak of the presence of MAO type B within the neurons (30) having a functional role (15,16).

In the rat brain, liver and gut, both tyramine and dopamine are considered substrates for both enzyme forms (24,30). This may be the reason why selective MAO inhibitors (clorgyline and l-deprenyl) hardly affect brain levels of dopamine in this animal (15). Furthermore, unlike the non-selective MAO inhibitors (pargyline and tranylcypromine) the above selective inhibitors do not induce the behavioural syndrome in response to levodopa. However, a combination of A and B inhibitors at their selective doses do so, with a concomitant increase of brain concentration of dopamine similar to that which is observed with tranylcypromine (15).

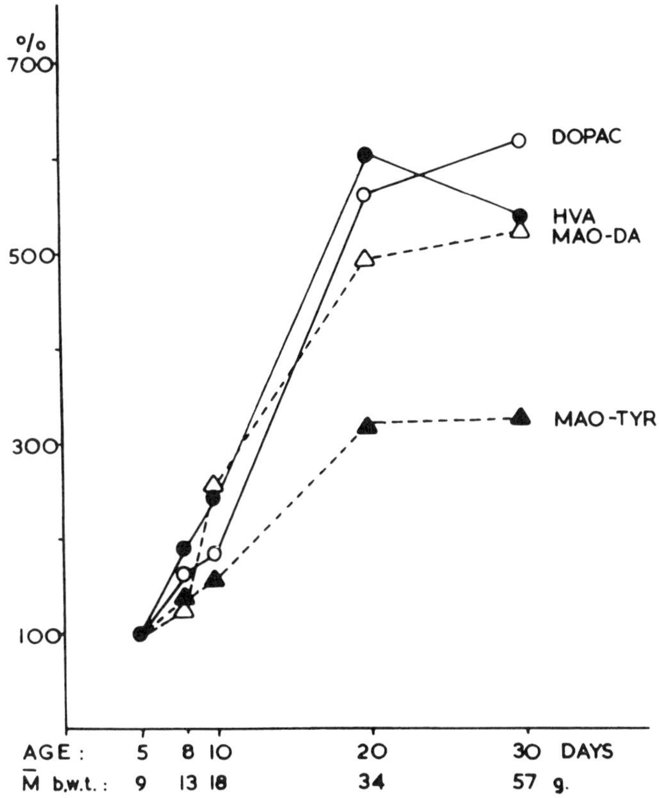

Fig. 1. Postnatal development of MAO activity towards dopamine (MAO-DA) and tyramine (MAO-TYR) and the appearance of dopamine metabolites in the rat striatum. DOPAC, dihydroxyphenylacetic acid; HVA, homovalinic acid (21).

In contrast, human brain (caudate nucleus, pallidum, substantia nigra, thalamus) MAO activity has repeatedly been shown to be predominantly type B. Both tyramine (32,33) and dopamine (34) are considered to be B substrates in this tissue (35). Furthermore, unlike that which has been observed in rat brain, the ratio of MAO A and MAO B varies significantly in the different regions of human brain (35).

MAO INHIBITORS AS ANTI-PARKINSON DRUGS

MAO inhibitors were among the first psychotropic drugs to be discovered and used clinically in the management of depressive illness (14). Considering their natural pharmacological action, namely inhibiton of MAO, iproniazid and isocarboxazid were used in combination with L-Dopa in the treatment of Parkinson's disease as early as 1961. However, the occurrence of side effects, including hypertensive reaction ("cheese effect") overrode their beneficial effectiveness. The "cheese effect", thus, was the main reason for the abandonment of non-selective MAO inhibitors as antidepressants (14) and anti-Parkinson drugs (36).

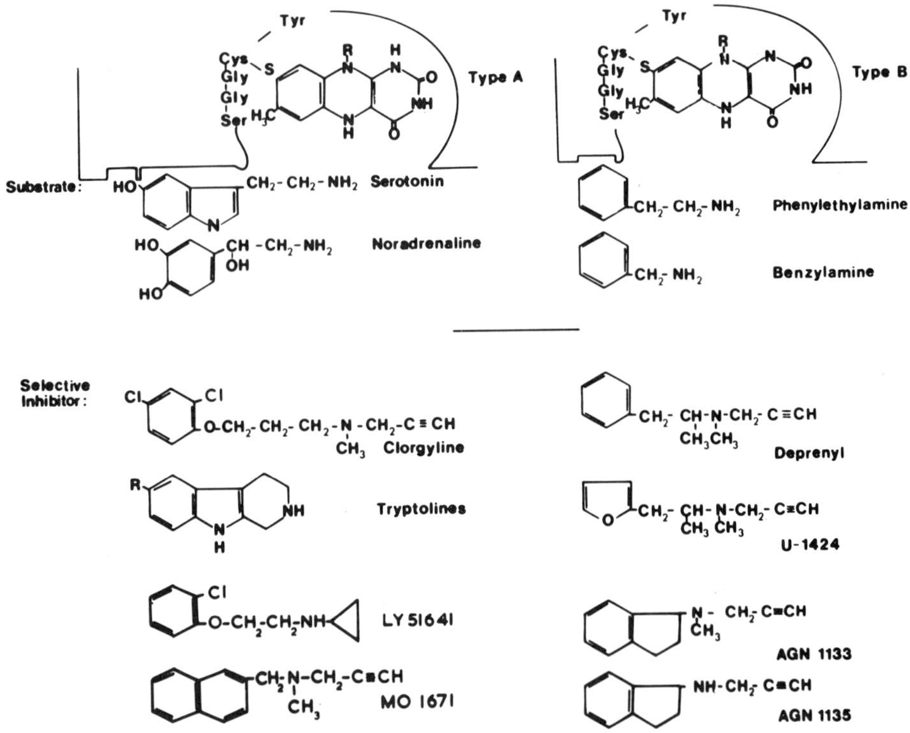

Fig. 2. MAO binding sites, their selective substrates and inhibitors. Note that dopamine and tyramine are substrates for both enzyme forms (14).

Selective MAO-B Inhibitors

The use of an MAO inhibitor to potentiate the action of dopamine formed from L-Dopa had always been considered logical considering the essential role of MAO for dopamine deamination either before or after release (15). The rationale implicit in this therapy was that the therapeutic effectiveness of MAO inhibitors in Parkinson patients would rely on a localized accumulation of dopamine at a specific site in the brain. The discovery of multiple forms of human brain MAO led Youdim et al. (37) to suggest that synthesis of specific MAO inhibitors without the "cheese effect" (potentiation of sympathomimetic action of tyramine) (14) tailored to an individual enzyme form at a particular site in the brain should be possible (37). Without exception, all non-selective and the newly developed selective MAO A inhibitors initiated the "cheese effect" in isolated pharmacological preparations, as well as *in vivo* (14,38). This is also evidenced in studies carried out in human volunteers (14,38). However, MAO B inhibitors, l-deprenyl (25) and AGN 1135 (Fig. 2.) (14,39), are devoid of this pharmacological side effect. This will be discussed in more detail later.

The original concept for the use of l-deprenyl in combination with levodopa for the management of Parkinson's disease was a logical consequence of studies showing a) human brain MAO in the extrapyramidal regions may be enriched with MAO type B and, therefore, susceptible to inhibition by l-deprenyl (Youdim and Riederer, 1974, unpublished observation). The studies of

Youdim et al. (37) on MAO activity in human brain regions obtained at autopsy from geriatric patients having terminal disease and treated with various MAO inhibitors for the depressive episodes lend credence to this concept. While therapeutic doses of tranylcypromine had fully inhibited the deamination of dopamine by MAO in hypothalamus, basal ganglia and centrum ovalis, the enzyme activity in the same regions was hardly affected by the MAO A inhibitor, clorgyline (37); b) l-deprenyl was shown to increase selectively but moderately dopamine levels in rat brain (40) and that inhibition curves with clorgyline and l-deprenyl using human brain mitochondrial fraction pointed to substantial presence of MAO type B (32,33) when using tyramine and kynuramine as substrates, and c) l-deprenyl did not cause "cheese effect" i.e. potentiation of sympathomimetic action of tyramine. The absence of the latter phenomenon was the major factor for its clinical use (25).

The first clinical trials with l-deprenyl indicated that the drug was effective in potentiating the anti-akinetic action of levodopa, reducing the incidence of "on-off" phenomen and recouping the beneficial effect of levodopa in patients who had lost their response to it (41,42,43). Although there is overwhelming evidence to support these original findings (11), the mechanism of l-deprenyl's action is not fully understood. It can best be explained by the inhibition of MAO B, the major enzyme form responsible for dopamine deamination in human brain, thus making more dopamine formed from levodopa available for neurotransmission. In the human extrapyramidal brain regions dopamine was shown to be an MAO B substrate (34). Further biochemical evidence supporting this has come from brain autopsy of Parkinsonian patients treated with l-deprenyl (44). The daily therapeutic dose of l-deprenyl (10 mg) is sufficient to inhibit fully dopamine deamination by MAO B and signficantly increase dopamine concentrations in caudate nucleus, putament, globus pallidus and substantia nigra (Fig. 3.) (44). MAO type A activity as measured by <u>ex vivo</u> deamination of serotonin is much less affected. Furthermore serotonin and its deaminated metabolite 5-hydroxyindoleacetic acid concentrations were unchanged in the same brain regions (44). The possibility that the anti-Parkinson action of l-deprenyl may be related to its amphetamine metabolite and property (45,46) has not received much support. Recent and earlier clinical trials with amphetamine have shown it to be ineffective in Parkinson patients on levodopa therapy (47). It is obvious that clinical trials with another selective MAO B inhibitor, such as AGN 1135, devoid of amphetamine activity and unlike l-deprenyl, not metabolized to amphetamine, is necessary to clarify this question. <u>In vitro</u> studies using human brain caudate nucleus mitochondrial preparations confirm that AGN 1135 is even more superior to l-deprenyl as a selective inhibitor of MAO B (44). Trials with this inhibitor and MDL 72145, another irreversible MAO B inhibitor, are being considered.

MPTP INDUCED PARKINSONISM AND MAO INHIBITORS

The most prominent pathological and biochemical feature of idiopathic Parkinsonism is the degeneration of nigrostrial dopaminergic neurons cell bodies in the substantia nigra with concomitant decrease of dopamine and its major metabolites HVA and DOPAC concentrations in the caudate nucleus and putamen. The reversal of clinical symptoms in Parkinsonian patients with levodopa, directly acting dopamine agonists, and selective monoamine oxidase B inhibitors, emphasize the importance of dopamine. Recently a syndrome similar to idiopathic Parkinsonism has been described in human subjects, and animals (rhesus monkey, squirrel monkey, dogs and mice) as a resultant administration of the elicit compound N-methyl-4-phenyl-1,2,5,6-tetrahydropyridine (MPTP) (6,7,8). The latter drug causes a severe loss of nerve cells in the pars compacta of the striatum in rhesus and squirrel monkeys (48,49). It is apparent that administration of levodopa and dopamine agonists can suppress the neurological and biochemical changes resulting from neurotoxicity of MPTP in human subjects and monkeys (50,51).

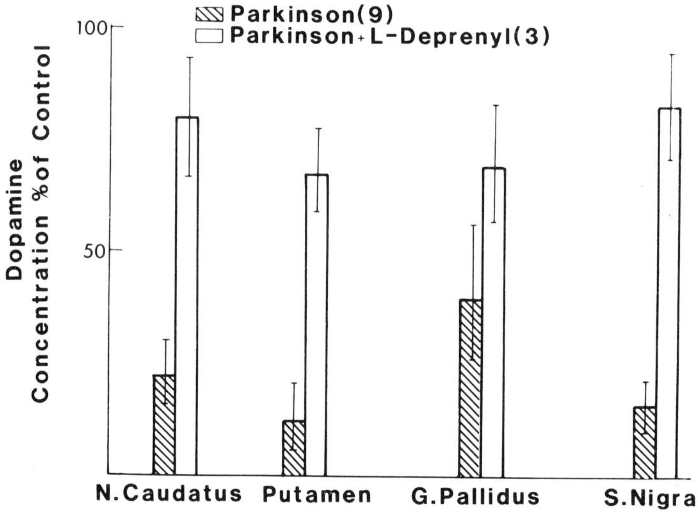

Fig. 3. Dopamine concentrations in brains of Parkinsonian patients treated with l-deprenyl (10 mg daily dose, 6-18 days before death) (44). □ per cent increase above that of ▧.

MPTP is a small lipid soluble, non-polar, molecule which can rapidly be taken up into the brain when administered intravenously or intraperitoneally. The mechanism by which MPTP is selectively accumulated in the dopamine terminals of caudate nucleus and putamen, and the biochemical processes by which it causes retrograde cell degeneration is not known. However, being a tertiary amine it is thought to interact with MAO (52) after being taken up by the dopamine neurons. Distribution of ^{3}H-MPTP in the rat or mouse brain shows close similarity to this enzyme. The recent exciting data from several laboratories indicate that MPTP could be a substrate for MAO. Thus, the non-selective MAO inhibitors, pargyline, iproniazid and tranylcypromine have been shown to inhibit the conversion of MPTP to N-methyl-4-phenylpyridinium ion (MPP^+) in vitro (13) and in vivo (48-51). Furthermore, MAO inhibitors prevent the neurotoxic effect of MPTP in the substantia nigra (12,48-51). Added to this excitement are the studies of Heikkila et al. (12,13), who showed that the MPTP induced neurotoxic effects and diminution of dopamine, HVA and DOPAC can be selectively blocked by the selective MAO B inhibitors, l-deprenyl and AGN 1135 and not by the selective MAO A inhibitor, clorgyline.

Looking at the structure of MPTP one should not be surprised that it might be a substrate for MAO B. Its close resemblance to phenylethylamine, a substrate for MAO B, is apparent. The oxidation of MPTP to MPP^+ involves a dehydrogenation process (53), which resembles the first step in the oxidative deamination of monoamines by MAO, namely the formation of an imine. Tetrazolium nitro blue (TNB) has been used not only for the histochemical demonstration of MAO but many other dehydrogenases. Taking advantage of this reaction, MPTP oxidation was coupled to the reduction of tetrazolium nitro blue in the presence of MAO preparation from rat brain. The apparent Km of TNB-reductase system is close to the Km of MAO-B for phenylethylamine

Table 1. The apparent Km values of MPTP-tetrazolium reductase, MAO-A and MAO-B activities in rat brain. 5-HT, 5-hydroxytryptamine; PEA, phenylethylamine; TNB, tetrazolium nitro blue. *MPTP-TNB reductase is selectively inhibited by 0.1μM 1-deprenyl or AGN 1135 but not by 0.1μM clorgyline.

	Km (uM)		
Fraction	MPTP-TNB Reductase*	PEA (MAO-B)	5-HT (MAO-A)
Microsomal	16	17	180
Mitchondrial	9	21	210

and not that of MAO A for serotonin (Table 1) in both rat brain microsomal and mitochondrial fractions. TNB-reductase system, namely the formation of formazan, can be selectively inhibited with 1-deprenyl and AGN 1135 but not by the same concentrations of clorgyline (53).

The inhibition of MPTP oxidation by MAO A and B inhibitors using mouse brain as measured by the decline of H_2O_2 production is shown in Table 2. A comparison of IC_{50} of MAO A (tryptamine) and MAO B (benzylamine) inhibition by a number of MAO inhibitors shows that inhibition of MPTP oxidation behaves more like an MAO B substrate. Thus its oxidation is far more susceptible to inhibition by selective MAO B inhibitors, 1-deprenyl and AGN 1135 (Table 2). In retrospect AGN 1135 appears to have even a greater selectivity than AGN 1133 and 1-deprenyl for inhibition of MAO B (13a). Similar data have been observed with this inhibitor using human brain mitochondrial preparation (Table 2) (44).

Like other MAO inhibitors, intraperitoneal injection of AGN 1135 and AGN 1133 (Fig. 2.) protect against MPTP induced decrements in nigrostrial content of dopamine and its metabolites (Table 3). The concentration (2.5mg/kg i.p.) at which these inhibitors protect against MPTP neurotoxicity is significantly lower than used (10mg/kg) for 1-deprenyl in similar experiments by Keikkila et al. (12). The greater MAO B (54) selectivity of AGN 1135, as compared to AGN 1133, may be the reason why the brain concentrations of dopamine metabolites and 3-methoxy-dopamine (3OMeDA) are not significantly affected in non-MPTP and MPTP treated mice. In the brain of mice, like that of rat, dopamine is a substrate for both enzyme forms (55). Thus when MAO B is inhibited, MAO A can still continue to deaminate dopamine (15). AGN 1133, in contrast, with poor selectivity for MAO B (Table 2) (54), caused significant reduction of dopamine metabolites and an increase in 3-OMeDA (Table 3) showing its non-selectivity.

The mechanism underlying the neurotoxicity of MPTP and its prevention by MAO B inhibitors is not known. The available information indicates that MPP^+ is the sole metabolite derived from MPTP and its formation is inhibited by MAO B inhibitors (56). The protective effect of MAO B inhibitors resulting in increased brain level of MPTP and decreased MPP^+ would indicate that

Table 2. IC_{50} values for several MAO inhibitors on the oxidation of benzylamine, MPTP and tryptamine in mouse brain mitochondrial preparations.

MAOI	IC50 (uM) Benzylamine (MAO-B)	MPTP	Tryptamine (MAO-A)	IC50 Ratio TRY/BZ	TRY/MPTP
AGN-1133	0.002	0.003	0.221	110	73
AGN-1135	0.014	0.039	339.0	24214	8692
Pargyline	0.008	0.009	2.85	356	316
l-Deprenyl	0.011	0.023	70.5	6409	3065
Clorgyline	4.39	9.71	0.011	0.003	0.001

the neurotoxicity may be due to the formation of MPP^+ itself and/or toxic intermediates (e.g. hydrogen peroxide, free radicals, superoxide, etc.) as a resultant of MAO reaction, which in turn could cause lipid peroxidation reactions damaging to the dopamine neurones. Although the conversion of MPTP to MPP^+ does not strictly follow the reaction of MAO, i.e. formation of aldehyde and ammonia, we have evidence that H_2O_2 is formed (see Table 2) during MPTP oxidation (13a).

IS PARKINSON'S DISEASE A NEUROTOXIC EVENT AND DO MAO B INHIBITORS RETARD ITS DEGENERATIVE PROGRESSION?

It is well established that long term levodopa therapy does not lead to the modification of the progression underlying pathology and the natural course of Parkinson's disease. In some cases levodopa may even accelerate the degeneration of dopamine neurons. Because we have used l-deprenyl as adjunct to levodopa for the past twelve years an attempt has been made to answer the question whether addition of l-deprenyl can retard the progression of the disease.

It is clear from our earlier studies (9,41,56), those of Yahr (8) and others (11) that the introduction of l-deprenyl into levodopa therapy can lead to recouping the loss of response to levodopa and patients having diminished incidents of "on-off" effects. Since it is known that the therapeutic doses of l-deprenyl fully inhibits dopamine deamination in Parkinsonian brain, leading to increased brain dopamine concentrations (Fig. 3) (44), the therapeutic features of l-deprenyl can be explained by the following: Brain MAO inhibition (a) makes it possible for a more sustained release of dopamine, (b) prevents accumulation of dopamine metabolites or dopamine-aldehyde condensation products such as tetrahydropapaveroline (57) which themselves could be inhibitory to postsynaptic dopamine receptor and (c) prevents hydrogen peroxide formation from the reaction of dopamine deamination. Hydrogen peroxide itself can bring about a lipidperoxidation reaction which in turn would damage the remaining dopamine neurons. This hypothesis appears to receive some support, since the dehydrogenation of MPTP by MAO results in the formation of hydrogen peroxide (13).

The neurotoxicity of MPTP can be effectively blocked in animals by selective MAO B inhibitors, l-deprenyl and AGN 1135 (Table 3) (12,13). The question whether long-term l-deprenyl treatment could retard or prevent the degeneration of dopaminergic neurons has been investigated by evaluating

Table 3. The effects of AGN 1133 and AGN 1135 on MPTP-induced decrements in the neostriatal content of dopamine and its metabolites. The mice were given the AGN 1133 or AGN 1135 at 2.5 mg/1g on day 1. On day 2 some of the mice were given 4 injections of MPTP, at two hour intervals. The dose of MPTP was 0.113 mMoles/kg for each injection (total dose equalled 0.453 mMoles/kg. The mice were sacrificed on days 8 and 9, and the neostriatal levels of dopamine and its metabolites determined. The data are expressed in ug/g of tissue ± SD. 3.OMeDA, 3-methoxy dopamine.

MAOI	MPTP	n	DA	DOPAC	HVA	3-OMeDA
				(ug/g tissue)		
-	-	8	12.5 ± 0.9	2.9 ± 0.5	1.3 ± 0.1	0.8 ± 0.1
AGN-1133	-	5	14.0 ± 1.6	1.5 ± 0.2	1.1 ± 0.1	1.0 ± 0.1
AGN-1135	-	5	13.2 ± 1.4	2.0 ± 0.3	1.4 ± 0.2	0.7 ± 0.1
-	+	9	1.9 ± 0.9	0.9 ± 0.4	0.7 ± 0.2	0.4 ± 0.2
AGN-1133	+	8	14.3 ± 1.1	1.4 ± 0.3	1.0 ± 0.1	0.9 ± 0.1
AGN-1135	+	8	13.2 ± 1.1	2.0 ± 0.3	1.3 ± 0.1	0.6 ± 0.1

1,200 patients treated with l-deprenyl for the past nine years and compared them to similar groups on levodopa therapy. The analysis of the data showed a significant prolongation of duration of Parkinson's disease, i.e. longevity of l-deprenyl-levodopa treated patients was substantially extended (Fig. 4). The results were interpreted by us in an earlier preliminary report (58) as being indicative of l-deprenyl's action in retarding the degeneration of dopamine neurons. This phenomenon so far has not been observed with any other anti-Parkinson drug. In the light of these findings and the fact that MAO B inhibitors (l-deprenyl and AGN 1135) prevent the dopaminergic-neurotoxicity of MPTP, can it be said that Parkinson's disease may not be due to a neurotoxic event (59). Whatever the mechanism of action of MAO B inhibitors in the treatment of Parkinson's disease or their prevention of MPTP induced loss of dopamine nerve cells in pars compacta of substantia nigra, it is apparent that inhibition of MAO B is all important. Therefore, these drugs represent a new approach to the treatment and understanding of the pathogenesis and origin of classical Parkinson's disease and that induced by MPTP.

PHARMACOLOGY OF MAO B INHIBITORS

MAO inhibitors, like other drugs, possess intrinsic pharmacological activity in addition to their MAO inhibiting property. These additional pharmacological actions may be reversible and short lasting, as opposed to their irreversible inactivation of MAO. They could very well contribute to their overall activity (14). The report that l-deprenyl did not potentiate, and even inhibited, the effects of tyramine in a number of pharmacological preparations (25) was confirmed in human subjects (60). At a dose of l-deprenyl which was adequate for selective inhibition of MAO type B, the pressor effect of orally administered tyramine was not potentiated. The non-potentiation of tyramine effects by l-deprenyl was attributed by

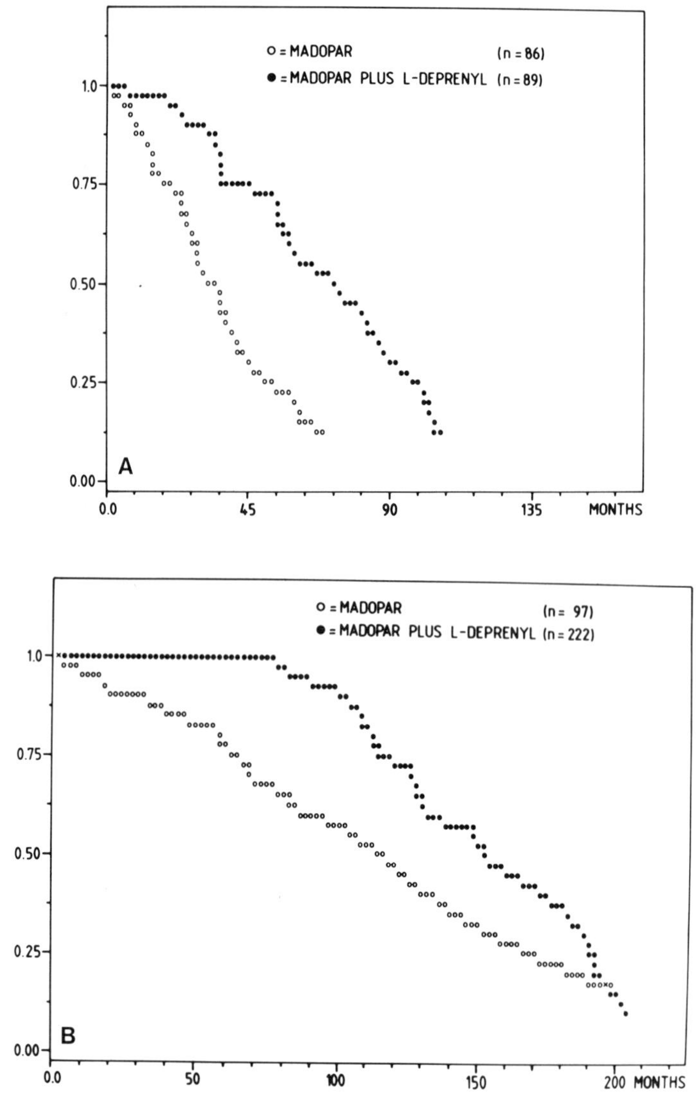

Fig. 4. Life expectancies of Madopar (l-dopa plus benzerazide, peripheral decarboxylase inhibitor) and Madopar l-deprenyl treated Parkinsonian patients with mean ages (A) 75 and (B) 65 years. Covariants included sex, age and duration of treatment using Breslow and Mantel-Cox test statistics.

Knoll to several factors: a) l-deprenyl does not inhibit intestinal MAO in man, which is of type A and thus tyramine can be deaminated, b) l-deprenyl blocks neuronal amine uptake and c) l-deprenyl blocks release of noradrenaline from storage vesicles. Finberg et al., (39) have investigated the tyramine antagonistic property of l-deprenyl and AGN 1135. While in isolated rat vas deferens both compounds antagonized tyramine responses, in whole animal they did not potentiate tyramine pressor responses at doses which selectively inhibited MAO B. However, at higher <u>in vivo</u> doses both l-deprenyl and AGN 1135 potentiated the pressor effects of tyramine, probably due to loss of MAO inhibitory selectivity. The inhibition of amine uptake system does not fully explain the results since neither drug was able to inhibit ^{3}H-metaraminol, ^{3}H-octopamine, ^{3}H-tyramine or ^{3}H-noradrenaline at concentrations of 10^{-4}-10^{-5}M in vas deferens while desmethylimipramine (10^{-6}M) did so (39). Tyramine antagonistic property of both l-deprenyl and AGN 1135 in isolated tissues is seen only at high inhibitor concentrations and may be related to α-adrenoreceptor antagonism (61).

It may not be necessary to look for a pharmacological mechanism for lack of "cheese effect" by l-deprenyl and AGN 1135 in view of the fact that neuronal MAO is mainly type A (62,63) and since all selective MAO A inhibitors (reversible and irreversible) do produce the "cheese effect" (14,38,64). Tyramine, an indirectly acting sympathomimetic amine must be taken up by sympathomimetic neurons in order to release noradrenaline which produces the effect on the adrenoreceptor. Release of noradrenaline by tyramine is not by an exocytatic process but by displacement into the neuronal cytosplasm so that such displaced noradrenaline is partially metabolized by MAO before egress from the neurons (39,65). Therefore, it follows that inhibition of MAO A would produce a profound affect on tyramine responsiveness by a) reducing metabolism of tyramine with the neurons, and b) protecting the released noradrenaline (substrate for MAO A) from metabolism by MAO within the neurone. To support this concept, Simpson (66) showed that the sympathomimetic action of amphetamine, an indirectly acting amine, itself not metabolized by MAO, was potentiated by clorgyline but not by l-deprenyl.

Regarding the lack of <u>in vivo</u> tyramine pressor potentiation by l-deprenyl and AGN 1135, it should be remembered that tyramine is a substrate for MAO A and well as MAO B. Thus the inhibition of type B would not prevent its metabolism by MAO A in the gut, lover or pulmonary circulation when given intravenously or orally. Thus selective inhibition of MAO in the gut and eeuron, which is predominantly MAO A (64), would facilitate tyramine uptake resulting in increased release of noradrenaline.

SUMMARY

The biochemical and pharmacological action of MAO B inhibitors lend themselves to be suitable drugs for potentiation of levodopa effects in Parkinson's disease. We believe they offer a new approach for the treatment of Parkinson's disease because:

1. l-Deprenyl potentiates the action of levodopa leading to a 30-50% reduction of daily dose of the latter, resulting in decreased incidents of side effects.

2. l-Deprenyl induces the recouping of levodopa action in those patients who have lost their response and diminishes the occurrence and duration of "on-off" effects.

3. In an open uncontrolled study, l-deprenyl has been shown to increase the life expectancy of Parkinsonian patients significantly. This suggests for the first time the course of Parkinson's disease can be altered by a drug, which may retard the degeneration of dopaminergic neurones. This hypothesis receives support from animal experimental studies with MPTP, a compound which causes Parkinsonism in human and animals clearly similar to classical Parkinson's disease.

REFERENCES

1. O. Hornykiewicz, Br. Med. Bull. 29:172 (1973)
2. D. B. Calne and J. K. Kebabian, J. Neural Transm. Suppl. 16, 1 (1980).
3. P. A. Le Witt and D. B. Calne, J. Neural Transm. 51:175 (1981).
4. S. Fahn, R. Comi, S.R. Snyder and A. L. N. Prasad, in: "Catecholamines: Basic and Clinical Frontiers," E. Usdin, I.J. Kopin and D. Barchas, eds., Pergamon Press, New York (1979). pp 225-230.
5. M. B. H. Youdim, J. P. M. Finberg and U. Wajsbort, in: "Progress in Medicinal Chemistry," G. P. Ellis and G. B. West, eds., Elsevier, Amsterdam (1985).
6. G. C. Davis, A. C. Williams, S. P. Markey, M. H. Ebert, E. D. Caine, C. M. Reichert and I. J. Kopin, Psychiat. Res. 1:249 (1979).
7. J. W. Langston, P. Ballard, J. W. Tetrud and I. Irwin, Science 219:979 (1983).
8. R. S. Burns, C. C. Chiuen, S. P. Markey, M. H. Ebert, D. M. Jacobowitz and I. J. Kopin, Proc. Natl. Acad. Sci. U.S.A. 80:4546 (1983).
9. W. Birkmayer, R. Riederer, L. Ambrozi and M. B. H. Youdim, Lancet 1:439 (1977).
10. M. Yahr, J. Neural Transm. 48:227 (1978).
11. U. K. Rinne, Acta Neurol. Scand. 68:7 (1983).
12. R. E. Heikkila, A. Hess and R. C. Duvoisin, Science 224:1451 (1984).
13. R. E. Heikkila, L. Manzio, F. S. Cabbat and R. C. Duvoisin, Nature 311: 467 (1984).

13a. R. E. Heikkila, J. P. M. Finberg and M. B. H. Youdim (1985) submitted.

14. M. B. H. Youdim and J. P. M. Finberg, in: "Psychopharmacology I," D. G. Grahame-Smith, ed., Excerpta Medica, Amsterdam (1982). pp 37-54.
15. A. R. Green, B. D. Mitchell, A. Tordoff and M. B. H. Youdim, Br. J. Pharmac. 60:343 (1977).
16. D. Kuhn, W. Wolf and M. B. H. Youdim, Br. J. Pharmac. (1985) in press.
17. A. Carlsson and M. Lindquist, Acta Pharmac.Tox. 20:140 (1963).
18. N. E. Anden, B. E. Roos and B. Werdinins, Life Sci. 3:149 (1964).
19. M. J. Beson, A. Cheramy, J. Glowinski and C. Gauchy, in: "Frontiers in Catecholamine Research," E. Usdin and S. Snyder, eds., Pergamon Press, New York (1973). pp 557-560.
20. M. B. H. Youdim, G. G. S. Collins and M. Sandler, Biochem. J. 34:121 (1971).
21. A. J. Davies, M. Holzbauer, D. F. Sharman and M. B. H. Youdim, Br. J. Pharmac. 55:558 (1975).
22. D. Blatchford, M. Holzbauer, D. G. Grahame-Smith and M. B. H. Youdim, Br. J. Pharmac. 57:279 (1976).
23. G. G. S. Collins, M. Sandler, E. D. S. Williams and M. B. H. Youdim, Nature (Lond) 225:817 (1970).
24. J. P. Johnston, Biochem. Pharmac. 17:1285 (1968).
25. J. Knoll and K. Magyar, Adv. Biochem. Psychopharmac. 5:352 (1972).
26. P. H. Yu, J. Pharm. Pharmac. 36:2 (1984).
27. N. H. Neff and J. A. Fuentes, in: "Monoamine Oxidase and Its Inhibition," Ciba Foundation Symposium No. 39 (New Series), Elsevier, Amsterdam (1976). pp 163-180.
28. H. Y. T. Yang and N. H. Neff, J. Pharmac. Exp. Ther. 187:365 (1973).
29. C. Goridis and N. H. Neff, Neuropharmacology 10:552 (1971).
30. P. Levitt, J. E. Pintar and X. O. Breakefield, Proc. Natl. Acad. Sci. (U.S.A.) 79:6385 (1982).
31. K. F. Tipton, M. D. Houslay and T. J. Mantle, in: "Monoamine Oxidase and Its Inhibition," Ciba Foundation Symposium No. 39 (New Series), Elsevier, Amsterdam (1976). pp 5-32.
32. R. Squires, Adv. Biochem. Psychopharmac. 5:355 (1972).
33. M. B. H. Youdim, in: " Neuroregulators and Psychiatric Disorders," E. Usdin, D. Hamburg and J. D. Barchas, eds., Oxford University Press, New York (1977). pp 57-67.

34. V. Glover, M. Sandler, F. Owen and G. J. Riley, Nature (Lond) 265:80 (1977).
35. A. M. O'Carroll, C. J. Fowler, J. P. Phillips, I. Tobbia and K. F. Tipton, Arch. Pharmac. 322:198 (1983).
36. H. Bernheimer, W. Birkmayer and O. Hornykiewicz, Wr. Klin. Wschr. 74: 558 (1962).
37. M. B. H. Youdim, G. G. S. Collins and M. Sandler, Nature (Lond) 236: 225 (1972).
38. M. B. H. Youdim and J. P. M. Finberg, in:"Psychopharmacology II," D. G. Grahame-Smith, ed., Excerpta Medica, Amsterdam (1985) in press.
39. J. P. M. Finberg, M. Tenne and M. B. H. Youdim, Br. J. Pharmac. 73:65 (1981).
40. N. H. Neff, H-Y. T. Yang and C. Goridis, in: "Frontiers in Catecholamines," E. Usdin and S. H. Snyder, eds., Pergamon Press, New York (1973). pp 133-138.
41. W. Birkmayer, P. Riederer, M. B. H. Youdim and W. Linauer, J. Neural Transm. 36:303 (1975).
42. W. Birkmayer, P. Riederer, L. Ambrozi and M. B. H. Youdim, Lancet 1, 439 (1977).
43. A. J. Lees, L. J. Kohout, K. M. Shaw, G. M. Stern, J. D. Elsworth, M. Sandler and M. B. H. Youdim, Lancet 2:791 (1977).
44. L. Riederer, G. Reynolds and M. B. H. Youdim, in: "Monoamine Oxidase Inhibitors - The State of the Art," M. B. H. Youdim and G. S. Paykel, eds., Wiley, Chichester (1980). pp 167-181.
45. G. M. Stern, A. J. Lees and M. Sandler, J. Neural Transm. 43:245 (1978).
46. J. D. Elsworth, M. Sandler, A. J. Lees and C. Ward, J. Neural Transm. 54:105 (1982).
47. G. M. Stern, A. J. Lees, R. J. Hardie and M. Sandler, Acta Neural. Scand. Suppl. 95, 68:113 (1983).
48. J. W. Langston, I. Irwin, E. B. Langston and L. S. Forno, Science 225: 1482 (1984).
49. R. S. Burns, S. P. Markey, J. M. Phillips and C. C. Chiuen, Can. J. Neurol. Sci. 11:166 (1984).
50. J. W. Langston and P. Ballard, Can. J. Neurol.Sci. 11:160 (198).pp1983.
51. P. A. Ballard, J. W. Tetrud and J. W. Langston, Neurology (1985) in press.
52. B. Parsons and T. Rainbow, Eur. J. Pharmacol. 102:375 (1984).
53. M. B. H. Youdim, Eur. J. Pharmacol. (1985) in press.
54. A. Kalir, A. Sabbagh and M. B. H. Youdim, Br. J. Pharmacol. 73:55 (1981).
55. M. B. H. Youdim, J. P. M. Finberg and K. F. Tipton, in: "Catecholamine II. Handbook of Experimental Pharmacology," N. Weiner and U. Trendlenburg, eds., Springer-Verlag, Berlin (1985) in press.
56. J. Wajsbort, K. Kartmazov, B. Oppenheim, R. Barkey and M. B. H. Youdim, J. Neurol Transm. 55:201 (1982).
57. M. Sandler, in: "Neuroregulators and Psychiatric Disorders, E. Usdin, D. Hamburg and J. Barchas, eds., Oxford University Press, New York (1977). pp 68-74.
58. W. Birkmayer, J. Knoll, P. Riederer and M. B. H. Youdim, Mod. Probl. Pharmacopsychiat. 19:170 (1983).
59. D. Calne and J. W. Langston, Lancet 11, 1457 (1983).
60. J. D. Elsworth, V. Glover, G. P. Reynolds, M. Sandler, A. J. Lees, P. Phuapradit, K. Shaw, G. M. Stern and P. Kumar, Psychopharmacology 57:33 (1978).
61. J. P. M Finberg and M. Tenne, Br. J. Pharmacol. 77:13 (1982).
62. N. H. Neff and C. Goridis, Adv. Biochem. Psycho. Pharmacol. 5:307 (1972).
63. B. Jarrott and L. L. Iversen, J. Neurochem. 18:1 (1971).
64. J. P. M. Finberg and M. B. H. Youdim, in: "Monoamine Oxidase and Disease," K. F. Tipton and M. Strolin-Benedetti, eds., Academic Press, London (1984). pp 479-486.

65. F. Brando, E. Rodrigues-Pereira, J. G. Monteiro and W. Osswald, Arch. Pharmacol. 311:9 (1980).
66. L. L. Simpson, J. Pharmacol. Exp. Ther. 205:392 (1978).

ALZHEIMER'S AND PARKINSON'S DISEASE: STRATEGIES IN RESEARCH AND DEVELOPMENT

GENERAL DISCUSSION

Moderated and summarized by

Israel Hanin

Department of Psychiatry
Western Psychiatric Institute and Clinic
University of Pittsburgh School of Medicine
Pittsburgh, Pennsylvania 15213, USA

The 30th OHOLO Biological Conference concluded with a stimulating and provocative general discussion, on the afternoon of the last day of the meetings. Eleven specific questions were posed to the audience, based on issues and topics which had been raised in the presentations and posters prior to this Discussion. The audience was asked to consider each question in turn, and to debate its pros and cons. Over three hours were dedicated to this General Discussion.

The following consists of a presentation of each of the eleven question which were posed, and a capsule of the discussions which followed. All attempts have been made to be as accurate as possible in the identification of the participants involved, and in the summary of their statements. The author extends his apology in advance, to those who may have been misrepresented or even worse, overlooked, in the following narrative.

QUESTION 1: WHY ARE PARKINSON'S DISEASE AND ALZHEIMER'S DISEASE PARTICULARLY EVIDENT IN AGING?

Dr. London initiated the discussion by wondering whether in fact these disease actually begin to occur in the individual prior to senescence. The symptoms however may not be evident until neurochemical losses which are known to occur in aging (e.g. reduction in tyrosine hydroxylase and choline acetyltransferase levels in the brain) are superimposed on the disease process. **Dr. Wisniewski** disagreed with the above suggestion. He indicated that, from a pathological point of view, Alzheimer's and Parkinson's Disease both generally appear to occur after the individual reaches the age of 50. He proposed, instead, that old age leads to loss of reserve, and makes us vulnerable to ubiquitous external factors which in turn induce these disease states. Those individuals who are more susceptible than others to the detrimental effects in the environment may be the ones who end up contracting Alzheimer's or Parkinson's Disease. **Dr. Korczyn** suggested, alternatively, that the reason that some individuals contract Parkinson's Disease and others do not may simply be due to the fact that, by natural variability, some individuals lose their dopaminergic cells faster than others. This may be purely an individual phenomenon which cannot be predicted in advance. Once the cause is known, however, steps could be taken to attempt to arrest or retard the degenerative process. **Dr. Cohen** wondered whether there are any records in the history of ancient medicine of cases which could be identified as Alzheimer's Disease or any other types of dementia. This provocative question was brought up in an attempt to enquire whether natural selection of our species may in any way have been affected/influenced in the past by cases of dementia of various types. **Dr. Leventhal** referred back to Dr. Wisnieski's earlier comments, and pointed out that AIDS, as well as some of the common autoimmune diseases (e.g. rheumatoid arthritis, lupus, thyroiditis, etc.) are not commonly seen in aged people. Hence, he questioned the possibility that there may be a loss in immune capacity with age that leads to the development of Alzheimer's Disease. **Dr. Wisniewski** added that although not all cancers are caused by viruses, there is an increase in the incidence of neoplastic diseases with age. He therefore suggested that there is a genetic component inherent in susceptibility of an individual to contracting Alzheimer's Disease; possibly a problem inherent in an "aging gene" that is more readily affected by external environmental factors.

QUESTION 2: WHAT IS THE ROLE OF THE BLOOD BRAIN BARRIER (BBB) IN THE ETIOLOGY OF PARKINSON'S AND ALZHEIMER'S DISEASE? IS THE BBB COMPROMISED OR ALTERED IN ANY WAY IN THE DISEASE STATE?

Dr. Growdon indicated that amino acids, and choline, both putative precursors of neurotransmitter substances in the brain, have been measured in the cerebrospinal fluid (CSF), as an index of the transport of these substances from the periphery into the central nervous system. There was essentially no difference in the content of various amino acids measured in CSF of normals and of patients with Parkinson's Disease; or of levels of CSF choline in normals versus patients with Alzheimer's Disease. These results were interpreted as indicating that, at least the transport of nutrients such as amino acids and choline, is not compromised in patients with either of the above two diseases. **Dr. Wisnieski** reminded the audience that he and his colleagues have shown, using polyclonal and monoclonal antibodies, that the BBB appears indeed to be compromised in Alzheimer's Disease. Moreover, he also suggested that small vessel pathology should also be considered in this disease state. To date people have concerned themselves primarily with multi-infarct dementia, which is the result of large vessel pathology. However, the BBB may actually in part be compromised as the result of extensive infiltration by amyloid of the wall of the microvessels. **Dr. Moss** pointed out that, unlike the other major transmitters, acetylcholine is not an amino acid or a simple modification of amino acids. Alzheimer's Disease therefore probably is not related in any way to nutrient transport. Rather, metabolic and therapeutic aspects of choline metabolism vis-a-vis the membrane would most likely be the direction to take in studying changes in membrane such as those involved in the BBB, in individual neurons, microtubules, etc.

QUESTION 3: WHY IS THE CHOLINERGIC SYSTEM SELECTIVELY TARGETED IN ALZHEIMER'S DISEASE? ARE THE EFFECTS SEEN ON OTHER NEUROTRANSMITTER SYSTEMS SECONDARY TO THIS INITIAL CHOLINERGIC DEFICIT?

Dr. Gamzu proposed that we focus on the question whether indeed the cholinergic deficit is primary in Alzheimer's Disease. Other neurotransmitter systems are also involved, and they too may be key elements in the etiology of the disease state. **Dr. Hanin** pointed out as an aside that very little had been said about somatostatin at this conference. He wondered about this apparent omission. **Dr. Korczyn** echoed Dr. Gamzu's feeling that the cholinergic system indeed may not be the primary neurotransmitter affected in Alzheimer's Disease, even if cholinergic agonists have been shown to be effective in improving memory in human subjects, controls included. With regards to somatostatin, he suggested that little has been said so far about this neurotransmitter simply because less is known about it at this stage. As more information is gained about the role of somatostatin as a neurotransmitter, more work and information regarding its role in the etiology of Alzheimer's Disease will be forthcoming. **Dr. Fisher** argued that a cholinergic deficit is always, and consistently, evident in Alzheimer's Disease, while other neurotransmitters are not always affected to a similar extent. This, he felt, plus the fact that the only known approaches (albeit not very effective) for the improvement of memory deficits in Alzheimer's Disease are with the use of cholinergic agonists, was strong evidence in favor of the cholinergic hypothesis in Alzheimer's Disease. **Dr. Growdon** asked whether the neuropathologists in the audience could help settle this question with regards to the central role of the cholinergic system in Alzheimer's Disease, in view of the fact that some evidence had been presented earlier at this meeting demonstrating actually an increase (rather than a decrease) in choline acetyltransferase activity in four patients treated for Alzheimer's Disease. **Dr. Bowen** responded by stating that he had studied a small group of relatively elderly demented patients with plaque and tangle formation of an intensity consistent with a diagnosis of Alzheimer's Disease which did not show reduced choline acetyltransferase activity in either neocortex or hippocampus. However, these brains generally did not have intense plaque or tangle formation, so the senile morphology could have been due to a change in aging, rather than indicative of Alzheimer's Disease. **Dr. Hanin** pointed out the diversity in the literature vis-a-vis the spelling of the abbreviation of choline acetyltransferase. Some use "CAT", and some use "ChAT" for this purpose. He suggested that a uniform abbreviation be adopted, and recommended that it be "ChAT", in line with the abbreviation of choline, which is accepted as "Ch". **Dr. Butcher** next offered two comments. First, with regards to somatostatin, he felt that the reason little has been said about it so far is that very little is known about its central function, or about its origins and projection pathways. In response to the question raised earlier regarding the selective sensitivity of cholinergic neurons in Alzheimer's Disease, he suggested that the reason may be in the size of the cholinergic neurons in the brain. Terry and colleagues have shown that large neurons are preferentially affected in Alzheimer's Disease. Virtually all choline acetyltransferase-positive, probably cholinergic, cells in the basal forebrain are large, not only in soma dimensions (25-40um) but also in total amount of protein and surface area. It is conceivable that such cells would be more likely, by virtue of their larger absorptive surface, to take up toxic substances (such as aluminum). Intraneuronal accumulation of the toxic substance to cytotoxic levels might occur more rapidly in the cholinergic neurons; therefore these neurons might die sooner. **Dr. Sarter** proposed an alternative explanation for the atrophic effects in Alzheimer's Disease. He pointed out that the basal forebrain neurons project in a very restricted way via collaterals to the cortex, and terminate in a very restricted cortical region. This is different from, for example, the raphe neurons, which innervate widespread cortical areas. Retrograde degeneration as a result of cortical atrophy may be more effective on basal forebrain nerve cell degeneration than on other subcortical structures. Thus, cortical atrophy may represent the major symptom, as Alzheimer stated originally, and basal forebrain degeneration may be the most striking consequence of this effect, in Alzheimer's Disease. **Dr. Mayeux** drew a parallelism between Parkinson's Disease and Alzheimer's Disease. Initially, dopamine was implicated as the key neurotransmitter affected in Parkinson's Disease. With time it was found that other neurotransmitters, e.g. norepinephrine and serotonin were also reduced in Parkinson's Disease. He suggested that, in a similar manner, in Alzheimer's Disease the cholinergic deficit might be primary, but that other neurotransmitters may also be implicated. **Dr. Rabey** suggested that one should try to gain more information about calcium availability in old age. He suggested that some of the degenerative effects observed in Alzheimer's Disease might be due to a reduction in calcium availability, coupled with excess aluminum and reduced glucose availability.

QUESTION 4: ARE ENDOTOXINS OR EXOTOXINS INVOLVED IN THE ETIOLOGY OF ALZHEIMER'S, OR PARKINSON'S DISEASE?

Dr. Munoz-Garcia pointed out that, in his opinion, the accumulation of a non-metabolizable exo- or endotoxin would be the simplest explanation for the observed increase in the incidence of Alzheimer's Disease in the aged population. **Dr. Youdim** referred to recent findings with MPTP, which provide a strong argument favoring the concept that, at least in Parkinson's Disease, the disorder may be caused as a result of an endogenous neurotoxin. **Dr. Perl** reminded the audience that there are a number of exogenous neurotoxins with very precise patterns of destruction. Three specific examples include: a) the selective destruction of the occipital cortex and cerebellum caused by methyl mercury; b) the precise destruction of hippocampus produced by trimethyl tin; and c) the selective destruction of globus pallidus neurons, demonstrated in the classic studies of Cotzias, related to exposure to manganese. The mechanisms for these selective patterns of neuronal destruction remain, however, unknown. **Dr. Fisher** reiterated the suggestion, elaborated on in his previous lecture (see chapter by Fisher and Hanin, this book), that the destruction seen in cholinergic nerve teminals in Alzheimer's Disease might be due to a cytotoxic complex of betaine aldehyde, generated <u>in vivo</u>, with aluminum, which is obtained <u>ex vivo</u>. **Dr. LeWitt** suggested that one should look at populations subjected to chronic hypoxia, to see whether they show a different incidence of dementia from that seen in individuals living under normoxic conditions. **Dr. Wisniewski** pointed out that the olfactory system is also affected in Alzheimer's Disease. This implies that some exogenous toxin may be penetrating into the individual via the olfactory pathway. He also indicated that he has found that the blood brain barrier is compromised in scrapie treated animals, and possibly also in animals injected with Alzheimer material. These findings would favor the infectious hypothesis for the etiology of Alzheimer's Disease. **Dr. Van Den Bosch**, added that some toxic substance apparently develops <u>in vivo</u> with aging. He is using the approach of implanting Alzheimer tissue into fetal material, and believes that this approach will eventually be extremely useful for the study of the development of this toxin. The identity of this toxin is as yet unknown, and is subject to further investigation at this time. **Dr. Spiegelstein** expressed his interest in knowing more about the possible involvement of an autoimmune disease in the etiology of Alzheimer's Disease. Due to a lack of time during this Round Table Discussion, it was felt that this subject should be returned to in much more detail, in the next conference on Alzheimer's Disease.

QUESTION 5: ARE THERE ADEQUATE CRITERIA TODAY, WHICH ENABLE ONE TO DISTINGUISH ALZHEIMER'S DISEASE FROM OTHER DEMENTIAS? FROM DEPRESSION?

Dr. Davous started out by asking the experts in the audience what were the criteria by which one could identify Alzheimer's Disease from the onset, and what were the best instruments with which one could do so. **Dr. Growdon** indicated that the criteria developed by the NINCDS were, in his opinion, the best available to date. He did add, however, that even with the best available instruments there is a chance of misdiagnosing by more than 15% of all cases. He therefore placed emphasis on the need for concurrent biological laboratory tests, to assist in the diagnosis and selective identification of Alzheimer's Disease. **Dr. Rozin** indicated, from his own clinical experience, that it is extremely difficult to pick up the early case of Alzheimer's Disease. Clinical signs of cognitive defect only occur after much tissue has actually been lost. Thus, he also spoke in favor of better biological antemortem diagnoses as an aid in the identification of the illness. Dr. Rozin further pointed out that other than cognitive defects also occur early on in the onset of ALzheimer's Disease, such as gait abnormalities, and that these should also be carefully considered in the early diagnosis of the illness, even though such neurological abnormalities are not selective for Alzheimer's Disease alone. **Dr. Salamone** proposed that we should be looking differentially at patients with early onset pre-senile dementia, versus senile dementia. There is evidence that younger demented individuals have more severe global neurochemical deficits than the older, demented subjects. **Dr. Korczyn** reminded the audience of the high incidence of infarcts, which confounds the diagnostic process in the clinic. **Dr. Rabey** added that scanning techniques have demonstrated a large incidence of vascular lesions in many of the patients. He therefore was interested in having an indication whether one should look carefully at the neuropathological picture, compare it with the vascular picture, and somehow be able, with this information, to separate "pure" Alzheimer patients from those suffering from "mixed dementia". An unidentified participant (who did not state his name for the tape recording of this discussion) provided an optimistic note to the effect that, over the past ten years, there has been a progressive improvement in the available tools to identify Alzheimer's Disease, with a current specificity of 90% accurate diagnosis of Alzheimer's Disease. Hence, we have a good prognosis for the future. **Dr. Hanin** expressed his surprise at the high (90%) statement of diagnostic accuracy mentioned by the previous seaker, and questioned this assertion. **Dr. LeWitt** stressed the importance of separating in our discussions dementia per se from the diagnosis of Alzheimer's Disease. He has treated nondemented patients with clear-cut Alzheimer pathology (determined with biopsy). Thus, the disease/pathology could be there even though the symptoms do not occur. Consequently, clinicians might actually be underdiagnosing those patients who have the pathology in them, as well as perhaps overdiagnosing people who have the accumulation of life time use of alcohol, of head trauma, of pseudodementia in depression, etc. He therefore stressed the importance of holding, for research purposes, to very strict criteria, such as the NINCDS criteria. **Dr. Oppenheim** expressed his concern that too much emphasis is being placed on the memory disturbances of Alzheimer's Disease. He reminded the audience that Alzheimer's Disease is expressed by a large constellation of other manifestations including severe behavioral disturbances, extreme disturbance in judgement, possibly delusions, sleep disorder, apathy in all areas, overeating combined with paradoxical weight loss, possibly dysphasia and dyspraxia, etc. He emphasized, therefore, the need to learn more about the neurochemical basis of the other integral symptoms of Alzheimer's Disease as well.

QUESTION 6: PHYSOSTIGMINE, BETHANECHOL, AND OTHER CHOLINERGIC AGONISTS. ARE THEY THE DRUGS OF CHOICE IN THE TREATMENT OF ALZHEIMER'S DISEASE?

Dr. Edery stated that physostigmine has been used extensively in humans, and its effects are well known. He suggested that it be administered in patients with Alzheimer's Disease directly into the ventricles, since there is a favorable precedent for such an approach with other agents, and since intraventricular administration will deliver the compound in the vicinity of the hippocampus. Alternatively, he suggested that physostigmine could be administered in patients by slow infusion, in the presence of a peripheral cholinesterase inhibitor. **Dr. Hanin** wondered whether slow infusion of a compound which is rapidly broken down _in vivo_, such as physostigmine, would be an effective approach. **Dr. Cohen** responded that, in order to attain a steady state level of a compound _in vivo_ one would best involve a slow infusion technique. On the other hand, however, he questioned the utility of using a cholinesterase inhibitor such as physostigmine for the purpose of activating cholinergic receptors. Cholinesterase inhibitors augment the lifetime of available stores of acetylcholine, which are known to be compromised in Alzheimer's Disease. On the other hand, a muscarinic agonist, such as bethanechol, would act directly on existing muscarinic receptors, which apparently are not severely compromised in this disease state. Thus the latter should be a more efficient tool in the treatment of Alzheimer's Disease. **Dr. Davous** next reported on preliminary studies which he has conducted using bethanechol, in Alzheimer patients. Using oral (75 mg) bethanechol for 6 months he did not observe any significant reduction of global dementia in his patients. On the other hand, when bethanechol was administered by the subcutaneous route to ten patients, it significantly reduced their reaction time within 15 minutes, with a rebound at 30 minutes. Thus, in summary, bethanechol had a slight effect compared to placebo in a short term trial. However, the results obtained were not better than those seen following physostigmine administration. **Dr. Oppenheim** expressed his concern about the recent report by Harbough et al. (Neurosurgery 15:514-518, 1984) regarding the intracranial infusion of bethanechol. The study was done only in four patients; it involved a craniotomy; the evaluation of the patients was done based upon family impressions of the patients' condition; and the study could not possibly have been double-blind, because of the side effects of bethanechol. Unfortunately, Dr. Harbough did not participate in this conference, and could not therefore respond to this criticism. **Dr. Middlemiss** asked whether anyone had tried the intranasal route of administration of cholinergic compounds. **Dr. Growdon** suggested that, as we begin to explore the role of different peptides in Alzheimer's Disease, the intraventricular route of administration might be more useful. Most of the peptides do not cross the blood brain barrier in sufficient quantities. As far as the intranasal administration is concerned, this approach is not very effective nor is it commonly used. **Dr. Lerer** posed a fundamental, yet provocative question. She wondered why encouraging results seen in experimental animals, utilizing nootropic agents and cholinesterase inhibitors etc, are not readily reproduced in the clinic. **Dr. Hanin** ventured that this might be inherent in the different drug histories of the human subjects involved, as well as in the individual variability among human subjects, unlike the inbred similarities that exist in our experimental animals, particularly rodents. **Dr. Munoz-Garcia** suggested that an alternative explanation might be inherent in the fact that, in the rat, we are assuming a cholinergic deficit. In the Alzheimer patient, however, the disease state might involve much more than a simple cholinergic deficit.

QUESTION 7: ARE THERE SPONTANEOUS MEMORY DEFICITS IN DOMESTIC ANIMALS?

Dr. Edery assured the audience that this question was not proposed in jest. We have ready access to two domestic animal species which have a long lifetime: the dog and the horse. Dogs, for instance, contract epilepsy similar to that seen in humans. Thus, there may be certain illnesses that are common to man and to one or the other of these species. If Alzheimer's Disease is caused by viral or exotoxic mechanisms, perhaps the same disease will be contracted by the dog or horse living in close proximity with its master. Therefore, Dr. Edery proposed that we look closer at this possibility, in conjunction with clinical veterinarians. **Dr. Gamzu** reminded the audience that within a regular population of experimental rats, one can discern those that learn better than others. In fact, poor performers and superior performers in certain behavioral tasks have been isolated and even bred. However, this condition is not necessarily age dependent, and is specific for the particular test/maze on which the animals are being evaluated. **Dr. Sanberg** suggested that interpretation of behavioral data in experimental animals is highly dependent on the test used. Hence one must be cautious when making inferences based on one or two behavioral tests. He also stressed the fact that rats are nocturnal animals, and that their behavior is considerably different at night than it is during the day. Thus, this is another confounding factor with which we should concern ourselves. Dr. Sanberg suggested, consequently, that we should start testing animals in a more analogous way that we test humans, especially if we will be making large inferences from animals to humans. **Dr. Butcher** informed the audience that old cats (17-24 years old) have difficulty learning in a classical conditioning paradigm. He referred in this comment to studies conducted previously by Dr. Jennifer Buchwald at UCLA. **Dr. Wisniewski** pointed out that, in an old dog, he has recently found neurofibrillary changes at the light microscopic level, including plaques and tangles, comparable to those seen in Alzheimer's Disease. At the electron microscopic level, however, he was not able to find paired helical filaments. Owners of aged dogs also have reported signs of mental deficiency in their pets, such as inability to identify their owners, inability to find their food, and incontinence. These symptoms appear to be remarkably similar to symptoms of dementia in man.

QUESTION 8: RECEPTOR DISTRIBUTION: DOES IT CHANGE IN ALZHEIMER'S DISEASE?

Dr. London stressed the importance of uniform brain area sampling techniques. Receptor changes may be specific for very discrete brain regions. For example, Dr. London, in collaboration with Drs. Ball and Waller have shown increased densities of muscarinic receptors in Alzheimer's Disease in specific cortical gyri. However, these observations are obliterated when one combines data from entire cortical lobes. Another important consideration is the drug history of the patients under study. Alzheimer patients frequently receive antidepressants, neuroleptics and other drugs, which can affect cholinergic systems either directly or indirectly. Dr. London suggested that such information is extremely important, yet often overlooked, and only anticholinergic medication is generally monitored in these patients.

QUESTION 9: AF64A (ETHYLCHOLINE MUSTARD AZIRIDINIUM): HOW SPECIFIC IS IT AS A CENTRAL CHOLINOTOXIN?

Dr. Sarter wondered whether there was any advantage in using AF64A over another behaviorally effective neurotoxin, e.g. ibotenic acid.

Dr. Fisher responded to the effect that AF64A is preferable to ibotenic or kainic acid due to the selective cholinotoxicity of the compound. The other two toxins have a general, more nonspecific locus of action. Of more importance, in his opinion, is the question of how much of a reduction of choline acetyltransferase activity is necessary, using any of these toxins, before one induces demonstrable behavioral deficits in an experimental animal. In response to the latter comment, **Dr. Lerer** related recent results in her lab showing that injection of only vehicle in the nucleus basalis will result in a 15% reduction in choline acetyltransferase activity, with no concurrent effect on the animals' behavior. Administration of kainic acid into the nucleus basalis, resulting in 18-20% in choline acetyltransferase loss does, on the other hand, result in significant behavioral deficits. She suggested, therefore, that the behavioral deficits might not be related to the decrease in choline acetyltransferase per se, but might in fact be due to some damage induced by the administration of the drug, or due to an effect on other neurotransmitters apart from the cholinergic system. **Dr. Levy** reiterated the selectivity of action of AF64A on cholinergic terminals. He did caution, however, that it is important to establish the appropriate dose and time relationships of action of the compound. Moreover, he stressed the importance of obtaining very careful histological data on the effect of AF64A *in vivo*, under the various conditions tested. **Dr. Heldman** pointed to several reported experimental facts, which strengthen the notion of a cholinotoxic action of AF64A. For example: the peripheral toxicity of AF64A is competitively antagonized by choline. Moreover, behavioral memory deficits induced by AF64A are reversed following cholinesterase inhibition. He did, on the other hand, caution potential users of AF64A that administration of the compound in very small volumes in essence represents local administration of extremely high, and hence toxic, concentrations of the compound. He suggested that we attempt to find different approaches to the effective administration of the compound, which would result in higher specificity of action of AF64A. **Dr. Schuurman** stated that, in his hands, 0.1 nmol AF64A in the nucleus basalis of rats showed some specificity for the cholinotoxicity of the compound, but no behavioral effects. Higher concentrations of AF64A resulted in behavioral effects, but also in some nonspecific lesions in the brain. He therefore suggested that a good animal model of Alzheimer's Disease has to meet three criteria: biochemical specificity, histological specificity, and behavioral effects - all with the same dosage. **Dr. Sanberg** reminisced about similar counterclaims on efficacy which were levelled on the use of kainic acid, during its initial use. The strain of animal, the batch of compound, even from the same company, and many other factors, contributed to differences in the efficacy of the compound in different laboratories. He suggested that AF64A is presently undergoing a similar evolution. **Dr. Youdim** next stated that many of the enzymes in the central nervous system are known to be in excess. Monoamine oxidase can be inhibited by up to 80%, and nothing appears to happen to neurotransmitter buildup or to the animal's behavior. Once the enzyme is inhibited further, however, one begins to see all the expected functional changes. **Dr. Reches** shared with the audience results which he had obtained vis-a-vis the effect of AF64A on dopaminergic transmission in the substantia nigra. In a dose and time study with AF64A he observed a toxic effect of AF64A on dopaminergic terminals in the striatum. He was not able to replicate earlier studies from Coyle's laboratories (Sandberg et al., Brain Res. 293:49-55, 1984) showing no adverse effects of AF64A administration on striatal tyrosine hydroxylase activity. **Dr. Levy** indicated that he has also seen lesions of the substantia nigra with AF64A administration. However, the behavior of these animals was different from those lesioned in the substantia nigra by other means. Hence, conceivably, the effect of AF64A may invoke some cholinergic component, in addition to the effect of the lesion, about which we do not, at present, have enough information. **Dr. Sarter** stated categorically that he prefers to work with ibotenic acid, because it is easier to handle than AF64A. **Dr. Hanin** summarized the various arguments around this question. He further suggested that the area of investigation with AF64A is currently undergoing the second of three phases through which all new toxins have had to endure. The first phase is one of disbelief in the effectiveness of the toxin. The second stage accepts the effectiveness of the toxin, but questions its mode of action and its specificity. The third and last stage is one of acceptance of the toxin by some investigators as a tool in their experimental approaches. Dr. Hanin was encouraged by the tremendous interest which has been generated by AF64A over the previous two years, and was pleased by the rational discussion on the topic which had transpired in this round table.

QUESTION 10: WHAT IS THE RELATIONSHIP BETWEEN BINDING TO CHOLINERGIC RECEPTORS AND ACTUAL FUNCTION?

Dr. London stated that we can indeed demonstrate functional activity of muscarinic receptors, by administering agonists and observing behavioral and metabolic changes. The question she asked, however, was whether tonic activation of muscarinic receptors (which appear intact in Alzheimer's Disease) would restore function in the same way as phasic transmitter release. If that is not the case, then administration of receptor stimulants in this disease state may not have much therapeutic benefit. **Dr. Nordberg** reviewed some of her recent findings using nicotine administration in animals. Nicotine generally increases acetylcholine release, alters passive avoidance behavior at low (0.125 mg/kg), but not at high (0.500 mg/kg) concentrations of administration, and binds with high affinity in the cerebral cortex. **Dr. Birdsall** pointed out that on the muscarinic receptor there is an allosteric binding site which is capable of "tuning up" or "tuning down" muscarinic receptor function. A drug interacting with that allosteric site would have no effect on its own. Rather, it would only come into action when there is neuronally released acetylcholine. The allosteric site is different in different parts of the brain, thus providing for selectivity as well. Dr. Birdsall suggested that a valuable drug in Alzheimer's Disease would be one that could "tune" the allosteric site in accordance with available acetylcholine released. **Dr. Cohen** asked where presynaptic muscarinic receptors would fit in the scheme of events regulating acetylcholine release and availability at the receptor site. **Dr. Birdsall** responded that they do apparently exist, but he did not feel that at the present time there is any indication of selective differences between presynaptic and postsynaptic receptors.

QUESTION 11: WHAT TYPES OF DRUGS SHOULD WE BE LOOKING FOR IN THE DEVELOPMENT OF TREATMENTS FOR ALZHEIMER'S DISEASE?

Dr. Moss felt that the most desirable drugs which one should develop for this purpose are effective, central nervous system - active irreversible cholinesterase inhibitors. He listed several advantages as well as disadvantages in the use of such agents. Finally, he stressed the importance of studying the effect of chronic administration of cholinesterase inhibitors in patients, in view of the fact that the disease is chronic, and would require repeated administration of the compound. **Dr. Giacobini** addressed his question to representatives of industry in the audience. He wondered what research directions academia should take, in order to generate further information for industry, thus helping in their effort to develop new drugs for the treatment of

Alzheimer's Disease. **Dr.Middlemiss** pointed out that what is really necessary from academia is clinical pharmacology, which would detect, acutely, the same sort of effects in human beings, which are observed in experimental animals. **Dr. Cook** took issue with those who objected to the use of animal models. Until more information is available regarding the clinical entity being modeled, the animal model, he felt, was "the only act in town". He stressed therefore that what is essential is that we have very sharp clinical criteria in terms of evaluating relevant pharmacological properties, and a sharper definition of the syndrome; definitions which could then be used effectively at the preclinical level. **Dr. Hanin** closed the Round Table by acknowledging the efforts of the technical crew and the superb organizational efforts of Drs. Fisher and Lachman. He felt that the conference could be summarized by three "W"s. It was warm, well organized, and made all the participants very welcome.

PARTICIPANTS

ABRAHAM, D.J., University of Pittsburgh, Pittsburgh, PA, U.S.A
ADOLFSSON, R., University of Umea, Umea, Sweden
AGRANAT, I., Hebrew University, Jerusalem, Israel
AHARONSON, E., Israel Institute for Biological Research, Ness-Ziona, Israel
AMIR, A., Israel Institute for Biological Research, Ness-Ziona, Israel
AMITAI, G., Israel Institute for Biological Research, Ness-Ziona, Israel
APPEL, S.H., Baylor College of Medicine, Houston, TX, U.S.A
APPEL, V., U.S.A.
ASHANI, L., Israel Institute for Biological Research, Ness-Ziona, Israel
ASHANI, Y., Israel Institute for Biological Research, Ness-Ziona, Israel
AVERICK, N., St. Francis Hospital, Blue Island, NY, U.S.A
AYALON, N., Kimron Veterinary Institute, Beit-Dagan, Israel
AZCONA, A., Sandoz Ltd., Basle, Switzerland
BALAN, A., Israel Institute for Biological Research, Ness-Ziona, Israel
BALL, S.M., Albany Medical College, Albany, NY, U.S.A
BARAK, D., Israel Institute for Biological Research, Ness-Ziona, Israel
BARAK, R., Israel Institute for Biological Research, Ness-Ziona, Israel
BARNESS, I., Israel Institute for Biological Research, Ness-Ziona, Israel
BARZILAI, R., Israel Institute for Biological Research, Ness-Ziona, Israel
BECHAR, M., Beilinson Medical Center, Petah-Tikva, Israel
BEN-DAVID, N., Israel Institute for Biological Research, Ness-Ziona, Israel
BIEGON, A., Weizmann Institute of Science, Rehovot, Israel
BIRDSALL, N.M.J., MRC National Institute for Medical Research, London, UK
BLANCHARD, J.-C., Rhone-Poulenc Sante Centre de Recherches, Vitry sur Seine, France

BLASS, J.P., The Burke Rehabilitation Center, White Plains, NY, U.S.A
BOLLIGER, G., Sandoz Ltd., Basle, Switzerland
BOSCH de AGUILAR van den, Ph., Universite Catholique de Louvain,
Louvain-La Neuve, Belgium
BOWEN, D.M., Institute of Neurology, London, UK
BRANDEIS, R., Israel Institute for Biological Research, Ness-Ziona,
Israel
BRUCKSTEIN-DAVIDOVICI, R., Israel Institute for Biological Research,
Ness-Ziona, Israel
BUTCHER, L.L., University of California, Los Angeles, CA, U.S.A
CHAPMAN, Y., Tel-Aviv University, Ramat-Aviv, Israel
COHEN, S., Tel-Aviv University, Ramat-Aviv, Israel
COOK, L., E.I. du Pont de Nemours & Co. Inc., Wilmington, DE, U.S.A
CORETT, R., Israel Institute for Biological Research, Ness-Ziona,
Israel
DACHIR, S., Israel Institute for Biological Research, Ness-Ziona,
Israel
DASBERG, H., Ezrath Nashim Hospital, Jerusalem, Israel
DASSA, C., Harzfeld Hospital for Chronic Diseases, Gedera, Israel
DAVIDSON, M., Mt. Sinai School of Medicine, New York, NY, U.S.A
DAVOUS, P., Hopital St. Anne, Paris, France
DE LEON, M., New York University Medical Center, New York, NY, U.S.A
DORSSER van, W., Continental Pharma, Inc., Mont-St-Guibert, Belgium
DUBNOV, B., Central Emek Hospital, Afula, Israel
DUCKLER, S., Tel-Aviv, Israel
DUVDEVANI, N., Israel Institute for Biological Research, Ness-Ziona,
Israel
EBSTEIN, R.P., Ezrath Nashim Hospital, Jerusalem, Israel
EDERY, H., Israel Institute for Biological Research, Ness-Ziona, Israel
Israel
EDWARDSON, C., Newcastle General Hospital, Newcastle Upon Tyne, England
EVENCHIK, Z., Israel Institute for Biological Research, Ness-Ziona,
Israel
FIELDING, S., Hoechst Roussel Pharmaceuticals, Inc., Somerville, N.J.
U.S.A
FINKELSTEIN, Y., Rambam Hospital, Haifa
FISHER, A., Israel Institute for Biological Research, Ness-Ziona,
Israel
FOLMAN, E., Forest Hills, NY, U.S.A
FRIEDMAN, E., New York University Medical Center, New York, NY, U.S.A
FROLICH, L., Institute for Pathochemistry & Gen. Neurochemistry,
Heidelberg, Germany
FUCHS, P., Israel Institute for Biological Research, Ness-Ziona, Israel
FUCHS, S., Weizmann Institute of Science, Rehovot, Israel
GABISON, D., Israel Institute for Biological Research, Ness-Ziona,
Israel
GADOTH, N., Beilinson Medical Center, Petah-Tikva, Israel
GAMZU, E., Hoffman La Roche, Inc., Nutley, NJ, U.S.A
GARTY, I., Central Emek Hospital, Afula, Israel
GERSHON, S., Wayne State University, Detroit, MI, U.S.A
GIACOBINI, E., South Illinois University School of Medicine,
Springfield, IL, U.S.A
GILAD, G., Weizmann Institute of Science, Rehovot, Israel
GILAD, V., Weizmann Institute of Science, Rehovot, Israel

GLICKFELD, P., Israel Institute for Biological Research, Ness-Ziona, Israel
GLOBUS, M., Bikur Cholim Hospital, Jerusalem, Israel
GOTLIEB-STEMATSKY, T., Sheba Medical Center, Tel-Hashomer, Israel
GRAUER, E., Israel Institute for Biological Research, Ness-Ziona, Israel
GRAVEH, D., Israel Institute for Biological Research, Ness-Ziona, Israel
GRONER, Y., Weizmann Institute of Science, Rehovot, Israel
GROWDON, J.H., Massachusetts General Hospital, Harvard Medical School, Boston, MA, U.S.A
GRUNWALD, J., Israel Institute for Biological Research, Ness-Ziona, Israel
GULYA, K., University of Arizona, Tucson, AZ, U.S.A
GUREVICH, D., Wayne State University, Detroit, MI, U.S.A
HABERMAN, F., Israel Institute for Biological Research, Ness-Ziona, Israel
HALPERIN, B., Israel Institute for Biological Research, Ness-Ziona, Israel
HALPERIN, G., Israel Institute for Biological Research, Ness-Ziona, Israel
HALMANN, M., Israel Institute for Biological Research, Ness-Ziona, Israel
HALMANN, M., Weizman Institute of Science, Rehovot, Israel
HANIN, I., University of Pittsburgh, Pittsburgh, PA, U.S.A
HEFTI, F., University of Miami Medical School, Miami, FL, U.S.A
HELDMAN, E., Israel Institute for Biological Research, Ness-Ziona, Israel
HEMLI, J.A., Medical School, Technion, Haifa, Israel
HERTMAN, I., Israel Institute for Biological Research, Ness-Ziona, Israel
HINZEN, D., Boehringer Ingelheim KG, Ingelheim, Germany
INOKE, T., Snow Brand Milk Products, Hamburg, Germany
ISRAEL, L., Centre Hospitalier de Grenoble, Grenoble, France
ISRAELI, E., Israel Institute for Biological Research, Ness-Ziona, Israel
JACOBS, R., University of California, Los Angeles, CA, U.S.A
JANSSENS de VAREBEKE, P., Continental Pharma Inc., Mont-St-Guibert, Belgium
KADAR, T., Israel Institute for Biological Research, Ness-Ziona, Israel
KAHANA, E., Barzilai Medical Center, Ashkelon, Israel
KAPLUN, A., Israel Institute for Biological Research, Ness-Ziona, Israel
KARTON, Y., Israel Institute for Biological Research, Ness-Ziona, Israel
KASA, P., Medical University Central Laboratory, Szeged, Hungary
KERANEN, A.J., Orion Pharmaceuticals, Espoo, Finland
KOPIN, I.J., National Health Institutes, Bethesda, MD., U.S.A
KORCZYN, A.D., Tel-Aviv University, Ramat-Aviv, Israel
KOTT, E., Meir Hospital, Kfar-Sava, Israel
KROFT, F., North York Branson Hospital, Toronto, Canada
KROFT, S.S., North York Branson Hospital, Toronto, Canada
KUHN, F.J., Boehringer Ingelheim KG, Ingelheim, Germany
KUSHNIR, M., Israel Institute for Biological Research, Ness-Ziona, Israel

LACHMAN, C., Israel Institute for Biological Research, Ness-Ziona, Israel
LAMOUR, Y., INSERM, Paris, France
LERER, B., E.I. du Ponte de Nemours & Co., Inc., Wilmington, DE, U.S.A
LEVENTHAL, C.M., NINCDS, NIH, Bethesda, MD, U.S.A
LEVY, A., Israel Institute for Biological Research, Ness-Ziona, Israel
LEVY, D., Israel Institute for Biological Research, Ness-Ziona, Israel
LeWITT, P., Lafayette Clinic, Detroit, MI, U.S.A
LINDBERG, U., Astra Lakemedel, Sodertalje, Sweden
LONDON, E.D., National Institute of Drug Abuse, Baltimore, MD, U.S.A
LUZ, S., Israel Institute for Biological Research, Ness-Ziona, Israel
MAYEUX, R., Neurological Institute, New York, NY, U.S.A
MELAMED, E., Hadasah University Hospital, Jerusalem, Israel
MELLON, V.H., U.S.A
MERVIS, R., Ohio State University, Columbus, OHIO, U.S.A
MIDDLEMISS, D., Merrell-Dow Research Institute, Strasbourg, France
MILDWORF, B., Hadassah University Hospital, Jerusalem, Israel
MILGRAM, N., Weizmann Institute of Science, Rehovot, Israel
MIZOBE, F., Snow Brand Milk Products, Tokyo, Japan
MOSS, D., University of El Paso, TX, U.S.A
MUNOZ-GARCIA, D., University of Vermont, Burlington, VT, U.S.A
NAVON, M., Israel Institute for Biological Research, Ness-Ziona, Israel
NEUMEYER, J.L., Research Biochemicals, Inc., Wayland, MA, U.S.A
NORDBERG, A., Uppsala University, Uppsala, Sweden
OPPENHEIM, Y., Shaare Zedek Medical Center, Jerusalem, Israel
OREN, R., Israel Institute for Biological Research, Ness-Ziona, Israel
ORGAD, U., Kimron Veterinary Institute, Beit-Dagan, Israel
ORON, H., Israel Institute for Biological Research, Ness-Ziona, Israel
ORON, U., Tel-Aviv University, Ramat-Aviv, Israel
PATCHORNIK, A., Weizmann Institute of Science, Rehovot, Israel
PELED, M., Israel Institute for Biological Research, Ness-Ziona, Israel
PERL, D., University of Vermont, Burlington, VT, U.S.A
PERLMAN, A., Israel Institute for Biological Research, Ness-Ziona, Israel
PINTO, M., Israel Institute for Biological Research, Ness-Ziona, Israel
PITEL, Z., Israel Institute for Biological Research, Ness-Ziona, Israel
PLATEL, A., Laboratoires Fournier, Dijon, France
PNIEL, R., Israel Institute for Biological Research, Ness-Ziona, Israel
PROHOVNIK, I., Columbia University, New York, NY, U.S.A
PUYMIRAT, J., Hopital Saint-Anne, Paris, France
RAAIJMAKERS, W.G.M., University of Nijmegen, The Netherlands
RABEY, J.M., Ichilov Hospital, Tel-Aviv, Israel
RACHAMAN,E., Israel Institute for Biological Research, Ness-Ziona, Israel
RASCHIG, A., Boehringer Ingelheim, KG, Ingelheim, Germany
RAVID, R., Netherlands Institute for Brain Research, Amsterdam, Holland
RECHES, A., Hadassah University Hospital, Jerusalem, Israel
REHAVI, M., Tel-Aviv University, Ramat-Aviv, Israel
RICHARDS, F.G., St. Catharines, Ontario, Canada
ROSIN, A.J., Shaare Zadek Medical Center, Jerusalem, Israel
ROUFA, D., Monsanto Co., St. Louis, MO, U.S.A
SAAR, M., Israel Institute for Biological Research, Ness-Ziona, Israel
SACHS, H., Children's Memorial Hospital, Glencoe, IL, U.S.A
SALAMONE, J., Merck Sharp & Dohme, UK
SAMUEL, D., Weizmann Institute of Science, Rehovot, Israel
SANBERG, P.R., Ohio University, Athens, OHIO, U.S.A
SANDMAN, P.O., Umea University, Umea, Sweden

SARA, S., CNRS, Gif-sur-Yvette, France
SARTER, M., Schering AG, Berlin, Germany
SCHEIN, J., Albert Einstein College of Medicine, Bronx, NY, U.S.A
SCHLOSSBERG, A., Mental Health Center, Beer-Yaacov, Israel
SCHOLTHOLT, J., Hoechst AG, Frankfurt, Germany
SCHREIBER, M., Kaplan Hospital, Israel
SCHUURMAN, T., The Netherlands
SEGAL, M., Weizmann Institute of Science, Rehovot, Israel
SEIDEL, P-R., Bayer, AG, Wuppertal, Germany
SELKOE, D.J., Harvard Medical School, Belmont, MA, U.S.A
SENNEF, C., Organon International, Oss, The Netherlands
SHAPIRA, S., Israel Institute for Biological Research, Ness-Ziona, Israel
SHAFFERMAN, A., Israel Institute for Biological Research, Ness-Ziona, Israel
SHINITZKY, M., Weizmann Institute of Science, Rehovot, Israel
SIEGEL, B., Beit-Rivka Geriatric Center, Petah Tikva, Israel
SIMON, G., Israel Institute for Biological Research, Ness-Ziona, Israel
SINAI, Y., Israel Institute for Biological Research, Ness-Ziona, Israel
SIVAN, Y., Israel Institute for Biological Research, Ness-Ziona, Israel
SPEISER, Z., Tel-Aviv University, Ramat-Aviv, Israel
SPIEGELSTEIN, M., Israel Institute for Biological Research, Ness-Ziona, Israel
STEFANOVICH, V., Hoechst AG Werk Albert, Wiesbaden, Germany
STEINMETZ, D., Central Emek Hospital, Afula, Israel
STERN, Y., Neurological Institute, New York, NY, U.S.A
STREIFLER, M.B., Tel-Aviv University, Ramat-Aviv, Israel
STROLIN-BENEDETTI, M., Laboratoires Fournier, Dijon, France
STUDLER, J.-M., France
TEICHBERG, V., Weizmann Institute of Science, Rehovot, Israel
TEITZ, Y., Tel-Aviv University, Ramat-Aviv, Israel
TESSE, B., Rego Park, NY, U.S.A
THOEN, G., Mayo Memorial Hospital, Minneapolis, MN, U.S.A
TORTEN, M., Israel Institute for Biological Research, Ness-Ziona, Israel
TRAUB, A., Israel Institute for Biological Research, Ness-Ziona, Israel
TROPPER, M.S., Zamenhof Outpatient Clinic & Geriatric Center, Rishon-Le-Zion, Israel
TURNER, I., Israel Institute for Biological Research, Ness-Ziona, Israel
VINCZE, A., Israel Institute for Biological Research, Ness-Ziona, Israel
WAEGEMANS, T., Psychiatric Institute, Leuven, Belgium
WALSH, T.J., NIH/NIEHS, Research Triangle Park, NC, U.S.A
WEINSTOCK-ROSIN, M., Hadassah University Hospital, Jerusalem, Israel
WISNIEWSKI, H.M., Inst. of Basic Research in Development Disabilities, Staten Island, NY, U.S.A
WOLFSON, S., JR., University of Pittsburgh, Pittsburgh, PA, U.S.A
WOOLF, N.J., University of California, Los Angeles, CA., U.S.A
WULFERT, E., UCB, Research & Development, Brussels, Belgium
WURTMAN, R.J., Massachusetts Institute of Technology, Cambridge, MA, U.S.A
WYSENBEEK, H., Tel-Aviv University, Ramat-Aviv, Israel
YOUDIM, M.B.H., Technion, Israel Institute of Technology, Haifa, Israel
ZEHAVI, J., Israel Institute for Biological Research, Ness-Ziona, Israel
ZUTRA, A., Weizmann Institute of Science, Rehovot, Israel

INDEX